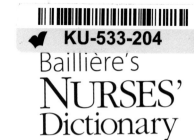

Baillière's
# NURSES'
Dictionary

*For Elsevier:*

*Commissioning Editor:* Mairi McCubbin
*Development Editor:* Sally Davies
*Project Manager:* Alan Nicholson
*Design Direction:* Stewart Larking
*Illustrations Manager:* Bruce Hogarth
*Illustrations:* Amanda Williams

# Baillière's
# NURSES'
## Dictionary

### For nurses and health care workers

EDITED BY

## Barbara F. Weller
BA MSc RGN RSCN RNT

Independent Nurse Consultant; Honorary Consultant
Lecturer, Thames Valley University, London;
Editor, *INFANT* (Journal for Neonatal and Paediatric
Healthcare Professionals); formerly Nursing Officer,
Department of Health and Chief Nursing Adviser,
British Red Cross Society, UK

FOREWORD BY

## Robert J. Pratt
CBE BA MSc RN RNT DN(Lond) FRCN
Professor of Nursing, Associate Dean for Research,
Director, Richard Wells Research Centre,
Thames Valley University, London, UK

ELSEVIER
BAILLIÈRE
TINDALL

Edinburgh   London   New York   Oxford   Philadelphia   St Louis   Sydney   Toronto   2009

# BAILLIÈRE
# TINDALL
### ELSEVIER

First published 1912
© Elsevier Science Ltd, 2002
24th edition 2005 (Main and international)
25th edition © 2009, (Main and international) Elsevier Limited. All rights reserved.

ISBN 978-0-7020-3233-2
International ISBN 978-0-7020-3234-9

**British Library Cataloguing in Publication Data**
A catalogue record for this book is available from the British Library

**Library of Congress Cataloging in Publication Data**
A catalog record for this book is available from the Library of Congress

**Notice**
Knowledge and best practice in this field are constantly changing. As new research and experience broaden our knowledge, changes in practice, treatment and drug therapy may become necessary or appropriate. Readers are advised to check the most current information provided (i) on procedures featured or (ii) by the manufacturer of each product to be administered, to verify the recommended dose or formula, the method and duration of administration, and contraindications. It is the responsibility of the practitioner, relying on their own experience and knowledge of the patient, to make diagnoses, to determine dosages and the best treatment for each individual patient, and to take all appropriate safety precautions. To the fullest extent of the law, neither the Publisher nor the Editor assumes any liability for any injury and/or damage to persons or property arising out of or related to any use of the material contained in this book.

The Publisher

**ELSEVIER** your source for books,
journals and multimedia
in the health sciences

**www.elsevierhealth.com**

Working together to grow
libraries in developing countries

www.elsevier.com | www.bookaid.org | www.sabre.org

ELSEVIER   BOOK AID International   Sabre Foundation

The publisher's policy is to use **paper manufactured from sustainable forests**

Printed in China

# Contents

# Contributors

**Nicola Bandaranayake** BSc(Hons) DipDiet RD
Diabetes Specialist Dietitian, Imperial College Healthcare NHS Trust, Hammersmith Hospital, London, UK

**Christine Bishop** BSc(Hons)
Managing Editor, *Journal of the Intensive Care Society*; Publisher, *Infant* (Journal for Neonatal and Paediatric Healthcare Professionals), Bishop's Stortford, Hertfordshire, UK

**Joanne Boyle** MSc RD
Specialist Dietitian, Obesity Management, Department of Nutrition and Dietetics, Imperial College NHS Trust, Charing Cross Hospital, London, UK

**Bob Brown** BSc(Hons) DNSc PGDip DipSocPsych RGN
Assistant Director of Nursing (Learning and Development) and Mental Health Services for Older People, South Eastern Health and Social Care Trust, Ulster Hospital, Belfast, UK

**Linda Carter** BSc(Hons) SRD
Senior Dietitian, formerly at Imperial College Healthcare NHS Trust, Hammersmith Hospital, London, UK

**Lindsay Creek** RGN ENB199, 998 ALS(I) EPLS(I)
Senior Resuscitation Officer, Resuscitation Services, Addenbrooke's Hospital, Cambridge, UK

**John Driscoll** BSc(Hons) DPSN Cert Ed(FE) RGN RMN
Professional Development Consultant and Coach, Norfolk, UK

**Chris Evans** BSc MA MRPharmS DMS
Chief Pharmacist, St George's Healthcare NHS Trust, London, UK

**Gary Frost** PhD SRD
Professor of Nutrition and Dietetics, Investigative Medicine, Investigative Science, Faculty of Medicine, Imperial College Healthcare NHS Trust, London, UK

**Jonathan Green** LLB(Hons)
Solicitor and Senior Legal Officer, Royal College of Nursing, Exeter, Devon, UK

**Sandra Horn**
Senior Administrative Assistant, School of Nursing and Midwifery, University of East Anglia, Norwich, UK

**Karen Johnson** RN SPDN Nurse Prescriber (V100)
District Nurse Team Leader, NHS Norfolk Primary Care Trust, Norfolk, UK

**Caroline King** BSc SRD
Specialist Neonatal and Paediatric Dietitian, Department of Dietetics, Imperial College Healthcare NHS Trust, Hammersmith Hospital, London, UK

**Carol Pellowe** EdD BA(Hons) MA(Ed) RN RNT
Deputy Director, Richard Wells Research Centre, Thames Valley University, London, UK

**Robert J. Pratt** CBE BA MSc RN RNT DN(Lond) FRCN
Professor of Nursing, Associate Dean for Research, Director, Richard Wells Research Centre, Thames Valley University, London, UK

**Judy Rivett** OHNCert PGDip SRN
Independent Consultant, Judy Rivett & Associates, Norfolk, UK

**Claire Smiter-Coe** RN DipHE (Nursing)
Senior Recovery Practitioner, Ipswich Hospital NHS Trust, Suffolk, UK

**Lorna Telford** BSc(Hons) MSc RN
Assistant Director, Safe and Effective Care, South Eastern Trust, Ulster Hospital, Belfast, UK

**Liesl Wandrag** BSc RD
Senior Critical Care Dietitian, Nutrition & Dietetic Department, Imperial College Healthcare NHS Trust, Charing Cross Hospital, London, UK

**Barbara F. Weller** BA MSc RGN RSCN RNT
Independent Nurse Consultant; Honorary Consultant Lecturer, Thames Valley University, London; Editor, *Infant* (Journal for Neonatal and Paediatric Healthcare Professionals); formerly Nursing Officer, Department of Health and Chief Nursing Adviser, British Red Cross Society, UK

# Foreword

Many professions and disciplines work together in the National Health Service (NHS) and the independent health care sector to ensure the provision of a comprehensive range of high-quality services. Nurses, as the largest group of health care professionals, deliver 80% of health care in the NHS. They have always been at the sharp edge of caring and their practice and presence makes the defining difference in the achievement of positive patient outcomes. Never has it been more exciting to be a nurse; never has it been more challenging.

All over the world, nursing continues to evolve within a matrix of radical changes in the organization and delivery of health care, shifting health priorities, new evidence for best practice, emerging technologies and increasing specialisms in nursing.

Although many forces drive change, one of the most important in the United Kingdom (UK) and many other European countries is an ever-expanding cultural and ethnic diversity in today's pluralistic societies. Reflective of our cosmopolitan communities, those who now access health services have a wide range of different expectations and needs, and nurses have to be responsive to the complexities involved in caring for people from diverse cultural backgrounds.

This diversity is also mirrored in the nurses, midwives, doctors and other health care workers from nations throughout the world who now work in the NHS. Professional nursing has always been an international qualification but now more than ever, nurses and midwives from the member states of the European Union (EU) are expanding their horizons and professional experience by periods of practice in other EU countries.

In addition, vast numbers of students from many different cultures and countries are currently studying in UK universities for academic and practice qualifications in nursing and midwifery and for vocational qualifications in health care. As an essential component of their educational programme, they will undertake periods of supervised clinical practice in NHS hospitals and in primary and community care settings.

This inevitable increasing cultural and ethnic diversity in society and in health care environments is both challenging and enriching. Cultural awareness provides unique opportunities for all of us to learn from each other and to grow and develop, both professionally and as individuals. In nursing, it has increased our sensitivity towards others, taught us greater tolerance, helped us to listen better and to become more flexible, patient and gentle with all who require care. Embracing and celebrating diversity, and capitalizing on the valuable opportunities it presents, is a hallmark of true professional maturity.

To ensure that we develop effective nursing care strategies that are culturally appropriate and responsive to the different needs of different patients from diverse backgrounds, nurses and other health care professionals need to be efficient communicators. We need to understand our patients and it is equally important that they understand us. We also need to be absolutely clear in our communications with our colleagues. As nurses coordinate the care of patients and liaise with various health services, they interact with a wide range of health care professionals and others who provide support services. Communication effectiveness, a core component of clinical governance, is essential in ensuring safe quality care.

One of the potential barriers to communication effectiveness is the language we use to communicate with each other and with our patients. In the scientific disciplines of medicine and nursing, quite specialized words and terminology have necessarily developed to describe observations, perceptions, activities, structures, diseases, events and outcomes. This is our scientific vocabulary and we use this to enhance the precision and clarity of our professional communications. It goes without saying that we need to understand the exact meaning of the words we use so that we communicate accurately with each other and with other health care disciplines. Equally importantly, we also need to have this comprehensive appreciation of our scientific vocabulary so that we can correctly interpret information for our clients and patients in culturally meaningful ways. For many of our patients, colleagues and students, English will not be their first language yet it is the language we use to communicate with each other. This makes it even more imperative that we are careful and clear in using professional language.

In a changing world, new words and terms evolve, meanings for old words often change as the context in which they are used changes and new concepts, phenomena, technology and resources need to be described. In any profession, it can be a daunting task to keep abreast of our changing scientific vocabulary and yet it is absolutely essential that we do if we are to continue to use communications effectively to support and provide safe, competent and culturally appropriate care for our clients and patients. Having access to and regularly using a comprehensive, good-quality and up-to-date dictionary of nursing and nursing-related scientific terms is one of the best ways to ensure that we understand and are correctly using our professional language.

Like many of my colleagues all over the world, I have relied upon *Baillière's Nurses' Dictionary* throughout my career in nursing. It has helped me to communicate well and to use professional language appropriately and with confidence. I used earlier editions of this dictionary as a student and I continue to use the latest edition as one of the key references in my work today. Barbara Weller is one of the most experienced and skilled nursing editors in the UK and once again she has developed and delivered to us a new edition of this greatly respected and well used resource. I congratulate her, her colleagues at Elsevier and everyone who has contributed to this excellent dictionary. I highly commend it to all student and qualified nurses and midwives and to others working in the health services.

*Robert J. Pratt*

# Preface

In today's professional world, our communication skills need to be inclusive of a whole raft of communication techniques and language definitions that we all share and use. By sharing usage and definition we have a common modality enabling us to work jointly towards the removal of jargon in communicating with our clients, patients and their families, as well as in our communications with our colleagues. Welcome, then, to the 25th edition of *Baillière's Nurses' Dictionary*. The aim of the team of contributors and the editor has been to maintain the high standards of past editions, but to push further the boundaries of our shared professional language for nurses and other health care professionals.

Health professionals today work as team members in an arena that is changing and evolving according to society's demands for its health care services. As the deliverers of a high-quality service we need to recognize the need not only to maintain standards of practice but to be constantly mindful of our individual obligations for updating and developing our own practice. Inevitably this has to be undertaken in a 'melee' of many and sometimes competing factors, such as the growing demand for resources, the expansion of medical and health care technology and the increasing shift to self-governed NHS Foundation Trusts. The aim for this dictionary is to project something of the challenge by assisting our readers to keep up-to-date with the enlarging knowledge base that underpins our practice.

Readers have in the past commentated on the practicality and usefulness of this dictionary (it fits into a pocket or a bag!) in its compact size and presentation. However, its convenient size is also constraining for an editor, and often compromises have had to be made with some definitions being reduced or omitted. As Editor, I have accepted the responsibility for these changes.

> 'I can no other answer make but thanks.
> And thanks and ever thanks.'

> *'Twelfth Night'*, W. Shakespeare

The production of the 25th edition of this dictionary has been made possible because of good teamwork combined with the enthusiasm and keenness of the contributors, together with many other colleagues who have been so generous with their time and commitment. I thank them all.

Producing a dictionary such as this also involves wide consultation and I am especially grateful to Sandra Horn who has used her talented secretarial skills in coming to my rescue when faced with computer tantrums, her calmness and step-by-step approach was always the effective therapy.

I am greatly indebted to Professor Robert Pratt both for his generous Foreword to the 24th as well as the 25th editions and for his professional support and friendship without which this task would have been much more difficult. The publishing team at Elsevier, led by Mairi McCubbin, Commissioning Editor has taken the edition smoothly from its concept through the publishing and printing process to our readers. Finally, I should like to acknowledge the support from my husband David Fisher in smoothing the path to ensure that all was completed according to schedule.

*Dereham, Norfolk 2009*                              *Barbara F. Weller*

# Acknowledgements

The figures and tables below have been reproduced or adapted with permission from the following publications:

Hatchett R, Thompson D R, 2001, *Cardiac Nursing,* Churchill Livingstone; Figure 12.6

Jennett S, *Dictionary of Sport and Exercise Science and Medicine,* 2008 Churchill Livingstone; Figures: pages 95 and 316

Porter S, *Dictionary of Physiotherapy,* 2005, Elsevier Butterworth Heinemann; Figures: pages 67 and 166

Symonds E M, Symonds I M, 1997, *Essential Obstetrics and Gynaecology* 3rd edition, Churchill Livingstone; Figure 6.15

Waugh A, Grant A, 2001, *Ross and Wilson Anatomy and Physiology in Health and illness* 9th edition, Churchill Livingstone; Figures 3.1, 3.37, 4.6, 4.9, 7.16, 7.27, 8.13, 12.36, 16.3, 16.15, 19.3, 19.10

Wilson J, 2001, *Infection Control in Clinical Practice* 2nd edition, Baillière Tindall; Figure 1.2

Winson N V & McDonald S, *Illustrated Dictionary of Midwifery,* 2005, Elsevier Butterworth Heinemann; Table: page 28

The NHS Confederation is thanked for permission to use extracts from their publication *The NHS in England 03/04.*

# Style Guide

**Subentries**
The term being sought may be a main entry or a subentry under the main entry. In subentries, the main entry is represented by its initial letter if it is singular, and by the addition of an apostrophe and *s* if it is plural. Subentries are listed alphabetically under the main entry. For example:

> **abdomen**…
> > *Acute a*….
> > *Pendulous a*….
> > *Scaphoid (navicular) a*….

**Cross-referencing**
Throughout the dictionary, cross-references are given within the text as SMALL CAPITALS. For example:

> **fibrin** an insoluble protein that is essential to CLOTTING of blood, formed from fibrinogen by action of thrombin.

There are also situations where it is simply more convenient to define the word in a different location, to which the reader is then referred.

**Translations**
Where a translation of a foreign term occurs, it is indicated in *italic type* immediately after the abbreviation for the language (which is in square brackets). For example:

> **acus** [L.] *a needle*

**Abbreviations Used in this Dictionary**
| | |
|---|---|
| *b.* born | L. Latin |
| Fr. French | *pl.* plural |
| Ger. German | *sing.* singular |

**Drug Names**
Where possible, only generic names are used; however, some proprietary drug names and names for preparations are included, with information (and sometimes cross-references) about the generic drug(s) involved. Inclusion of a drug in the dictionary does not imply endorsement.

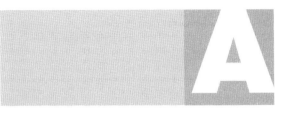

**A** accommodation; adenine; anode (anodal); anterior; axial; symbol for *ampere* and *mass number*.

**abatement** a decrease in the severity of a pain or a symptom.

**abdomen** The cavity between the diaphragm and the pelvis, lined by a serous membrane, the peritoneum, and containing the stomach, intestines, liver, gallbladder, spleen, pancreas, kidneys, suprarenal glands, ureters and bladder. For descriptive purposes, its area can be divided into nine regions (*see* Figure). *Acute a.* any abdominal condition urgently requiring treatment, usually surgical. *Pendulous a.* a condition in which the anterior part of the abdominal wall hangs down over the pubis. *Scaphoid (navicular) a.* a hollowing of the anterior wall commonly seen in grossly emaciated people.

**abdominal** pertaining to the abdomen. *A. aneurysm* a dilatation of the abdominal aorta. *A. aorta* that part of the aorta below the diaphragm. *A. breathing* deep breathing; hyperpnoea. *A. examination* a systematic examination of the abdomen by inspection, palpation and auscultation carried out by midwives during pregnancy and after delivery. The purpose is to determine the equality of uterine size with the calculated period of gestation and later in the pregnancy to determine the position of the fetus. Postnatally the

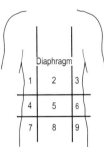

1. Right hypochondriac region
2. Epigastric region
3. Left hypochondriac region
4. Right lumbar region
5. Umbilical region
6. Left lumbar region
7. Right iliac fossa
8. Hypogastric region
9. Left iliac fossa

REGIONS OF THE ABDOMEN

examination is used to ascertain that the uterus is regaining its former non-pregnant size and position. *A. reflex* reflex contraction of abdominal wall muscles observed when skin is lightly stroked. *A. section* incision through the abdominal wall. *A. thrust see* HEIMLICH MANOEUVRE. *See* Appendix 2.

**abdominoperineal** pertaining to the abdomen and the perineum.

*A. excision* an operation performed through the abdomen and the perineum for the excision of the rectum or bladder. Often done as a synchronized operation by two surgeons, one working at each approach.

**abduce** to abduct or to draw away.

**abducent** leading away from the midline. *A. muscle* the external rectus muscle of the eye, which rotates it outward. *A. nerve* the cranial nerve that supplies this muscle.

**abductor** a muscle that draws a limb away from the midline of the body. The opposite of adductor.

**aberrant** taking an unusual course. Used of blood vessels and nerves.

**aberration** deviation from the normal. In optics, failure to focus rays of light. *Mental a.* mental disorder of an unspecified kind.

**ability** the power to perform an act, either mental or physical, with or without training. *A. test* a test that measures a person's level of performance or estimates future performance. Sometimes also known as an intelligence test, achievement test or aptitude test. *Innate a.* the ability with which a person is born.

**ablation** removal or destruction, by surgical or radiological means, of neoplasms or other body tissue.

**abnormal** varying from what is regular or usual.

**ABO system** *see* BLOOD GROUPS.

**abort** 1. to terminate a process or disease before it has run its normal course. 2. to remove or expel from the womb an embryo or fetus before it is capable of independent existence.

**abortifacient** an agent or drug that may induce abortion.

**abortion** 1. premature cessation of a normal process. 2. emptying of the pregnant uterus before the end of the 24th week. 3. the product of such an abortion. *Complete a.* one in which the contents of the uterus are expelled intact. *Criminal a.* the termination of a pregnancy for reasons other than those permitted by law (i.e. danger to mental or physical health of mother or child or family) and without medical approval. *Incomplete a.* one in which some part of the fetus or placenta is retained in the uterus. *Induced a.* the intentional emptying of the uterus. *Inevitable a.* abortion where bleeding is profuse and accompanied by pains, the cervix is dilated and the contents of the uterus can be felt. *Missed a.* one where all signs of pregnancy disappear and later the uterus discharges a blood clot surrounding a shrivelled fetus, i.e. a carneous mole. *Septic a.* abortion associated with infection. *Therapeutic (legal) a.* one induced on medical advice because the continuance of the pregnancy would involve risk to the life of the pregnant woman, or injury to the physical or mental health of the pregnant woman or any existing children of her family, greater than if the pregnancy were terminated; or because there is a substantial risk that if the child were born it would suffer from such physical or mental abnormalities as to be seriously handicapped (1967 Abortion Act, as amended by the Human Fertilization and Embryology Act Amendments 1991). *Threatened a.* the appearance of signs of premature expulsion of the fetus; bleeding is slight, the cervix is closed. *Tubal a.* the termination of a tubal pregnancy caused by rupture of the uterine tube.

**abrasion** a superficial injury, where the skin or mucous membrane is rubbed or torn. *Corneal a.* this can occur when the surface of the cornea has been removed, e.g. by a scratch or other injury.

**abreaction** the reliving of a painful experience, with the release of repressed emotion.

**abruptio placentae** premature detachment of the placenta, causing maternal shock.

**abscess** a collection of pus in a cavity. Caused by the disintegration and replacement of tissue damaged by mechanical, chemical or bacterial injury. *Alveolar a.* an abscess in a tooth socket. *Brodie's a.* a bone abscess, usually on the head of the tibia. *Cold a.* the result of chronic tubercular infection and so called because there are few, if any, signs of inflammation. *Psoas a.* a cold abscess that has tracked down the psoas muscle from caries of the lumbar vertebrae. *Subphrenic a.* one situated under the diaphragm.

**absorbent** 1. able to take in, or suck up and incorporate. 2. a tissue structure involved in absorption. 3. a substance that absorbs or promotes absorption.

**absorption** 1. in physiology, the taking up by suction of fluids or other substances by the tissues of the body. 2. in psychology, great mental concentration on a single object or activity. 3. in radiology, uptake of radiation by body tissues.

**abstinence** a refraining from the use of or indulgence in food, stimulants or coitus. *A. syndrome* withdrawal symptoms.

**abstract** A brief, comprehensive summary of a research study or other academic report.

**abuse** misuse, maltreatment – may be physical, sexual, psychological or neglect. Can apply to any group of people, e.g. the vulnerable, children, women, people with learning disabilities or the elderly. May also apply to the misuse of power, authority, drugs and other substances, e.g. solvents and equipment.

**Acarus** a genus of small mites. *A. scabiei* (*Sarcoptes scabiei*) the cause of scabies.

**acataphasia** loss of the ability to express connected thought, resulting from a cerebral lesion.

**acceleration** 1. An increase in the speed or velocity of an object or reaction. 2. An increase in the fetal heartbeat of at least 15 beats per minute over the baseline rate for at least 15 seconds.

**access to health care records** The Act of 1990 allows the patient access to paper and computerized health care records made after 1991, unless it is considered that serious physical or mental harm to the patient may result. Where the patient has died, application to access the health care records can be made by the patient's representative or by any person who may have a claim arising out of the patient's death.

**accessory** supplementary. *A. nerve* the 11th cranial nerve. It is made up of two portions: the cranial and the spinal.

**accident and emergency** sometimes referred to as casualty or trauma medicine. A setting for dealing with problems which require immediate attention and where patients can be directed or referred by a general practitioner or the emergency services.

**accident form** a form known as also 'Untoward Incident form' which provides a record of any accident to any person on NHS Trust and other health care premises. Employers require that the form is completed as soon after the accident as possible.

**accommodation** adjustment. In ophthalmology, the term refers specifically to adjustment of the ciliary muscle, which controls the shape of the lens. *Negative a.* the ciliary muscle relaxes and the lens becomes less convex, giving long-distance vision. *Positive a.* the ciliary muscle contracts and the lens becomes more convex, giving near vision.

**accountable** liable to be held responsible for a course of action. A qualified nurse has a duty of care according to law; in nursing, being accountable refers to the responsibility the qualified nurse takes for prescribing and initiating nursing care. Nurses are accountable to their patients, their peers and their employing authority, according to the Code of Professional Conduct. Registered practitioners (nurses, midwives or health visitors) are accountable at all times for their actions, on or off duty and whether engaged in current practice or not. Accountability is also identified as one of the three foundations of public service. Everything done by those who work in the NHS must be able to stand the test of parliamentary scrutiny, public judgements on propriety and professional codes of conduct.

**accreditation** 1. to give someone official status within an organization, e.g. an approved and acknowledged representative of a union or professional organization. 2. the official system used in some countries for the licensing of a hospital or health care facility by government agencies which meet agreed standards following initial assessment and regular appraisal that they meet a satisfactory level of organizational achievement. *A. for Prior Experiential Learning* abbreviated APEL. Credit gained for non-academic work (clinical or work experience) that can be used to give credit to academic course work and programmes of study in colleges and universities. *A. for Prior Learning* abbreviated APL. A system used by academic institutions and other establishments to grant credit for previous academic achievements. Usually used to gain credit transfer between institutions leading to academic qualifications.

**accretion** growth. The accumulation of deposits, e.g. of salts to form a calculus in the bladder. In dentistry, the growth of tartar on the teeth.

**acculturation** the process by which a person absorbs the beliefs, values and customs of another culture, usually through direct contact, e.g. migrants resident in another country.

**ACE inhibitors** a group of drugs used in the treatment of hypertension. Their name, angiotensin converting enzyme inhibitors, explains part of their mode of action, although it is thought that some of their other actions may also be important in reducing blood pressure.

**acet-** combining form denoting acid. From the Latin *acetum*, vinegar.

**acetabuloplasty** an operation performed to improve the depth and shape of the hip socket in correcting congenital dislocation of the hip or in treating osteoarthritis of the hip (*see* Figure).

**acetabulum** the cup-like socket in the innominate bone, in which the head of the femur moves.

**acetate** a salt of acetic acid.

**acetoacetic acid** diacetic acid. A product of fat metabolism. It occurs in

ACETABULOPLASTY

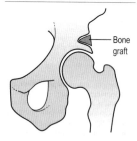

Bone graft

excessive amounts in diabetes and starvation, giving rise to acetone bodies in the urine.

**acetonaemia** the presence of acetone bodies in the blood.

**acetone** a colourless inflammable liquid with a characteristic odour. Traces are found in the blood and in normal urine. *A. bodies* ketones found in the blood and urine of uncontrolled diabetic patients and also in acute starvation as a result of the incomplete breakdown of fatty and amino acids.

**acetonuria** the presence of an excess quantity of acetone bodies in the urine, giving it a peculiar sweet smell.

**acetylcholine** a chemical transmitter that is released by some nerve endings at the synapse between one neurone and the next or between a nerve ending and the effector organ it supplies. These nerves are said to be cholinergic, e.g. the parasympathetic nerves and the lower motor neurones to skeletal muscles. Acetylcholine is rapidly destroyed in the body by cholinesterase.

**acetylcoenzyme A** active form of acetic acid, to which carbohydrates, fats and amino acids not needed for protein synthesis are converted.

**achalasia** failure of relaxation of a muscle sphincter causing dilatation of the part above, e.g. of the oesophagus above the cardiac sphincter (*see* Figure).

**ache** a dull continuous pain.

**Achilles** Greek mythological hero who could be wounded only in the heel. *A. tendon* tendo calcaneus, connecting the soleus and gastrocnemius muscles of the calf to the heel bone (os calcis). Tapping the Achilles tendon normally produces the Achilles reflex or ankle jerk.

**achlorhydria** the absence of free hydrochloric acid in the stomach. May be found in pernicious anaemia, pellagra and gastric cancer.

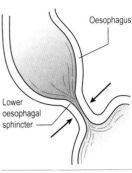

ACHALASIA

**acholia** lack of secretion of bile.

**acholuria** deficiency or lack of bile in the urine.

**acholuric** pertaining to acholuria. *A. jaundice* jaundice without bile in the urine.

**achondroplasia** an inherited condition in which there is early union of the epiphysis and diaphysis of long bones. Growth is arrested resulting in short stature.

**achromasia** 1. lack of colour in the skin. 2. absence of normal reaction to staining in a tissue or cell.

**achromatopsia** complete colour-blindness caused by disease or trauma. It may be congenital.

**achylia** absence of hydrochloric acid and enzymes in the gastric secretions. *A. gastrica* a condition in which gastric secretion is reduced or absent.

**acid** 1. sour or sharp in taste. 2. a substance which, when combined with an alkali, will form a salt. Any acid substance will turn blue litmus paper red. Individual acids are given under their specific names. *A. alcohol-fast* descriptive of stained bacteria that are resistant to decolorization by both acid and alcohol. *A.–base balance* the normal ratio between the acid ions and the basic or alkaline ions required to maintain the pH of the blood and body fluids. Most of the body's metabolic processes produce acids as their end products, but a somewhat alkaline body fluid is required as a medium for vital cellular activities. Therefore chemical exchanges of hydrogen ions must take place continuously in order to maintain a state of equilibrium. An optimal pH (hydrogen ion concentration) between 7.35 and 7.45 must be maintained; otherwise, the enzyme systems and other biochemical and metabolic activities will not function normally.

**acidaemia** abnormal acidity of the blood, which contains an excess of hydrogen ions in which the pH of the blood falls below 7.35.

**acidity** 1. sourness or sharpness of taste. 2. the state of being acid.

**acidosis** a pathological condition resulting from accumulation of acid or depletion of the alkaline reserve (bicarbonate content) in the blood and body tissues, and characterized by increase in hydrogen ion concentration (decrease in pH to below 7.30). *Metabolic a.* acidosis resulting from accumulation in the blood of ketoacids (derived from fat metabolism) at the expense of bicarbonate, thus diminishing the body's ability to neutralize acids. Occurs in diabetic ketoacidosis, lactic acidosis and failure of renal tubules to reabsorb bicarbonate. *Respiratory a.* acidosis resulting from ventilatory impairment and subsequent retention of carbon dioxide. Carbon dioxide accumulates in the blood and unites with water to form carbonic acid. Occurs with severe birth asphyxia and other respiratory conditions affecting the newborn.

**acidotic** 1. pertaining to acidosis. 2. a person suffering from acidosis.

**acinus** a minute saccule or alveolus of a compound gland, lined by secreting cells. The secreting portion of the mammary gland consists of acini.

**acme** 1. the highest point. 2. the crisis of a fever when the symptoms are fully developed.

**acne** an inflammatory condition of the sebaceous glands in which blackheads (comedones) are usually present together with papules and pustules. *A. keratitis* inflammation of the cornea associated with acne rosacea. *A. rosacea* a redness of the forehead, nose and cheeks due to chronic dilatation of the subcutaneous capillaries, which becomes permanent with the formation of pustules in the affected areas. *A. vulgaris* form that occurs commonly in adolescents and young adults, affecting the face, chest and back.

**acneiform** resembling acne.

**acousma** the hearing of imaginary sounds.

**acoustic** relating to sound or the sense of hearing.

**acquired** pertaining to disease, habits or immunity developed after birth; not inherited.

**acquired immune deficiency syndrome** abbreviated AIDS. *See* AIDS.

**acrocephalia** a malformation of the head, in which the top is pointed. Oxycephaly.

**acrocyanosis** persistent cyanosis, coldness of the hands and feet and profuse sweating of the digits, often associated with a vasomotor defect.

**acromegaly** a chronic condition producing gradual enlargement of the hands, feet, and bones of the head and chest. Associated with overactivity of the anterior lobe of the pituitary gland in adults.

**acromioclavicular** pertaining to the joint between the acromion process of the scapula and the lateral aspect of the clavicle.

**acromion** the outward projection of the spine of the scapula, forming the point of the shoulder.

**acroparaesthesia** condition in which pressure on the nerves of the brachial plexus causes numbness, pain and tingling of the hand and forearm.

**acrophobia** morbid terror of being at a height.

**acrosclerosis** a type of scleroderma that affects the hands, feet, face or chest.

**acrosome** part of the head of a spermatozoon containing enzymes that break down the cell membrane of the ovum and allow penetration.

**ACTH** adrenocorticotrophic hormone; corticotrophin.

**actin** the protein of myofibrils responsible for contraction and relaxation of muscles.

**actinodermatitis** inflammation of the skin due to the action of ultraviolet or X-rays.

**Actinomyces** a genus of branching, spore-forming, vegetable parasites, which may give rise to actinomycosis and from which many antibiotic drugs are produced, e.g. streptomycin.

**actinomycosis** a chronic infective disease of cattle that is also found in humans. Granulated tumours occur, chiefly in the lung and jaw, and more rarely the intestine.

**actinotherapy** treatment of disease by rays of light, e.g. artificial sunlight.

**action** the accomplishment of an effect, whether mechanical or chemical, or the effect so produced. *A. research* a method of undertaking social research that incorporates the researcher's involvement as a direct and deliberate part of the research, i.e. the researcher acts as a change agent. *Cumulative a.* the sudden and markedly increased action of a drug after administration of several doses. *Reflex a.* an involuntary response to a stimulus conveyed to the nervous system and reflected to the periphery, passing below the level of consciousness (*see also* REFLEX).

**activator** a substance, hormone or enzyme that stimulates a chemical change, although it may not take part in the change. In chemistry, a catalyst. For example, yeast is the activator in the process by which sugar is converted into alcohol; the digestive secretions are activated by hormones to carry out normal digestion.

**active** causing change; energetic. *A. immunity* an immunity in which individuals have been stimulated to produce their own antibodies. *A. labour* the normal progress of the birth process, including uterine contractions, dilation of the cervix to at least 3–4 cm and the descent of the fetus into the birth canal. *A. listening* the act of alert, intentional hearing and demonstration of an interest in what a person has to say through verbal signs, nonverbal gestures and body language. *A. movements* movements made by the patient, as distinct from passive movements. *A. principle* the ingredient in a drug that is primarily responsible for its therapeutic action. *A. transport* the movement of ions or molecules across the cell membranes and epithelial layers, usually against a concentration gradient, resulting directly from the expenditure of metabolic energy. Under normal circumstances more potassium ions are present within the cell and more sodium ions extracellularly. The process of maintaining these normal differences in electrolytic composition between the intracellular fluids is active transport. The process differs from simple diffusion or osmosis in that it requires the expenditure of metabolic energy.

**activities of daily living** abbreviated ADL. Those activities usually performed in the course of a person's normal daily routine, such as eating, cleaning teeth, washing and dressing.

**activities of living (ALs)** those activities which meet the physical, psychological and social needs of the individual, e.g. eating, elimination, communication, breathing, expressing sexuality, working, play, etc.

**activity theory** describes a psychosocial process whereby ageing people disengage from some activities of their earlier life and replace these with other hobbies and pastimes, according to their changing physical abilities and economic situation.

**activity tolerance** the amount of physical activity tolerated by a patient. It may be assessed in patients with cardiac or chronic respiratory disease. Graded exercise, including walking, cycling and going up and down stairs, may be used to rebuild confidence during the convalescent phase after any serious illness or injury as an important part of any rehabilitation programme.

**actomysin** muscle protein complex; the myosin component acts as an enzyme which causes the release of energy.

**acuity** sharpness. *A. of hearing* an acute perception of sound. *A. of vision* clear focusing ability.

**acupressure** a system of complementary medicine in which pressure is applied to various points on the body to stimulate the innate self-healing capacity of the individual. *See* ACUPUNCTURE, SHIATSU.

**acupuncture** a Chinese medical system which aims to diagnose illness and promote health by stimulating the body's self-healing powers. The insertion of special needles into specific points along the 'meridians' of the body is used

for the production of anaesthesia, the relief of pain and the treatment of certain conditions.

**acute** a term applied to a disease in which the attack is sudden, severe and of short duration.

**acute respiratory distress syndrome** abbreviated ARDS. A severe form of acute lung function failure which occurs after an event such as trauma, inhalation of a toxic substance or septic shock. There is severe breathlessness and a dangerous reduction in the supply of oxygen to the blood.

**acute stress disorder** an anxiety disorder that is usually transient which occurs within 4 weeks following exposure or involvement to a traumatic event. The staff of the emergency services may be affected, e.g. following a major road traffic incident.

**acyclic** occurring independently of a natural cycle of events (such as the menstrual cycle).

**Adam's apple** the laryngeal prominence, a protrusion of the front of the neck formed by the thyroid cartilage.

**adamantine** pertaining to the enamel of the teeth.

**adaptation** 1. the process of modification that a living organism undergoes when adjusting itself to new surroundings or circumstances. 2. a function of the stimulus to which the individual is exposed and of the individual's accommodation to the situation. The adaptation response may relate to physiological needs, role, 'self' concept and interdependence. 3. the process of overcoming difficulties and adjusting to changing circumstances. Neuroses and psychoses are often associated with failure of adaptation. 4. used in ophthalmology to mean the adjustment of visual function according to the ambient illumination. *Colour a.* 1. changes in visual perception of colour with prolonged stimulation. 2. adjustment of vision to degree of brightness or colour tone of illumination. *Dark a.* adaptation of the eye to vision in reduced illumination. *Light a.* adaptation of the eye to vision in bright illumination (photopia), with reduction in the concentration of the photosensitive pigments of the eye.

**addict** a person exhibiting addiction.

**addiction** 1. the taking of drugs or alcohol leading to physiological and psychological dependence with a tendency to increase use. 2. the state of being devoted to a particular activity or interest, e.g. gambling or computer games to the exclusion of the normal activities of daily living. *See* DEPENDENCE and DRUG (ADDICTION).

**Addison's disease** *T. Addison, British physician, 1793–1860.* Deficiency disease of the suprarenal cortex; often tuberculous. There is wasting, brown pigmentation of the skin and extreme debility.

**additives** substances added to improve, enhance or preserve something. *Food additives.* used in the food industry to preserve and make the food look more attractive; these are given serial numbers, e.g. E102 (tartrazine) E476 (soya lecithin). Some additives may produce an allergic reaction in some people and a few are thought to be implicated in behavioural problems in children.

**adducent** leading towards the midline. *A. muscle* the medial rectus muscle of the eye, which turns it inwards.

**adductor** a muscle that draws a limb towards the midline of the body. The opposite of abductor.

**adenine** one of the purine bases found in DNA.

**adenitis** inflammation of a gland.

**adenoid** resembling a gland. Generally applied to abnormal lymphoid growth in the nasopharynx.

**adenoidectomy** the surgical removal of adenoid tissue from the nasopharynx.

**adenomyoma** an innocent new growth involving both endometrium and muscle tissue; found in the uterus or uterine ligaments.

**adenopathy** enlargement of any gland, especially those of the lymphatic system.

**adenosine** a nucleoside consisting of adenine and D-ribose (a pentose sugar). *A. triphosphate* abbreviated ATP. A compound containing three phosphoric acids. It is present in all cells and serves as a store for energy.

**adenovirus** a virus of the Adenoviridae family. Many types have been isolated, some of which cause respiratory tract infections, while others are associated with conjunctivitis, epidemic keratoconjunctivitis or gastrointestinal infection.

**ADH** antidiuretic hormone. Vasopressin.

**adhesion** union between two surfaces normally separated. Usually the result of inflammation when fibrous tissue forms, e.g. peritonitis may cause adhesions between organs. A possible cause of intestinal obstruction.

**adipose** of the nature of fat. Fatty.

**adiposity** the state of being too fat. Obesity.

**aditus** an opening or passageway; often applied to that between the middle ear and the mastoid antrum.

**adjustment** in psychology, the ability of a person to adapt to changing circumstances or environment.

**adjuvant** 1. any treatment used in conjunction with another to enhance its efficacy. 2. a substance administered with a drug to enhance its effect.

**ADL** activities of daily living.

**Adler's theory** *A. Adler, Austrian psychiatrist, 1870–1937.* The theory that neuroses develop as a compensation for feelings of inferiority, either social or physical.

**adolescence** the period between puberty and maturity. In the male, 14–25 years. In the female, 12–21 years.

**adopt** 1. to take a person, especially another's child, into a legal relationship as one's own. 2. to choose to follow a course of action.

**adoption** the legal procedure by which a child is transferred from its natural parents to adopting parents. The child's welfare is paramount and the Adoption Acts 1976 and 1978 (Scotland), with amendments in the Children Act 1989, detail clearly how and when an adoption can take place and who can adopt. Local authorities offer advice and social work support and may act as an adoption agency, and there are also private and charitable organizations which must be registered with the local authority.

**adrenal** 1. near the kidneys. 2. a triangular endocrine gland situated above each kidney.

**adrenalectomy** surgical excision of an adrenal gland.

**adrenaline** a hormone secreted by the medulla of the adrenal gland. Has an action similar to normal stimulation of the sympathetic nervous system: (a) causing dilatation of the bronchioles; (b) raising the blood pressure by constriction of surface vessels and stimulation of the cardiac output; (c) releasing glycogen from the liver. It is therefore used to treat such conditions as asthma, collapse and hypoglycaemia. It acts as a haemostat in local anaesthetics.

**adrenergic** pertaining to nerves that release the chemical transmitter noradrenaline in order to stimulate the muscles and glands they supply.

**adrenocorticotrophin** adrenocorticotrophic hormone (ACTH);
secreted by the anterior lobe of the pituitary body. Stimulates the adrenal cortex to produce cortisol. *See* CORTICOTROPHIN.

**adrenogenital** relating to both the adrenal glands and the gonads. *A. syndrome* a condition of masculinization caused by overactivity of the adrenal cortex resulting in precocious puberty in the male infant and masculinization in the female. Both sexes are liable to Addisonian crises.

**adrenolytic** a drug that inhibits the stimulation of the sympathetic nerves and the activity of adrenaline.

**adsorbent** a substance that has the power of attracting gas or fluid to itself, e.g. charcoal.

**adsorption** the power of certain substances to attach gases or other substances in solution to their surface and so concentrate them there. This is made use of in chromatography.

**adult** mature. A mature person.

**adulteration** addition of an impure, cheap or unnecessary ingredient to cheat with, cheapen or falsify a preparation.

**advance directive or statement** a written declaration made by a mentally competent person, which sets out their wishes with regard to life-prolonging medical interventions if they are incapacitated by an irreversible disease or are terminally ill which prevents them making their wishes known to health professionals at the time. *See* LIVING WILL.

**advanced life support (ALS)** resuscitation techniques used during a cardiac arrest that follows on from basic life support. They include defibrillation and the administration of appropriate drugs. Paediatric advanced life support (PALS) is a structured and algorithm method of life support for children with severe medical emergencies. *See* Appendix 2.

**advanced trauma life support (ALS)** a set of protocols recommended for use by doctors and paramedics when dealing with seriously injured people at the scene of an accident. The immediate treatment of shock from reduced blood volume by the infusion of fluids is an integral component of the life support regime.

**advancement** in surgery, an operation to detach a tendon or muscle and reattach it further forward. Used in the treatment of strabismus and plastic surgery.

**adventitia** the outer coat of an artery or vein.

**advocacy** the process whereby a nurse provides a patient and/or the family with information to enable them to make informed decisions relating to the care situation. The nurse is then able to support the patient's decision vis-à-vis other professionals and also to incorporate the informed decisions into care planning.

**aeration** supplying with air. Used to describe the oxygenation of blood which takes place in the lungs.

**aerobe** an organism that can live and thrive only in the presence of oxygen.

**aerobic exercise** physical exercises for which the degree of effort is such that it can be maintained for long periods without undue breathlessness. The aim of this form of exercising is to increase the effectiveness of the heart and lungs and the supply of oxygen to the tissues of the body.

**aeropathy** commonly called 'the bends' (decompression sickness).

**aerophagy** the excessive swallowing of air.

**aerosol** finely divided particles or droplets. *A. sprays* used in medicine to humidify air or oxygen, or for the administration of drugs by inhalation.

**Æsculapius** the god of healing in Roman mythology.

**aetiology** the science of the causes of disease.

**afebrile** without fever.

**affect** in psychiatry, the feeling experienced in connection with an emotion or mood.

**affection** 1. a morbid condition or disease state. 2. a warm feeling for someone or something.

**affective** pertaining to the emotions or moods. *A. psychoses* major mental disorders in which there is grave disturbance of the emotions.

**afferent** conveying towards the centre. *A. nerves* the sensory nerve fibres that convey impulses from the periphery towards the brain. *A. paths* or *tracts* the course of the sensory nerves up the spinal cord and through the brain. *A. vessels* arterioles entering the glomerulus of the kidney, or lymphatics entering a lymph gland. *See* EFFERENT.

**affiliation** the judicial decision about the paternity of a child with a view to the issue of a maintenance order.

**affinity** in chemistry, the attraction of two substances to each other, e.g. haemoglobin and oxygen.

**afibrinogenaemia** absence of fibrinogen in the blood. The clotting mechanism of the blood is impaired as a result.

**African tick fever** disease caused by a spirochaete, *Borrelia duttonii*. Transmitted by ticks. *See* RELAPSING FEVER.

**afterbirth** a lay expression used to describe the placenta, cord and membranes expelled after childbirth.

**aftercare** social, medical or nursing care provided after a period of hospital treatment.

**afterimage** a visual impression that remains briefly after the cessation of sensory stimulation.

**afterpains** the pains due to uterine contraction after childbirth.

**afunctional** lacking function.

**agammaglobulinaemia** a condition in which there is no gammaglobulin in the blood. The patients are therefore susceptible to infections because of an inability to form antibodies.

**agar** a gelatinous substance prepared from seaweed. Used as a culture medium for bacteria and as a laxative because it absorbs liquid from the digestive tract and swells, so stimulating peristalsis.

**age** 1. the duration, or the measure of time, of the existence of a person or object. 2. to undergo change as a result of the passage of time. *Achievement a.* 1. *see* DEVELOPMENTAL (MILESTONES). 2. proficiency in study expressed in terms of the chronological age of a normal child showing the same degree of attainment. 3. acquirement of a new skill or interest in old age or a praiseworthy accomplishment by an aged person. *A. spots* with increasing age skin blemishes appear; most commonly they are seborrhoeic keratoses which are brown or yellow and can occur anywhere on the body. Also common with increasing age are freckles, red pinpoint blemishes on the trunk and solar keratoses due to overexposure to the sun. Treatment is usually unnecessary except occasionally for solar keratoses which may eventually progress to skin cancer. *Chronological a.* the actual measure of time elapsed since a person's birth. *Gestational a.* an expression of age of a developing fetus, usually given in weeks. It is measured from the date of the mother's last menstrual period, and so is approximately 2 weeks longer than time from conception. *Mental a.* the age level of mental ability of a person as gauged by standard intelligence tests.

**age-associated memory impairment** with age short-term memory declines; most elderly people learn to overcome and compensate for this deficit. However, for some it may be a considerable problem in daily living. Memory loss associated with dementia is often due to Alzheimer's disease or cerebral vascular disease. *See* DEMENTIA and ALZHEIMER'S DISEASE.

**ageing** the structural changes that take place with time and are not caused by accident or disease. Heredity is an important determinant of life expectancy, but factors such as smoking, an excessive intake of alcohol, obesity, poor diet and insufficient exercise can all contribute to physical and mental deterioration. *A. population* as the number of older people increase, the demand for health care increases. Expectations for health care delivery and provision too are changing as patients become increasingly knowledgeable about their health. Current ageist practices in health care provision are likely to be challenged with subsequent implications for health care services.

**ageism** the systematic discrimination against people on the grounds of age, based on stereotyping of the elderly as helpless, infirm, confused, requiring health care and supportive social services.

**agenesis** failure of a structure to develop properly.

**agent** any substance or force capable of producing a physical, chemical or biological effect. *Alkylating a.* a cytotoxic preparation. *Chelating a.* a chemical compound that binds metal ions. *Wetting a.* a substance that lowers the surface tension of water and promotes wetting.

**agglutination** collecting into clumps, particularly of cells suspended in a fluid and of bacteria affected by specific immune serum. *A. test* a means of aiding diagnosis and identification of bacteria. If serum containing known agglutinins comes into contact with the specific bacteria, clumping will take place (*see* WIDAL REACTION). *Cross a.* a simple test to decide the group to which blood belongs (*see* BLOOD GROUPS).

**agglutinin** any substance causing agglutination (clumping together) of cells, particularly a specific antibody formed in the blood in response to the presence of an invading agent. Agglutinins are proteins (IMMUNOGLOBULIN) and function as part of the immune mechanism of the body. When the invading agents that bring about the production of agglutinins are bacteria, the agglutinins produced bring about agglutination of the bacterial cells.

**agglutinogen** any substance that, when present in the bloodstream, can cause the production of specific antibodies or agglutinins.

**aggregation** the massing together of materials, as in clumping. *Familial a.* the increased incidence of cases of a disease in a family compared with that in control families. *Platelet a.* the clumping together of platelets, which may be induced by a number of agents, such as thrombin and collagen.

**aggression** animosity or hostility shown towards another person or object as a response to opposition or frustration.

**agitation** 1. shaking. 2. mental distress causing extreme restlessness.

**aglutition** difficulty in the act of swallowing. Dysphagia.

**agnosia** an inability to recognize objects because the sensory stimulus cannot be interpreted, in spite of the presence of a normal sense organ.

**agonist** the prime mover. A muscle opposed in action by another (the antagonist).

**agony** extreme suffering, either mental or physical.

**agoraphobia** a fear of open spaces.

**agranulocyte** a white blood cell without granules in its cytoplasm. The term includes monocytes and lymphocytes.

**agranulocytosis** a condition in which there is a marked decrease or complete absence of granular leukocytes in the blood, leaving the body defenceless against bacterial invasion. May result from: (a) the use of toxic drugs; (b) irradiation. Characterized by a sore throat, ulceration of the mouth and pyrexia. It may result in severe prostration and death.

**agraphia** absence of the power of expressing thought in writing. It arises from a lack of muscular coordination or as a result of a cerebral lesion.

**ague** malaria.

**AHF** antihaemophilic factor (clotting factor VIII).

**AHG** antihaemophilic globulin (clotting factor VIII).

**AID** artificial insemination of a woman with donor semen.

**AIDS** acquired immunodeficiency syndrome. The late symptomatic stage of chronic disease caused by human immunodeficiency virus (HIV) infection which progressively impairs the body's cell-mediated immune responses to infections and cancers. This results in serious 'opportunistic infections' caused by microorganisms that do not usually cause illness in people with a healthy immune system, e.g. *Pneumocystis carinii* pneumonia (PCP), or cancers such as Kaposi's sarcoma (KS) and lymphoma. Additionally, this late stage of HIV disease is characterized by a high and rising level (viral load) of HIV and a progressively decreasing number (less then 200 cells/mm$^3$) of CD4$^+$ T lymphocytes in the plasma. Prior to AIDS, many HIV-infected people experience a variety of recurrent signs and symptoms, including lymphadenopathy, night sweats, diarrhoea, weight loss, malaise, oropharyngeal or vaginal candidiasis (thrush), and herpes zoster (shingles). Formerly known as the AIDS-related complex, this stage is now generally referred to as early symptomatic HIV disease (as opposed to AIDS which is also known as late symptomatic HIV disease).

**AIH** artificial insemination of a woman with her husband's semen.

**ailment** any minor disorder of the body.

**air** a mixture of gases that make up the earth's atmosphere. It consists of: non-active nitrogen 79%; oxygen 21%, which supports life and combustion; traces of neon, argon, hydrogen, etc.; and carbon dioxide 0.03%, except in expired air, when 6% is exhaled as a result of diffusion that has taken place in the lungs. Air has weight and exerts pressure, which aids in syphonage from body cavities. *A.-bed* a rubber mattress inflated with air. *A. embolism* an embolism caused by air entering the circulatory system. *A. encephalography* radiological examination of the brain after the injection of air into the subarachnoid space. *A. hunger* a form of dyspnoea in which there are deep sighing respirations, characteristic of severe haemorrhage or acidosis. *Complemental a.* additional air that can be inhaled with inspiratory effort. *Residual a.* air remaining in the lungs after deep expiration. *Stationary a.* that retained in the lungs after normal expiration. *Supplemental a.* the extra air forced out of the lungs with expiratory effort. *Tidal a.* that which passes in and out of the lungs in normal respiratory action.

**airway** 1. the passage by which the air enters and leaves the lungs. 2. a mechanical device (tube) used

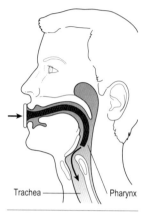

Trachea — Pharynx

OROPHARYNGEAL AIRWAY

for securing unobstructed respiration during general anaesthesia or on other occasions when the patient is not ventilating or exchanging gases properly. It may be passed through the mouth or nose. The tube prevents a flaccid tongue from resting against the posterior pharyngeal wall and causing obstruction of the airway (*see* Figure).

**akinesia** loss of muscle power. This may be the result of a brain or spinal cord lesion or, temporarily, of anaesthesia.

**akinetic** relating to states or conditions where there is lack of movement.

**alalia** loss or impairment of the power of speech due to muscle paralysis or a cerebral lesion.

**alanine** an amino acid formed by the ingestion of dietary protein.

**albinism** a condition in which there is congenital absence of pigment in the skin, hair and eyes. It may be partial or complete.

**albino** a person affected with albinism.

**albumin** 1. any protein that is soluble in water and moderately concentrated salt solutions and is coagulable by heat, e.g. egg white. 2. serum albumin; a plasma protein, formed principally in the liver and constituting about four-sevenths of the 6–8% protein concentration in the plasma. Albumin is a very important factor in regulating the exchange of water between the plasma and the interstitial compartment (space between the cells). A drop in the amount of albumin in the plasma results in an increase in tissue fluid, which, if severe, becomes apparent as oedema. Albumin serves also as a transport protein.

**albuminuria** the presence of albumin in the urine, occurring e.g. in renal disease, in most feverish conditions and sometimes in pregnancy. *Orthostatic* or *postural a.* a non-pathological form that affects some individuals after prolonged standing but disappears after bedrest for a few hours.

**alcohol** a volatile liquid distilled from fermented saccharine liquids and forming the basis of wines and spirits. The official (British Pharmacopoeia) preparation of ethyl alcohol (ethanol) contains 95% alcohol and 5% water. Used: (a) as an antiseptic; (b) in the preparation of tinctures; (c) as a perspective for anatomical specimens. Taken internally, it acts as a temporary heart stimulant, and in large quantities as a depressant poison. It has some value as a food, 30 ml brandy producing about 400 J. *Absolute a.* that which contains not more than 1% by weight of water. *A.-fast* pertaining to bacteria that, once having been stained, are resistant to decolorization by alcohol. *A. related disorders* A variety of physical and mental disorders associated with prolonged and excessive consumption of alcohol including hepatitis, cirrhosis, some cancers, e.g. of the oesophagus, larynx and throat. Heavy alcohol consumption in pregnancy increases the risk of miscarriage and fetal alcohol syndrome. Alcoholics are more likely to suffer from personality changes, depression and to develop dementia. Many alcoholics suffer from a poor diet and are prone to nutritional deficiency. See Wernicke–Korsakoff syndrome. *A. withdrawal syndrome* a group of symptoms that develop in a person suffering from alcoholism within 6–24 hours of taking the last drink of alcohol. The symptoms include restlessness, tremors, loss of appetite, nausea, vomiting, insomnia, disorientation, seizures and delirium tremens. Treatment involves sedation, improving nutrition, counselling and social support.

**alcoholic** 1. pertaining to alcohol. 2. a person addicted to excessive, uncontrolled alcohol consumption. This results in loss of appetite and vitamin B deficiency, leading to peripheral neuritis with eye changes and cirrhosis of the liver and to progressive deterioration in the personality.

**alcoholism** the state of poisoning resulting from alcoholic addiction.

**aldosterone** a compound, isolated from the adrenal cortex, that aids the retention of sodium and the excretion of potassium in the body, and by so doing aids the maintenance of electrolyte balance. *A. antagonists* a group of drugs which block the action of aldosterone.

**aldosteronism** an excess secretion of aldosterone caused by an adrenal neoplasm. The serum potassium is low and the patient has hypertension and severe muscular weakness.

**aleukaemia** an acute condition in which there is an absence or deficiency of white cells in the blood.

**Alexander technique** *F.M. Alexander, Australian actor and physiotherapist, 1869–1955.* A process of psychophysical postural re-education. Body posture is believed to affect physical and psychological wellbeing and the postural re-education process aims to assist individuals in monitoring how they consciously use their bodies to promote good health.

**alexia** a form of aphasia in which there is an inability to recognize written or printed words. Word blindness.

**algorithm** a process or set of rules used in calculations, e.g. of medications, or for other problem solving. Computer programs are the most familiar examples of algorithms in everyday use.

**alienation** a feeling of estrangement or separation from others or from self. A symptom of schizophrenia. Sufferers often believe that they are under the control of someone else. See DEPERSONALIZATION.

**alignment** the state of being arranged in a line, i.e. in the correct anatomical position.

**aliment** food or nourishment.

**alimentary** relating to the system of nutrition. *A. canal* alimentary tract. The passage through which the food passes, from mouth to anus. *A. system* the alimentary tract together with the liver and other organs concerned in digestion and absorption. *A. tract* alimentary canal.

**alimentation** the giving or receiving of nourishment. The process of supplying the patient's need for nutrition.

**alkalaemia** an increase in the alkali content of the blood. See ALKALOSIS.

**alkali** a substance capable of uniting with acids to form salts, and with fats and fatty acids to form soaps. Alkaline solutions turn red litmus paper blue. *A. reserve* the ability of the combined buffer systems of the blood to neutralize acid. The pH of the blood is normally slightly on the alkaline side, between 7.35 and 7.45. The principal buffer in the blood is bicarbonate; the alkali reserve is essentially represented by the plasma bicarbonate concentration.

**alkaline** having the reactions of an alkali. *A. phosphatase* an enzyme localized on cell membranes that hydrolyses phosphate esters, liberating inorganic phosphate, and has an optimal pH of about 10.0. Serum alkaline phosphatase activity is elevated in obstructive jaundice and bone disease.

**alkalinity** 1. the quality of being alkaline. 2. the combining power of a base, expressed as the maximum number of equivalents of acid with which it reacts to form a salt.

**alkaloid** one of a group of active nitrogenous compounds that are alkaline in solution. They usually have a bitter taste and are characterized by powerful physiological activity. Examples are morphine, cocaine, atropine, quinine, nicotine and caffeine. The term is also applied to synthetic substances that have structures similar to plant alkaloids, such as procaine.

**alkalosis** an increase in the alkali reserve in the blood. It may be confirmed by estimation of the blood carbon dioxide content and treated by giving normal saline or ammonium chloride intravenously to encourage the excretion of bicarbonate by the kidneys.

**alkylating agent** a drug that damages the deoxyribonucleic acid (DNA) molecule of the nucleus of the cell. Many are nitrogen mustard preparations and may be termed chromosome poisons; they are used in cancer chemotherapy.

**all-or-none law** principle that states that in individual cardiac and skeletal muscle fibres there are only two possible reactions to a stimulus: either there is no reaction at all or there is a full reaction, with no gradation of response according to the strength of the stimulus. Whole muscles can grade their response by increasing or decreasing the *number* of fibres involved.

**allantois** a membranous sac projecting from the ventral surface of the fetus in its early stages. It eventually helps to form the placenta.

**allele** allelomorph. One of a pair of genes that occupy the same relative positions on homologous chromosomes and produce different effects on the same process of development.

**allelomorph** allele.

**allergen** a substance that can produce an allergy or manifestation of an immune response.

**allergy** a hypersensitivity to some foreign substances that are normally harmless but which produce a violent reaction in the patient. Asthma, hay fever, angioneurotic oedema, migraine and some types of urticaria and eczema are allergic states. *See* ANAPHYLAXIS.

**allocate** to assign for a particular purpose.

**allocation** the act of allocating. *Clinical a.* a period of time spent in ward/department/unit where there are patients/clients. *Patient a.* one nurse is designated as responsible for the care of one patient or a group of patients for a spell of duty. *Task a.* patient care in a ward/unit is provided by a group of nurses. Each nurse is allocated a specific nursing activity task. As this system of providing care does not take into account the patients' personal interests, individualized care is preferred.

**allograft** an organ or tissue transplanted from one person to another of a dissimilar genotype but of the same species. *Non-viable a.* skin, taken from a cadaver, which cannot

regenerate. *Viable a.* living tissue transplanted. *See* HOMOGRAFT.

**alloimmunization** the immune response to donated blood, bone marrow or transplanted organ; rhesus-negative pregnant women with a rhesus-positive fetus can become alloimmunized following a sensitizing event, e.g. antepartum haemorrhage or miscarriage, through the development of antibodies that target the foreign material, causing haemolytic disease of the newborn.

**allopathy** the practice of conventional medicine, i.e. with drugs having opposite effects to the symptoms.

**alopecia** baldness. Loss of hair. The cause of simple baldness is not yet fully understood, although it is known that the tendency to become bald is limited almost entirely to males, runs in certain families and is more common in certain racial groups than in others. Baldness is often associated with ageing. *A. areata* hair loss in sharply defined areas, usually the scalp or beard. *Cicatricial a., a. cicatrisata* irreversible loss of hair associated with scarring, usually on the scalp. *Male-pattern a.* loss of scalp hair, genetically determined and androgen-dependent, beginning with frontal recession and progressing symmetrically to leave ultimately only a sparse peripheral rim of hair.

**alpha** the first letter of the Greek alphabet, a. *A. cells* cells found in the islet of Langerhans in the pancreas. They produce the hormone glucagon. *A. fetoprotein* abbreviated AFP. A plasma protein originating in the fetal liver and gastrointestinal tract. The serum AFP level is used to monitor the effectiveness of cancer treatment; the amniotic fluid AFP level is used in the prenatal diagnosis of neural tube defects.

*A. receptors* tissue receptors associated with the stimulation (contraction) of smooth muscle.

**alternative medicine** a form of medicine differing from conventional health care. Consists of a range of treatments essentially based upon a holistic approach to health and wellbeing, including homeopathy, aromatherapy, hypnosis, acupuncture and others. These therapies fall into three categories: touch and movement medicinal and psychological. Commonly called complementary therapies (*see* COMPLEMENTARY).

**altitude sickness** condition caused by hypoxia that occurs as a result of lower oxygen pressure at high altitudes before acclimatization to the increased altitude.

**altruism** a sense of unconditional concern for the welfare of others.

**aluminium** *symbol* Al. A silver-white metal with a low specific gravity, compounds of which are astringent and antiseptic. *A. hydroxide* compound used as an antacid in the treatment of gastric conditions.

**alveolar** concerning an alveolus, or air sac of the lung. *A. air* air found in the alveoli.

**alveolitis** inflammation of the alveoli. *Extrinsic allergic a.* inflammation of the alveoli caused by inhalation of an antigen, such as pollen.

**Alzheimer's cells** *A. Alzheimer, German neurologist, 1864–1915.* 1. giant astrocytes with large prominent nuclei found in the brain in hepatolenticular degeneration and hepatic comas. 2. degenerated astrocytes.

**Alzheimer's disease** a progressive form of neuronal degeneration in the brain and the most common cause of dementia in people of all ages. It is more common in older than younger people and is not just a form of presenile dementia, as was originally thought. The degeneration of neu-

rones is accompanied by changes in the brain's biochemistry. At the moment this condition is irreversible and there is no effective treatment.

**amalgam** a compound of mercury and other metals. *Dental a.* now rarely used for filling teeth.

**amaurosis** loss of vision, sometimes following excessive blood loss, especially after prolonged bleeding, e.g. haematuria. The visual loss may be partial or complete, temporary or permanent.

**ambidextrous** equally skilful with either hand.

**ambivalence** the existence of contradictory emotional feelings towards an object, commonly of love and hate for another person. If these feelings occur to a marked degree they lead to psychological disturbance.

**amblyopia** dimness of vision without any apparent lesion of the eye. Uncorrectable by optical means.

**ambulant** able to walk.

**ambulatory** having the capacity to walk. *A. treatment* or *care* health services provided on an outpatient or day care basis.

**amelioration** improvement of symptoms; a lessening of the severity of a disease.

**amenorrhoea** absence of menstruation. *Primary a.* the non-occurrence of the menses. *Secondary a.* the cessation of the menses, after they have been established, owing to disease or pregnancy.

**ametropia** defective vision. A general word applied to incorrect refraction.

**amino acid** a chemical compound containing both $NH_2$ and COOH groups. The end product of protein digestion. *Essential a.* one required for replacement and growth but which cannot be synthesized in the body in sufficient amounts and must be obtained in the diet (*see* Table on p. 19). Histidine is also essential

| Essential amino acids | |
|---|---|
| 1 | Threonine |
| 2 | Lysine |
| 3 | Methionine |
| 4 | Valine |
| 5 | Phenylalanine |
| 6 | Leucine |
| 7 | Tryptophan |
| 8 | Isoleucine |

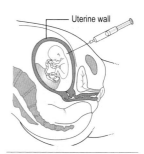

AMNIOCENTESIS

in childhood. ***Non-essential a. a.*** one necessary for proper growth but that can be synthesized in the body and is not specifically required in the diet.

**aminoglycoside** any of a group of bacterial antibiotics, derived from various species of *Streptomyces*, that interfere with the function of bacterial ribosomes. The aminoglycosides include gentamicin, netilmicin, streptomycin, tobramycin, amikacin, kanamycin and neomycin. They are used to treat infections caused by Gram-negative organisms and are classified as bactericidal agents because of their interference with bacterial replication. All the aminoglycoside antibiotics are highly toxic, requiring monitoring of blood serum levels and careful observation of the patient for early signs of toxicity, particularly ototoxicity and nephrotoxicity.

**amitosis** multiplication of cells by simple division or fission.

**ammonia** $NH_3$. A colourless pungent gas that dissolves in water. It is a naturally occurring compound of nitrogen and hydrogen.

**amnesia** partial or complete loss of memory. ***Anterograde a.*** loss of memory of events that have taken place since an injury or illness. ***Retrograde a.*** loss of memory for events prior to an injury. It often applies to the time immediately preceding an accident.

**amniocentesis** the withdrawal of fluid from the uterus through the abdominal wall by means of a syringe and needle (*see* Figure). It is primarily used in the diagnosis of chromosome disorders in the fetus and in cases of hydramnios. Mothers who are rhesus-negative should be given a reduced dose of anti-D immunoglobulin after the procedure to prevent then making antibodies.

**amniography** radiography of the gravid uterus.

**amnion** the innermost membrane enveloping the fetus and enclosing the liquor amnii, or amniotic fluid.

**amniotic** pertaining to the amnion. ***A. fluid*** the albuminous fluid contained in the amniotic sac. Liquor amnii.

**amoeba** a minute unicellular protozoon. It is able to move by pushing out parts of itself (called pseudopodia). Capable of reproduction by amitotic fission. Infection of the intestines by *Entamoeba histolytica* causes 'amoebic dysentery'.

**amoebiasis** infection with amoeba, particularly *Entamoeba histolytica*.

**amoebic** pertaining to, caused by, or of the nature of an amoeba. ***A. abscess*** an abscess cavity of the liver resulting from liquefaction necrosis due to entrance of *Entamoeba histolytica* into the portal circulation in amoebiasis; amoebic abscesses may affect the lung, brain and spleen. *A. dysentery* a form of dysentery caused by *Entamoeba histolytica* and spread by contaminated food, water and flies; called also amoebiasis. Amoebic dysentery is mainly a tropical disease but many cases occur in temperate countries. Symptoms are diarrhoea, fatigue and intestinal bleeding. Complications include involvement of the liver, liver abscess and pulmonary abscess.

**amoeboid** resembling an amoeba in structure or movement.

**amorphous** without definite shape. The term may be applied to fine powdery particles, as opposed to crystals.

**amphiarthrosis** a form of joint in which the bones are joined together by fibrocartilage, e.g. the junctions of the vertebrae.

**amphoric** pertaining to a bottle. Used to describe the sound sometimes heard on auscultation over cavities in the lungs, which resembles that produced by blowing across the mouth of a bottle.

**ampoule** a small glass or plastic phial in which sterile drugs of specified dose for injection are sealed.

**ampulla** the flask-like dilatation of a canal, e.g. of a uterine tube.

**amputation** surgical removal of a limb or other part of the body, e.g. the breast.

**amputee** a person who has had one or more limbs amputated.

**amylase** an enzyme that reduces starch to maltose. Found in saliva (ptyalin) and pancreatic juice (amylopsin).

**amyloid** 1. pertaining to starch. 2. a waxy starch-like material that is a complex protein forming in tissues and organs leading to disturbance of function, called amyloidosis.

**amylopsin** an enzyme found in the pancrease. Amylase.

**amylum** [L.] *starch*.

**amyotonia** atonic condition of the muscles. *A. congenita* any of several rare congenital diseases marked by general hypotonia of the muscles; called also Oppenheim's disease or floppy baby syndrome.

**anabolic** relating to anabolism. *A. compound* a substance that aids in the repair of body tissue, particularly protein. Androgens may be used in this way.

**anabolism** the building up or synthesis of cell structure from digested food materials. *See* METABOLISM.

**anacidity** decrease in normal acidity.

**anaclitic** denoting the dependence of the infant on the mother or mother substitute for its sense of wellbeing. *A. choice* a psychoanalytical term for the adult selection of a loved one who closely resembles one's mother (or another adult on whom one depended as a child). *A. depression* severe and progressive depression found in children who have lost their mothers and have not found a suitable substitute.

**anacrotism** an abnormal pulse wave tracing embodying a secondary expansion.

**anaemia** deficiency in either quality or quantity of red corpuscles in the blood that reduces the oxygen carrying capacity of the blood, giving rise especially to symptoms of anoxaemia. There is pallor, breathlessness on exertion, with palpitations, lassitude, headache, giddiness and often a history of poor resistance to infection. Anaemia may be due to many different causes. Increasingly, with the advent of electronic cell counters, anaemia is now classified according to the morphological characteristics of the erythrocytes. *Aplastic a.* the bone marrow is unable to produce red blood corpuscles. A rare condition. *Deficiency a.* any type that is due to the lack of the necessary factors for red cell formation, e.g. hormones or vitamins. *Haemolytic a.* a variety in which there is excessive destruction of red blood corpuscles caused by antibody formation in the blood (*see* RHESUS FACTOR), by drugs or by severe toxaemia, as in extensive burns. *Iron-deficiency a.* the most common type of anaemia, due to a lack of absorbable iron in the diet. It may also be due to excessive or chronic blood loss, or to poor absorption of dietary iron. *Macrocytic a.* a type in which the cells are larger than normal; present in pernicious anaemia. *Microcytic a.* a variety in which the cells are smaller than normal, as in iron deficiency. *Pernicious a.* a variety caused by the inability of the stomach to secrete the intrinsic factor necessary for the absorption of vitamin $B_{12}$ from the diet. *Sickle-cell a.* a hereditary haemolytic anaemia seen most commonly in black people living in or originating from the Caribbean islands, Africa, Asia, the Middle East and the Mediterranean. The red blood cells are sickle-shaped. *Splenic a.* a congenital, familial disease in which the red blood cells are fragile and easily broken down.

**anaerobe**  a microorganism that can live and thrive in the absence of free oxygen. These organisms are found in body cavities or wounds where the oxygen tension is very low. Examples are the bacilli of tetanus and gas gangrene.

**anaesthesia**  loss of feeling or sensation in a part or in the whole of the body, usually induced by drugs. *Basal a.* basal narcosis. Loss of consciousness, although supplemental drugs have to be given to ensure complete anaesthesia. *Epidural a.* injection into the extradural space between the vertebral spines and beneath the ligamentum flavum. *General a.* unconsciousness produced by inhalation or injection of a drug. *Inhalation a.* drugs or gas are administered by a face mask or endotracheal tube to cause general anaesthesia. *Intravenous a.* unconsciousness is produced by the introduction of a drug into a vein. *Local a.* local analgesia. Nerve conduction is blocked by injection of a local anaesthetic, or by freezing with ethyl chloride or by topical application. *Spinal a.* injection of anaesthetic agent into the spinal subarachnoid space.

**anaesthetic**  a drug causing anaesthesia.

**anaesthetist**  a person who is medically qualified to administer an anaesthetic and in the techniques of life support for the critically ill or injured.

**anal**  pertaining to the anus. *A. eroticism* sexual pleasure derived from anal functions. *A. fissure see* FISSURE. *A. fistula see* FISTULA. *A. stage* the second stage of a child's psychosexual development, characterized by the child's sensual interest in the anal area and the passing retention of faeces.

**analeptic**  a drug that stimulates the central nervous system.

**analgesia**  insensibility to pain, especially the relief of pain without causing unconsciousness. *Patient-controlled a.* a preset dose of analgesic, which the patient controls according to need. In-built safety measures prevent accidental overdose.

**analgesic**  1. relating to analgesia. 2. a remedy that relieves pain. *A. cocktail* an individualized mixture of drugs used to control pain.

**analogue**  1. an organ with a different structure and origin to but the same function as another one. 2. a compound with a similar structure to another but differing in respect of a particular element.

**analysis** 1. the act of determining the component parts of a substance. 2. in psychiatry, a method of trying to understand the complex mental processes, experiences and relationships with other individuals or groups of individuals to determine the reasons for an individual's behaviour. *A. of covariance (ANCOVA)* a statistic that measures differences among group means and uses a statistical technique to equate the groups under study in relation to another given variable. *A. of variance (ANOVA)* a statistic that tests whether groups differ from each other, rather than testing each pair of means separately. ANOVA considers the variation among all groups.

**anaphase** part of the process of mitosis or meiosis.

**anaphylaxis** anaphylactic shock. A severe reaction, often fatal, occurring in response to drugs, e.g. penicillin, but also to bee stings and food allergy, e.g. nuts in sensitive individuals. The symptoms are severe dyspnoea, rapid pulse, profuse sweating and collapse.

**anaplasia** a change in the character of cells, seen in tumour tissue.

**anarthria** inability to articulate speech sounds owing to a brain lesion or damage to peripheral nerves innervating articulatory muscles.

**anastomosis** 1. in surgery, any artificial connection of two hollow structures, e.g. gastroenterostomy. 2. in anatomy, the joining of the branches of two blood vessels.

**anatomy** the science of the structure of the body.

*Ancylostoma* hookworm. A genus of nematode roundworms which may inhabit the duodenum and cause extreme anaemia and malnutrition. *A. duodenale* a hookworm very widespread in tropical and subtropical areas.

**androgen** one of a group of hormones secreted by the testes and adrenal cortex. They are steroids which can be synthesized and produce the secondary male characteristics and the building up of protein tissue.

**android** resembling a man. *A. pelvis* a female pelvis shaped like a male pelvis with a wedge-shaped entrance and narrow anterior segment.

**anergy** 1. specific immunological tolerance in which T cells and B cells fail to respond normally. The state can be reversed. 2. tiredness, lethargy, lack of energy.

**aneurine** thiamin. An essential vitamin involved in carbohydrate metabolism. The main sources are unrefined cereals and pork. Vitamin $B_1$.

**aneurysm** a local dilatation of a blood vessel, usually an artery. Atherosclerosis is responsible for most arterial aneurysms; any injury to the arterial wall can predispose to the formation of a sac. Other diseases that can lead to an aneurysm include syphilis, certain non-specific inflammations, and a congenital defect in the artery. The pressure of blood causes it to increase in size and rupture is likely. Sometimes excision of the aneurysm or ligation of the artery is possible. *Dissecting a.* a condition in which a tear occurs in the aortic lining when the middle coat is necrosed and blood gets between the layers, stripping them apart. *Fusiform a.* a spindle-shaped arterial aneurysm. *Saccular a.* a dilatation of only a part of the circumference of an artery (*see* Figure on p. 23).

**angina** 1. a tight strangling sensation or pain. 2. an inflammation of the throat causing pain on swallowing. *A. cruris* intermittent claudication. Severe pain in the leg after walking. *A. pectoris* cardiac pain that occurs on exertion owing to insufficient blood supply to the heart muscles. *Vincent's a.* infection and ulceration of the tonsils by

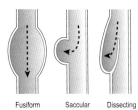

Fusiform    Saccular    Dissecting

TYPES OF ANEURYSM

a spirochaete, *Borrelia vincentii*, and a bacillus, *Fusiformis fusiformis*.

**angiocardiography** radiological examination of the heart and large blood vessels by means of cardiac catheterization and an opaque contrast medium.

**angiography** radiological examination of the blood vessels using an opaque contrast medium.

**angioma** a benign tumour composed of dilated blood vessels.

**angioedema** A type of reaction; most commonly caused by an allergy, characterized by well defined swellings or weals of sudden and rapid onset in the skin, throat, mouth, eyes and other areas. Fatal oedema of the glottis may occur resulting in a medical emergency. *See* OEDEMA.

**angioplasty** surgery of a narrowed artery to promote the normal flow of blood. ***Balloon a.*** technique in which a catheter with an elastic, flexible (balloon-like) tip that can be inflated is passed into a narrowed blood vessel, e.g. in the heart. The balloon is inflated to widen the stenosed area and increase the blood flow.

**angiosarcoma** a malignant vascular growth.

**angiospasm** a spasmodic contraction of an artery, causing cramping of the muscles.

**angiotensin** a substance that raises the blood pressure. It is a polypeptide produced by the action of renin on plasma globulins. Hypertensin.

**anhidrosis** marked deficiency in the secretion of sweat.

**anhidrotic** an agent that decreases perspiration. An adiaphoretic.

**anhydraemia** deficiency of water in the blood.

**aniline** a chemical compound derived from coal tar, used for making antiseptic dyes. It is an important cause of serious industrial poisoning associated with bone marrow depression as well as methaemoglobinaemia.

**anima** 1. the soul. 2. Jung's term for the unconscious, or inner being, of the individual, as opposed to the personality presented to the world (persona). In Jungian psychoanalysis, the more feminine soul or feminine component of a man's personality.

**anion** a negatively charged ion which travels towards the anode, e.g. chloride ($Cl^-$), carbonate ($CO_3^{2-}$). *See* CATION.

**aniridia** lack of part or the whole of the iris.

**anisocoria** inequality of diameter of the pupils of the two eyes.

**anisocytosis** inequality in the size of the red blood cells.

**anisometropia** a marked difference in the refractive power of the two eyes.

**ankle** the joint between the leg and foot, formed by the tibia and fibula articulating with the talus.

**ankle-brachial pressure index (ABPI)** The measurement of the ratio of systolic blood pressure at the ankle measured by a Doppler ultrasound probe to that measured at the brachial artery to quantify the degree of arterial occlusion in the leg. Forms an important part of a leg ulcer assessment regarding the patient's suitability for compression bandaging.

**ankyloblepharon** adhesions and scar tissue on the ciliary borders of the eyelids, giving the eye a distorted appearance.

**ankylosis** consolidation, immobility and stiffness of a joint as a result of disease.

**annular** ring-shaped.

**anoci-association** the exclusion of pain, fear and shock in surgical operations, brought about by means of local anaesthesia and basal narcosis.

**anodyne** 1. pain-relieving or relaxing. 2. a drug or other treatment that relieves pain.

**anomaly** considerable variation from normal.

**anomie** a feeling of hopelessness and lack of purpose.

*Anopheles* a genus of mosquito. Many are carriers of the malarial parasite and by their bite infect humans. Other species transmit filariasis.

**anophthalmia** congenital absence of a seeing eye. Some portion of the eye, e.g. the conjunctiva, is always present.

**anorexia** loss of appetite for food. *A. nervosa* a condition in which there is complete lack of appetite, with extreme emaciation. It is due to psychological causes and most commonly occurs in young women with poor self esteem, fear of obesity associated with a distorted body image, leading them to perceive themselves as fat and to take extreme forms of dietary control in order to lose weight.

**anosmia** loss of the sense of smell.

**anovular** applied to the absence of ovulation. Usually refers to uterine bleeding when there has been no ovulation, the result of taking contraceptive pills.

**anoxaemia** complete lack of oxygen in the blood.

**anoxia** lack of oxygen to an organ or tissue.

**antacid** a substance neutralizing acidity, particularly of the gastric juices.

**antagonist** 1. a muscle that has an opposite action to another, e.g. the biceps to the triceps. 2. in pharmacology, a drug that inhibits the action of another drug or enzyme, e.g. methotrexate is a folic acid antagonist. 3. in dentistry, a tooth in one jaw opposing one in the other jaw.

**anteflexion** a bending forward, as of the body of the uterus. *See* RETROFLEXION.

**antenatal** before birth. *A. care* care provided by midwives and obstetricians during pregnancy to ensure that the fetal and maternal health are satisfactory. Deviations from normal can be detected and treated early. The mother can be prepared for labour and parenthood and health education offered.

**antepartum** shortly before birth, i.e. in the last 3 months of pregnancy. *A. haemorrhage* bleeding occurring before parturition. *See* PLACENTA PRAEVIA.

**anterior** situated at or facing towards the front. The opposite of posterior. *A. capsule* the anterior covering of the lens of the eye. *A. chamber of the eye* the space between the cornea in front and the iris and lens behind.

**anterograde** extending or moving forwards.

**anteversion** the forward tilting of an organ, e.g. the normal position of the uterus. *See* RETROVERSION.

**anthelmintic (anthelminthic)** 1. destructive to worms. 2. an agent destructive to worms.

**anthracosis** a disease of the lungs, caused by inhalation of coal dust. A form of pneumoconiosis. 'Miner's lung'.

**anthrax** an acute, notifiable, infectious disease due to *Bacillus anthracis*, acquired through contact with infected animals or their by-products. A worldwide zoonosis, anthrax is now very uncommon in the UK.

**anthropoid** resembling man. *A. pelvis* female pelvis in which the antero-posterior diameter exceeds the transverse diameter.

**anthropology** the study of human beings that focuses on origins, historical and cultural development, and races. *Cultural a.* that branch of anthropology that is concerned with individuals and their relationship to others and to their environment. *Medical a.* biocultural discipline concerned with both the biological and sociocultural aspects of human behaviour, and the ways in which the two interact to influence health and disease. *Physical a.* that branch of anthropology that concerns the physical and evolutionary characteristics of human beings.

**anthropometry** the science that deals with the comparative measurement of parts of the human body, such as height, weight, body fat, etc.

**anti-D immunoglobulin** anti-rhesus antibody which is given by intramuscular injection to a rhesus-negative woman within 72 hours of delivery of her infant or following termination of her pregnancy, miscarriage or invasive investigations such as amniocentesis, to prevent haemolytic disease of the newborn in the next pregnancy. Anti-D is also available to all rhesus-negative women as antenatal prophylaxis. *See* RHESUS FACTOR.

**anti-inflammatory** a drug that reduces or acts against inflammation. May belong to one of several groups.

**antibacterial** a substance that destroys or suppresses the growth of bacteria.

**antibiotic** substances (e.g. penicillin), produced by certain bacteria and fungi, that prevent the growth of, or destroy, other bacteria. *A. resistance* the evolution and survival, as a result of worldwide antibiotic misuse, of bacteria undergoing the process of natural selection, despite the use of antibiotics to which they were once sensitive.

**antibody** also known as immunoglobulin, an antibody is one of a group of these glycoprotein molecules found either on the cell surface of B lymphocytes (membrane antibody) where they act as antigen receptors, or produced and secreted by B lymphocytes that have been stimulated and transformed by an antigen into plasma cells. Secreted antibodies are found in blood, serum and in other body fluids and tissues. Antibodies react and combine with a specific antigens during humoral immune responses, forming immune complexes. Antibodies are an important component of acquired (learned) immunity. There are five different types, or classes of antibody, each named by the abbreviation for immunoglobulin (Ig) and a letter of the alphabet, i.e. IgM, IgG, IgA, IgD, IgE. IgG (also called GAMMA-GLOBULIN) is the most abundant of the five classes of antibody and is the major immunoglobulin in the secondary humoral immune response.

**anticholinergic** a drug that inhibits the action of acetylcholine.

**anticholinesterase** an enzyme that inhibits the action of the enzyme acetylcholinesterase, thereby potentiating the action of acetylcholine at postsynaptic receptors in the parasympathetic nervous system, thus allowing return of normal muscle contraction.

**anticoagulant** a substance that prevents or delays the blood from clotting, e.g. heparin.

**anticonvulsant** a substance that will arrest or prevent convulsions. Anticonvulsant drugs such as phenytoin are used in the treatment of epilepsy and other conditions in which convulsions occur.

**antidepressant** one of a group of drugs which elevate mood, often diminish anxiety and increase coping behaviour. Tricyclic antidepressants are the most commonly used in treatment of depression. Monoamine oxidase inhibitors (MAOIs) are less commonly used because of the dietary restriction necessary and the toxic side-effects.

**anti-discriminatory practice** the professional policies, practice and provisions that actively seek to reduce institutional discrimination experienced by individuals and groups, particularly on the grounds of age, race, gender, disability, social class or sexual orientation. Anti-discriminatory practice can utilize particular legislation, such as the Sex Discrimination Act (1975) and the Disability Discrimination Act (1995), to challenge discrimination.

**antidiuretic** a substance that reduces the volume of urine excreted. *A. hormone* abbreviated ADH. A hormone which is secreted by the posterior pituitary gland. Vasopressin.

**antidote** an agent that counteracts the effect of a poison.

**antiembolic** against embolism. Anti-embolic hose/stockings are worn to prevent the formation or decrease the risk of deep vein thrombosis, especially in patients after surgery or those confined to bed.

**antiemetic** a drug that prevents or overcomes nausea and vomiting.

**antifungal** a preparation effective in treating fungal infections.

**antigen** any substance, bacterial or otherwise, which in suitable conditions can stimulate the production of an immune response.

**antihaemophilic** 1. effective against the bleeding tendency in haemophilia. 2. an agent that counteracts the bleeding tendency in haemophilia.

*A. factor* abbreviated AHF. One of the clotting factors, deficiency of which causes classic, sex-linked haemophilia; called also factor VIII and antihaemophilic globulin (AHG). It is available in a preparation for preventive and therapeutic use.

**antihistamine** any one of a group of drugs which block the tissue receptors for histamine. They are used to treat allergic conditions, e.g. drug rashes, hay fever and serum sickness, and include promethazine.

**antihypertensive** 1. effective against hypertension. 2. an agent that reduces high blood pressure.

**antimalarial** against malaria. Drugs that are used both in the treatment of an attack and for prophylaxis. All visitors to malarial countries should take preventative anti-malarial drugs. Expert advice should be sought regarding the appropriate drug and dose. *See* MALARIA.

**antimetabolite** one of a group of chemical compounds which prevent the effective utilization of the corresponding metabolite, and interfere with normal growth or cell mitosis if the process requires that metabolite.

**antineoplastic** effective against the multiplication of malignant cells.

**antiperistalsis** contrary contractions which propel the contents of the intestines backwards and upwards.

**antiperspirant** a substance applied to the body as a lotion, cream or spray to reduce sweating. Use can sometimes result in irritation especially if the skin is broken.

**antipruritic** an external application or drug that relieves itching.

**antipyretic** an agent that reduces fever.

**antisepsis** the prevention of infection by destroying or arresting the growth of harmful microorganisms.

**antiseptic** 1. preventing sepsis. 2. any substance that inhibits the growth of bacteria, in contrast to a germicide, which kills bacteria outright.

**antiserum** animal or human blood serum which contains antibodies to infective organisms or to their toxins. The serum donor must have previously been infected with the identified organism.

**antisocial** against society. *A. behaviour* in psychiatry, the refusal of an individual to accept the normal obligations and restraints imposed by the community upon its members.

**antispasmodic** any measure used to prevent or relieve the occurrence of muscle spasm.

**antitoxin** a substance produced by the body cells as a reaction to invasion by bacteria, which neutralizes their toxins. *See* IMMUNITY.

**antitussive** 1. effective against cough. 2. an agent that suppresses coughing.

**antivenin** an antitoxic serum to neutralize the poison injected by the bite of a snake or insect.

**antiviral** 1. acting against viruses. 2. a drug that is effective against viruses causing disease, e.g. acyclovir.

**antrum** a cavity in bone. *Mastoid a.* the tympanic antrum, which is an air-conditioning cavity in the mastoid portion of the temporal bone. *Maxillary a.* antrum of Highmore. The air sinus in the upper jawbone.

**anuria** cessation of the secretion of urine.

**anus** the extremity of the alimentary canal, through which the faeces are discharged. *Imperforate a.* one where there is no opening because of a congenital defect.

**anxiety** a chronic state of tension, which affects both mind and body. *A. neurosis see* NEUROSIS.

**anxiolytic** a substance, such as diazepam, used for relief of anxiety. Anxiolytics may quickly cause dependence and are not suitable for long-term administration. Also called anti-anxiety agent and minor tranquillizer.

**aorta** the large artery rising out of the left ventricle of the heart and supplying blood to all the body. *Abdominal a.* that part of the artery lying in the abdomen. *Arch of the a.* the curve of the artery over the heart. *Thoracic a.* that part which passes through the chest.

**aortic** pertaining to the aorta. *A. incompetence* owing to previous inflammation the aortic valve has become fibrosed and is unable to close completely, thus allowing backward flow of blood (*a. regurgitation*) into the left ventricle during diastole. *A. stenosis* a narrowing of the aortic valve. *A. valve* the valve between the left ventricle of the heart and the ascending aorta, which prevents the backward flow of blood through the artery.

**aortography** radiographic examination of the aorta. A radio-opaque contrast medium is injected into the blood to render visible lesions of the aorta or its main branches.

**APACHE** abbreviation for Acute Physiology And Chronic Health Evaluation. A classification system for indicating severity of illness in intensive care patients.

**apathy** an appearance of indifference, with no response to stimuli or display of emotion.

**aperient** a drug that produces an action of the bowels. A laxative.

**aperistalsis** lack of peristaltic movement of the intestines.

**Apert's syndrome** *E. Apert, French paediatrician, 1868–1940.* A congenital abnormality in which there is fusion at birth of all the cranial sutures, in addition to syndactyly (webbed fingers).

**apex** the top or pointed end of a cone-shaped structure. *A. beat* the

| APGAR SCORE | | | |
|---|---|---|---|
| **Sign** | **Score** | | |
| | **0** | **1** | **2** |
| Heart rate | Absent | Slow – below 100 | Fast – above 100 |
| Respiratory effort | Absent | Slow, irregular | Good, crying |
| Muscle tone | Limp | Some flexion of the extremities | Active |
| Reflex irritability | No response | Grimace | Crying, cough |
| Colour | Blue, pale | Body pink, extremities blue | Completely pink |

beat of the heart against the chest wall which can be felt during systole. *A. of the heart* the end closing the left ventricle. *A. of the lung* the extreme upper part of the organ.

**Apgar score** *V. Apgar, American anaesthetist, 1909–1974.* A system used in the assessment of the newborn: reflex irritability and colour. The Apgar score is assessed 1 minute after birth and again at 5 minutes. Most healthy infants score 9 at birth. A score below 7 would indicate cause for concern (*see* Table).

**APEL** *see* ACCREDITATION.

**APH** antepartum haemorrhage.

**aphagia** loss of the power to swallow.

**aphakia** absence of the lens of the eye. Aphacia.

**aphasia** a communication disorder due to brain damage; characterized by complete or partial disturbance of language comprehension, formulation or expression. Partial disturbance is also called dysphasia. *Broca's a.* disorder in which verbal output is impaired, and in which verbal communication may be affected as well. Speech is slow and laboured and writing is often impaired. *Developmental a.* a childhood failure to acquire normal language when deafness, learning difficulties, motor disability or severe emotional disturbance are not causes.

**aphonia** inability to produce sound. The cause may be organic disease of the larynx or may be purely functional.

**aphrodisiac** a drug which excites sexual desire.

**aphthae** small ulcers surrounded by erythema on the inside of the mouth (aphthous ulcers).

**apical** pertaining to the apex of a structure.

**apicectomy** excision of the root of a tooth. Root resection.

**APL** *see* ACCREDITATION.

**aplasia** incomplete development of an organ or tissue or absence of growth.

**aplastic** without power of development. *A. anaemia see* ANAEMIA.

**apnoea** cessation of respiration. *A. mattress* a mattress designed to sound an alarm if the infant lying on it ceases breathing. *A. monitor* designed to give an audible signal when a certain period of apnoea has occurred. *A. of prematurity* apnoeic periods occurring in the respiration of newborn infants in whom the respiratory centre is immature or depressed. *Cardiac a.* the temporary cessation of breathing caused by a reduction of the carbon dioxide tension in the blood, as seen in Cheyne–Stokes respiration. *Sleep a.* transient attacks of failure of autonomic control of respiration, becoming more pronounced during sleep.

**apocrine** pertaining to modified sweat glands that develop in hair follicles, such as are mainly found in the axillary, pubic and perineal areas.

**aponeurosis** a sheet of tendon-like tissue which connects some muscles to the parts that they move.

**apophysis** a prominence or excrescence, usually of a bone.

**apoplexy** a sudden fit of insensibility, usually caused by rupture of a cerebral blood vessel or its occlusion by a blood clot. Rarely used term.

**apparition** a hallucinatory vision, usually the phantom appearance of a person. A spectre.

**appendectomy** appendicectomy.

**appendicectomy** removal of the vermiform appendix.

**appendicitis** inflammation of the vermiform appendix.

**appendix** a supplementary or dependent part. *A. epiploicae* small tag-like structures of peritoneum containing fat, which are scattered over the surface of the large intestine, especially the transverse colon. *Vermiform a.* a worm-like tube with a blind end, projecting from the caecum in the right iliac region. It may be from 2.5 to 15 cm long.

**apperception** conscious reception and recognition of a sensory stimulus.

**appetite** the desire for food. It is stimulated by the sight, smell or thought of food, and accompanied by the flow of saliva in the mouth and gastric juice in the stomach. The stomach will also receives an extra blood supply in preparation for its digestive activity. Appetite is psychological, dependent on memory and associations, as compared with hunger, which is physiologically aroused by the body's need for food. Appetite can be discouraged by unattractive food, surroundings or company, and by emotional states such as anxiety, irritation, anger and fear.

**apposition** the bringing into contact of two structures, e.g. fragments of bone in setting a fracture.

**appraisal** a formal review, usually annually of a health care professional's performance by a trained appraiser in order to provide feedback on past performance, identifying progress made and together agreeing future goals.

**apprehension** a feeling of dread or fear.

**approved name** the non-proprietary or generic name for a drug. The approved name should always be used in prescribing except where the bioavailability may vary between brands.

**apraxia** the inability to perform correct movements because of a brain lesion and not because of sensory impairment or loss of muscle power in the limbs. *Oral a.* inability to perform volitional movements of the tongue and lips in the absence of paralysis or paresis. Involuntary movements may, however, be observed, e.g. patients may purse their lips in order to blow out a match.

**aptitude** the natural ability or capacity to acquire mental and physical skills. *A. test* the evaluation of a person's ability for learning certain skills or carrying out specific tasks.

**apyrexia** the absence of fever.

**aqua** [L.] *water. A. destillata* distilled water.

**aqueduct** a canal for the passage of fluid. *A. of Sylvius* the canal connecting the third and fourth ventricles of the brain.

**aqueous** watery. *A. humour* the fluid filling the anterior and posterior chambers of the eye.

*Arachis* a genus of leguminous plants used in various preparations such as earwax softeners and skin medications.

**arachnodactyly** abnormally long and thin fingers and toes. A congenital condition.

**arachnoid** 1. resembling a spider's web. 2. a web-like membrane covering the central nervous system between the dura and pia mater.

**arborization** the branching terminations of many nerve fibres and processes.

**arbovirus** one of a large group of viruses transmitted by insect vectors (anthropod-borne), e.g. mosquitoes, sandflies or ticks. The diseases caused include many types of encephalitis, also yellow, dengue, sandfly and Rift Valley fevers.

**arcus** [L.] *bow, arch. A. senilis* an opaque circle appearing round the edge of the cornea in old age.

**ARDS** acute respiratory distress syndrome.

**areola** 1. a space in connective tissue. 2. a ring of pigmentation, e.g. that surrounding the nipple.

**arginase** an enzyme of the liver that splits arginine into urea and ornithine.

**arginine** an essential amino acid produced by the digestion of protein. It forms a link in the excretion of nitrogen, being hydrolysed by the enzyme arginase.

**Argyll Robertson pupil** *D. Argyll Robertson, British ophthalmologist, 1837–1909. See* PUPIL.

**Arnold–Chiari malformation** *J. Arnold, German pathologist, 1835–1915; H. Chiari, German pathologist, 1851–1916.* Herniation of the cerebellum and elongation of the medulla oblongata; occurs in hydrocephalus associated with spina bifida.

**aromatherapy** the therapeutic use of specially prepared essential or aromatic oils obtained from the different parts of plants, including the flowers, leaves, seeds, wood,

roots and bark. The oils may be diluted for use in massage, baths or infusions.

**arousal** a state of alertness and increased response to stimuli.

**arrector pili** a small muscle attached to the hair follicle of the skin. When contracted it causes the hair to become erect, producing the appearance known as gooseflesh.

**arrest** a cessation or stopping. *Cardiac a.* cessation of ventricular contractions. *Developmental a.* discontinuation of a child's mental or physical development at a certain stage. *Respiratory a.* cessation of breathing.

**arrhythmia** variation from the normal rhythm, e.g. in the heart's action. *Sinus a.* an abnormal pulse rhythm due to disturbance of the sinoatrial node, causing quickening of the heart on inspiration and slowing on expiration.

**art therapy** the use of the creative arts as a medium to encourage patients to express their feelings when unable to do so verbally.

**artefact** something that is man-made or introduced artificially.

**arterial blood gases (ABGs)** normally present in arterial blood include oxygen, carbon dioxide and nitrogen. Measurements of the partial pressures of oxygen and carbon dioxide together with the blood's pH provide important information on the oxygen saturation of the haemoglobin and acid-base state of the blood indicating the adequacy of ventilation in critical care situations.

**arteriectomy** the removal of a portion of artery wall, usually followed by anastomosis or a replacement graft. *See* ARTERIOPLASTY.

**arteriography** radiography of arteries after the injection of a radio-opaque contrast medium.

**arterioplasty** the reconstruction of an artery by means of replacement or plastic surgery.

**arteriosclerosis** a gradual loss of elasticity in the walls of arteries due to thickening and calcification. It is accompanied by high blood pressure, and precedes the degeneration of internal organs associated with old age or chronic disease.

**arteriotomy** an incision or puncture into an artery.

**arteriovenous** both arterial and venous; pertaining to both artery and vein, e.g. an arteriovenous aneurysm, fistula or shunt for haemodialysis.

**arteritis** inflammation of an artery. *Giant cell a.* a variety of polyarteritis resulting in partial or complete occlusion of a number of arteries. The carotid arteries are often involved. *Temporal a.* occlusion of the extracranial arteries, particularly the carotid arteries.

**artery** a tube of muscle and elastic fibres, lined with endothelium, which distributes blood from the heart to the capillaries throughout the body.

**arthralgia** neuralgic pains in a joint.

**arthrectomy** excision of a joint.

**arthritis** inflammation of one or more joints. Movement in the joint is restricted, with pain and swelling. Arthritis and the rheumatic diseases in general constitute the major cause of chronic disability in the UK, where it is estimated that 20 million persons have a rheumatic disease, of whom between 6 and 8 million are severely affected. *Acute rheumatic a.* rheumatic fever. *Osteo-a.* (DJD) a degenerative condition attacking the articular cartilage and aggravated by an impaired blood supply, previous injury or overweight, mainly affecting weight-bearing joints and causing pain. *Rheumatoid a.* a chronic inflammation, usually of unknown origin. The disease is progressive and incapacitating, owing to the resulting ankylosis and deformity of the bones. Usually affects the elderly. A juvenile form is known as STILL'S DISEASE.

**arthroclasia** the breaking down of adhesions in a joint to produce freer movement.

**arthrodesis** the fixation of a movable joint by surgical operation.

**arthrography** the examination of a joint by means of X-rays. An opaque contrast medium may be used.

**arthrogryposis** 1. a congenital abnormality in which fibrous ankylosis of some or all of the joints in the limbs occurs. 2. a tetanus spasm.

**arthroplasty** plastic surgery for the reorganization of a joint. *Charnley's a. see* MCKEE FARRAR A. *Cup a.* reconstruction of the articular surface, which is then covered by a vitallium cup. *Excision a.* excision of the joint surfaces affected, so that the gap thus formed then fills with fibrous tissue or muscle. *Girdlestone a.* an excision arthroplasty of the hip. *McKee Farrar a.* replacement of both the head and the socket of the femur; *Charnley's a.* is similar. *Replacement a.* partial removal of the head of the femur and its replacement by a metal prosthesis.

**arthroscope** an endoscope for examining the interior of a joint.

**articular** pertaining to a joint.

**articulation** 1. a junction of two or more bones. 2. the enunciation of words.

**artificial** not natural. *A. feeding* 1. the giving of food other than by placing it directly in the mouth. It may be provided via the mouth, using an oesophageal tube; the food may be introduced into the stomach through a fine tube via the nostril (the nasal route); an opening through the abdominal wall into the stomach (i.e. a gastrostomy) may allow direct introduction; or food may be injected intravenously (*see* PARENTERAL). 2. in reference to the feeding of infants, giving food other than human milk. *A. insemination* the insertion of sperm into the uterus by means of syringe and cannula instead of coitus. The husband's (AIH) or donor (AID) semen may be used. *A. kidney* a dialysis machine to remove unwanted waste materials from the patient with acute or chronic renal failure. *See* HAEMODIALYSIS. *A. respiration* a means of resuscitation from asphyxia. *A. tears* sterile solutions designed to maintain the moisture of the cornea when the latter is abnormally dry due to inadequate tear production. Methylcellulose is a common ingredient.

**arytenoid** resembling the mouth of a pitcher. *A. cartilages* two cartilages of the larynx; their function is to regulate the tension of the vocal cords attached to them.

**asbestos** a fibrous non-combustible silicate of magnesium and calcium that is a good non-conductor of heat. There are three types of asbestos fibre – white, brown and blue – that were widely used in the building industry. White fibre was the most commonly used and brown fibre the most dangerous to health. In many countries there are now strict regulations controlling the decline of asbestos (which has declined), including its removal from buildings. Contact with asbestos over a prolonged period may result in asbestosis, bronchial and laryngeal cancer and mesothelioma.

**asbestosis** a form of pneumoconiosis (chronic lung disease), due to the inhalation of asbestos fibres causing scarring of the lung tissue. It results in breathlessness and leads to respiratory failure. It may be latent for many years. *See* MESOTHELIOMA

**ascariasis** the condition in which roundworms are found in the gastrointestinal tract. Treatment is with anthelmintic drugs to eliminate the infestation.

**ascites** free fluid in the peritoneal cavity. It may be the result of local inflammation or venous obstruction, or be part of a generalized oedema.

**ascorbic acid** vitamin C. This acid is found in many vegetables and fruits and is an essential dietary constituent for humans. Vitamin C is destroyed by heat and deteriorates during storage. It is necessary for connective tissue and collagen fibre synthesis and promotes the healing of wounds. Deficiency causes scurvy.

**asepsis** freedom from pathogenic microorganisms.

**aseptic** free from sepsis. *A. technique* a method of carrying out sterile procedures so that there is a minimum risk of introducing infection. Achieved by the sterility of equipment and a non-touch technique.

**asexual** without sex. *A. reproduction* the production of new individuals without sexual union, e.g. by cell division or budding.

**asparaginase** an enzyme that catalyses the deamination of asparagine; used as an antineoplastic agent against cancers, e.g. acute lymphocytic leukaemia, in which the malignant cells require exogenous asparagine for protein synthesis.

**aspartame** a synthetic compound of two amino acids (L-aspartyl-L-phenylalanine methyl ester) used as a low-calorie sweetener. It is 180 times as sweet as sucrose (table sugar); the amount equal in sweetness to a teaspoon of sugar contains 0.1 calorie (4.2J). Aspartame does not promote the formation of dental caries. It should be avoided by patients with phenylketonuria.

**aspect** that part of a surface facing in a particular direction. *Dorsal a.*

that facing and seen from the back. *Ventral a.* that facing and seen from the front.

**aspergillosis** a bronchopulmonary disease in which the mucous membrane is attacked by the fungus *Aspergillus*.

**Aspergillus** a genus of fungi. *A. fumigatus* a common cause of aspergillosis, found in soil and manure.

**aspermia** absence of sperm.

**asphyxia** a deficiency of oxygen in the blood and an increase in carbon dioxide in the blood and tissues. Symptoms include irregular and disturbed respirations, or a complete absence of breathing, and pallor or cyanosis. Asphyxia may occur whenever there is an interruption in the normal exchange of oxygen and carbon dioxide between the lungs and the outside air. Common causes are drowning, electric shock, lodging of a foreign body in the air passages, inhalation of smoke and poisonous gases and trauma to or disease of the lungs or air passages. Treatment includes immediate remedy of the situation (*see* RESPIRATION (ARTIFICIAL)) and removal of the underlying cause whenever possible.

**aspiration** 1. the act of inhaling. 2. the drawing off of fluid from a cavity by means of suction.

**assault** unlawful personal attack or trespass upon another person even if only with menacing words.

**assay** a quantitative examination to determine the amount of a particular constituent of a mixture, or of the biological or pharmacological potency of a drug.

**assent** agreement to undergo medical care and treatment that is obtained from an adult or child who is legally incompetent to consent.

**assertiveness** a form of behaviour characterized by a confident declaration or affirmation of a statement without need of proof.

To assert oneself is to compel recognition of one's rights or position without either aggressively transgressing the rights of another and assuming a position of dominance, or submissively permitting another to deny one's rights or rightful position. *A. training* instruction and practice in techniques for dealing with interpersonal conflicts and threatening situations in an assertive manner, avoiding the extremes of aggressive and submissive behaviour.

**assessment** 1. the critical analysis and valuation or judgement of the status or quality of a particular condition, situation or other subject of appraisal. In the nursing process, assessment involves the gathering of information about the health status of the patient/client, analysis and synthesis of the data, and the making of a clinical nursing judgement (*see* NURSING (PROCESS)). The outcome of the nursing assessment is the establishment of a nursing DIAGNOSIS, the identification of the nursing problems. 2. an examination set by an examining authority to test a candidate's skills and knowledge.

**assimilation** the process of transforming food so that it can be absorbed and utilized as nourishment by the tissues of the body.

**associate nurse** a nurse who, as a member of the primary nursing team, is responsible for effecting a patient's care plans on behalf of the primary nurse. *See* PRIMARY NURSING.

**association** coordination of function of similar parts. *A. fibres* nerve fibres linking different areas of the brain. *A. of ideas* a mental impression in which a thought or any sensory impulse will call to mind another object or idea connected in some way with the former. *Free a.* a method employed in psychoanalysis in which the patient is encouraged to express freely whatever comes to mind. By this method material that is in the unconscious can be recalled.

**associative play** a form of play in which a group of children participate in similar activities without formal organization or direction.

**asthenia** want of strength. Debility. Loss of tone.

**asthenic** description of a type of body build: a pale, lean, narrowly built person with poor muscle development.

**asthenopia** eye strain likely to arise in long-sighted people when continual effort of accommodation is required for close work.

**asthma** paroxysmal dyspnoea characterized by wheezing and difficulty in expiration. The illness often commences in childhood but can commence at any age and in about half of the children affected it may be outgrown. *Bronchial a.* attacks of dyspnoea in which there is wheezing and difficulty in expiration due to muscular spasm of the bronchi. The attacks may be precipitated by hypersensitivity to foreign substances, air pollution, exertion or infection, or associated with emotional upsets. There is often a family history of asthma or other allergic condition. Management involves avoidance of known allergens and treatment is with bronchodilators with or without corticosteroids, usually via an aerosol. Other drug therapies used include sodium cromoglycate useful in preventing exercise-induced asthma and inhaled anticholinergic drugs may also be used to assist bronchodilation. An asthmatic person with an acute attack that does not respond to initial drug therapy should be referred to hospital for immediate assessment and treatment. *Cardiac a.* attacks of dyspnoea and palpitation, arising most often at night,

associated with left-sided heart failure and pulmonary congestion. Treatment is with diuretic therapy.

**astigmatism** inequality of the refractive power of an eye, due to curvature of its corneal meridians. The curve across the front of the eye from side to side is not quite the same as the curve from above downwards. The focus on the retina is then not a point but a diffuse and indistinct area. May be congenital or acquired.

**astringent** an agent causing contraction of organic tissues, thereby checking secretions, e.g. silver nitrate.

**astrocytoma** a malignant tumour of the brain or spinal cord. It is slow-growing. A glioma.

**asymmetry** inequality in size or shape of two normally similar structures or of two halves of a structure normally the same.

**asymptomatic** without symptoms.

**asynergy** lack of coordination of structures which normally act in harmony.

**asystole** absence of heartbeat. Cardiac arrest.

**at risk** whereby an individual or population may be vulnerable to a particular disease, hazard or injury. At risk situations are those involving possible problems that may be preventable with appropriate intervention, or, if they should occur, treatment.

**ataraxia** a state of detached serenity with depression of mental faculties or impairment of consciousness.

**ataxia, ataxy** failure of muscle coordination resulting in irregular jerky movements, and unsteadiness in standing and walking from a disorder of the controlling mechanisms in the brain, or from inadequate input to the brain from joints and muscles. *Hereditary a.* Friedreich's ataxia.

**atelectasis** a collapsed or airless state of the lung, which may be acute or chronic and may involve all or part of the lung: (a) from imperfect expansion of pulmonary alveoli at birth (*congenital a.*); (b) as the result of disease or injury.

**atheroma** an abnormal mass of fatty or lipid material with a fibrous covering, existing as a discrete, raised plaque within the intima of an artery.

**atherosclerosis** a condition in which the fatty degenerative plaques of atheroma are accompanied by arteriosclerosis, a narrowing and hardening of the vessels.

**athetosis** a recurring series of slow, writhing movements of the hands, usually due to a cerebral lesion.

**athlete's foot** a fungal infection between the toes, easily transmitted to other people. *See* TINEA.

**atlas** the first cervical vertebra, articulating with the occipital bone of the skull.

**atmosphere** 1. the gases that surround the earth, extending to an altitude of 16 km. 2. the air or climate of a particular place, e.g. a smoking atmosphere. 3. mental or moral environment, tone or mood.

**atmospheric pressure** pressure exerted by the air in all directions. At sea level it is about 100 kPa.

**atom** the smallest particle of an element that retains all the properties of that element. It is made up of a central positively charged nucleus and, moving around it in orbit, negatively charged electrons.

**atomizer** an instrument by which a liquid is divided to form a fine spray or vapour (nebulizer).

**atony** lack of tone, e.g. in the muscle detrusor of the bladder resulting in incontinence.

**atopy** a state of hypersensitivity to certain antigens. There is an inherited tendency that includes asthma, eczema and hay fever.

**ATP** adenosine triphosphate.

**atresia** absence of a natural opening or tubular structure, e.g. of the anus or vagina; usually a congenital malformation.

**atrial** relating to the atrium. *A. fibrillation* overstimulation of the atrial walls so that many areas of excitation arise and the atrioventricular node is bombarded with impulses, many of which it cannot transmit, resulting in a highly irregular pulse. *A. flutter* rapid regular action of the atria. The atrioventricular node transmits alternative impulses or one in three or four. The atrial rate is usually about 300 beats per minute. *A. septal defect* the non-closure of the foramen ovale at the time of birth, giving rise to a congenital heart defect.

**atrioventricular** pertaining to the atrium and ventricle. *A. bundle see* BUNDLE OF HIS. *A. node* a node of neurogenic tissue situated between the atrium and ventricle and transmitting impulses. *A. valves* the bicuspid and tricuspid valve on the left and right sides of the heart respectively.

**atrium** *pl.* atria. 1. a cavity, entrance or passage. 2. one of the two upper chambers of the heart. Formerly called auricle.

**atrophy** wasting of any part of the body, due to degeneration of the cells, from disuse, or lack of nourishment or nerve supply. *Progressive muscular a.* (motor neurone disease) degeneration of the motor neurones with wasting of muscle tissue.

**atropine** the active principle of belladonna. An alkaloid which inhibits respiratory and gastric secretions, relaxes muscle spasm and dilates the pupil.

**attack** an episode or onset of illness. *A. rate* number of cases of a disease in a particular group, e.g. a school, over a given period, related to the population of that group. *Transient ischaemic a.* brief attack (a few hours or less) of cerebral dysfunction of vascular origin, without lasting neurological deficit.

**attention deficit syndrome** a disorder of childhood characterized by marked failure of attention, impulsiveness and increased motor activity. Affects more boys than girls. Treatment involves medication, behaviour therapy and social support. Also known as attention deficit hyperactivity disorder (ADHD).

**attenuation** a bacteriological process by which organisms are rendered less virulent by culture in artificial media through many generations, exposure to light, air, etc.; it is used for vaccine preparations.

**attitude** 1. a posture or position of the body; in obstetrics, the relation of the various parts of the fetal body to one another. 2. a pattern of mental views established by cumulative prior experience.

**atypical** irregular; not conforming to type.

**audiogram** a graph produced by an audiometer.

**audiologist** an allied health professional specializing in audiology, who provides services that include: (a) evaluation of hearing function to detect hearing impairment and, if there is a hearing disorder, to determine the anatomical site involved and the cause of the disorder; (b) selection of appropriate hearing aids; and (c) training in lip reading, hearing aid use and maintenance of normal speech.

**audiology** the science concerned with the sense of hearing, especially the evaluation and measurement of impaired hearing and the rehabilitation of those with impaired hearing.

**audiometer** an instrument for testing hearing, whereby the threshold of the patient's hearing can be measured.

**audit** systematic review and evaluation of records and other data to determine the quality of the services or products provided in a given situation. It is also now a government requirement for the financial review of NHS Trusts. *A. Monitor* an adaptation for the UK of the USA Rush Medicus system of assessing quality of nursing care. It consists of 'checklists' for quality, leading to a scoring system. *A. trail* the process in which careful documentation of the research process makes it possible for students and other researchers to understand how any particular finding was reached. *Medical a.* the systematic critical analysis of the quality of medical treatment and care, including the procedures for diagnosis and treatment, the use of resources, outcomes and the resultant quality of life for the patient. *Nursing a.* an evaluation of structure, process and outcome as a measurement of the quality of nursing care. *Concurrent audits* are conducted at the time the care is being provided to clients/patients. They may be conducted by means of observation and interview of clients/patients, review of open charts, or conferences with groups of consumers and providers of nursing care. *Retrospective audits* are conducted after the patient's discharge. Methods include the study of closed patient's charts and nursing care plans, questionnaires, interviews and surveys of patients and families.

**Audit Commission** an independent body established in 1983 to appoint and regulate external auditors of local authorities in England and Wales. In 1990 its responsibilities were extended to include the NHS. The main duties of the Audit Commission include the promotion of 'best practice' in local government and NHS bodies, encouraging economy, efficiency and effectiveness in both the management and delivery of services. It appoints external auditors to all local government authorities and to NHS purchasers and providers including Primary Care Trusts to monitor stewardship of public finances.

**auditory** relating to the ear or to the sense of hearing

**aura** the premonition, peculiar to an individual, which often precedes an epileptic fit.

**aural** referring to the ear.

**auricle** 1. the external portion of the ear. 2. obsolete term for the atrium.

**auriscope** an instrument for examining the drum of the ear. An otoscope.

**aurum** [L.] gold.

**auscultation** examining the internal organs by listening to the sounds that they give out. In *direct* or *immediate a.* the ear is placed directly against the body. In *mediate a.* a stethoscope is used.

**autism** self-absorption. Abnormal dislike of the society of others. *Infantile a.* failure of a child to relate to people and situations, leading to complete withdrawal into a world of private fantasies.

**autistic** pertaining to autism.

**autoagglutination** 1. clumping or agglutination of cells by an individual's own serum, as in autohaemagglutination. Autoagglutination occurring at low temperatures is called cold agglutination. 2. agglutination of particulate antigens, e.g. bacteria, in the absence of specific antigens.

**autoantibody** an antibody formed in response to and reacting against the individual's own tissues.

**autoantigen** a tissue constituent that stimulates production of autoantibodies in the organism in which it occurs.

**autoclave** a steam-heated sterilizing apparatus in which the temperature is raised by reducing the air pressure inside; steam is injected under pressure, bringing

about efficient sterilization of instruments and dishes treated in this way.

**autodigestion** dissolution of tissue by its own secretions. Autolysis.

**autoeroticism** sexual pleasure derived from self-stimulation of erogenous zones (the mouth, the anus, the genitals and the skin). *See* MASTURBATION.

**autogenic therapy** a complementary therapy combining self-hypnosis and relaxation.

**autogenous** generated within the body and not acquired from external sources.

**autograft** the transfer of skin or other tissue from one part of the body to another to repair some deficiency.

**autoimmune disease** condition in which the body develops antibodies to its own tissues, e.g. in autoimmune thyroiditis (Hashimoto's disease).

**autoimmunization** the formation of antibodies against the individual's own tissue.

**autoinfection** self-infection, transferred from one part of the body to another by fingers, towels, etc.

**autoinoculation** inoculation with a microorganism from the body itself.

**autointoxication** poisoning by toxins generated within the body itself.

**autologous** related to self; belonging to the same organism. *A. blood transfusion* abbreviated ABT. The patient donates blood before elective surgery for transfusion postoperatively. ABT may also be obtained as a blood salvage procedure during operation or postoperatively. Avoids cross-matching, compatibility and transfusion infection problems.

**autolysis** a breaking up of living tissues, e.g. as may occur if pancreatic ferments escape into surrounding tissues. It also occurs after death.

**automated auditory brainstem response (AABR)** one of two hearing tests in the Newborn

Hearing Screening Programme that records brain activity in response to clicking sounds via sensors placed on the infant's head. Those infants who fail to respond to this test are referred for a full auditory diagnostic assessment.

**automatic** performed without the influence of the will.

**automatism** performance of non-reflex acts without apparent volition, and of which the patient may have no memory afterwards, as in somnambulism. *Post-epileptic a.* automatic acts following an epileptic fit.

**autonomic** self-governing. *A. nervous system* the sympathetic and parasympathetic nerves that control involuntary muscles and glandular secretion, over which there is no conscious control.

**autonomy** the right of personal freedom of action, which is regarded as one of the hallmarks of a profession.

**autoplasty** 1. replacement of missing tissue by grafting a healthy section from another part of the body. 2. in psychoanalysis, instinctive modification within the psychic systems in adaptation to reality.

**autopsy** postmortem examination of a body to determine the cause of death.

**autosome** any chromosome other than the sex chromosomes. In humans there are 22 pairs of autosomes and one pair of sex chromosomes.

**autosuggestion** suggestion arising in one's self. Uncritical acceptance of an idea arising in the individual's own mind.

**autotransfusion** reinfusion of a patient's own blood.

**autotransplantation** transfer of tissue from one part of the body to another part.

**avascular** not vascular. Bloodless. *A. necrosis* death of bone owing to deficient blood supply, usually following an injury.

**average** 1. the value or score that is typical of a group. The result is obtained by adding several amounts together and then dividing the total by the number of amounts. Sometimes also referred to as the mean. 2. A colloquial term used to mean 'usual' or 'ordinary'.

**aversion** intense dislike. *A. therapy* a method of treating addictions by associating the craving for what is addictive with painful or unpleasant stimuli. It is rarely used.

**avian influenza** commonly known as bird flu, a disease of poultry and other birds caused by strains of the influenza virus that can occasionally infect people who are in close contact with infected birds. The severity of the disease depends upon the strain of the virus involved; the strain caused by the H5N1 virus is particularly virulent. At the present time, normal influenza vaccines do not protect against the H5N1 virus. *See* ORTHOMYXOVIRUS and SWINE INFLUENZA.

**aviation medicine** the medical speciality concerned with the effects of air travel and with the causes and treatment of health problems that may occur in flight.

**avitaminosis** a condition resulting from an insufficiency of vitamins in the diet. A deficiency disease.

**avoidance** a conscious or unconscious defence mechanism whereby an individual seeks to escape or avoid certain situations, feelings or conflicts.

**avulsion** the tearing away of one part from another. *Phrenic a.* a tearing away of the phrenic nerve. It paralyses the diaphragm on the affected side.

**axilla** an armpit.

**axiom** a statement or proposition that can be accepted without evidence as it is obviously true.

**axis** 1. a line through the centre of a structure. 2. the second cervical vertebra.

**axon** the process of a nerve cell along which electrical impulses travel. The nerve fibre.

**axonotmesis** nerve injury characterized by disruption of the axon and myelin sheath but with preservation of the connective tissue fragments, resulting in degeneration of the axon distal to the injury site; regeneration of the axon is spontaneous.

**azoospermia** absence of spermatozoa in the semen.

**azygos** something that is unpaired.

**azygous vein** an unpaired vein that ascends the posterior mediastinum and enters the superior vena cava.

**Ba** symbol for *barium*.

**Babinski's reflex or sign** *J.F.F. Babinski, French neurologist, 1857–1932.* On stroking the sole of the foot, the great toe bends upwards instead of downwards (dorsal instead of plantar flexion). Present in disease or injury to the upper motor neurone. Babies who have not walked react in the same way, but normal flexion develops later.

**baby** an infant or young child who is not yet walking. *B. blues* the transient feelings of unhappiness and tearfulness that affect many women after the birth of their baby. *B. Friendly Initiative* abbreviated BFI. Part of a global campaign by the World Health Organization and the United Nations Children's Fund to ensure that all mothers are facilitated in breast feeding to enable babies to benefit from the health and social advantages. *Battered b.* one suffering from the result of continued violence; extensive bruising, fractures of limbs, rib and skull, or an internal trauma may be found. *See* ABUSE. *Blue b.* one suffering from cyanosis at birth as a result of atelectasis or congenital heart malformation.

**Bach flower remedies** a system of complementary medicine, devised by Dr Edward Bach and based on homeopathic principles. Flower remedies can be used to treat emotional and psychological disorders.

There are 38 flower remedies. *See also* HOMEOPATHY.

**bacillaemia** the presence of bacilli in the blood.

**bacilluria** the presence of bacilli in the blood.

**bacillus** loosely, the cause of any bacterial infection by a rod-shaped microorganism, e.g. *Escherichia coli*, the colon bacillus.

**Bacillus** a genus of aerobic, spore-bearing Gram-positive bacteria. *B. anthracis* the causative agent of ANTHRAX.

**back** dorsum. Posterior trunk from neck to pelvis. Posterior vertebral column. *B. slab* plaster or plastic splint in which a limb is supported. *Hunch b.* kyphosis.

**backache** any pain in the back, usually the lower part. The pain is often dull and continuous, but sometimes sharp and throbbing. Backache, or lumbago, is one of the most common ailments and can be caused by a variety of disorders. Health care workers are at particular risk and one in six nurses is thought to experience back pain.

**bacteraemia** the presence of bacteria in the blood-stream.

**bacterial** pertaining to bacteria.

**bactericidal** capable of killing bacteria, e.g. disinfectants, great heat, intense cold or sunlight.

**bacteriologist** one who is qualified in the science of bacteriology.

**bacteriology** the scientific study of bacteria.

**bacteriolysin** an antibody produced in the blood to assist in the destruction of bacteria. The action is specific.

**bacteriolysis** the dissolution of bacteria by a bacteriolytic agent.

**bacteriophage** a virus that only infects bacteria. Many strains exist, some of which are used for identifying types of staphylococci and salmonellae.

**bacteriostat** an agent that inhibits the growth of bacteria.

**bacteriostatic** inhibiting the growth of bacteria.

**bacteria** a general name given to a minute vegetable organism which may live on organic matter. There are many varieties, only some of which are pathogenic to humans, animals and plants. Each bacteria consists of a single cell and, given favourable conditions, multiplies by subdivision. Bacteria are classified according to their shape (a) *bacilli*, rod-shaped and (b) *cocci*, spherical (see Figure on p. 42), subdivided into (i) streptococci, in chains; (ii) staphylococci, in groups; (iii) diplococci, in pairs; (c) *spirilla*, *spirochaetes*, spiral. *Pathogenic b.* one whose growth in the body gives rise to disease, either by destruction of tissue or by formation of toxins, which circulate in the blood. Pathogenic bacteria thrive on organic matter in the presence of warmth and moisture.

**bag** a sac or pouch. *B. of waters* the membranes enclosing the AMNIOTIC (FLUID) and the developing fetus in utero. *Colostomy b.* a receptacle worn over the stoma by the patient, to receive the faecal discharge. *Douglas b.* a receptacle for the collection of expired air, permitting measurement of respiratory gases. *Ileostomy b.* any of various plastic or latex pouches attached to the stoma for the collection of faecal material after ILEOSTOMY. *Politizer b.* a soft bag of rubber for inflating the pharyngotympanic tube. *Urine b.* a receptacle used for urine by ambulatory patients with urinary incontinence.

**balance** the ability to remain upright and to move without falling over. In physiological terms the harmonious relationship between parts and organs of the body and their functions or between substances in the body. *See* ACID-BASE BALANCE. *B. of probabilities* the standard of proof required in civil proceedings.

**balanced diet** a varied diet that contains all the nutritional elements in the correct quantities required for growth and repair of body tissues.

**balanced salt solution (BSS)** a solution that is made to a physiological pH with appropriate concentrations of salts and electrolytes. Used during intraocular surgery to replace intraocular fluids.

**balanitis** inflammation of the glans penis and of the prepuce, usually associated with phimosis. Balanoposthitis.

**baldness** absence of hair, especially from the scalp. Alopecia.

**ballottement** [Fr.] a method of testing for a floating object, e.g. abdominal palpation of the uterus when testing for pregnancy. The uterus is pushed upward by a finger in the vagina, and if a fetus is present it will fall back again like a heavy body in water.

**bandage** 1. a strip or roll of gauze or other material for wrapping or binding any part of the body. 2. to cover by wrapping with such material. Bandages may be used to stop the flow of blood, to provide a safeguard against contamination, or to hold a dressing in place. They may also be used to hold a splint in position or otherwise immobi-

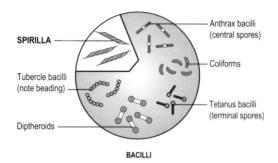

**SPIRILLA**

Anthrax bacilli (central spores)

Coliforms

Tubercle bacilli (note beading)

Tetanus bacilli (terminal spores)

Diptheroids

**BACILLI**

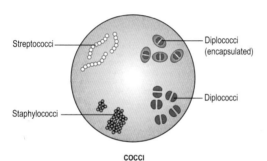

Streptococci

Diplococci (encapsulated)

Diplococci

Staphylococci

**COCCI**

BACTERIA: BACILLI (ROD-SHAPED) AND COCCI (SPHERICAL)

lize an injured part of the body to prevent further injury and to facilitate healing.

**banding** placing a band round a vessel to restrict the flow from it. *Pulmonary arterial b.* a palliative operation used in treating infants with ventricular septal defects.

**bank** an institution offering services, or a store of donated human tissues for use in the future by other individuals, e.g. *blood b., human milk b., sperm b.* **Nurse b.** a group of nurses who are known to the employing authority and available for employment on an on-call basis.

**Bankhart's operation** *A.S.B. Bankhart, British orthopaedic surgeon, 1879–1951.* An operation to repair a defect in the glenoid cavity that causes repeated dislocation of the shoulder joint.

**barbiturates** a large group of sedative and hypnotic drugs derived from barbituric acid, e.g. phenobarbitone, amylobarbitone. Prolonged use may lead to addiction.

**barium** *symbol* Ba. A soft silvery metallic element. *B. sulphate* a heavy mineral salt that is comparatively impermeable to X-rays and can therefore be used as a contrast medium, given as a meal or as an enema. Used to demonstrate abnormality in the stomach or intestines, and to show peristaltic movement. *B. sulphide* the chief constituent of depilatory preparations, i.e. those which remove hair.

**baroreceptors** the sensory branches of the glossopharyngeal and vagus nerves that influence the blood pressure. The receptors are situated in the walls of the carotid sinus and aortic arch.

**barotrauma** injury due to pressure, such as to structures of the ear, owing to differences between atmospheric and intratympanic pressures. May affect air travellers or scuba divers.

**Barr body** M.L. Barr, *Canadian anatomist, 1908–1995*. Small, dark-staining area underneath the nuclear membrane of female cells. Represents an inactive X chromosome.

**Barré–Guillain syndrome** *see* GUILLAIN–BARRÉ SYNDROME.

**barrier** an obstruction. *B. contraceptive* mechanical barrier preventing the sperm from entering the cervical canal, e.g. diaphragm, sheath. *B. cream* a cream used to protect the skin against irritant substances and water, e.g. hand cream. *B. nursing* precautions taken by nurses to prevent infection from a patient spreading to other patients and/or staff. This normally involves nursing the patient in a separate room or cubicle. *Blood–brain b.* the selective barrier which separates the circulating blood from the cerebrospinal fluid. *Placental b.* semipermeable membrane between maternal and fetal blood. *Protective b.* radiation-absorbing shield, e.g. lead, concrete, to protect the body against ionizing radiations. *Reverse b. nursing* an isolation technique used to prevent the transmission of infection to the patient who may be especially vulnerable, e.g. the immunosuppressed patient. *See* UNIVERSAL PRECAUTIONS.

**Bartholin's glands** *C.T. Bartholin, Danish anatomist, 1655–1738*. Two glands situated in the labia majora, with ducts opening inside the vulva.

**basal** 1. fundamental. 2. referring to a base. *B. cell carcinoma* a common type of skin cancer. Generally occurs in later life, most usually on the face, scalp or neck and is caused by skin damage from the ultraviolet irradiation in sunlight over many years. Without treatment the carcinoma invades and destroys the surrounding tissues but rarely invades other parts of the body. Treatment is usually with surgery. People who have had a basal cell carcinoma should be alert to any changes in their skin as they may develop new tumours. The risk of further tumours is also further reduced by avoiding overexposure to sunlight, wearing protective clothing and a sunscreen preparation on the skin. Also known as a rodent ulcer or BCC. *B. ganglia* the collections of nerve cells or grey matter in the base of the cerebrum. They consist of the caudate nucleus and putamen, forming the corpus striatum, and the globus pallidus. Such cells are concerned with modifying and coordinating voluntary muscle movements. *B. metabolic rate* abbreviated BMR. An indirect method of estimating the rate of metabolism in the body by measuring the oxygen intake and carbon dioxide output on breathing. The age, sex, weight and size of the patient have to be taken into account.

**base** 1. the lowest part or foundation. 2. the main constituent of a compound. 3. an alkali or other substance that can unite with an acid to form a salt.

**basement membrane** a thin layer of modified connective tissue supporting layers of cells, found at the base of the epidermis and underlying mucous membranes.

**basic life support (BLS)** a protocol of resuscitation of a collapsed patient which comprises initial assessment, airway maintenance, expired air ventilation and chest compression. BLS implies that no equipment is available to be used. Its purpose is to maintain adequate ventilation and circulation until further means are available to reverse the underlying condition. *See* Appendix 2 Resuscitation.

**basilar** situated at the base. *B. artery* midline artery at the base of the skull, formed by the junction of the vertebral arteries.

**basilic** prominent. *B. vein* a large vein on the inner side of the arm.

**basophil** adj. *basophilic.* 1. any structure, cell or histological element staining readily with basic dyes. 2. a granular leukocyte with an irregularly shaped, relatively pale-staining nucleus that is partially constricted into two lobes, and with cytoplasm containing coarse bluish-black granules of variable size. 3. a beta cell of the adenohypophysis.

**basophilia** 1. an affinity of cells or tissues for basic dyes. 2. the reaction of relatively immature erythrocytes to basic dyes whereby the stained cells appear blue, grey or greyish-blue, or bluish granules appear. 3. abnormal increase of basophilic leukocytes in the blood. 4. basophilic leukocytosis.

**bath** 1. a medium, e.g. water, vapour, sand or mud, with which the body is washed or in which the body is wholly or partially immersed for therapeutic or cleansing purposes; application of such a medium to the body. 2. the equipment or apparatus in which a body or object may be immersed. *Bed b.* washing a patient in bed. *Emollient b.* a bath in a soothing and softening liquid, used in various skin disorders. It is prepared by adding soothing agents such as gelatin or similar emollient substances to the bathwater, for the purpose of relieving skin irritation and pruritus. The patient is dried by patting rather than rubbing the skin. Care must be taken to avoid chilling. *Hot b.* one taken in water at 36–44°C. Care must be taken to avoid faintness. *Sponge b.* one in which the patient's body is not immersed but is wiped with a wet cloth or sponge. Sponge baths are most often employed for reduction of body temperature in the presence of a fever, in which case the water used is tepid and may contain alcohol to increase evaporation of moisture from the skin. *Tepid b.* one taken in water at 30–33°C. *Warm b.* one taken in water at 32–40°C. *Whirlpool b.* (Jacuzzi) one in which the water is kept in constant motion by mechanical means. It has a gentle massaging action that promotes relaxation.

**B cell** *see* IMMUNITY.

**BCG vaccine** bacille Calmette–Guérin vaccine, a tuberculosis vaccine prepared from artificially weakened stain of bovine tubercle bacillis (*Mycobacterium bovis*). BCG is given to those at risk of tuberculosis and for whom a tuberculin test is negative. This includes health care workers, close contacts of people with tuberculosis and immigrants and their families from countries with a high rate of tuberculosis. *See* Appendix 9.

'**bearing down**' 1. the expulsive pains in the second stage of labour. 2. a feeling of heaviness and downward strain in the pelvis, present with some uterine growths or displacements.

**beat** pulsation of the heart or an artery. *Apex b.* pulsation of the heart felt over its apex. The beat of the heart is felt against the chest wall. *Dropped b.* the occasional loss of a ventricular beat. *Ectopic b.* one that originates somewhere other than the sinoatrial node.

**Beck inventory of depression** abbreviated BID. A self-scoring system used to determine the presence and severity of depression.

**Beck scale for suicide ideation (BSS)** an assessment tool used to identify the potential and risk of suicide in vulnerable patients.

**becquerel** abbreviated Bq. The SI unit of radioactivity equal to the quantity of material undergoing one disintegration per second; $3.7 \times 10^{10}$ becquerels is equal to 1 curie.

**bed** 1. a supporting structure or tissue. 2. a couch or support for the body during sleep. *B. cradle* a frame placed over the body of a bed patient. *See* CRADLE. *Capillary b.* the capillaries of a tissue, area or organ considered collectively, and their volume capacity. *Fracture b.* a bed for the use of patients with broken bones. *King's Fund b.* a bed fitted with jointed springs, which may be adjusted to various positions. *See also* KING'S FUND. *Nail b.* the area of modified epidermis beneath the nail over which the nail plate slides as it grows.

**bedboard** a rigid board placed beneath the mattress of a bed to give firm support to the patient lying upon it.

**bedbug** a bug of the genus *Cimex*, a flattened, oval, reddish insect that inhabits houses, furniture and neglected beds, and feeds on humans, usually at night.

**bedpan** a shallow vessel used for defecation or urination by patients confined to bed.

**bedrest** limiting the patient to staying in bed for a prescribed period for therapeutic reasons.

**bedsore** an ulcer-like sore caused by prolonged pressure of the patient's body. Pressure sore is now the preferred term, as these sores are primarily due to pressure and can also occur in patients who are not confined to bed. A decubitus ulcer. *See* PRESSURE SORE.

**bed-wetting** enuresis; involuntary voiding of urine. *See also* ENURESIS.

**bee sting** injury caused by the venom of a bee. Symptoms of a severe allergic reaction, such as collapse or swelling of the body, indicate anaphylaxis and require that medical help be sought.

**behaviour** the way in which an organism reacts to an internal or external stimulus. *B. disorders* may take many forms, such as truancy, stealing, temper tantrums. *B. modification* an approach to correction of undesirable behaviour that focuses on changing observable actions. Modification of the behaviour is accomplished through systematic manipulation of the environmental and behavioural variables related to the specific behaviour to be changed. *B. therapy* a therapeutic approach in which the focus is on the patient's observable behaviour, rather than on conflict and unconscious processes presumed to underlie the maladaptive behaviour. This is accomplished through systematic manipulation of the environmental and behavioural variables related to the specific behaviour to be modified; operant conditioning, systematic desensitization, token economy, aversive control, flooding and implosion are examples of techniques that may be used in behaviour therapy. *Incongruous b.* behaviour that is out of keeping with the person's normal reaction or has the opposite effect to that consciously desired.

**behavioural sciences** the application of scientific principles to the study of the behaviour of organisms, e.g. sociology, psychology and anthropology, etc.

**behaviourism** the purely objective study and observation of the behaviour of individuals.

**Behçet's syndrome** *H. Behçet, Turkish dermatologist, 1889–1948.* A chronic condition of unknown origin, resulting in painful, recurring mouth and genital ulcers, arthritis, skin lesions and inflammation of the eyes.

**bejel** a non-venereal but infectious form of syphilis caused by a treponema indistinguishable from that causing syphilis. Occurs mainly in children of Africa and the Middle East. The primary lesion is on the mouth, spreading to the trunk, arms and legs. Treated with penicillin.

**belching** the noisy expulsion of gas from the stomach through the mouth. Eructation.

**beliefs** thoughts, ideas and concepts developed by an individual over a period of time from cultural influences, education, religion, parents and family. *Health b.* those beliefs held by an individual regarding the maintenance of his or her state of physical wellbeing, which may be at variance with those beliefs held by the health care practitioner, possibly leading to conflict and non-compliance with prescribed treatment.

**belle indifference** [Fr.] an indication of conversion hysteria, in which the patient describes symptoms, appearing not to be distressed by them.

**Bell's palsy** *Sir C. Bell, British physiologist, 1774–1842.* Facial paralysis due to oedema of the facial nerve.

**bench marking** comparing 'like with like' in order to identify best practice; or a process whereby organizations identify the best performers in order to improve their own performance. A scoring system is used which enables one hospital, department or other health care facility to compare their practices and services with another similar to their own. A quality-assurance technique.

**bends** a colloquial term for caisson disease. Decompression sickness.

**beneficence** the duty to do good, to avoid harm to other people and to protect the weak and the vunerable. In the health care setting this involves the staff acting in the best interests of their patients, and if necessary acting as advocate for them.

**benign** 1. the opposite to malignant. 2. describes a non-invasive condition or illness that is not serious even though treatment may be required for health or cosmetic reasons.

**bereavement** the experience of suffering loss, usually of a loved one by death or separation, but may also include the loss of previous good health, position or wealth. Produces a psychological reaction that has recognized 'stages' that may overlap; these include anger, denial, disbelief and finally acceptance. Collectively recognized as mourning or grieving. There are specialist voluntary groups that provide help and support to those who have lost a family member or loved one from a specific disease, e.g. *Terence Higgins Trust* for those who have lost a friend or family member to AIDs, or *Epilepsy Bereaved*, which provides a similar service to families and friends of those who have died from epilepsy.

**beriberi** a deficiency disease due to insufficiency of vitamin B$_1$ in the diet. The disease is more common in areas where refined rice is the main staple in the diet. It is a form of neuritis, with pain, paralysis and oedema of the extremities.

**berylliosis** an industrial lung disease due to the inhaling of the metallic element beryllium. Interstitial fibrosis arises, impairing lung function.

**beta** the second letter in the Greek alphabet, β. *B. blockers* drugs used to block the action of adrenaline on beta-adrenergic receptors in cardiac muscle, thus decreasing the workload of the heart. *B. cells* insulin-producing cells found in the islets of Langerhans in the pancreas. *B. rays* electrons used therapeutically for treatment of lesions of the cornea and iris. *B. receptors* associated with the inhibition (relaxation) of smooth muscle. They also bring an increase in the force of contraction and rate of the heart.

**bias** in research, any tendency for results to differ from the true value in some consistent way. It is always associated with some systematic, non-random usually undesirable phenomenon.

**bicarbonate** any salt containing the HCO$_3$ anion. *Blood b., plasma b.* the bicarbonate of the blood plasma, an important parameter of acid–base balance (*see* ACID) measured in blood gas analysis.

**bicellular** composed of two cells.

**biceps** a muscle with two heads; a flexor of the arm; one of the hamstring muscles of the thigh.

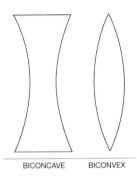

BICONCAVE    BICONVEX

**biconcave** pertaining to a lens or other structure with a hollow or depression on each surface (*see* Figure).

**biconvex** pertaining to a lens or other structure that protrudes on both surfaces (*see* Figure).

**bicornuate** having two horns. *B. uterus* a congenital malformation in which there is a partial or complete vertical division into two parts of the body of the uterus.

**bicuspid** having two cusps or projections. *B. teeth* the premolars. *B. valve* the mitral valve of the heart between the left atrium and ventricle.

**bifid** divided or cleft into two parts.

**Bifidus factor** present in human milk; promotes growth of Grampositive bacteria in gut flora, particularly *Lactobacillus bifidus*, which prevents the multiplication of pathogens.

**bifocal** having two foci, as with spectacles in which the lenses have two different foci.

**bifurcate** to divide into two branches; arteries bifurcate frequently, thereby getting smaller.

**bifurcation** the junction where a vessel divides into two branches, e.g. where the aorta divides into the right and left iliac vessels.

**bigeminal** double. **B. pulse** two pulse beats which occur together, regular in time and force. A regular irregularity.

**biguanides** oral hypoglycaemic agents for treating diabetes. They exert their effect by decreasing gluconeogenesis in muscle tissue. Only effective in those diabetics with functioning islet of Langerhans cells. Most commonly used in non-insulin-dependent diabetics, especially those who are overweight.

**bilateral** pertaining to both sides.

**bile** a secretion of the liver, greenish-yellow to brown in colour. It is concentrated in the gallbladder and passes into the small intestine, where it assists digestion by emulsifying fats and stimulating peristalsis. **B. ducts** the canals or passageways that conduct bile. The hepatic and cystic ducts join to form the common bile duct. **B. pigments** bilirubin and biliverdin, produced by haemolysis in the spleen. Normally these colour the faeces only, but in jaundice the skin and urine may also become coloured. **B. salts** sodium taurocholate and sodium glycocholate, which cause the emulsification of fats.

*Bilharzia* T.M. Bilharz, German physician, 1825–1862. A genus of blood fluke now known as *Schistosoma*.

**bilharziasis** schistosomiasis.

**biliary** pertaining to bile, the bileducts and gallbladder. **B. colic** spasm of muscle walls of the bile duct causing excruciating pain when gallstones are blocking the tube. Pain is in the right upper quadrant of the abdomen and referred to the shoulder. **B. fistula** an abnormal opening between the gallbladder and the surface of the body.

**biliousness** a symptom complex comprising nausea, abdominal discomfort, headache and constipation.

**bilirubin** an orange bile pigment produced by the breakdown of haem and reduction of biliverdin; it normally circulates in plasma and is taken up by liver cells and conjugated to form bilirubin diglucuronide, the water-soluble pigment excreted in the bile. Bilirubin may be classified as indirect ('free' or unconjugated) while en route to the liver from its site of formation by reticuloendothelial cells, and direct (diglucuronide) after its conjugation in the liver with glucuronic acid. Normally the body produces a total of about 260 mg of bilirubin per day. Almost 99% of this is excreted in the faeces; the remaining 1% is excreted in the urine as UROBILINOGEN. The typical yellowness of jaundice is caused by the accumulation of bilirubin in the blood and body tissues.

**bilirubinaemia** the presence of bilirubin in the blood.

**Billings method** a method of contraception, now rarely used. Ovulation time is estimated by observing changes in the cervical mucus that occur during the menstrual cycle.

**bimanual** using both hands. **B. examination** examination with both hands. Used chiefly in gynaecology, when the internal genital organs are examined between one hand on the abdomen, and the other hand or a finger within the vagina.

**binary** made up of two parts. **B. fission** the multiplication of cells by division into two equal parts. **B. scale** one used in calculating, in which only two digits, 0 and 1, are used. Digital computers use this scale.

**binaural** pertaining to both ears. **B. stethoscope.** See STETHOSCOPE.

**Binet's test** A. Binet, French physiologist, 1857–1911. A method of ascertaining the mental age of children or young persons by using a series of questions standardized on the capacity of normal children at various ages.

**Bing test** *A. Bing, German otologist, 1844–1922.* A vibrating tuning fork is held to the mastoid process and the auditory meatus is alternately occluded and left open; an increase and decrease in loudness (positive Bing) is perceived by the normal ear and in sensorineural hearing impairment, but in conductive hearing impairment no difference in loudness is perceived (negative Bing).

**binge–purge syndrome** an alternative term for bulimia.

**binocular** relating to both eyes.

**binovular** derived from two ova. *B. twins* twins, who may or may not be of different sexes.

**bioassay** biological assay. The use of animals or an isolated organ preparation to determine the effect of the active power of a sample of a drug. Comparison is made with the effect of a standard preparation.

**bioavailability** the proportion of a drug that reaches the target organs of the body. Bioavailability is dependent upon metabolism, diet and administrative route. Intravenous administration results in 100% bioavailability. Orally administered drugs have a much lower bioavailability.

**biochemistry** the chemistry of living matter.

**biofeedback** visual or auditory evidence provided to an individual of the satisfactory performance of an autonomic body function, e.g. sounding a tone when blood pressure is at a satisfactory level, so that, through conditioning, the patient may assert control over that function.

**biogenesis** 1. the origin of life. 2. the theory that living organisms can originate only from those already living and cannot be artificially produced.

**biohazard** any hazard arising from inadvertent human biological processes, e.g. accidental inoculation, needle-stick injury.

**biology** the science of living organisms, dealing with their structure, function and relations with one another.

**biomechanical engineering** the application of engineering knowledge and methods to the functions of the body. Used both as a means of explanation of bodily function and in the treatment of disorders of the body. Practical applications include the use of artifical joints, electronic hearing aids and pacemakers.

**biometrics, biometry** 1. anthropometry. 2. the use of statistics in biological science.

**biomicroscopy** a microscopic examination of living tissues, e.g. of the structures of the anterior of the eye during life. *See* SLIT LAMP.

**biophysical profile** a non-invasive test of fetal wellbeing using ultrasound to measure fetal heart rate, fetal tone, somatic movements, breathing movements and amniotic fluid volume. Each factor is scored to obtain a total biophysical score, which is an accurate predictor of fetal death in high-risk pregnancies. The score may be affected by gestation, maternal illness, therapeutic medication, substance abuse or fetal abnormality.

**biopsy** the removal of some tissue or organ from the living body, e.g. a lymph gland, for examination to establish a diagnosis. *Aspiration b.* biopsy in which the tissue is obtained by suction through a needle and syringe. *Cone b.* biopsy in which an inverted cone of tissue is excised, as from the uterine cervix. *Excisional b.* removal of an entire lesion and significant portion of normal-looking tissue for examination. *Needle b.* tissue obtained by the puncture of a lesion with a needle. Rotation of the needle removes tissue within the lumen of the needle.

**biorhythm** any cyclic biological event, e.g. sleep cycle and menstrual cycle, affecting daily life.

**biosensors** non-invasive instruments that measure the result of biological processes, e.g. body temperature.

**biostatistics** that branch of biometry that deals with the data and laws of human mortality, morbidity, natality and demography; called also vital statistics.

**biosynthesis** the creation of a compound within a living organism.

**biotin** formerly termed vitamin H, now part of the vitamin B complex and present in all normal diets.

**biparietal** pertaining to both parietal eminences or bones.

**biparous** giving birth to two infants at a time.

**bipolar** with two poles. *B. nerve cells* cells having two nerve fibres, e.g. ganglionic cells.

**birth** the act of being born. *B. certificate* statement issued by the registrar for births, marriages and deaths for the district in which the baby is born, which certifies details of parentage, name and sex of child, and date and place of birth. This certificate must be obtained by the parents or, failing them, anyone present at the delivery within 42 days of birth in England (21 days in Scotland). It gives legal status to the child and is necessary before Child Benefit can be paid. A birth certificate is issued to any baby born alive, irrespective of the period of gestation. *B. control* limiting the size of the family by abstention from sexual intercourse or the use of contraceptives. *B. mark* a naevus present from birth. *B. notification* a person present, or in attendance, at the birth or up to 6 hours afterwards must notify the district medical officer within 36 hours (Public Health Act 1936).

This responsibility is accepted by the midwife when in attendance. *B. plan* a plan prepared by the expectant mother, usually in conjunction with her partner and midwife, which records her preferences for care during and after labour. *B. rate* the number of births during one year per 1000 total estimated mid-year population (crude birth rate), per 1000 estimated mid-year female population (refined birth rate), or per 1000 estimated mid-year female population of child-bearing age (true birth rate) – that is, between the ages of 15 and 45. *B. registration* either parent must register the birth within 42 days at the registrar's office in the district in which the birth took place in England and Wales or within 21 days in Scotland. Failure to do so incurs a fine. The responsibility rests with the midwife if the parents default. *Premature b.* one taking place before term.

**birthing chair** a specially designed chair for use in labour and delivery to promote greater mobility for the mother.

**birthing pool** a specially designed pool allowing mothers to give birth underwater.

**bisexual** 1. having gonads of both sexes. 2. hermaphrodite. 3. having both active and passive sexual interests or characteristics. 4. capable of the function of both sexes. 5. both heterosexual and homosexual. 6. an individual who is both heterosexual and homosexual. 7. of, relating to or involving both sexes, as in bisexual reproduction.

**bite** 1. to seize with the teeth. 2. a wound made by biting. 3. an impression made by the teeth on a thin sheet of malleable material such as wax.

**Bitot's spots** *P.A. Bitot, French physician, 1822–1888.* Collections of dried epithelium, microorganisms, etc., forming shiny, greyish spots on the cornea. A sign of vitamin A deficiency.

**bivalve** 1. having two valves, as the shells of molluscs such as oysters. 2. to cut a plaster cast into an anterior and a posterior section. *B. speculum* a vaginal speculum with two blades that can be adjusted for easy insertion.

**blackhead** a comedo.

**blackout** momentary failure of vision and unconsciousness due to cerebral circulatory insufficiency.

**blackwater fever** a form of malignant malaria in which severe haemolysis causes a dark discoloration of the urine. *See* MALARIA.

**bladder** a membranous sac for holding fluid or gas. *Atonic b.* a condition in which there is lack of tone in the urinary bladder wall, which may be the result of incomplete emptying over a long period. *B. retraining* a process of education used by nurses to reduce urgency of micturition and episodes of urinary incontinence by increasing the time intervals between emptying the bladder. *B. worm* a cysticercus. *Irritable b.* a condition in which there is frequent desire to micturate. *Urinary b.* the reservoir for urine.

**Blalock–Taussig operation** *A. Blalock, American surgeon, 1899–1964; H.B. Taussig, American paediatrician, 1898–1986.* Operation in which the subclavian artery is anastomosed to the pulmonary artery.

**bland** non-stimulating. *B. fluids* mild and non-irritating fluids such as barley water and milk.

**blast** 1. an immature cell. 2. a wave of high air pressure caused by an explosion.

**blastocyst** blastula.

**blastoderm** the germinal cells of the embryo consisting of three layers: the ectoderm, mesoderm and entoderm.

**blastolysis** the destruction of germ substance.

**blastomycosis** a fungal infection, which, after invasion of the skin, may cause granulomatous lesions in the mouth, pharynx and lungs.

**blastula** blastocyst. An early stage in the development of the fertilized ovum. This stage precedes the gastrula.

**bleb** a blister.

**bleeder** 1. a colloquial name for one who suffers from haemophilia. 2. a vessel that is difficult to seal at operation.

**bleeding** 1. escape of blood from an injured vessel. 2. venesection. *B. time* the time taken for oozing to cease from a sharp prick of the finger or ear lobe. The normal value is 1–3 minutes. *Functional b.* bleeding from the uterus when no organic lesion is present.

**blennorrhagia** an excessive discharge of mucus, e.g. leukorrhoea. 2. gonorrhoea.

**blennorrhoea** blenorrhagia.

**blepharitis** inflammation of the eyelids. *Allergic b.* that associated with response to drugs or cosmetics applied to the eye or eyelids. *Squamous b.* that associated with dandruff of the scalp.

**blepharon** the eyelid.

**blepharophimosis** abnormal narrowing of the aperture between the eyelids. Usually congenital but may arise from chronic inflammation.

**blepharospasm** prolonged spasm of the orbicular muscles of the eyelids.

**blind** without sight. *B. spot* the point where the optic nerve leaves the retina, which is insensitive to light.

**blind loop syndrome** a condition of stasis in the small intestine, which aids bacterial multiplication, leading to diarrhoea and salt deficiencies. The cause may be intestinal obstruction or surgical anastomosis.

**blindness** lack or loss of ability to see; lack of perception of visual stimuli. Blindness is defined as less than 6/60 vision with glasses (vision of 6/60 is the ability to see only at 6 metres what the normal eye can see at 60 metres). A person with this level of vision may be registered as 'Blind'. A person may also be registered as 'Partially Sighted' if they are substantially and permanently handicapped by defective vision caused by congenital defect, illness or injury.

**blister** a bleb or vesicle. A collection of serum between the epidermis and the skin. *Blood b.* a blister containing blood, usually caused by a pinch or bruise.

**block** a stoppage or obstruction. The term is used to describe: (a) various forms of regional anaesthesia, e.g. epidural block; (b) obstruction to the passage of a nervous impulse due to disease, e.g. heart block (*see* HEART); (c) an interruption of mental function.

**blood** the fluid that circulates through the heart and blood vessels, supplying nutritive material to all parts of the body and carrying away waste products. Blood is a red viscid fluid and consists of plasma in which are suspended erythrocytes (red blood cells), leukocytes (white blood cells) and lymphocytes, and platelets or thrombocytes. (a) The red corpuscles or ERYTHROCYTES contain haemoglobin, which combines with oxygen in passing through the lungs. This oxygen is released into the tissues from the capillaries and oxidation takes place. (b) The white corpuscles or LEUKOCYTES defend against invading microorganisms, which they have power to destroy. (c) Blood platelets or thrombocytes are concerned with the clotting of blood. Plasma also contains many other specialized substances that have important roles to play in immunity and clotting of blood.

**blood bank** 1. a place of storage for blood. 2. an organization that collects, processes, stores and transfuses blood. In most hospitals the blood bank is located in the pathology laboratory.

**blood-borne viruses** viruses that are transmitted by blood and some other body fluids (e.g. semen, amniotic fluid), such as hepatitis B virus, hepatitis C virus and human immunodeficiency viruses (HIV-1, HIV-2).

**blood–brain barrier** abbreviated BBB. The membranous barrier separating the blood from the brain. It is permeable to water, oxygen, carbon dioxide, glucose, alcohol, general anaesthetics and some drugs.

**blood casts** casts of coagulated red blood cells formed in the renal tubules and found in the urine.

**blood clotting** coagulation. The formation of a jelly-like substance over the ends or within the walls of a blood vessel, with resultant stoppage of the blood flow. Clotting is one of the natural defence mechanisms of the body when injury occurs. A clot will usually form within 5 minutes of a blood vessel being damaged. The exact process of clotting is not known but it is believed that the mechanism is triggered by the platelets, which disintegrate as they pass over rough places in the injured surface. If normal amounts of calcium, platelets and tissue factors are present (*see* Figure on p. 53), prothrombin will be converted to thrombin. Thrombin then acts as a catalyst for the change of fibrinogen into a mesh of insoluble fibrin, in which are embedded erythrocytes and leukocytes and small amounts of fluid (serum). Plasma coagulation factors are:

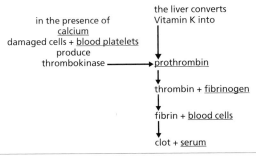

in the presence of <u>calcium</u>
damaged cells + <u>blood platelets</u>
produce
thrombokinase ⟶ <u>prothrombin</u>

the liver converts
Vitamin K into

↓

thrombin + <u>fibrinogen</u>

↓

fibrin + <u>blood cells</u>

↓

clot + <u>serum</u>

CLOTTING OF BLOOD
Underlined substances are normally present in blood

I      Fibrinogen
II     Prothrombin
III    Tissue thromboplastin
IV     Calcium ions
VII    Factor VII
VIII   Antihaemophilic factor (AHF)
IX     Christmas factor
X      Stuart factor (Power factor)
XI     Plasma thromboplastin antecedent (PTA)
XII    Hageman factor
XIII   Fibrin stabilizing factor

**blood count** the number of blood cells in a given sample of blood, usually expressed as the number of cells per litre of blood (as the red blood cell, white blood cell or platelet count). A differential white cell count determines the number of various types of leukocyte in a sample of blood. For the range of normal values, *see* Appendix 8.

**blood dyscrasia** any abnormality of the blood cells or of the clotting elements.

**blood gas analysis** laboratory studies of arterial and venous blood for the purpose of measuring oxygen and carbon dioxide levels and pressure or tension, and hydrogen ion concentration (pH). Analyses of blood gases provide the following information: $Pao_2$ – partial pressure ($P$) of oxygen ($O_2$) in the arterial blood ($a$); $SaO_2$ – percentage of available haemoglobin that is saturated (Sa) with oxygen ($O_2$); $Paco_2$ – partial pressure ($P$) of carbon dioxide ($CO_2$) in arterial blood ($a$); pH – an expression of the extent to which the blood is alkaline or acidic; $HCO_3$ – the level of plasma bicarbonate; an indicator of the metabolic acid–base status.

**blood groups** ABO system (*see* Table on p. 54). In clinical practice there are four main blood types: A, B, O and AB. In addition to this major grouping there is a rhesus (Rh) system that is important in the prevention of haemolytic disease of the newborn resulting from incompatibility of blood groups in mother and fetus. In determining blood group, a sample of blood is taken and mixed with specially prepared sera. One serum, anti-A agglutinin, causes blood of

| ABO SYSTEM | | |
|---|---|---|
| Group | Antigen present in red cell | Antibody present in plasma |
| AB | A and B | — |
| A | A | Anti-B (β) |
| B | B | Anti-A (α) |
| O | — | Anti-A and Anti-B (α and β) |

group A to agglutinate; another serum, anti-B agglutinin, causes blood of group B to agglutinate. Thus, if anti-A serum alone causes clumping, the blood is group A; if anti-B serum alone causes clumping, the blood group is B. If both cause clumping, the blood group is AB, and if it is not clumped by either, it is identified as group O. Transfusion with an incompatible ABO group will cause severe haemolytic reaction and death may occur.

**blood pressure** abbreviated BP. The pressure exerted on the artery walls by the blood as it flows through them. It can be measured in milligrams of mercury using a sphygmomanometer. Two readings are made. Arterial pressure fluctuates with each heart beat and one measure records the pressure while the heart is in systole (when the heart is ejecting blood into the arteries) and is the higher, or systolic, pressure. The other records the pressure while the heart is in diastole (when the aortic and pulmonary valves are closed and the heart is relaxed) and is the lower, or diastolic, pressure. The range of normal blood pressure recording varies according to age and body size, but in the normal young adult is approximately 100–120/70–80 mmHg.

**blood sugar** the amount of glucose present in the blood. The normal range is 2.5–4.7 mmol/litre. When the amount exceeds 10 mmol/litre, glucose is excreted in the urine, as in diabetes mellitus.

**blood transfusion** introduction of blood from the vein of one person (donor) or from a blood bank into the vein of another (recipient) in cases of severe loss of blood, trauma, septicaemia, etc. It is used to supplement the volume of blood and also to introduce constituents, such as clotting factors or antibodies, that are deficient in the patient. *Autologous b.t.* the use of a person's own blood donated earlier for transfusion. The patient's blood may also be salvaged during surgery, filtered and returned to the circulation, thus reducing the need for donated blood transfusion.

**blood urea** excretory product of protein present in the blood. The normal range is 3–7 mmol/litre; this increases in renal failure when the kidneys cease to function normally.

**'blue baby'** *see* BABY and FALLOT'S TETRALOGY.

**blush** growing redness of the face, usually a reaction to emotion or heat.

**BMI** body mass index.

**BMR** basal metabolic rate.

**Bobath technique** an approach to the treatment of neurological conditions developed by Dr and Mrs Bobath. It aims to facilitate movement by inhibiting abnormal tone, abnormal patterns of movement and abnormal balance reactions.

**body** 1. the trunk, or animal frame, with its organs. 2. the largest and most important part of any organ. 3. any mass or collection of material.

**body image** the total concept of the body, including conscious and unconscious feelings, thoughts and perceptions that a person has of it as an object in space, which is dependent and apart from other objects.

**body language** the expression of thoughts or emotions by means of posture or gestures. Body language may include unintended 'signs' as well as intended communication. Detailed studies of human nonverbal communication have been documented by several observers.

**body mass index** abbreviated BMI. The weight (kg) divided by the square of the height (m). A BMI of 18.5–24.9 is an ideal weight; below 18.4 is underweight; a BMI of 25–29.9 is overweight, a BMI of 30–39.9 is classified as obese and over 40 very obese. These figures apply to adults under the age of 60 years only and are not applicable to children, people over 60 years, those with chronic health problems, athletes or to pregnant or breast-feeding women.

**Body Substance Isolation** abbreviated BSI. An INFECTION CONTROL system, developed in 1987, that further elaborated UNIVERSAL PRECAUTIONS and focused on the isolation of all moist and potentially infectious body substances (blood, faeces, urine, sputum, saliva, wound drainage and other body fluids) from all patients, regardless of their presumed infection status, primarily through the use of gloves. This concept has now been further developed and is known by the term STANDARD PRECAUTIONS. *See* TRANSMISSION-BASED PRECAUTIONS. *See also* Appendix 12.

**boil** an acute staphylococcal inflammation of the skin and subcutaneous tissues round a hair follicle. It causes a painful swelling with a central core of dead tissue (SLOUGH), which is eventually discharged. A furuncle.

**bolus** 1. a large pill. 2. a rounded mass of masticated food immediately before being swallowed or one passing through the intestines. 3. a quantity of a drug injected directly to raise its concentration in the blood to a therapeutic level.

**bonding** the attachment process that occurs between an infant and its parents, especially the mother, during the first hours and days following birth. Bonding is a reciprocal process and is a biological need for the future development, both physical and emotional, of the infant. **B. dental** The use of plastic resins, acrylic or porcelain to repair, restore or improve the appearance of damaged or defective teeth.

**bone** the dense connective tissue forming the skeleton. It is composed of cartilage or membrane impregnated with mineral salts, chiefly calcium phosphate and calcium carbonate. This is arranged as an outer hard compact tissue and an inner network of cells (CANCELLOUS tissue), in the spaces of which is red bone marrow. In the shaft of long bones is a medullary cavity containing yellow marrow. Microscopically, the bone tissue is perforated with minute HAVERSIAN CANALS containing blood vessels and lymphatics for the maintenance and repair of the cells (*see* Figure on p. 56). Bone is covered by a fibrous membrane, the PERIOSTEUM, containing blood vessels and by which the bone grows in girth. **B. age** a measure of skeletal development in assessing physical maturity in children by using X-rays to show how much the bones have grown in a particular body area. **B. graft** transplantation of a healthy piece of bone to replace missing or repair defective bone. **B. marrow** substance which fills the marrow cavities of bones. Basically there are

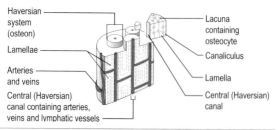

Haversian system (osteon)

Lamellae

Arteries and veins

Central (Haversian) canal containing arteries, veins and lymphatic vessels

Lacuna containing osteocyte

Canaliculus

Lamella

Central (Haversian) canal

STRUCTURE OF COMPACT BONE

two types: yellow and red marrow. The red marrow is responsible for producing the blood cells. The yellow is mostly fatty connective tissue. *B. marrow transplantation* a procedure used to treat aplastic anaemia, acute leukaemia and some rare congenital disorders, with varying success. Healthy bone marrow is taken from the donor and infused into the bloodstream of the recipient; from here it 'homes' in on the bone marrow, where it will grow. Histocompatibility between the donor (usually a sibling) and recipient is essential.

**bong** a water pipe used for smoking cannabis and other drugs.

**borborygmus** a rumbling sound caused by gas in the intestines.

*Bordetella* a genus of bacteria. *B. pertussis* the causal agent of whooping cough.

**Bornholm disease** an epidemic myalgia with pleural pain and fever due to Coxsackie virus infection. It is named after the Danish island of Bornholm where there was an outbreak in 1930.

**botulism** an extremely severe form of food poisoning due to a neurotoxin (botulin) produced by *Clostridium botulinum*, sometimes found in improperly canned or preserved foods. The symptoms include vomiting, abdominal pain, headache, weakness, constipation and nerve paralysis, which causes difficulty in seeing, breathing and swallowing. Death is usually due to paralysis of the respiratory organs.

**bougie** a flexible cylindrical instrument used to dilate a stricture, as in the oesophagus or urethra.

**bovine** relating to the cow or ox. *B. tuberculosis* that caused by infection from infected cows' milk, usually affecting glands and bones.

**bowel** the intestine. *B. sounds* relatively high-pitched abdominal sounds caused by the propulsion of the intestinal contents through the lower alimentary canal.

**bowleg** deformity where there is an outward curvature of one or both legs near the knee. This results in a gap between the knees on standing. Genu varum.

**Bowman's capsule** *Sir W.P. Bowman, British physician, 1816–1892.* The expanded end of the kidney tubule, which surrounds the glomerulus.

**brace** 1. a support used in orthopaedics to hold parts of the body in their correct positions. 2. an orthodontic appliance to correct the alignment of teeth.

**brachial** relating to the arm. *B. artery* the continuation of the axillary artery along the inner side of the upper arm. *B. plexus* a network of nerves at the root of the neck supplying the upper limb.

**brachytherapy** radiotherapy delivered into or adjacent to a tumour by means of an intracavitary or interstitial radioactive source.

**Braden scale** *See* PRESSURE ULCER ASSESSMENT SCALES.

**bradycardia** abnormally low rate of heart contractions and consequent slow pulse.

**bradykinesia** excessive slowness of voluntary movements and speech; a characteristic of Parkinsonism and some other nervous system disorders.

**bradykinin** peptide formed from the degradation of protein by enzymes. It is a powerful vasodilator that also causes contraction of smooth muscle.

**braille** a method of printing developed by *Louis Braille (1809–1852)* for the blind. Letters of the alphabet are represented by patterns of raised dots. These dots are read by passing the fingertips over them.

**brain** that part of the central nervous system contained in the skull. It consists of the cerebrum, midbrain, cerebellum, medulla oblongata and pons varolii.

**brainstem** the lower part of the brain which links with the spinal cord and controls the automatic functions of the body, e.g. heart and respiratory rate. This consists of the midbrain, pons varolii and medulla oblongata.

**brainstorming** or 'thought showering' is an approach to problem-solving through the encouragement of intensive discussion in a group, generating ideas and solutions about an issue.

**bran** the husk of grain, i.e. the coarse outer coat of cereals. High in roughage and vitamins of the B complex, bran is frequently recommended as a dietary component both for those with alimentary disorders and for those in normal health.

**branchial** relating to the clefts (branchia) that are present in the neck and pharynx in the developing embryo. Normally they disappear. *B. cyst* a cystic swelling arising from a branchial remnant in the neck. *B. sinus* (*lateral cervical sinus*) a tract leading from the posterior cervical region which opens in the lower neck in front of the sternomastoid muscle.

**Braun's frame** *H.F.W. Braun, German surgeon, 1862–1934.* A metal frame which incorporates one or more pulleys and is used to elevate the lower limb and to apply skeletal traction for a compound fracture of tibia and fibula.

**Braxton Hicks contractions** *J. Braxton Hicks, British gynaecologist, 1823–1897.* Painless uterine contractions occurring during pregnancy, becoming increasingly rhythmic and intense during the third trimester. Sometimes called 'false labour'.

**breast** 1. the anterior or front region of the chest. 2. the mammary gland. *B. access* formation of pus in the mammary gland. *B. bone* the sternum. *B. cancer* the breast is a common site of cancer in women and occurs occasionally in men. In the UK one in nine women will develop this disease and although the survival rates for breast cancer continue to increase, the incidence of the disease in the Western world is also increasing. Improvement in these survival rates has come from increased public awareness, breast self-examination, breast screening programmes and improved methods of treatment. Women should train themselves to perform a simple self-examination of the breasts (*see* Figure on p. 58). The best time

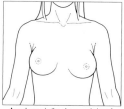

Any change in the shape and size of
either breast or nipple should first be
noted by looking in the mirror

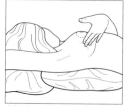

Lying down with a pillow or towel placed
under the shoulder helps to spread the
breast tissue for easier self-examination

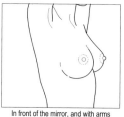

In front of the mirror, and with arms
raised, view the breasts from
different angles

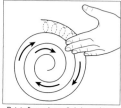

Rotate fingers in small circles and trace
a spiral route around the breast to check
for any lumps or unusual thickening

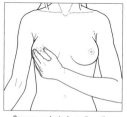

Squeeze each nipple gently, noting
any discharge or bleeding

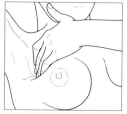

Finally, examine the armpits using
the spiral technique and note any
unusual findings

BREAST SELF-EXAMINATION

**TEN STEPS TO SUCCESSFUL BREAST FEEDING**

- Breast feeding policy available which is communicated to all staff.
- All health care staff trained to implement the policy.
- All pregnant mothers informed of the benefits and management of breast feeding.
- Mothers assisted to commence breast feeding within half an hour of delivery.
- Education of mothers re breast feeding and maintenance of lactation even if they are separated from their babies.
- Neonates to be given nothing other than breast milk unless medically necessary.
- 24-hour rooming-in.
- On-demand breast feeding.
- No teats or pacifiers to be given to breast feeding babies.
- Establishment of breast feeding support groups.

Source: UNICEF UK Baby Friendly Initiative.

for this is just after menstruation when the breasts are normally soft but should also be continued after the menopause on a regular basis. If any lump in the breast can be felt, a doctor should be consulted immediately. More than 90% of breast cancers are discovered by the patients themselves. *B. feeding* the method of feeding a baby with milk directly from the mother's breasts. Midwives and paediatricians agree that breast feeding is better for the baby and the mother, both physically and emotionally (*see* Table). *B. pump* an apparatus for removal of milk from the breast.

**breath** the air taken in and expelled by the expansion and contraction of the thorax. *B. holding* when a young child cries, holds its breath and goes blue. *B. sounds* the sounds heard when a stethoscope is placed over the lungs during respiration. *B. test* using a Breathalyser to analyze a person's breath in order to determine the level of alcohol consumed within a certain period of time. Used to test drivers to assess if the person is within or above the legal limit of alcohol consumption.

**breathing** the alternate inspiration and expiration of air into and out of the lungs (*see also* RESPIRATION).

**breech** the buttocks. *B. presentation* a position of the fetus in the uterus such that the buttocks present.

**bregma** the anterior fontanelle. The membranous junction between the coronal and sagittal sutures.

**bridge** in dentistry, an irremovable prosthesis carrying false teeth that bridges gaps left when natural teeth are extracted.

**British National Formulary** abbreviated BNF. A publication produced twice a year by the British Medical Association and the Pharmaceutical Society of Great Britain, containing details of nearly all the drugs currently available on prescription in the UK. The Nurse Prescribers' formulary is published as an addendum to the BNF. *See also* Appendix 3.

**British Pharmacopoeia** abbreviated BP. The official publication containing the list of drugs and other medicinal substances in use in the UK. The book gives details of how these substances are obtained or prepared, and their dosages and methods of administration. It is compiled under the auspices of the General Medical Council and is regularly revised and brought up to date.

**broad ligaments** folds of peritoneum extending from the uterus to the sides of the pelvis, and supporting the blood vessels to the uterus and uterine tubes.

**Broca's area of speech** *P.P. Broca, French surgeon, 1824–1880.* The motor centre for speech, situated in the left cerebral hemisphere. Damage to the nerve cells contained in it can impair speech.

**Brodie's abscess** *Sir B.C. Brodie, British surgeon, 1783–1862.* See ABSCESS.

**bromhidrosis** offensive and fetid sweat.

**bronchi** plural of bronchus.

**bronchiectasis** chronic dilatation of the bronchi and bronchioles with secondary infection, usually involving the lower lobes of the lung. The condition may occur as a congenital malformation of the alveoli with resultant dilatation of the terminal bronchi and is associated with cystic fibrosis. Most often it is an acquired disease secondary to partial obstruction of the bronchi with necrotizing infection. The symptoms include a chronic cough and purulent sputum. May lead to respiratory failure.

**bronchiole** one of the smallest of the subdivisions of the bronchi.

**bronchiolitis** inflammation of the bronchioles.

**bronchitis** inflammation of the bronchi. *Acute b.* a short-lived infection, common in young children and the elderly. It is a descending infection from the common cold, influenza, measles and other upper respiratory conditions. *Chronic b.* a chronic infection, usually associated with infection of the upper respiratory tract. It may in time lead to emphysema.

**bronchodilator** any agent that causes dilatation of the bronchi.

**bronchography** radiography of the bronchial tree after introduction of a radio-opaque medium.

**bronchomycosis** A general term used to cover a variety of fungal infections of the bronchi aspergillosis and pulmonary candiasis.

**bronchophony** resonance of the voice as heard in the chest over the bronchi on auscultation.

**bronchopneumonia** a descending infection starting around the bronchi and bronchioles. *See also* PNEUMONIA.

**bronchopulmonary** relating to the lungs, bronchi and bronchioles. *B. dysplasia* abbreviated BPD. A chronic respiratory condition occurring in babies who have been ventilated for long periods or have needed prolonged oxygen therapy. It results in serious disruption of lung growth. Examination of radiographs and lung specimens reveals patches of collapse and fibrosis. Following ventilation, these babies usually require supplementary oxygen for several weeks or even months to keep the arterial oxygen tension above 55 kPa.

**bronchorrhoea** an excessive discharge of mucus from the bronchi.

**bronchoscope** an endoscope that enables the operator to see inside the bronchi. It can also be used to wash out the bronchi, to remove foreign bodies or to take a biopsy.

**bronchoscopy** examination of the bronchi by means of a bronchoscope.

**bronchospasm** difficulty in breathing caused by the sudden constriction of plain muscle in the walls of the bronchi. This may arise in asthma or chronic bronchitis.

**bronchospirometer** an instrument used to measure the capacity of one lung or of one lobe of the lung, or of each lung separately.

**bronchotracheal** relating to both the trachea and the bronchi.

*B. suction* the removal of mucus with the aid of suction.

**bronchus** *pl.* bronchi. any of the larger passages conveying air to (right or left principal bronchus) and within (lobar and segmental bronchi) the lungs.

**brow** the forehead. *B. presentation* a position of the fetus such that the forehead appears at the cervix first.

**brown fat** special type of adipose tissue found in the newborn infant, and which is widely distributed throughout the body. The tissue is highly vascular and owes its colour to the large number of mitochondria found in the cytoplasm of its cells. It allows the infant to increase its metabolic rate and thus its heat production when subjected to cold. At the same time the fat itself is used up.

**browser** a computer program used to access the internet, e.g. Netscape, Navigator or Microsoft Internet Explorer.

*Brucella* a genus of bacteria primarily pathogenic in animals but which may affect humans.

**brucellosis** a rare generalized infection involving primarily the reticuloendothelial system, marked by remittent undulant fever (*see* below), malaise, headache and anaemia. It is caused by various species of *Brucella* and is transmitted to humans from domestic animals such as pigs, goats and cattle, especially through infected milk or contact with the carcass of an infected animal. The disease is also called undulant fever because one of the major symptoms in humans is a fever that fluctuates widely at regular intervals. Prevention is best accomplished by the pasteurization of milk and a programme of testing, vaccination and elimination of infected animals. Also called Malta fever, abortus fever and Mediterranean fever.

**Brudzinski's sign** *J. Brudzinski, Polish physician, 1874–1917.* 1. passive flexion of one thigh causing spontaneous flexion of the opposite thigh. 2. flexion of the neck causing bilateral flexion of the hips and knees. These signs are indicative of meningeal irritation.

**bruise** a superficial injury to tissues produced by sudden impact in which the skin is unbroken. A contusion.

**bruit** [Fr.] an abnormal sound or murmur heard on auscultation of the heart and large vessels.

**bruxism** teeth clenching, particularly during sleep. This occurs in persons under tension and may cause headaches as a result of muscle fatigue.

**bubo** inflammation of the lymphatic glands of the axilla or groin. Typical of bubonic plague (*see* PLAGUE) and venereal infections.

**buccal** pertaining to the cheek or to the mouth.

**Budd–Chiari syndrome** *G. Budd, British physician, 1808–1882; H. Chiari, Austrian pathologist, 1851–1916.* A condition in which thrombosis of the hepatic vein causes vomiting, jaundice, enlargement of the liver and ascites.

**Buerger's disease** *L. Buerger, American physician, 1879–1943.* Thromboangiitis obliterans.

**buffer** 1. a physical or physiological system that tends to oppose change within that system, e.g. the reflexes involved in blood pressure homeostasis. 2. a chemical system that acts to prevent change in the concentration of another chemical substance. Sodium bicarbonate is the chief buffer of the blood and tissue fluids. 3. anything that is used to reduce shock or jarring upon contact.

**buggery** anal intercourse, either heterosexual or homosexual. In law the term also includes sexual contact with an animal. Also known as sodomy.

**bulbar** pertaining to the medulla oblongata. *B. paralysis see* PARALYSIS.

**bulbourethral** relating to the bulb of the urethra (bulb of the penis). *B. glands* small glands opening into the male urethra. Cowper's glands.

**bulimia** abnormal increase in the sensation of hunger. *B. nervosa* a pattern of 'binge eating', or episodes of uncontrolled and compulsive overeating occurring in response to stress. Bulimic 'binges' often occur in anorexia nervosa.

**bulk-forming agent** an antidiarrhoeal agent that makes the faeces less fluid by absorbing water.

**bulla** a large, fluid-containing blister.

**bullying** the tormenting of others through verbal harassment, physical assault or other subtle methods of coercion such as manipulation or sending hurtful or scary messages or phone calls, SMS text or emails. Bullying is widespread and occurs in settings where people interact. This includes schools and workplaces. These settings have a responsibility to create an environment where children and adults feel safe. In recent years steps have been taken to develop policies against bullying. *See also* HARASSMENT.

**bundle** a collection of nerve fibres all running in the same direction. *B. branch block* the delay in conduction along either branch of the atrioventricular bundle of the heart. The abnormality is detected by an ECG recording.

**bundle of His** *L. His Jr, German physiologist, 1863–1934.* The band of neuromuscular fibres which, passing through the spectrum of the heart, divides at the apex into two parts, these being distributed into the walls of the ventricles. The impulse of contraction is conducted through the structure. Atrioventricular bundle.

**bunion** a prominence of the head of the metatarsal bone at its junction with the great toe, caused by inflammation and swelling of the bursa at that joint. Usually due to shoes that distort the natural shape of the foot.

**buphthalmos** abnormal enlargement of the eyes in congenital GLAUCOMA.

**burden of proof** the duty to establish the facts; usually associated with litigation including insurance claims and criminal proceedings.

**Burkitt's tumour** *D.P. Burkitt, Irish surgeon, b. 1911.* African lymphoma. A lymphosarcoma, frequently of the jaw, occurring almost exclusively in children living in low-lying moist areas. Occurs in New Guinea and Central Africa. The Epstein–Barr virus (EB virus), a herpes virus, has been isolated from Burkitt's lymphoma cells in culture, and has been implicated as a causative agent.

**burn** an injury to tissues caused by: (a) physical agents, the sun, excess heat or cold, friction, nuclear radiation; (b) chemical agents, acids or caustic alkalis; (c) electrical current. Burns are described as being partial thickness (involving only the epidermis) or full thickness (involving the dermis and underlying structures). Clinically, emphasis is placed on the percentage of the body affected by the burn. The treatment of shock and prevention of infection and malnutrition need special attention.

**burnout** a term used to describe the result of chronic stress amongst workers and commonly in members of the helping professions. Burnout is characterized by chronic low energy, defensiveness and emergence of manoeuvres designed to create distance between helper and patient/client. Dissatisfaction and tension may be carried over from the work situation into the personal one and self-esteem and confidence may suffer badly.

**burr** a bit for a surgical drill, used for cutting bone or teeth. *B. hole* a circular hole drilled in the cranium to permit access to the brain or to release raised intracranial pressure.

**bursa** a small sac of fibrous tissue, lined with synovial membrane and containing synovial fluid. It is situated between parts that move upon one another at a joint to reduce friction.

**bursitis** inflammation of the bursa. It produces pain and may impede movement of the joint. *Prepatellar b.* housemaid's knee.

**buttock** either of the two prominences formed by the flesh-covered gluteal muscles at either side of the lower spine.

**bypass** diversion of flow. Formation of a shunt. *Aortocoronary b.* diversion of flow from the aorta to the coronary arteries via a saphenous vein or artificial graft. *Femoropopliteal b.* diversion of flow from the femoral to the popliteal artery to overcome an occlusion.

**byssinosis** an industrial disease caused by inhalation of cotton or linen dust in factories. A type of pneumoconiosis.

**byte** the storage space in the memory of a computer allocated to one character or letter, usually composed of a sequence of six or eight bits.

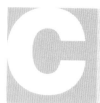

**C** symbol for *carbon*; *centigrade* or *celsius*; *cytosine*.

**Ca** symbol for *calcium*.

**cachexia** a condition of extreme debility. The patient is emaciated, the skin being loose and wrinkled from rapid wasting, but shiny and tense over bone. The eyes are sunken, the skin yellowish, and there is a grey 'muddy' complexion. The mucous membranes are pale and anaemia is extreme. The condition is typical of the late stages of chronic diseases.

**cadaver** a corpse. The dead body used for dissection.

**caecum** the blind pouch forming the beginning of the large intestine. The vermiform appendix is attached to it.

**caesarean section** delivery of a fetus by an incision through the abdominal wall and uterus. Performed for the safety of either the mother or the infant. Tradition has it that Julius Caesar was born in this way.

**caesium** *symbol* Cs. A metallic element. *C.-137* radioactive caesium; a fission product from uranium.

**café-au-lait spot** pigmented macules of a distinctive light-brown colour, like coffee with milk, as in neurofibromatosis and Albright's syndrome.

**caffeine** an alkaloid of tea and coffee which acts as a nerve stimulant and diuretic.

**caffeinism** an agitated state due to the excessive ingestion of caffeine.

**caisson disease** decompression sickness. *See* BENDS.

**calcaneum** the heel bone. Calcaneus.

**calcareous** chalky. Containing lime.

**calciferol** the chemical name for vitamin D.

**calcification** 1. the deposit of lime in any tissue, e.g. in the formation of callus. 2. the deposit of lime salts in cartilage as part of the normal process of bone formation. *Dystrophic c.* the deposition of calcium in abnormal tissue, such as scar tissue or atherosclerotic plaques, without abnormalities of blood calcium.

**calcitonin** a polypeptide hormone, produced by the parafollicular or C cells of the thyroid gland, which regulates blood calcium levels.

**calcium** *symbol* Ca. A metallic element necessary for the normal development and functioning of the body. Calcium is the most abundant mineral in the body; it is a constituent of bones and teeth. Deficiency or excess of serum calcium causes nerve and muscle dysfunctions and abnormalities in blood clotting. The correct concentration is regulated by hormones. *C. carbonate* chalk. *C. gluconate* used as an antacid. A compound that is easily absorbed and can be given by intramuscular or intravenous route to raise the blood

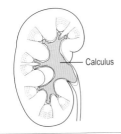

STAGHORN OR MANY-
BRANCHED CALCULUS IN
THE RENAL PELVIS

calcium. *C. lactate* a compound
that increases the coagulability
of blood; used orally as a calcium
supplement.

**calculus** 1. a stony concretion
which may be formed in any of
the secreting organs of the body or
their ducts (*see* Figure). 2. a calcified deposit that forms on the surface of the teeth leading to tooth
decay and gum disease.

**Caldicott guardian** all NHS organizations must appoint a Caldicott
guardian to safeguard the confidentiality of patient information,
as do all local councils with a social
services responsibility. They must
be either: a member of the organization's management board or
a senior health professional with
responsibility for promoting clinical governance in the organization.
The Caldicott principles apply in
addition to the requirements of the
Data Protection Act 1998. *See also*
GUARDIAN CALDICOTT.

**calibrator** 1. an instrument for measuring the size of openings. 2. an
instrument used to dilate a tube,
e.g. in urethral stricture.

**caliper** a two-pronged instrument
that may be used to exert traction
on a part. *Walking c.* an appliance

fitted to a boot or shoe to give
support to the lower limb. It may
be used when the muscles are
paralysed or in the repair stage of
fractures.

**calipers** compasses for measuring diameters and curved surface.
*Skinfold c.* an instrument used in
nutritional assessment for determining the amount of body fat.
A fold of skin and subcutaneous tissue, usually over the triceps muscle,
is pinched away from the underlying muscle using the thumb and
forefinger.

**callisthenics** mild gymnastics for
developing the muscles and producing a graceful carriage.

**callosity** the plaques of thickened
skin often seen on the soles of the
feet or the palms of the hand, areas
subject to friction.

**callous** hard and thickened.

**callus** 1. a callosity. 2. the tissue
that grows round fractured ends of
bone and develops into new bone
to repair the injury.

**calor** [L.] *heat*; one of the signs of
inflammation.

**caloric** pertaining to heat or calories.

**calorie** *symbol* cal. A unit of heat.
Used to denote physiological values of various food substances,
estimated according to the amount
of heat they produce on being oxi-
dized in the body. *See* OXIDIZATION.
A calorie (or kilocalorie) represents the heat required to raise 1 kg
(1000 g) of water by 1°C. A small
calorie equals the heat produced in
raising 1 g of water by 1°C. In the
SI system the calorie is replaced by
the joule (1 cal = 4.18 kJ).

**calorific** heat-producing.

**calorimeter** an apparatus for measuring the heat that is produced or
lost during a chemical or physical
change.

**calyx** any cup-shaped vessel or
part. *C. of kidney* the cup-like terminations of the ureter in the renal

pelvis surrounding the pyramids of the kidney.

*Campylobacter* a genus of bacteria, family Spirillaceae, made up of Gram-negative, non-spore-forming, motile, spirally curved rods. Causes an acute intestinal illness lasting several days. Usually associated with unpasteurized milk, partially cooked meat and poultry.

**canal** a tubular passage. *Alimentary c.* the passage along which the food passes on its way through the body. *C. of Schlemm* that which drains the aqueous humour. *Cervical c.* that through the cervix of the uterus. *Semicircular c.* one of the three canals in the middle ear responsible for maintenance of balance.

**canaliculus** a small channel or canal.

**cancellous** being porous or spongy. Applied to the honeycomb type of bone tissue in the ends of long bones and in flat and irregular bones.

**cancer** a general term to describe malignant growths in tissue, of which CARCINOMA is of epithelial and SARCOMA of connective tissue origin, as in bone and muscle that is parasitic and flourishes at the expense of the host. The basic aetiology of cancer remains unknown but many potential causes are now recognized, e.g. cigarette smoking, ionizing radiation, exposure to certain chemicals and overexposure to the sun. Hereditary factors also play an important part in its development. A cancerous growth is one that is not encapsulated, but infiltrates surrounding tissues, the cells of which it replaces by its own. It is spread by the lymph and blood vessels and causes metastases in other parts of the body. Death is caused by destruction of organs to a degree incompatible with life, by extreme debility and anaemia, or by haemorrhage. For early warning signs of cancer, *see* Table. *C. phobia* an irrational fear of cancer. *C. staging* is a measure of how much a cancer has grown and spread. A common method of cancer staging is based on the measurement of the primary tumour (T) any spread to lymph nodes (N) rate of metastases (M) and is known as the TNM classification. There are also other staging systems and some use a number system such as stage 1, 2, 3 or 4 (or stage I, II, III or IV).

*C.* **units** specialist wards and clinics in district general hospitals that support the work of the Regional

---

## EARLY WARNING SIGNS OF CANCER

- Any lump or thickening, especially in the breast, lip or tongue.
- Any irregular or unexplained bleeding. Blood in the urine or bowel movements. Blood or bloody discharge from the nipple or any body opening. Unexplained vaginal bleeding or discharge, or any bleeding after the menopause.
- A sore that does not heal, particularly around the mouth, tongue or lips, or anywhere on the skin.
- Noticeable changes in the colour or size of a wart, mole or birthmark.
- Loss of appetite or continual indigestion.
- Persistent hoarseness, cough or difficulty in swallowing.
- Persistent change in normal elimination (bowel habits).

*Special note:* Pain is not usually an early warning sign of cancer.

Cancer Centres, which provide a national network of services for the treatment and care of patients with cancer. *C. screening See* SCREENING.

**cancrum oris** gangrenous stomatitis. An ulceration of the mouth which is a rare complication of measles in debilitated children. Noma.

*Candida* a genus of small fungi, formerly called *Monilia*. *C. albicans* the variety that causes candidiasis.

**candidiasis** infection by the *Candida* fungus. Occurs particularly in moist areas, such as mouth, vagina and skinfolds. Popularly known as thrush. Candidiasis can occur as a result of a debilitating illness or immunosuppressive therapy and/or cytotoxic drugs. The infection may also occur as a result of disturbed intestinal flora, and in pregnancy. Oral infection may be due to poor hygiene, carious teeth or badly fitting dentures.

**canine** 1. pertaining to a dog. 2. an 'eye tooth'. There are two in each jaw between the incisors and the molars.

**cannabis** an illegal drug (class B) which may be swallowed or smoked. It produces hallucinations and a temporary sense of wellbeing, followed by extreme lethargy. Alternative terms for cannabis include marijuana, spliff, hashish, blow, hash, grass, pot, the weed, ganja and bob hope.

**cannula** a hollow tube for insertion into the body by which fluids are introduced or removed. Usually a trocar is fitted into it to facilitate its introduction.

**canthus** the angle formed by the junction of the upper and lower eyelids.

**CAPD** continuous ambulatory peritoneal dialysis.

**capillarity** the action by which a liquid will rise upwards in a fibrous substance or in a fine tube. Capillary attraction.

**capillary** 1. hair-like. 2. a minute vessel connecting an arteriole and a venule. 3. a minute vessel of the lymphatic system.

**capsular** relating to a capsule. *C. ligaments* those that completely surround a movable joint, forming a capsule which loosely encloses the bones and is lined with synovial membrane which secretes a fluid for lubrication of the articular surfaces. Also called articular capsule.

**capsule** 1. a fibrous or membranous sac enclosing an organ. 2. a small soluble case of gelatin in which a nauseous medicine may be enclosed. 3. the gelatinous envelope which surrounds and protects some bacteria.

**capsulotomy** the incision of a capsule, particularly that of a joint or of the lens of the eye.

**caput** head. *C. succedaneum* a transient soft swelling on an infant's head, due to pressure during labour, which disappears within the first few days of life.

**carbaminohaemoglobin** a compound of carbon dioxide and haemoglobin, present in the blood.

**carbohydrate** a compound of carbon, hydrogen and oxygen. Carbohydrates are classified into mono-, di-, tri-, poly- and heterosaccharides. In food they are an important and immediate source of energy for the body; 1 g of carbohydrate yields 17 kJ (14 kcal). They are synthesized by all green plants. In the body they are absorbed immediately or stored in the form of glycogen.

**carbon** *symbol* C. A non-metallic element. *C. dioxide* a gas which, dissolved in water, forms weak carbonic acid. As a product of metabolism by the oxidation of carbon, it leaves the body via the lungs. It can be compressed until it freezes, and then forms a solid (carbon dioxide snow, also known as dry ice) used as an escharotic in various skin conditions. Inhalations of the gas in a 5–7% mixture with oxygen are useful for stimulating the depth of respiration. *C. monoxide* a colourless gas that is very poisonous. It is a major constituent of coal gas and is usually present in the exhaust gases from petrol and diesel engines. In poisoning there is vertigo, flushed face with very red lips, loss of consciousness, and convulsions. The blood is bright red because of the formation of carboxyhaemoglobin. *C. tetrachloride* a powerful anthelmintic used in treating hookworm and whipworm. Also used in cleaning fluids; the inhalation of its vapours in solvent abuse can depress central nervous system activity and cause degeneration of the liver and kidneys.

**carbonic anhydrase** an enzyme that catalyses the decomposition of carbonic acid into carbon dioxide and water, facilitating transfer of carbon dioxide from tissues to blood and from blood to alveolar air.

**carboxyhaemoglobin** the combination of carbon monoxide with haemoglobin in the blood in carbon monoxide poisoning.

**carbuncle** an acute staphylococcal inflammation of subcutaneous tissues, which causes local thrombosis in the veins and death of tissue with several discharging sinuses. In appearance it resembles a collection of boils.

**carcinogen** any substance or agent that can produce a cancer.

**carcinogenic** pertaining to substances or agents that produce or predispose to cancer.

**carcinoid syndrome** a rare condition associated with certain bowel tumours, which spread to other parts of the body. Marked by attacks of severe cyanotic flushing of the skin and by diarrhoea, bronchoconstrictive attacks, pain,

serious heart damage, sudden drops in blood pressure, oedema and ascites. Symptoms are caused by serotonin, prostaglandins and other biologically active substances secreted by the tumour.

**carcinoma** a malignant growth of epithelial tissue. Microscopically the cells resemble those of the tissue in which the growth has arisen. *Adenoic c.* adenocarcinoma. *Basal cell c.* a rodent ulcer (*see* ULCER). *Epithelial c.* epithelioma. *Squamous cell c.* one arising from the squamous epithelium of the skin.

**carcinomatosis** the condition in which a carcinoma has given rise to widespread metastases.

**cardia** the cardiac orifice of the stomach.

**cardiac** 1. pertaining to the heart. 2. pertaining to the cardia. *C. arrest* the cessation of the heart beat. *C. asthma see* ASTHMA. *C. atrophy* fatty degeneration of the heart muscle. *C. bed* one that can be manipulated to form a chair shape for those who are comfortable only when sitting up. *C. catheterization* a procedure whereby a radio-opaque catheter is passed from an arm vein to the heart. Its passage through the heart can be watched on a screen. Also blood pressure readings and specimens can be taken, thus aiding diagnosis of heart abnormalities. *C. cycle* the sequence of events, lasting about 0.8 seconds, during which the heart completes one contraction. *C. massage* rhythmic compression of the heart performed in order to re-establish circulation of the blood in cardiac arrest. *C. monitor* (cardiorator) equipment used to monitor and visually record the cardiac cycle. *C. pacemaker* an electrical device that stimulates the heart muscle to maintain myocardial contractions. *See* PACEMAKER. *C. stimulant* a pharmacological agent that increases the action of the heart. Cardiac glycosides, e.g. digoxin and digitalis, increase myocardial contractions and decrease the heart rate and conduction velocity, thus allowing more time for the ventricles to relax and fill with blood.

**cardialgia** pain in the region of the heart. Cardiodynia.

**cardiogenic** originating in the heart. *C. shock* shock caused by disease or failure of heart action.

**cardiography** the recording of the force and movements of the heart producing a tracing on paper (a cardiogram) or monitor.

**cardiologist** a medically qualified person skilled in the diagnosis of heart disease.

**cardiology** the study of the heart: how it works and its diseases.

**cardiomyopathy** a chronic disorder of the heart muscle not resulting from atherosclerosis.

**cardiopulmonary** relating to the heart and lungs. *C. bypass* the use of the heart–lung machine to oxygenate and pump the blood round the body while the surgeon operates on the heart. *C. resuscitation (CPR)* whereby life-saving measures are commenced to maintain the respiration and circulation of a patient who has sustained a cardiac arrest. *See* Appendix 2 Resuscitation.

**cardioscope** a flexible instrument with a lens and illumination attachment; used for examining the inside of the heart.

**cardiospasm** spasm of the sphincter muscle at the cardiac end of the stomach. It may result in dilatation of the oesophagus, difficulty in swallowing solids and liquids, and regurgitation of undigested food. Achalasia.

**cardiothoracic** pertaining to the heart and thoracic cavity. A specialized branch of surgery.

**cardiotocography** the simultaneous recording of the fetal heart rate, fetal movements and uterine contractions in order to discover possible lack of oxygen (hypoxia) to the fetus. Fetal monitoring.

**cardiotomy** surgical incision into the heart or the cardia. *C. syndrome* an inflammatory reaction after heart surgery. There is pyrexia, pericarditis and pleural effusion.

**cardiotoxic** anything that has a deleterious or poisonous effect on the heart.

**cardiovascular** concerning the heart and blood vessels. *C. system* the heart together with the two chief networks of blood vessels: the systemic circulation and the pulmonary circulation.

**cardioversion** a method of restoring an abnormal heart rhythm to normal (as in atrial fibrillation) by means of an electric shock.

**carditis** inflammation of the heart.

**care** the provision of welfare and protection to children, the elderly in need, the sick and other vulnerable people. An important component of nursing practice (and that of other health care professionals) that extends the concept to include psychosocial and physical care interventions. *C. contract* an agreement whereby the care giver and the patient commit themselves, usually in writing, to a defined course of action. This document specifies certain behaviours that are to occur and the conditions under which they are met. Rewards and penalties are established and agreed appropriate to the outcomes. *C. pathway* an integrated approach or pathway which determines and utilizes locally agreed multidisciplinary practice based on guidelines and evidence for a specific patient or client group. It may form part or all of the clinical record; it documents the care given and facilitates the evaluation of outcomes.

*C. plan* An individualized plan for the care of a patient. Nursing information in this document includes data from the patient assessment regarding the patient's needs, the specific nursing interventions are outlined, the desired goals stated and the priorities set. *See* NURSING (CARE PLAN).

**Care Programme Approach (CPA)** ensures that all Primary Care Trusts and Social Services Departments have systematic arrangements in place for assessing the health and social care needs of mentally ill people, and that people referred to secondary services get appropriate care, including an individual treatment plan.

**Caregiver Strain Index** abbreviated CSI. Measure used by community and mental health nurses to assess caregiver strain for those carers who are providing care for a family member or partner in the home. The results of the questionnaire answered by the caregiver provide a crude analysis of how well the carer is coping in the care situation.

**care in the community** policy whereby patients with continuing medical and social care needs are cared for in a community or domestic, rather than institutional, setting. Care in the community is part of the UK Government agenda to give patients and clients more right to choose and be involved in their care.

**carer** a non-professional who provides care for someone in need at home; most commonly a member of the individual's family or partner.

**Carers (Recognition and Services) Act 1995** gives people who provide substantial care on a regular basis the right to ask for an assessment from social services.

**caries** suppuration and subsequent decay of bone, corresponding to

ulceration in soft tissues. In caries, the bone dissolves; in necrosis it separates in large pieces and is thrown off. *Dental c.* decay of the teeth due to penetration of bacteria through the enamel to the dentine. *Spinal c.* tuberculosis of the spine. Pott's disease.

**Caring about Carers** a national strategy supporting an estimated 6 million carers in England and Wales. Its main features are: (a) grants to allow English local authorities to help carers take a break; (b) credits towards a second pension; (c) council tax reductions for more disabled people and their carers; (d) more carer-friendly employment policies; and (e) support for young carers, including those at school.

**carminative** an aromatic drug that relieves flatulence and associated colic. Cloves, ginger, cardamon and peppermint are examples.

**carneous** fleshy. *C. mole* a tumour of organized blood clot surrounding a dead fetus in the uterus. *See* ABORTION.

**carotene** the colouring matter in carrots, tomatoes and other yellow foods and in fats. It is a provitamin capable of conversion into vitamin A in the liver.

**carotid** the principal artery on each side of the neck. *C. bodies* chemoreceptors in the bifurcation of both carotid arteries which monitor the oxygen content of the blood. *C. sinuses* dilated portions of the internal carotids containing the baroreceptors that monitor blood pressure.

**carpal** relating to the carpus or wrist. *C. tunnel syndrome* compression of the median nerve at the wrist causing numbing and tingling in the fingers.

**carpopedal** relating to the wrist and foot. *C. spasm* spasm of the hands and feet such as occurs in tetany.

**carpus** the eight bones forming the wrist and arranged in two rows: (a) scaphoid, lunate, triquetral, pisiform; (b) trapezium, trapezoid, capitate, hamate.

**carrier** 1. a person who harbours the microorganisms of an infectious disease but is not necessarily affected by it, although that person may infect others. 2. one who carries and passes on a hereditary abnormality.

**cartilage** a specialized, fibrous connective tissue present in adults and forming most of the temporary skeleton in the embryo. The three most important types are hyaline cartilage, elastic cartilage and fibrocartilage. Also, a general term for a mass of such tissue in a particular site in the body. *Elastic c.* cartilage containing elastic fibres and forming the pinna of the ear, the epiglottis and part of the nasal septum. *Fibro-c.* cartilage in which bundles of white fibres predominate, forming the intervertebral discs and costal cartilages. *Hyaline c.* flexible, somewhat elastic, semitransparent cartilage with an opalescent bluish tint, composed of a basophilic fibril-containing substance with cavities in which the chondrocytes occur.

**cartilaginous** of the nature of cartilage.

**caruncle** a small fleshy swelling. *Lacrimal c.* a small reddish body situated at the medial junction of the eyelids. *Urethral c.* a small fleshy growth occurring at the urinary orifice in females and giving rise to great pain on micturition.

**case** a particular instance of disease, as in a case of leukaemia; sometimes used incorrectly to designate the patient with the disease. *C. conference* a meeting of professionals involved in the care of a particular person (often a child), to agree patterns of action and to monitor progress. *C.-control study* an epidemiological study in which the characteristics of cases of disease are compared with a matched control group of persons without the disease. Also called retrospective study, case referent study. *C. fatality rate* the number of persons dying of a particular disease expressed as a proportion of the total contracting the disease; usually expressed as a percentage. *C. history* the collected data concerning an individual and that person's family and environment, including the medical history and any other information that may be useful in analysing and diagnosing the health issues or for instructional or research purposes. *C. load* a system of care whereby a nurse, midwife or health visitor is responsible for a group of patients or clients. *C. mix database* computerized record system which combines all the data received from patient administration systems and operational systems to provide a comprehensive set of information about all the treatment and services received by each patient/client during an episode of care. The information helps to develop normal care profiles for different groups, to analyse and compare different treatment regimes, to produce comparative costings for different treatments, etc. It may also be used as part of the medical audit process.

**caseation** degeneration of diseased tissue into a cheesy mass.

**casein** the chief protein of milk. It forms a curd from which cheese is made. *C. hydrolysate* a predigested concentrated protein; a useful supplement for a high-protein diet.

**cast** 1. a positive copy of an object, e.g. a mould of a hollow organ (a renal tubule, bronchiole, etc.), formed of effused plastic matter and extruded from the body, as in a urinary cast; named, according to constituents, as epithelial, fatty, waxy, etc. 2. a positive copy of the tissues of the jaws, made in an impression, over which denture bases or other restorations may be fabricated. 3. to form an object in a mould. 4. a stiff dressing or casing, usually made of plaster of Paris, used to immobilize body parts. 5. strabismus.

**castor oil** a vegetable oil. Internally it is a purgative. Externally it is protective and soothing and may be used in zinc ointment to protect the skin from excoriation.

**castration** the removal of the testes in the male or the ovaries in the female.

**CAT** computerized axial tomography.

**cat-scratch disease (fever)** a benign, subacute, regional lymphadenitis with fever, resulting from a scratch or bite of a cat or a scratch from a surface contaminated by a cat. Three quarters of all cases occur in children. The fever is due to a small bacterium called *Rochalimaea henselae*. Treatment is mainly palliative with analgesic drugs to relieve any headache and fever.

**catabolism** the chemical breakdown of complex substances in the body to form simpler ones, with a release of energy. *See* METABOLISM.

**catalase** an enzyme found in body cells, including red blood cells and liver cells.

**catalyst** a substance that hastens or brings about a chemical change without itself undergoing alteration; for example, enzymes act as catalysts in the process of digestion.

**cataplexy** sudden recurrent loss of muscle power without unconsciousness, often associated with narcolepsy. It may be produced by any strong emotion.

**cataract** opacity of the crystalline lens of the eye causing partial or complete blindness. It may be congenital or may be due to degenerative changes, injury or diabetes.

**catarrh** chronic inflammation of a mucous membrane accompanied by an excessive discharge of mucus.

**catatonia** a syndrome of motor abnormalities occurring in schizophrenia, but less commonly in organic cerebral disease, characterized by stupor and the adoption of strange postures, or outbursts of excitement and hyperactivity. The patient may change suddenly from one of these states to the other.

**catchment area** a specific geographical area for which an NHS Trust or health centre is responsible for providing the health care services.

**catecholamines** a group of compounds that have the effect of sympathetic nerve stimulation. They have an aromatic and an amine portion and include dopamine, adrenaline and noradrenaline.

**catgut** a substance prepared from the intestines of sheep and used in surgery for sutures and ligatures. It is gradually absorbed in the body at a variable rate, according to the preparation.

**catharsis** 1. a cleansing or purgation. 2. the bringing into consciousness and the emotional reliving of a forgotten (repressed) painful experience as a means of releasing anxiety and tension.

**catheter** a tubular, flexible instrument, passed through body channels for withdrawal of fluids from (or introduction of fluids into) a body cavity. Catheters are made of a variety of materials including plastic, metal, rubber and gum-elastic. *Angiographic c.* one through which a contrast medium is injected for visualization of the vascular system of an organ. *Arterial c.* one inserted into an artery and utilized as part of a catheter–transducer–monitor system to continuously observe the BLOOD PRESSURE of critically ill patients. An arterial catheter also may be inserted for radiological studies of the arterial system and for delivery of chemotherapeutic agents directly into the arterial supply of malignant tumours. *Cardiac c.* a long, fine catheter especially designed for passage, usually through a peripheral blood vessel, into the chambers of the heart under fluoroscopic control. *Central venous c.* a long, fine catheter inserted into a vein for the purpose of administering, through a large blood vessel, parenteral fluids (as in parenteral NUTRITION), antibiotics and other therapeutic agents. This type of catheter is also used in the measurement of central venous pressure (*see* CENTRAL (VENOUS PRESSURE)). *Self-retaining c.* a catheter made in such a way that after introduction the blind end expands so that it can remain in the bladder. Useful for continuous or intermittent drainage or where frequent specimens are required. *Ureteric c.* a fine gum-elastic catheter passed up the ureter to the renal pelvis and used to insert a contrast medium in retrograde urography.

**catheterization** the insertion of a catheter into a body cavity.

**cauda** a tail-like appendage. *C. equina* the bundle of coccygeal, sacral and lumbar nerves with which the spinal cord terminates.

**caudal** referring to a cauda. *C. block* a local anaesthetic agent injected into the sacral canal so that operations may be carried out in the peritoneal area without a general anaesthetic.

**caul** the amnion, which occasionally does not rupture but envelops the infant's head at birth.

**causalgia** an intense burning pain which persists after peripheral nerve injuries.

**caustic** a substance, usually a strong acid or alkali, capable of burning organic tissue. Silver nitrate (*lunar c.*) and carbon dioxide snow are those most commonly used, e.g. silver nitrate to destroy warts.

**cauterization** the destruction of tissue with cautery.

**cautery** 1. the application of searing heat by a hot instrument, an electric current or other means such as a laser. 2. an agent so used. *Cold c.* cauterization by carbon dioxide, called also cryocautery.

**cavernous** having caverns or hollows. *C. breathing* sounds heard on auscultation over a pulmonary cavity. *C. sinus* a venous channel lying on either side of the body of the sphenoid bone through which pass the internal carotid artery and several nerves. *C. sinus thrombosis* a serious complication of any infection of the face, the veins from the orbit draining into the sinus and carrying the infection into the cranium.

**cavitation** the formation of cavities, e.g. in the lung in tuberculosis.

**cavity** a confined space or hollow or potential hollow within the body or one of its organs, e.g. the abdominal cavity or a decayed hollow in a tooth.

**CCU** critical care unit; coronary care unit.

**cell** 1. the basic structural unit of living organisms (*see* Figure p. 74). A microscopic mass of protoplasm, consisting of a nucleus surrounded by cytoplasm and enclosed in a cell membrane, from which all organic tissues are constructed. Each cell can reproduce itself by mitosis. 2. a small, more or less enclosed space. *C. division* the processes by which cells multiply. *See* MITOSIS and MEIOSIS.

**cellulitis** a diffuse inflammation of connective tissue, especially of subcutaneous tissue, which

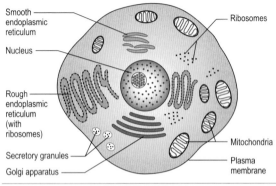

Smooth endoplasmic reticulum

Nucleus

Rough endoplasmic reticulum (with ribosomes)

Secretory granules

Golgi apparatus

Ribosomes

Mitochondria

Plasma membrane

MAJOR PARTS OF THE CELL

causes a typical brawny, oedematous appearance of the part; local abscess formation is not common.

**cellulose** a carbohydrate forming the covering of vegetable cells, i.e. vegetable fibres. Not digestible in the alimentary tract of humans but gives bulk and, as 'roughage', stimulates peristalsis.

**Celsius scale** *A. Celsius, Swedish astronomer, 1701–1744.* A temperature scale with the melting point of ice set at 0° and the boiling point of water at 100°. The normal temperature of the human body is 36.9°C. Formerly known as the centigrade scale. *See* FAHRENHEIT SCALE.

**cementum** cement. Connective tissue with a bone-like structure which covers the root of a tooth and supports it within the socket.

**censor** 1. a member of a committee on ethics or for critical examination of a medical or other society. 2. the psychic influence that prevents unconscious thoughts and wishes coming into consciousness.

**censorship** in psychiatry, the process of selecting, accepting or rejecting conscious ideas, memories and impulses arising from the individual's subconscious.

**census** enumeration of a population. The national census was first introduced in England and Wales in 1801 and has since been repeated every 10 years (except in 1941). It usually records name, address, age, sex, occupation, marital status and other social information.

**Centers for Disease Control** abbreviated CDC. An agency of the US Department of Health and Human Services, located in Atlanta, Georgia, which serves as a centre for the control, prevention and investigation of diseases. A similar function is performed in England and Wales by the Communicable Diseases Surveillance Centre and in Scotland by the Communicable Diseases (Scotland) Unit.

**centigrade** *see* CELSIUS SCALE.

**centile** *see* PERCENTILE.

**central** pertaining to the centre or midpoint. *C. nervous system* abbreviated CNS. The brain and spinal cord. *C. venous pressure* the pressure recorded by the introduction of a catheter into the right atrium in order to monitor the condition of a patient after a major operative procedure, such as heart surgery.

**Central Sterile Supplies and Disinfection Unit (CSSD)** A hospital sterilization and disinfection unit or department.

**central venous catheter/line** a special catheter that is inserted into a large central vein either through a peripheral vein or a skin tunnel for the administration of drugs, the infusing of hypertonic fluids and to measure pressures. The catheter/line also allows long-term access for the administration of medications, nutritional support and blood products.

**centrifugal** conveying away from a centre, such as from the brain to the periphery. Efferent; the reverse of centripetal.

**centrifuge** an apparatus that rotates at high speed. If a test tube, for example, is filled with a fluid such as blood or urine and rotated in a centrifuge, any bacteria, cells or other solids in it are precipitated.

**centripetal** conveying from the periphery to the centre. Afferent; the reverse of centrifugal.

**centromere** the region(s) of the chromosomes which become(s) allied with the spindle fibres at mitosis and meiosis.

**centrosome** a body in the cytoplasm of most animal cells, close to the nucleus. It divides during mitosis, one half migrating to each daughter cell.

**centrosphere** the cell centre, in an area of clear cytoplasm near the nucleus.

**cephalhaematoma** a swelling beneath the pericranium, containing blood, which may be found on the head of the newborn infant. Caused by pressure during labour. Gradually reabsorbed within the first few days of life.

**cephalocele** cerebral hernia. *See* HERNIA.

**cephalography** radiographic examination of the contours of the head.

**cephalometry** measurement of the dimensions of the head of a living person either directly or by radiography. *See also* PELVIMETRY.

**cerclage** [Fr.] encircling of a part with a ring or loop, as for correction of an incompetent cervix uteri or fixation of the adjacent ends of a fractured bone. *See* SHIRODKAR'S SUTURE.

**cerebellum** the portion of the brain below the cerebrum and above the medulla oblongata. Its functions include the coordination of fine voluntary movements and posture.

**cerebral** relating to the cerebrum. *C. cortex* the outer layer of the cerebrum, composed of neurones. *C. haemorrhage* rupture of a cerebral blood vessel. Likely causes are aneurysm or hypertension. *See* APOPLEXY. *C. hernia see* HERNIA. *C. irritation* a condition of general nervous irritability and abnormality, often with photophobia, which may be an early sign of meningitis, tumour of the brain, etc. It is also associated with trauma. *C. palsy* a condition caused by injury to the brain during or immediately after birth. Coordination of movement is affected, and may cause the child to be flaccid or athetoid, in which condition there is constant random and uncontrolled movement. *See* SPASTIC.

**cerebration** mental activity.

**cerebrospinal** relating to the brain and spinal cord. *C. fluid* abbreviated CSF. The fluid made in the choroid plexus of the ventricles of the brain and circulating from them into the subarachnoid space around the brain and spinal cord.

**cerebrovascular** pertaining to the arteries and veins of the brain. *C. accident* a disorder (also called stroke) arising from an embolus, thrombus or haemorrhage in the cerebrum; may vary in severity from a transient weakness or tingling in a limb to profound paralysis, coma and death. *C. disease* any disorder of the blood vessels of the brain and its meninges.

**cerebrum** the largest part of the brain, occupying the greater portion of the cranium and consisting of the right and left hemispheres divided by the longitudinal fissure (*see* Figure). Each hemisphere contains a lateral ventricle. The internal substance is white and the convoluted surface is grey. The centre of the higher functions of the brain.

**cerumen** a waxy substance secreted by the ceruminous glands of the auditory canal. Earwax.

**cervical** pertaining to the neck or the constricted part of an organ, e.g. uterine cervix. *C. canal* the passage through the uterine cervix. *C. cancer* cancer of the uterine cervix. *C. collar* a rigid or semirigid immobilizing support for the neck. *C. rib* a short, extra rib, often bilateral, which sometimes occurs on the seventh cervical vertebra and may cause pressure on an artery or nerve. *C. smear* a test for disorders of the cervical cells; material is scraped from the uterine cervix and examined microscopically. *C. spondylosis* a degenerative disease of the intervertebral joints and discs of the neck. *C. vertebra* one of the seven bones forming the neck portion of the spinal column.

**cervicitis** inflammation of the neck of the uterus.

**cervix** a constricted portion or neck. *C. uteri* the neck of the uterus; it is about 2 cm long and projects into the vagina. Capable of wide dilatation during childbirth.

**CESDI** Confidential Enquiry into Stillbirths and Deaths in Infancy. *See* CONFIDENTIAL ENQUIRY.

**cestode** tapeworm.

**chafe** irritation of the skin as caused by the friction between skinfolds. Occurs particularly in moist areas.

**chalazion** a meibomian or tarsal cyst. A swollen sebaceous gland in the eyelid. A small, hard tumour may develop.

**chancre** 1. the initial lesion of syphilis developing at the site of inoculation. 2. a papular lesion occurring at the site of infection in tuberculosis or in sporotrichosis.

**chancroid** soft chancre. A venereal ulceration, due to *Haemophilus ducreyi*, accompanied by inflammation and suppuration of the local glands.

**character** 1. the combination of traits and qualities distinguishing the unique nature of the individual. 2. a letter, mark or numeral seen on a computer screen or printed. *C. change* indicates alteration in a person's recognized behaviour to one alien to the person's normal manner of conduct. *C. disorder* a chronic state in which the person exhibits maladaptive and unacceptable forms of behaviour and social response.

CEREBRUM

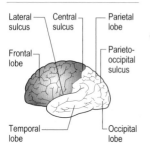

Lateral sulcus — Central sulcus — Parietal lobe — Parieto-occipital sulcus — Frontal lobe — Temporal lobe — Occipital lobe

**Charcot's disease or joint** *J.M. Charcot, French neurologist, 1825–1893.* A chronic progressive, degenerative disease of the stress-bearing portion of one or more joints. The disease is the result of an underlying neurological disorder, e.g. tabes dorsalis from syphilis or diabetic neuropathy or leprosy.

**Charcot's triad** nystagmus, intention tremor and scanning speech. A trio of signs of disseminated sclerosis.

**chart** a record in graphic or tabular form. *Genealogical c.* a graph showing various descendants of a common ancestor, used to indicate those affected by genetically determined disease. *Reading c.* a chart with material printed in gradually increasing type sizes, used in testing acuity of near vision. *Reuss' c's* charts with coloured letters printed on coloured backgrounds, used in testing colour vision. *Snellen's c.* a chart printed with block letters in gradually decreasing sizes, used in testing visual acuity.

**charting** the keeping of a clinical record of the important facts about a patient and the progress of their illness. The patient's chart usually contains a medical history, a nursing history, results of physical examinations, laboratory reports, results of special diagnostic tests, and the observations of the nursing staff. Medical treatments, medications and nursing approaches to problems are recorded on the chart, as are the patient's response to treatment. *See also* PROBLEM-ORIENTED RECORD.

**cheilosis** maceration at the angles of the mouth; fissures may also occur. It may be associated with general debility or riboflavin deficiency.

**chelating agent** a drug that has the power of combining with certain metals and so aiding excretion, to prevent or overcome poisoning. *See* DIMERCAPROL and PENICILLAMINE.

**chemical change** this differs from physical change in that a profound alteration in properties results, usually permanently and usually accompanied by use of energy in a new substance, e.g. hydrogen (two atoms) plus oxygen produces water.

**chemical compound** any substance produced by chemical change which may then be broken up into its components only by chemical means, unlike a mixture, which can usually be separated mechanically.

**chemistry** the science that deals with the elements, the atoms which compose them and the compounds that they form.

**chemoprophylaxis** the prevention of an acute or recurrent attack of a specific disease by the administration of chemotherapeutic agents, e.g. antibiotics to treat infections or the use of antitubercular drugs for tuberculosis.

**chemoreceptor** a sensory nerve ending or group of cells that is sensitive to chemical stimuli in the blood.

**chemosis** swelling of the conjunctiva due to the presence of fluid; an oedema of the conjunctiva.

**chemotaxis** the reaction of living cells to chemical stimuli. These are either attracted (*positive c.*) or repelled (*negative c.*) by acids, alkalis or other substances.

**chemotherapy** the specific treatment of disease by the administration of chemotherapeutic agents administered by the oral, intramuscular and intravenous routes and occasionally directly into a body cavity, e.g. the bladder. Used to arrest the progress of or eradicate a specific pathological condition in the body without causing irreversible harm to healthy tissue; widely used in the treatment of cancer.

**chest** the thorax. *Barrel c.* one more rounded than usual, with raised ribs and, usually, kyphosis. It is often present in emphysema. *C. leads* leads applied to the chest during the course of an electrocardiographic recording. *Flail c.* one where part of the chest wall moves in opposition to respiration as a result of multiple fractures of the ribs. *Pigeon c.* a chest with the sternum protruding forwards.

**Cheyne–Stokes respiration** *J. Cheyne, British physician, 1776–1836; W. Stokes, British physician, 1804–1878.* Tidal respiration. A form of irregular but rhythmic breathing with temporary cessations (apnoea). It is likely to be present in cerebral tumour, in narcotic poisoning and in advanced cases of arteriosclerosis and uraemia.

**chiasma** a crossing point. *Optic c.* the crossing point of the optic nerves.

**chickenpox** *see* VARICELLA.

**chilblain** a condition resulting from defective circulation when exposure to cold causes localized swelling and inflammation of the hands or feet, with severe itching and burning sensations.

**child** the human young, from infancy to puberty. *C. abuse* the non-accidental use of physical force or the non-accidental act of omission by a parent or other custodian responsible for the care of a child. Child abuse encompasses malnutrition and other kinds of neglect through ignorance, as well as deliberate withholding from the child of the necessary and basic physical care, including the medical and dental care necessary for the child to grow. Examples of physical abuse range from burns and exposure to extreme cold, to beating, poisoning, strangulation, and withholding food and water. If a child is seen to be in danger of suffering significant harm, from physical, sexual, emotional or neglectful causes, the child may be registered on the Child Protection Register. If a nurse, health visitor or midwife has reasonable cause to suspect the abuse of a child, appropriate action must be taken in order to protect that child. *See also* CHILDREN ACT 1989. *Deprived c.* a vague term usually implying that the child in question has been raised in a situation lacking in love, affection and consistent parenting responses from adults. Sometimes used to suggest that the child has experienced a generalized deficit of life opportunities, both interpersonal and social. *C. protection register* a listing of children considered to be at risk of deprivation or neglect. This register is used throughout the UK in inter-agency child-protection work. *C. sexual abuse* the subjection of a child to sexual activity likely to cause physical or psychological harm. *C. surveillance* the assessment of a (usually preschool) child's progress at defined ages by a health visitor, general practitioner or a community paediatrician to identify any developmental or physical concerns.

**child care** any matter associated with the upbringing and welfare of children, both familial and in relation to welfare and social services. *C.C. officer* a social worker who has a responsibility to investigate any situation where a child is thought to be at risk of harm due to neglect, injury or desertion, and in those situations where the child is considered 'beyond control' by the parents/guardians or is offending.

**child development** The stages of physical, psychological and social growth and attainment that occur from birth to adulthood.

**child health clinic** a centre which infants and preschool children attend on a regular basis to ensure normal progress and development. Immunizations against infectious diseases, screening and health promotion information are also provided.

**childbirth** the act or process of giving birth to a child. Parturition. *Natural c.* the act of giving birth without medical intervention. Relaxation and other complementary techniques are used to minimize pain and discomfort, allowing the mother and her partner to remain in control of events which are allowed to progress naturally.

**childminder** a person who is registered with the local authority social services department and who is approved by the department to mind an agreed number of children aged from birth to 5 years during the day.

**Children Act 1989** the main principles of this legislation for the care and welfare of children are as follows. (a) The welfare of children is the prime consideration and wherever possible they should be cared for within their own families. Parents with children in need should be helped and supported by the local authorities, and in partnership with other agencies, to bring up their children themselves. Parents should be informed of their right to complain if they are not satisfied with the services offered. (b) Children should be kept safe and protected by effective intervention if they are in danger but this should be open to parental challenge through the courts. (c) The courts, when dealing with children, should avoid any delays when processing their cases, and should only make an order if to do so is better for the child than making no order at all. (d) Children should be kept informed of any decisions taken in

their interests and should participate as far as possible in any decisions or actions taken. (e) Parents continue to have responsibility for their children, even when they are no longer living with them. Parents should be kept informed of and invited to participate in any decisions about their children's future. (f) Local authorities are required to take account of children's racial origins, culture, linguistic background and religion when making decisions about them.

**Children's Charter for Health and Social Care** introduced in 2004 by the Department of Health as part of the National Service Framework (NSF) to help parents and children have a better understanding of their rights in terms of health care and treatment.

**Chinese medicine** a traditional system based on the principles of Yin and Yang, combining acupuncture with a range of medications from herbal and animal sources.

**Chinese restaurant syndrome** transient arterial dilatation due to ingestion of monosodium glutamate, which is used in seasoning Chinese food; marked by throbbing head, light-headedness, tightness of the jaw, neck and shoulders, and backache.

**chiropody** podiatry, the study and care of the feet and the treatment of minor foot complaints.

**chiropractic** a system of treatment employing manipulation of the spine and other bony structures.

**chi-squared test** a statistical test to determine whether two or more groups of observations differ significantly from one another, i.e. more than would be expected by chance.

*Chlamydia* a genus of bacteria comprising three species: *C. psittacosis*, the cause of psittacosis (parrot fever); *C. pneumoniae* which causes chlamydia pneumonia (especially in children and in young adults); and *C. trachomatis* which includes 15 serotypes and causes many illness, including pneumonia acquired through maternal transmission, acute and chronic conjunctivitis (e.g. adult and neonatal inclusion conjunctivitis), trachoma and adult pharyngitis. Several serotypes of *C. trachomatis* are the most common cause of sexually transmitted diseases in the UK, many EU countries and the USA, including non-gono-coccal urethritis and epididymitis in men, cervicitis, urethritis and pelvic inflammatory disease in women, Reiter's syndrome, and lymphogranuloma venereum.

**chloasma** a condition in which there is brown, blotchy discoloration of the skin of the face, especially during pregnancy.

**chlorine** *symbol* Cl. A yellow, irritating poisonous gas. A powerful disinfectant, bleach and deodorizing agent. Used in hypochlorites for sterilization purposes.

**cholangiography** radiography of the hepatic, cystic and bile ducts after the insertion of a radio-opaque contrast medium.

**cholangitis** inflammation of the bile ducts.

**cholecystectomy** excision of the gall-bladder.

**cholecystitis** inflammation of the gallbladder.

**cholecystoduodenostomy** an anastomosis between the gallbladder and the duodenum.

**cholecystography** radiography of the gallbladder after administration of a radio-opaque contrast medium.

**cholecystolithiasis** the presence of stones in the gallbladder.

**cholecystotomy** an incision into the gallbladder, usually to remove gallstones.

**choledocholithiasis** the presence of stones in the bile duct.

**cholelithiasis** presence of gallstones in the bladder or bile ducts.

**cholera** an acute, notifiable, infectious enteritis endemic and epidemic in Asia and also in Africa. Caused by *Vibrio cholerae*, associated with faecal contamination of water supplies, overcrowding and poor hygienic conditions. It is marked by profuse diarrhoea, muscle cramp, suppression of urine with severe dehydration; it is often fatal but with rehydration affected people make a full recovery. Oral cholera vaccination is available to travellers to areas where cholera is endemic, though this only provides partial immunity. The local drinking water should be boiled or sterilized and uncooked foods avoided.

**cholestasis** arrest of the flow of bile due to obstruction of the bile ducts.

**cholesteatoma** a rare small tumour containing cholesterol. It may occur in the middle ear or in the meninges, central nervous system or bones of the skull.

**cholesterol** a sterol found in nervous tissue, red blood corpuscles, animal fat and bile. It is a precursor of bile acids and steroid hormones, and occurs in the most common type of gallstone, in atheroma of the arteries, in various cysts and in carcinomatous tissue. Most of the body's cholesterol is synthesized, but some is obtained in the diet. Blood cholesterol levels are influenced by diet, weight, heredity and metabolic diseases, e.g. diabetes mellitus, and can be measured by blood tests. Levels below 5.0 mmol/L are acceptable. Dietary measures to lower cholesterol include reducing the saturated fat intake and increased exercise.

**choline** an essential amine, found in the blood, cerebrospinal fluid and urine, which aids fat metabolism. Formerly classified as a vitamin of the B complex.

**cholinergic** pertaining to nerves that release acetylcholine as the chemical stimulator at their nerve endings. *C. drugs* drugs that inhibit cholinesterase and so prevent the destruction of acetylcholine.

**cholinesterase** an enzyme that rapidly destroys acetylcholine.

**chondroblast** an embryonic cell that forms cartilage.

**chondroma** an innocent new growth arising in cartilage.

**chondromalacia** a condition of abnormal softening of cartilage.

**chorda** a sinew or cord.

**chordee** downward curvature of the penis caused by congenital anomaly (common in hypospadias) or urethral infection.

**chorditis** inflammation of the vocal or spermatic cords.

**chordotomy** an operation on the spinal cord to divide the anterolateral nerve pathways for relief of intractable pain. Cordotomy.

**chorea** a symptom of disease of the basal ganglia when the individual suffers from spasmodic, involuntary, rapid movements of the face, shoulders and hips. *Huntington's c.* (or Huntington's disease) a rare hereditary disorder which manifests itself in early middle age. The individual also suffers from progressive dementia, which often precedes a premature death. *Sydenham's c.* St Vitus's dance. Occurs in childhood and is associated with rheumatic fever.

**choreiform** resembling chorea.

**choriocarcinoma** formerly known as chorioepithelioma. A highly malignant neoplasm usually arising from the trophoblast of a hydatidiform mole (*see* HYDATIDIFORM MOLE). It may develop after an abortion or the evacuation of a hydatidiform mole or even in normal pregnancy. Metastases usually develop rapidly but the disease normally carries a good prognosis if early treatment is given.

**chorion** the outer membrane enveloping the fetus; the placenta.

**chorionic** pertaining to the chorion. *C. gonadotrophin* human chorionic gonadotrophin (HCG). *C. villi* small protrusions on the chorion from which the placenta is formed. They are in close association with the maternal blood and, by diffusion, interchange of nutriment, oxygen and waste matters is effected between the maternal and the fetal blood. *C. villus biopsy* tissue removed from the gestational sac early in pregnancy so that chromosomal and other inherited disorders can be identified. Can be carried out at an earlier stage than amniocentesis but is less safe for the pregnancy.

**chorioretinitis** choroidoretinitis.

**choroid** the pigmented and vascular coat of the eyeball, continuous with the iris and situated between the sclera and retina. It reduces the amount of light that falls upon the retina. *C. plexus* specialized cells in the ventricles of the brain that produce cerebrospinal fluids. There is one choroid plexus in each ventricle.

**choroiditis** inflammation of the choroid.

**choroidoretinitis** an inflammatory condition of both the choroid and retina of the eye.

**Christmas disease** a hereditary bleeding disease similar to haemophilia but is due to a deficiency of clotting factor IX; also called haemophilia B. The name is derived from that of the first patient to be studied.

**chromatography** a method of chemical analysis by which substances in solution can be separated as they percolate down a column of powdered absorbent or ascend an absorbent paper by capillary traction. A definite pattern is produced and substances may be recognized by the use of appropriate colour reagents. Amino acids can be identified in this way.

**chromatometry** the measurement of colour perception.

**chromosome** in animal cells, a structure in the nucleus, containing a linear thread of DEOXYRIBONUCLEIC ACID (DNA), which transmits genetic information and is associated with RIBONUCLEIC ACID (RNA) and histones. During cell division the material composing the chromosome is compactly coiled. Each organism of a species is normally characterized by the same number of chromosomes in its somatic cells, 46 being the number usually present in humans: 22 pairs of autosomes, and two sex chromosomes (XX or XY), which determine the sex of the organism. In the mature GAMETE (ovum or spermatozoon) the number of chromosomes is halved as a result of MEIOSIS.

**chronic** of long duration; the opposite of acute. *C. fatigue syndrome* extreme fatigue for the patient over a long period, often years. The cause of this condition is not fully understood, although some cases have been reported following recovery from a viral infection. Most commonly affects women between 25 and 45 years age. The main symptom is constant tiredness but other symptoms may include poor concentration, sore throat, tender lymph nodes, muscle and joint pain. Also known as myalgic encephalomyelitis (ME). *C. obstructive pulmonary disease* a combination of chronic bronchitis and emphysema in which there is disruption of air flow into or out of the lungs. Dyspnoea, wheezing and cough predominate, often made worse by any exertion or pollution in the environment. Patients may be severely disabled and require oxygen for long periods.

**chronological** the recording of a number of events starting with the earliest and following the order in which they occurred. *C. age* the age of an individual expressed as a period of time that has elapsed since birth. In infants this may be given in hours, days or weeks but for children and adults it is expressed in years.

**Chvostek's sign** *F. Chvostek, Austrian surgeon, 1835–1884.* A spasm of the facial muscles which occurs in tetany. It can be elicited by tapping the facial nerve.

**chyle** digested fats which, as a milky fluid, are absorbed into the lymphatic capillaries (lacteals) in the villi of the small intestine.

**chylothorax** the presence of effused chyle in the pleural cavity.

**chyme** the semiliquid acid mass of food that passes from the stomach to the intestines.

**chymotrypsin** an enzyme secreted by the pancreas. It is activated by trypsin and aids in the breakdown of proteins.

**Ci** symbol for KELOID.

**cicatrix** the scar of a healed wound (*see* KELOID).

**cilia** 1. the eyelashes. 2. microscopic filaments projecting from some epithelial cells, known as ciliated membranes, as in the bronchi, where cilia wave the secretion upwards.

**ciliary** hair-like. *C. body* a structure just behind the corneoscleral margin, composed of the ciliary muscle and processes. *C. muscle* the circular muscle surrounding the lens of the eye. *C. processes* the fringed part of the choroid coat arranged in a circle in front of the lens.

*Cimex* a genus of blood-sucking bugs. *C. lectularius* the common bedbug.

**CINAHL** Abbreviation for Cumulative Index to Nursing and Allied Health Literature. *See* entry.

**cineangiocardiography** angiography using a cine camera to show the movements of the heart and blood vessels.

**circadian** denoting a period of 24 hours. *C. rhythm* the rhythm of certain biological activities that take place daily.

**circinate** having a circular outline. *Tinea circinata* is ringworm.

**circle of Willis** *T. Willis, British physician and anatomist, 1621–1675.* An anastomosis of arteries at the base of the brain, formed by the branches of the internal carotid and the basilar arteries.

**circulation** movement in a circular course, as of the blood (*see* Figure). *Collateral c.* enlargement of small vessels establishing adequate blood supply when the main vessel to the part has been occluded. *Coronary c.* the system of vessels that supplies the heart muscle itself. *Extracorporeal c.* 1. removal of the blood by intravenous cannulae, passing it through a machine to oxygenate it, and then pumping it back into circulation. 2. the 'heart–lung' machine or pump respirator, used in cardiac surgery. *Lymph c.* the flow of lymph through lymph vessels and glands. *Portal c.* the passage of blood from the alimentary tract, pancreas and spleen, via the portal vein and its branches through the liver and into the hepatic veins. *Pulmonary c.* passage of the blood from the right ventricle via the pulmonary artery through the lungs and back to the heart by the pulmonary veins. *Systemic c.* the flow of blood throughout the body. The direction of flow is from the left atrium to the left ventricle and through the aorta, with its branches and capillaries. Veins then carry it back to the right atrium, and so into the right ventricle.

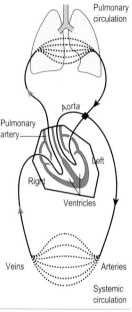

CIRCULATION

**circumcision** excision of the prepuce or foreskin of the penis. An operation performed for religious reasons, or sometimes for phimosis or paraphimosis. *Female c.* excision of the labia minora and/ or labia majora, and sometimes the clitoris; still performed ritualistically in certain countries, the extent of the surgery varying from one culture to another. Prior to pregnancy it may cause problems with micturition and intercourse. Special care will be required during labour and delivery, and excision

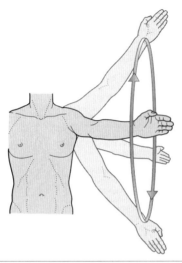

CIRCUMDUCTION

and separation of the tissues may be needed; alternatively a caesarian section may be considered. Female circumcision is illegal in some countries.

**circumduction** moving in a circle, e.g. the circular movement of the upper limb (*see* Figure).

**circumoral** around the mouth. *C. pallor* a pale area around the mouth contrasting with the flushed cheeks, e.g. in scarlet fever.

**cirrhosis** a degenerative change that can occur in any organ, but especially in the liver. May be due to viruses, microorganisms or toxic substances (*portal c.*). Fibrosis results and interferes with the working of the organ. In the liver it causes portal obstruction, with consequent

ascites, jaundice, splenomegaly, oesophageal varices and episodes of bleeding and bruising. Digital clubbing may be present.

**cisterna** a space or cavity containing fluid. *C. chyli* the dilated portion of the thoracic duct containing chyle. *C. magna* the subarachnoid space between the cerebellum and medulla oblongata.

**cisternal** concerning the cisterna. *C. puncture* insertion of a hollow needle into the cisterna magna to withdraw cerebrospinal fluid.

**citric acid** acid found in the juice of lemons, limes, etc. An antiscorbutic.

**CJD** *See* CREUTZFELDT–JAKOB DISEASE.

**Cl** symbol for *chlorine*.

**clairvoyance** extrasensory perception. The act or power of knowing about objects or events without the use of the senses.

**clang association** rhyming speech. A way of speaking where words are associated that are similar in sound. Observed in some mental disorders.

**clapping** in physiotherapy, rhythmic beating with cupped hands. Frequently used over the chest to aid expectoration.

**class** 1. a system that divides members of a society into sets based upon social or economic status and is based upon cultural characteristics in common. 2. a group of objects that have a common characteristic.

**claudication** lameness. *Intermittent c.* limping, accompanied by severe pain in the legs on walking, which disappears with rest. A sign of occlusive arterial disease.

**claustrophobia** fear of confined spaces, such as small rooms.

**clavicle** the collar bone. A long bone, part of the shoulder girdle.

**clawfoot** a deformity in which the longitudinal arch is abnormally raised. Pes cavus.

**clawhand** a deformity in which the fingers are bent and contracted, giving a claw-like appearance.

**cleft** a fissure or longitudinal opening. *C. lip* a congenital fissure in the upper lip, often accompanied by cleft palate. *C. palate* a congenital defect in the roof of the mouth due to failure of the medial plates of the palate to meet. Often associated with cleft lip.

**client** 1. a recipient of a professional service. 2. a recipient of health care, regardless of the person's state of health and where the service is delivered. 3. a patient.

**climacteric** the period of the menopause in women. Also used to denote the decline in sexual drive in men.

**climax** 1. the stage when a disease is at its greatest intensity. 2. the

stage in sexual intercourse when orgasm occurs.

**clinic** 1. instruction of students at the bedside. 2. a department of a hospital devoted to the treatment of a particular type of disease or a place which patients attend for a consultation with a medical or nurse practitioner.

**clinical** relating to bedside observation and the treatment of patients. *C. audit* a cyclical measurement and evaluation by health professionals of the clinical standards they are achieving. *C. Data Standards Board* the organization that mandates professionally agreed standards for clinical data throughout the NHS. *C. governance* a framework through which NHS organizations are accountable for continuously improving the quality of their services and for safeguarding high standards of care by creating an environment in which excellence in care will flourish (see Appendices). *C. nurse specialist* a qualified nurse who has acquired advanced knowledge and skills in a specific area of clinical nursing. *C. risk index for babies* abbreviated CRIB. A professional scoring tool used in assessing the initial neonatal risks for babies, and also for comparing the performance of one neonatal intensive care unit with another. *C. risk management* the means by which adverse events occurring in organizations and usually related to the delivery of patient care are systematically assessed and reviewed in order to seek ways for prevention of future incidents. *C. skills* skills required by clinicians (doctors, nurses, dentists and other clinical professions). Clinical skills vary depending on specialty but core skills remain constant, e.g. communication skills, history-taking skills, record-keeping, basic physical examination, etc. *C. supervision* an exchange between practising professionals to enable the development of professional skills. Has a vital role in sustaining and developing professional practice in nursing, midwifery and health visiting. *C. trial* a research investigation designed to provide objective information on the therapeutic efficacy of a particular drug or therapy.

**clip**  a metal device for holding the two edges of a wound together or for controlling the flow of liquid through a tube.

**clitoridectomy**  excision of the clitoris. *See* CIRCUMCISION (FEMALE).

**clitoris**  a small organ, formed of erectile tissue, situated at the anterior junction of the labia minora in the female.

**clone**  cells which are genetically identical to each other and have descended by asexual reproduction from the parent cell, to which they are also genetically identical.

**clonic**  having the character of clonus. The second stage of a grand mal fit; also referred to as a tonic–clonic seizure. *See* EPILEPSY.

**clonus**  muscle rigidity and relaxation which occurs spasmodically. *Ankle c.* spasmodic movements of the calf muscles when the foot is suddenly pushed upwards, the leg being extended.

**Clostridium**  a genus of anaerobic spore-forming bacteria, found as commensals of the gut of animals and humans and saprophytes of the soil. Pathogenic species include *C. botulinum* (botulism), *C. tetani* (tetanus) and *C. perfringens* (also known as *C. welchii*) (gas gangrene).

**Clostrium difficile (C. difficile)**  is a spore-forming bacterium that is present in the gut of some adults and children and normally does not cause any problems in healthy people. However, sometimes antibiotics are given to a patient to treat an infection which can interfere with the balance of the 'good bacteria' present in the gut. When this happens, *C. difficile* bacteria can multiply and cause symptoms such as diarrhoea and pyrexia. Most cases occur in a health care environment such as a hospital or care home. Generally, people with *C. difficile* infection make a full recovery, but the infection can sometimes be fatal especially in the elderly. A particularly virulent form of *C. difficile*, known as type 027, is associated with severe hospital outbreaks. The risks of transmitting *C. difficile* amongst patients during health care episodes can be minimized by prudent antimicrobial prescribing, the isolation of those with *C. difficile* diarrhoea with enhanced environmental cleansing, and especially hand hygiene. Care should be taken not to rely on alcohol hand gels which do not destroy bacterial spores. *See* Appendix 12.

**clot**  a semisolid mass formed in a liquid, such as blood or lymph, by coagulation.

**clotting**  coagulation. The formation of a clot (*see* BLOOD CLOTTING). *C. time* coagulation time. The length of time taken for shed blood to coagulate.

**clubbing**  broadening and thickening of the tips of the fingers (and toes) due to bad circulation. It occurs in chronic diseases of the heart and respiratory system, such as congenital cardiac defect and tuberculosis.

**clubfoot**  talipes.

**clumping**  the collecting together into clumps. The reaction of bacteria and blood cells when agglutination occurs.

**Co**  symbol for *cobalt*.

**coagulase**  an enzyme formed by pathogenic staphylococci that causes coagulation of plasma. Such bacteria are termed *c. positive*.

**coagulation** clotting. *See* BLOOD CLOTTING.

**coagulum** the mass of fibrin and cells formed when blood clots; the mass formed when other masses coagulate, e.g. milk curd.

**coal tar** a by-product obtained in the destructive distillation of coal; used in ointment or solution in the treatment of eczema and psoriasis.

**coarctation** a condition of contraction or stricture. *C. of aorta* a congenital malformation characterized by deformity of the aorta, causing narrowing, usually severe, of the lumen of the vessel. Surgical resection of the stricture may be performed.

**cobalt** *symbol* Co. A metallic element, traces of which are necessary in the diet to prevent anaemia. *Radioactive c.* cobalt-60, used as a source of gamma irradiation in radiotherapy.

**cocaine** a colourless alkaloid, obtained from coca leaves, which has a powerful but brief stimulant action. Formerly used as a local anaesthetic, cocaine has been replaced by less addictive preparations like procaine, lignocaine and amethocaine. It is now a major 'recreational' drug, producing euphoria with many undesirable behavioural and social effects. It is addictive and usually taken by snorting. Regular inhaling of the drug can damage the lining of the nose. Overdose can cause seizures and cardiac arrest. Also known, in its various forms, as 'crack', 'coke', 'snow', 'flake', 'nose candy' or 'rocks'.

**cocainism** addiction to cocaine. Long-term abuse is associated with a toxic psychosis.

**coccus** a bacterium of spheroidal shape.

**coccydynia** persistent pain in the region of the coccyx.

**coccyx** the terminal bone of the spinal column, in which four rudimentary vertebrae are fused together to form a triangle.

**cochlea** the spiral canal of the internal ear.

**Cochrane database** *A. Cochrane, 1909–1988.* Database of systematic reviews of published research. An international multidisciplinary collaboration of health professionals, consumers and researchers who review randomized controlled clinical trials.

**cod liver oil** purified oil from the liver of the codfish; valuable source of vitamins A and D.

**code** 1. a set of rules governing one's conduct. 2. a system by which information can be communicated. *Genetic c.* the arrangement of nucleotides in the DNA of the chromosomes and in the RNA of the protein transcription apparatus in the cell. *Professional c.* a code of professional conduct for the nurse, midwife and health visitor. Revised periodically, this code is intended to provide definite standards of practice and conduct that are essential to the ethical discharge of the nurse's and midwife's responsibility and to inform the public, other professions and employers of the standard of professional conduct expected of a registered practitioner. (*See* Appendix 5.) Many other professional groups have their own standards of conduct, performance and ethics. Some of these groups are regulated by the Health Professions Council and include arts therapists, biomedical scientists, chiropodists and podiatrists, clinical scientists, dietitians, occupational therapists, orthoptists, paramedics, physiotherapists, prosthesists, orthotists, radiographers and speech and language therapists.

**coeliac** relating to the abdomen. *C. disease* an inflammatory condition of the gastrointestinal tract due to a hypersensitivity to gluten (found in barley, wheat, oats and rye) in the diet. Damage to the gut causes malabsorption leading to weight loss and vitamin and mineral deficiencies that may cause anaemia and ill health. Diagnosis is made by blood, urine and faecal testing together with jejunal biopsies. Treatment involves a lifelong gluten-free diet. Coeliac disease can affect all ages and runs in some families. The incidence in the UK is 1:1000. *C. plexus* nerve complex that supplies the abdominal organs.

**coenzyme** an organic molecule activator to a larger protein enzyme.

**cognition** the action of knowing. Cognitive function of the conscious mind in contrast to the effective (feeling) and conative (willing).

**cognitive behavioural therapy** a method of treating psychological disorders based on the approach that the client's problems arise from a faulty way of looking at the world and oneself. In cognitive therapy the client is helped to identify negative or false cognitions and then encouraged to try out new thought strategies in daily living.

**cohabit** 1. to live together and have a sexual relationship without being married. 2. to coexist.

**cohort** a group of people possessing a common characteristic, such as being born in the same year or of the same sex, used in research to make generalizations derived from quantitative data. *C. study* concerning a specific group or subpopulation in a research study.

**coitus** sexual intercourse between male and female. *C. interruptus* a method of contraception in which the erect penis is removed from the vagina before ejaculation occurs.

**cold** 1. of low temperature. 2. a viral infection affecting the membranes of the nose and throat and the bronchial tubes. *C. sore* herpes simplex. *See* HERPES.

**colic** acute paroxysmal abdominal pain. *Biliary c.* pain due to the presence of a gallstone in a bile duct. *Infantile c.* excessive crying due to pain and distress. Most common in the first 3 months of life. The infant may pull up its legs and expel gas from the anus or 'belch'. May be due to air swallowing, milk intolerance or natural hyperactivity. *Intestinal c.* severe griping spasmodic abdominal pain which may be a symptom of food poisoning or of intestinal obstruction. *Renal c.* pain due to the presence of a stone in the ureter. *Uterine c.* spasmodic pain originating in the uterus, as in dysmenorrhoea.

**coliform** resembling the bacillus *Escherichia coli*.

**colitis** inflammation of the colon. It may be due to a specific organism, as in dysentery, but the term *ulcerative c.* denotes a chronic disease, often of unknown cause, in which there are attacks of diarrhoea, with the passage of blood and mucus.

**collagen** a fibrous structural protein that constitutes the protein of the white (collagenous) fibres of skin, tendon, bone, cartilage and all other connective tissues. It also occurs dispersed in a gel to provide stiffening, as in the vitreous humour of the eye. *C. diseases* a group of diseases having in common certain clinical and histological features that are manifestations of involvement of connective tissues (*see* CONNECTIVE (TISSUES)).

**collapse** 1. a state of extreme prostration due to defective action of the heart, severe shock or haemorrhage. 2. falling in of a structure.

**collar bone** the clavicle.

**collateral** accessory to. *C. circulation see* CIRCULATION.

**Colles' fracture** *A. Colles, Irish surgeon, 1773–1843.* Fracture of the lower end of the radius at the wrist following a fall on the outstretched hand. Typically, it produces the 'dinner fork' deformity.

**colloid** 1. glue-like. 2. the translucent, yellowish, gelatinous substance resulting from colloid degeneration. 3. a chemical system composed of a continuous medium of small particles which do not settle out under the influence of gravity and will not pass through a semipermeable membrane, as in DIALYSIS.

**coloboma** a congenital fissure of the eye affecting the choroid coat and the retina.

**colon** the large intestine, from the caecum to the rectum (*see* Figure). *Ascending c.* that part rising up to the right of the abdomen to in front of the liver. *Descending c.* that part running down from in front of the spleen to the sigmoid colon. *Giant c.* megacolon. *Irritable c. see* IRRITABLE (BOWEL SYNDROME). *Pelvic c., sigmoid c.* that part lying in the pelvis and connecting the descending colon with the rectum. *Transverse c.* that part lying across the upper abdomen connecting the ascending and descending portions.

**colonic** pertaining to the colon. *C. irrigation* colonic LAVAGE.

**colonoscope** a fibreoptic instrument, passed through the anus, for examining the interior of the colon.

**colony** a mass of bacteria formed by multiplication of cells when bacteria are incubated under favourable conditions.

**colostomy** an artificial opening (stoma) in the large intestine brought to the surface of the abdomen for the purpose of evacuating the bowel.

**colostrum** the fluid secreted by the breasts in the last few weeks of pregnancy and for the first 3 or 4 days after delivery, until lactation begins. Colostrum is high in protein and initially low in lactose; its fat content is equivalent to breast milk. It is an important source of passive antibody.

COLON

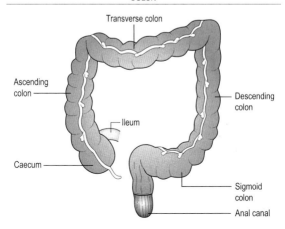

COLON

Transverse colon

Ascending colon

Ileum

Caecum

Descending colon

Sigmoid colon

Anal canal

**colour index** an index of the amount of haemoglobin in red blood cells. In normal blood the figure is 1, in iron deficiency anaemia it is less than 1 and in megaloblastic anaemia it is more than 1. *See* BLOOD.

**colour vision deficiency** any abnormality in colour vision that causes difficulty distinguishing between certain colours. The most common types of colour vision deficiency are reduced discrimination between red and green. A total absence of colour vision is very rare.

**colpocele** a hernia of either bladder or rectum into the vagina. Vaginocele.

**colphysterectomy** removal of the uterus through the vagina.

**colpoperineorrhaphy** the repair by suturing of an injured vagina and torn perineum.

**colpopexy** suture of a prolapsed vagina to the abdominal wall.

**colporrhaphy** repair of the vagina. *Anterior c.* repair for cystocele. *Posterior c.* repair for retrocele.

**colposcope** a speculum for examining the vagina and cervix by means of a magnifying lens; used for the early detection of malignant changes.

**coma** a state of unconsciousness from which the patient cannot be aroused. Characterized by an absence of both spontaneous eye movements and response to painful stimuli. *See* GLASGOW COMA SCALE.

**comatose** in the condition of coma.

**comedo** a blackhead. A plug of keratin and sebum within the dilated orifice of a hair follicle.

**comfort** to provide relief of or freedom from pain, depression or anxiety. *C. eating* eating at inappropriate times or eating unusual amounts for the relief of distress or anxiety. *C. measure* a specific action taken to promote the comfort of the patient, e.g. rearranging pillows or providing a change of position.

**comforter** a baby's dummy or pacifier.

**commensal** living on or within another organism, and deriving benefit without harming or benefiting the host individual.

**comminuted** broken into small pieces, as in a comminuted FRACTURE.

**Commission for Healthcare Audit and Inspection** abbreviated CHAI. Organization that from 2004 has brought together the previous work of the Commission for Health Improvement (CHI), the Mental Health Act Commission, the NHS 'Value for Money' for the Audit Commission and the independent health care work of the National Care Standards Commission. The Commission for Healthcare Audit and Inspection (a) is responsible for inspection of management and the provision of health care against national standards and priorities; (b) investigates serious service failures in the NHS, publishes reports and identifies lessons to be learnt by health care staff and provides independent scrutiny of the NHS complaints procedure (c) reports annually to Parliament on the progress on health care delivery and the use of resources; (d) replaces the Mental Health Act Commission; (e) licenses private health care provision. *See* Appendix 14.

**Commission on Human Medicines Expert Advisory Group on Paediatric Medicines (PMEAG)** was established to advise the Commission of Human Medicines on the safety, quality and efficacy of medicines for paediatric use, and on the implementation of the Department of Health/Medicines and Health Care Products Agency (MHRA), the EU paediatric work sharing project and the European regulation on medicines for paediatric use.

**Commission for Social Care Inspection** organization that from 2004 has provided a single comprehensive inspectorate for social care, bringing together the inspection functions of the Social Services Inspectorate and the National Care Standards commission. The Commission provides an annual report to Parliament on social care services and will identify poor performance in the services provided.

**commissioning** the process by which health needs of the population are delivered and priorities determined. It is a strategic, long-term activity that frames service development within the NHS. Commissioning is a cyclical process involving: assessment of health need, auditing of current service provision, setting priorities, service and practice development, with contracting and the evaluation of services. The commissioning process is undertaken in partnership with other agencies.

**commissure** a site of union of corresponding parts, as the angle of the lips or eyelids.

**commode** a bedside chair with a cutaway seat that allows a receptacle to be fitted underneath for the collection of urine and faeces. Used by a patient who is unable to reach the lavatory.

**communicable disease** an infectious disease caused by microorganisms that may be transmitted from a person, animal or the environment to susceptible persons, either directly or indirectly.

**communication skills** in the broadest sense involve listening, speaking, writing and reading. In the context of health care, they generally focus on listening and giving information to patients. Communication skills cover both verbal and nonverbal forms of communication. Communication skills may extend to communicating with other clinicians, communicating at conferences or formal meetings, and presenting material in class settings.

**community** a group of individuals living in an area, having a common interest, or belonging to the same organization. *C. care* the care of individuals within the community, as an alternative to institutional or long-stay residential care. *C. health services* services provided in the community by staff who are not employed by general practices but may work from the same premises as general practitioners. Staff groups involved include district nurses, health visitors, physiotherapists, speech therapists, podiatrists and school nurses. Such staff now work for Primary Care Trusts. *C. nurse* a nurse who is based within the community with a responsibility for providing nursing services within the patient's own home or environment and may come from a variety of specialized backgrounds, e.g. psychiatry. All community nurses have a strong commitment towards health promotion and the prevention of ill health. *C. safety partnership* aims to create safer places for people to live, work and visit. Involves different agencies to tackle issues such as antisocial behaviour, domestic violence, crime, and reducing accidents and injuries. *Therapeutic c.* any treatment setting (usually psychiatric) which provides a living–learning situation through group processes emphasizing social, environmental and personal interactions.

**compatibility** mutual suitability. The mixing together of two substances without chemical change or loss of power. *See* BLOOD GROUPS.

**compensation** 1. making good a functional or structural defect. 2. mental mechanism (unconscious) by which a person covers up a weakness by exaggerating a more desirable characteristic.

**compensatory techniques** assistance for patients/clients in developing new skills to compensate for a recognized handicap or deficit.

**competence** a set of professionally agreed deliverables, outputs and roles that the health care professional must be able to perform in a particular post.

**competency** a set of behaviour patterns, knowledge and skill that the holder needs to bring to a position in order to perform the required role and functions with competence.

**complaint** an act of expressing dissatisfaction with a service or individual; may be written or verbal. *C. management* the policies and procedures in place within an NHS Trust to respond to and learn from complaints received from patients, their families and members of the public regarding care, treatment and services.

**complement** a substance present in normal serum which combines with the antigen–antibody complex to destroy bacteria. *C. fixation test* measurement of the amount of complement with antigen–antibody complex. Complement fixation tests are used to detect antibodies for infectious diseases.

**complement system** a series of small inactive plasma proteins that are an important part of the innate immune response to infection. When stimulated by the presence of either an antibody–antigen complex or certain microbial products or antigens, complement proteins act as a biochemical cascade, with one protein activating the next. This results in the formation of activated complement which, by various means, attacks and destroys pathogenic micro-organisms, dissolves and removes immune complexes.

**complementary** pertaining to that which completes or makes perfect. *C. feed* feed given to infants to supplement breast feeding when

the mother has insufficient milk. *C. therapies* a range of treatments, including yoga, reflexology, homeopathy, acupuncture and others, which may be combined with traditional medicine. *See also* ALTERNATIVE MEDICINE.

**complex** a grouping of various things, as of signs and symptoms, forming a syndrome. In psychology, a grouping of ideas of emotional origin which are completely or partially represented in the unconscious mind. *Inferiority c.* a compensation by assertiveness or aggression to cover a feeling of inadequacy. *See* ELECTRA COMPLEX and OEDIPUS COMPLEX.

**compliance** the degree to which a patient follows medical or nursing advice.

**complication** an accident or second disease process arising during the course of or following the primary condition; may be fatal.

**compos mentis** [L.] *of sound mind.*

**compound** composed of two or more parts or substances. *C. fracture* a fracture in which a wound through to the skin has also occurred.

**comprehension** mental grasp of the meaning of a situation.

**compress** folded material, e.g. lint (wet or dry), applied to a part of the body for the relief of swelling and pain.

**compression** 1. the act of pressing upon or together; the state of being pressed together. 2. in embryology, the shortening or omission of certain developmental stages.

**compression bandages** are used in the treatment of leg ulcers to improve venous return and reduce venous hypertension. Following successful healing of the leg ulcer compression hose are worn to prevent reoccurrence.

**compression garments** these may be fitted and used following burns or for a patient with lymphoedema.

They work by exerting pressure on the tissues thus preventing the build up of fluid in the tissues.

**compulsion** an overwhelming urge to perform an irrational act or ritual.

**computed axial tomography** abbreviated CAT. The utilization of a computerized technique to examine a cross-section of the entire body. The CAT scanner produces an image of tissue density in a complete cross-section of the part of the body being scanned.

**computerized records** many health records are now held on computer systems which are required by law to be secure and to maintain confidentiality, usually achieved by limiting access. Most systems currently also provide a paper printout which is stored as a manual record. *See also* DATA PROTECTION ACT.

**conation** a striving in a certain direction. *See* COGNITION.

**concept** an image or idea held in the mind.

**conception** 1. the act of becoming pregnant, by the fertilization of an ovum. 2. a concept.

**conceptual framework** a group of concepts that are broadly defined and organized to provide a rationale or structure for the interpretation of information.

**concussion** a violent jarring shock. *C. of the brain* temporary loss of consciousness produced by a fall or a blow on the head. There may be amnesia, slow respiration and a weak pulse.

**conditioned response** a response that does not occur naturally but may be developed by regular association of some physiological function with an unrelated outside event, such as the ringing of a bell or flashing of a light. Soon the physiological function starts whenever the outside event occurs. Also

called conditioned reflex. *See also* UNCONDITIONED RESPONSE

**conditioning** a form of learning in which a response is elicited by a neural stimulus that had previously been repeatedly presented in conjunction with the stimulus that originally elicited the response. Also called classical and respondent conditioning.

**condom** a contraceptive sheath worn during sexual intercourse and affording some protection for both partners against sexually transmitted diseases. Now available for both males and females.

**conductive deafness** deafness caused by the faulty conduction of sound from the outer to the inner ear.

**conductor** 1. a substance through which electricity, light, heat or sound can pass. 2. any part of the nervous system that conveys impulses.

**condyle** a rounded eminence occurring at the end of some bones, and articulating with another bone.

**condylomata** *sing.* condyloma. An elevated wart-like lesion of the skin. *C. acuminata* small, pointed papillomas of viral origin, usually occurring on the skin or mucous surfaces of the external genitalia or perianal region. *C. lata* wide, flat, syphilitic condylomata occurring on most skin, especially about the genitals and anus.

**cone** a solid figure with a rounded base, tapering upwards to a point. *C. biopsy* the removal of a cone-shaped section from the cervix of the uterus. It is performed for confirmation of the diagnosis when a cervical smear test result suggests the presence of pre-cancerous cells. *Retinal c.* the cone-shaped end of a light-sensitive cell in the retina, used for acute vision and for distinguishing colours.

**confabulation** the production of fictitious memories, and the relating of experiences which have no relation to truth, to fill in the gaps due to loss of memory. A symptom of Korsakoff's syndrome.

**confidence** self-assurance arising from a belief in one's own ability to achieve. *C. interval* in statistics, a range of values that has some specified probability. By convention 95% and 99% confidence intervals are the most used. *C. limits* the bounds of the confidence interval.

**confidential enquiry** a unique form of audit in which case notes are scrutinized by relevant professionals to identify substandard care and make recommendations for future practice. The triennial Confidential Enquiry into Maternal Deaths and the Confidential Enquiry into Stillbirths and Deaths in Infancy (CESDI) is directly related to maternity care, and midwives may be involved in providing appropriate information. The Confidential Enquiry into Perioperative Deaths is also available.

**confidentiality** spoken, written or given in confidence.

**conflict** a mental state arising when two opposing wishes or impulses cause emotional tension and often cannot be resolved without repressing one of the impulses into the unconscious. Conflict situations may be associated with an anxiety neurosis.

**confluent** running together.

**confusion** disturbed orientation in regard to time, place or person, sometimes accompanied by disordered consciousness.

**congenital** present at and existing from the time of birth. *C. dislocation of the hip* failure in position of the head of the femur and development of the acetabulum. *C. heart defect* a structural defect of the heart or great vessels or both. *C. infection* an infection which takes place in utero. The most important congenital infections are rubella, cytomegalovirus, herpes simplex, human immunodeficiency virus (HIV), syphilis and toxoplasmosis.

**Congenital Disabilities (Civil Liabilities) Act 1976** this Act is applicable in England, Wales and Northern Ireland and provides for a child to be entitled to recover damages where the child has suffered as result of a breach in a duty of care owed to the mother or the father unless that breach of duty of care occurred before the child was conceived and either or both parents knew of the occurrence. In Scottish law the same provisions are made. The accuracy and preservation of records is therefore essential.

**congestion** an abnormal accumulation of blood in any part. *Pulmonary c.* congestion of the lung, as in pneumonia and congestive heart failure.

**conjugate** to join or yoke together as, in the liver, bilirubin is combined with albumin by the activity of glucuronyl transferase to render it water-soluble so that it may be excreted via the gut. *See also* ICTERUS *and* JAUNDICE.

**conjunctiva** the mucous membrane covering the front of the eyeball and lining the eyelids.

**conjunctivitis** inflammation of the conjunctiva. 'Pink eye' ophthalmia. *Catarrhal c.* a mild form, usually due to cold or irritation. *Granular c.* trachoma. *Phlyctenular c.* marked by small vesicles or ulcers on the membrane. *Purulent c.* caused by virulent organisms, with discharge of pus.

**connective** joining together. *C. tissues* those that develop from the mesenchyme and are formed of a matrix containing fibres and cells. Areolar tissue, cartilage and bone are examples.

**consanguinity** blood relationship.

**conscious** the state of being awake or aware. Levels of consciousness are loosely defined states of awareness of and response to stimuli, essential for the assessment of an individual's neurological status. The level of consciousness is an accurate indicator of the degree of brain (dys)function.

**consent** in law, voluntary agreement with an action proposed by another. Consent is an act of reason; the person giving consent must be of sufficient mental capacity and in possession of all essential information in order to give valid and informed consent. It is a legal requirement that doctors or researchers inform patients about to undergo surgery or invasive tests or to be a subject involved in a clinical trial of the risks and probable outcomes of the treatment or research. *C. forms* in non-emergency situations, written informed consent is generally required before many clinical procedures, such as surgery (including biopsies), endoscopy and radiographic procedures involving catheterization. The doctor must explain to the patient the diagnosis, the nature of the procedure, including the risks involved and the chances of success, and the alternative methods of treatment that are available. It is recommended that consent forms should contain a signed declaration that the doctor has explained the nature of the procedure to the patient in non-technical words. Nurses or other members of the health care team may be involved in filling out the consent form and witnessing the signature of the patient. *Informed c.* a process whereby patients, parents or guardians and research participants are kept fully informed of the procedures that they will be undertaking; enabling them to make an informed choice for consent. Ensuring informed consent is a moral and legal duty for all health care professionals.

**conservative treatment** the use of non-radical methods to restore health and preserve function.

**consolidation** a state of becoming solid. *C. of lung* in pneumonia the infected lobe becomes solid with exudate.

**constipation** incomplete or infrequent action of the bowels, with consequent filling of the rectum with hard faeces. *Atonic c.* constipation due to lack of muscle tone in the bowel wall. *Spastic c.* a form of constipation where spasm of part of the bowel wall narrows the canal.

**Consultant in Public Health Medicine** Responsible for functions such as promoting health, preventing disease and fostering co-operation between the health and social services.

**consumer** in health care, may be the user, client, patient or carer, in terms of the services being provided.

**consumption** 1. the act of consuming, or the process of being consumed. 2. a wasting away of the body; once applied to pulmonary tuberculosis.

**contact** 1. a mutual touching of two bodies or persons. 2. an individual known to have been in association with an infected person or animal or a contaminated environment. *C. dermatitis* a skin mark marked by itching, swelling, blistering, oozing and scaling. It is caused by direct contact between the skin and a substance to which the person is allergic or sensitive. (*See* LATEX) *C. lens* a glass or plastic lens worn under the eyelids in the front of the eye. It may be worn for therapeutic or for cosmetic reasons. *C. tracer* a health care worker who visits people known to have an infectious disease and their partners and family to encourage them to attend a clinic for health care in an attempt to prevent the spread of the infection in the community. *C. tracing* a public health measure taken to limit the spread of infectious disease, e.g. sexually transmitted diseases, tuberculosis.

**contagion** 1. the communication of disease from one person to another by direct contact. 2. an infectious disease.

**containment** a term used in communicable disease control, meaning prevention of spread of disease from a focus of infection. *C. isolation* a patient suspected of having or suffering from a communicable disease is separated from others to prevent the spread of the infection.

**content analysis** a research technique for the objective, systematic and quantitative description of communications and documentary evidence.

**continent** 1. able to control urination and defaecation. 2. exercising self-restraint, especially abstaining from sexual activity.

**continuing care** ongoing care of the physically, mentally and emotionally handicapped, and those suffering from chronic incapacitating illness.

**continuing education** further study and learning after the attainment of basic qualifications. This is vital for all professional practitioners so that they may keep up to date within their field and is accomplished in the form of organized study days or courses, or by individual reading and study. The Nursing and Midwifery Council regulations require nurses, midwives and health visitors to undertake periodic updating and refreshment in order to provide research-based care to their patients and clients. The Health Professions Council (UK) requires all its registered health care

professionals to regularly update their practice. See Appendix 5.

**continuity of care** the concept of a health care provider (general practitioner, health visitor or midwife, etc.) being continually involved with a patient throughout treatment over a period which may extend over years.

**continuous ambulatory peritoneal dialysis** abbreviated CAPD. Treatment in which the patient is ambulant while receiving peritoneal dialysis.

**continuous positive airway pressure** abbreviated CPAP. Medical gas is delivered to the patient at positive pressure to hold open alveoli that would normally close at the end of expiration, thereby increasing oxygenation and reducing the work of breathing.

**contraception** the prevention of conception and pregnancy.

**contraceptive** an agent used to prevent conception, e.g. condom, cap that occludes the cervix, spermicidal pessary or cream, intrauterine device (IUD) and oral contraceptives (hormone pills).

**contract** 1. to make or to enter into an agreement with a person, authority or company to deliver services or goods. 2. in health care, an agreement, usually between two people with differing interests and concerns. *See* CARE CONTRACT.

**contraction** a shortening or drawing together, especially applied to muscle action. *Uterine c's* those occurring during labour.

**contracture** fibrosis causing permanent contraction. *Dupuytren's c.* contraction of the palmar fascia causing permanent bending and fixation of one or more fingers. *Volkmann's ischaemic c.* contraction resulting from impairment of the blood supply. May occur in upper or lower limbs.

**contraindication** any condition that makes a particular line of treatment impracticable or undesirable.

**contralateral** occurring on the opposite side.

**contrast medium** a substance used in radiography to make visible or more visible certain organs.

**contrecoup** [Fr.] an injury occurring on the opposite side or at a distance from the site of the blow, e.g. brain damage on the opposite side of the skull to the blow.

**control** 1. restraint or command of objects or events. 2. a standard for testing where the procedure is identical in all respects to the experiment but the factor being studied is absent. *Birth c.* contraception. *C. group* a group of subjects who in the course of an experimental research project do not experience the factor under consideration. This enables the researcher to make a comparison with the effects produced on the experimental group. *C. of infection* standards and procedures within the health care service that provide guidelines for all staff to control infection within hospitals and in all health care facilities, e.g. ambulances and the community. *See* INFECTION.

**Control of Substances Hazardous to Health** abbreviated COSHH. Regulations that require the assessment of risk and action to be taken regarding the use of substances that may be hazardous to health within the workplace. An example within the health care environment is glutaraldehyde.

**controlled drugs** preparations subject to the Misuse of Drugs Act (1971), Misuse of Drugs (Notification of and Supply to Addicts) Regulations (1973) and the Misuse of Drugs Regulations (1985), which regulate the prescribing and dispensing of psychoactive drugs, including narcotics, hallucinogens, depressants and stimulants.

**controlled trial** a research method in which one group of subjects in a trial are not exposed to the experimental treatment or investigation, in an attempt to decrease the possibility of error and increase the possibility that the findings of the study are an accurate reflection of reality.

**controls assurance** a process designed to enable NHS organizations to do their reasonable best to protect patients, staff, the public and other stakeholders against all kinds of risk. The controls assurance set standards covering: buildings, land, plant and non-medical equipment; catering and food hygiene; decontamination of reusable medical devices; emergency planning; environmental management; financial management; fire safety; fleet and transport management; governance; health and safety management; human resources; infection control; information management and technology; management of purchasing and supply; medical devices management; medicines management; professional and product liability; records management; risk management; security management; waste management.

**contusion** a bruise.

**convalescence** period of recovery following illness, injury or operation.

**convection** a method of transmission of heat by the circulation of warmed molecules of a liquid or a gas.

**conversion** 1. the act of changing into something of different form or properties. 2. the transformation of emotions into physical manifestations. 3. manipulative correction of malposition of a fetal part during labour.

**convolution** a fold or coil, e.g. of the cerebrum or renal tubules.

**convulsion** involuntary contractions of the voluntary muscles. Convulsive seizures are symptomatic of some neurological disorders; they are not in themselves a disease entity. *Clonic c.* a convulsion marked by alternative contracting and relaxing of the muscles. *Febrile c.* a convulsion occurring almost exclusively in children aged 6 months to 5 years of age, and associated with a fever of 40°C or higher. *Tonic c.* prolonged contraction of the muscles, as a result of an epileptic discharge. *See* EPILEPSY.

**Coombs' test** *R.R.A. Coombs, British immunologist, b. 1921 d. 2006.* A test to detect the presence of any antibody on the surface of the red blood cell. Used to detect rhesus incompatibility in maternal or fetal blood and in the diagnosis of haemolytic anaemia.

**coordination** harmony of movement between several muscles or groups of muscle so that complicated manoeuvres can be made.

**coping** the process of contending with life difficulties in an effort to overcome or work through them. *C. mechanisms* conscious or unconscious strategies or mechanisms that a person uses to cope with stress or anxiety.

**copper** *symbol* Cu. A metallic element, traces of which are present in all human tissues.

**coprolalia** the uncontrolled use of obscene speech.

**coprolith** a mass of hard faeces in the rectum or colon.

**copulation** coitus. Sexual intercourse between male and female.

**cord** a long cylindrical flexible structure. *Spermatic c.* that which suspends the testicle in the scrotum, and contains the spermatic artery and vein and vas deferens. *Spinal c.* the part of the central nervous system enclosed in the spinal column. *Umbilical c.* the connection between the fetus and the placenta, through which the fetus receives nourishment. *Vocal c's* folds of mucous membrane in the larynx, which vibrate to produce the voice.

**corn** a local hardening and thickening of the skin from pressure or friction, occurring usually on the feet.

**cornea** the transparent portion of the anterior surface of the eyeball continuous with the sclerotic coat.

**corneal** pertaining to the cornea. *C. graft* a means of restoring sight by grafting healthy transparent cornea from a donor in place of diseased tissue. Keratoplasty.

**corneoscleral** relating to both the cornea and sclera. *C. junction* the point where the edge of the cornea joins the sclera. The limbus.

**cornu** a horn. *C. of the uterus* one of the two horn-shaped projections where the uterine tubes join the uterus at the upper pole on either side.

**coronal** relating to the crown of the head. *C. suture* the junction of the frontal and parietal bones.

**coronary** encircling. Crown-like. *C. arteries* the vessels that supply the heart. *C. artery bypass* an operation carried out to bypass a coronary artery narrowed by atheroma using a graft from a healthy saphenous vein or an internal mammary artery. *C. care unit* a ward or unit within a hospital which provides for the monitoring and intensive care by a specialist team of staff of patients who have suffered an attack of coronary thrombosis and of those who are in the immediate postoperative period following heart surgery. *C. circulation* see CIRCULATION. *C. thrombosis* see THROMBOSIS.

**coronaviruses** members of a family (Coronaviridae) of large, enveloped, positive-stranded RNA viruses. Human coronaviruses (HCoVs) are a major cause of mild respiratory illnesses, e.g. the common cold (coryza), but they can occasionally cause serious infections of the lower respiratory tract in children and adults and necrotizing enterocolitis in newborns. In early 2003, a new variant of coronavirus (SARS CoV) was discovered, which causes the severe acute respiratory syndrome (SARS).

**coroner** a public official (e.g. a barrister, solicitor or doctor) who holds inquests concerning sudden, violent or suspicious deaths.

**corporate governance** the accountability of an NHS Trust to meet standards in corporate management working within the need to meet statutory financial objectives and targets.

**corporate working** system in which managers and practitioners work within a team ethos, sharing a designated workload and providing an equity of service.

**corpse** a dead body; cadaver.

**corpulent** obese.

**corpus** a body. *C. albicans* the scar tissue on the surface of the ovary which replaces the corpus luteum before the recommencement of menstruation. *C. callosum* the mass of white matter that joins the two cerebral hemispheres together. *C. cavernosum* either of the two columns of the erectile tissue forming the body of the clitoris or the penis. *C. luteum* the yellow body left on the surface of the ovary and formed from the remains of the Graafian follicle after the discharge of the ovum. If it retrogresses, menstruation occurs, but it persists for several months if pregnancy supervenes. *C. striatum* a mass of grey and white matter in the base of each cerebral hemisphere.

**corpuscle** a small protoplasmic body or cell, as of blood or connective tissue.

**corrosive** a substance that erodes and destroys.

**cortex** [L.] an outer layer, as the bark of the trunk or root of a tree, or the outer layer of an organ or other structure, as distinguished from its inner substance. *Adrenal c.* the tissue surrounding the medulla or core of the adrenal gland. *Cerebral c.* the grey matter covering the two cerebral hemispheres. *Renal c.* the outer covering of the kidney.

**corticospinal** relating to the cerebral cortex and the spinal cord. *C. tract* the pyramidal tract. The nerve fibres making up the main pathway for rapid voluntary movement.

**corticosteroid** any of the hormones produced by the adrenal cortex or their synthetic substitutes. Glucocorticoids are responsible for carbohydrate, fat and protein metabolism. They have powerful anti-inflammatory properties. Mineralocorticoids, e.g. aldosterone, are responsible for salt and water regulation.

**corticotrophin** Adrenocorticotrophic hormone (ACTH).

**cortisol** the naturally occurring hormone of the adrenal cortex. Hydrocortisone.

**cortisone** a naturally occurring corticosteroid. Inactive in humans until converted into cortisol.

*Corynebacterium* a genus of slender, rod-shaped, Gram-positive and non-motile bacteria. *C. diphtheriae* Klebs–Löffler bacillus, the causative agent of diphtheria.

**coryza** acute infection of the upper respiratory tract, characterized by perfuse discharge from nasal mucous membranes, sneezing and watering of the eyes. The medical name for the common cold.

**cosmetic** 1. improving something outwardly. 2. relating to treatment intended to improve a person's appearance. *C. dentistry* treatment to improve the appearance of the teeth or to prevent further damage to teeth or gums, e.g. the whitening of teeth or fitting a crown to a damaged tooth.

*C. surgery* an operation to improve a person's appearance, e.g. mammoplasty to reduce or enhance the breasts or the removal of skin blemishes or excess body fat and tissue.

**cost effectiveness** a concept which relates cost to the effectiveness of a service and thus provides value for money, e.g. screening programmes to detect cervical cancer, rate of detection, and cost of the service and of treatment.

**costal** relating to the ribs. *C. cartilages* those that connect the ribs to the sternum directly or indirectly.

**cot death** *see* SUDDEN INFANT DEATH SYNDROME.

**cotyledon** A cup-shaped depression. Applied to the subdivisions of the placenta.

**cough** voluntary or reflex explosive expulsion of air from the lungs. Its purpose is usually to expel a foreign body or accumulations of mucus. *Dry c.* one where no expectoration occurs. *Wet c.* one where expectoration of mucus or foreign body occurs. *Whooping c.* infectious disease caused by *Bordetella pertussis*.

**Council for the Regulation of Healthcare Professionals** works with health professional regulatory bodies, such as the General Medical Council and the Nursing and Midwifery Council to build and manage a strong system of self-regulation which puts patients' interests first. *See* Appendix 5.

**counselling** a process of consultation and discussion in which one individual (the counsellor) listens actively and offers guidance to another who is experiencing difficulties (the client). The counsellor does not direct or make decisions for the client. The general aim is to solve problems and increase awareness. The emphasis is on clients finding their own solutions. *Disaster c.* specialized counselling offered to victims of a major disaster, e.g. an aircraft crash or terrorist attack, or a natural event, e.g. an earthquake. The survivors of such disasters often experience psychological problems and post-traumatic stress disorder resulting in ill health.

**counterextension** 1. the holding back of the upper fragment of a fractured bone while the lower is pulled into position. 2. the raising of the foot of the bed in such a way that the weight of the body counteracts the pull of the extension apparatus on the lower part of the limb. Used especially for fracture of the femur.

**counterirritant** a substance that produces mild inflammation of the skin when applied to it, but relieves pain and congestion.

**countertraction** the reduction of fractures by traction from two opposing directions at once.

**coupling** in cardiology, the frequent occurrence of a normal heart beat followed by an extraventricular one. May be found as a result of digitalis overdose.

**couvade** the experiencing of the symptoms of pregnancy and childbirth by the father. This psychosomatic phenomenon is common in many societies.

**coxa** the hip joint. *C. valga* a deformity of the hip in which there is an increase in the angle between the neck and the shaft of the femur. *C. vara* a deformity in which the angle between the neck and the shaft of the femur is smaller than normal.

**Coxiella** a genus of microorganisms of the order Rickettsiales. *C. burnetii* the causative agent of Q fever.

**Coxsackie virus** one of a group of enteroviruses that may give rise to a variety of illnesses, including meningitis, pleurodynia, acute myocarditis and acute pericarditis.

**crab louse** *Phthirus pubis. See* LOUSE.

**crack** purified form of cocaine, produced by a technique known as 'freebasing'. *See* COCAINE.

**cradle** 1. a frame placed over the body or limb of a bed patient for protecting injured parts and preventing them from coming into contact with the bedclothes. 2. an infant's bed with protective sides and, in the past, often on rockers. 3. to support, hold, comfort in the arms. *C. cap* an oily crust sometimes seen on the scalp of infants; also called milk crust (crusta lactea). Caused by excessive secretion of the sebaceous glands in the scalp.

**cramp** a painful spasmodic muscular contraction which may result from fatigue. *Occupational c.* occurs in miners and stokers; it is associated with intense heat and dehydration.

**cranial** relating to the cranium. *C. nerves* the 12 pairs of nerves arising directly from the brain.

**craniopharyngioma** a cerebral tumour arising in the craniopharyngeal pouch just above the sella turcica.

**craniosacral therapy** a form of osteopathic treatment in which very gentle manipulation of the cranium attempts to release tensions within the skull which are thought to be the cause of various problems. The therapy has been successfully used to treat babies fractious after difficult forceps or vacuum extraction deliveries, colic and hyperactivity in older infants.

**craniostenosis** premature closure of the suture lines of the skull in an infant. Surgery may be required to relieve raised intracranial pressure.

**craniosynostosis** premature closure of the cranial sutures.

**craniotabes** a patchy thinning of the bones of the vault of the skull of an infant; associated with rickets.

**craniotomy** a surgical opening of the skull made to relieve pressure, arrest haemorrhage or remove a tumour.

**cranium** 1. the skull. 2. the bony cavity that contains the brain.

**creatine** a nitrogenous compound present in muscle. It is also found in the urine in conditions in which muscle is rapidly broken down, e.g. acute fevers and starvation. *C. phosphate* a high-energy phosphate store in muscle.

**creatinine** a normal constituent of urine; a product of protein metabolism.

**creatinuria** increased concentration of creatine in the urine.

**credentialing** review and examination of the credentials of health care professionals to ensure that they have training and the qualifications necessary to deliver care and support to the patient and the family.

**credibility** a criteria for evaluating the data of qualitative research study, referring to the amount of confidence in the truth of the given information.

**Credit Accumulation and Transfer System** abbreviated CATS. Learning points or credits awarded by an academic institution to an individual for prior academic learning and/or evidence of the acquisition of professional expertise demonstrated, e.g. through a personal professional profile, contributing towards academic or professional awards. Originally developed to provide flexibility between academic institutions. *See* APEL and APL.

**crepitation** the grating sound caused by friction of the two ends of a fractured bone.

**crepitus** 1. the discharge of flatus from the bowels. 2. crepitation. 3. a crepitant râle.

**cretinism** congenital hypothyroidism. A condition caused by lack of thyroid secretion, characterized by arrested physical and mental development, dull facial expression with dry skin and lack of coordination.

**Creutzfeldt–Jakob disease** *H.G. Creutzfeldt, German physician, 1885– 1964; A. Jakob, German physician, 1884–1931.* Abbreviated CJD or known as prion disease. A rapidly progressive disease of the nervous system affecting middle-aged and elderly people. The disease has been reported in younger people treated in the past with human pituitary extract for short stature – now no longer used. It is a spongiform encephalopathy similar to the bovine form (BSE) popularly known as 'mad cow disease', and is known to be associated with an abnormal protein or prion. There is no effective treatment. A new variant of CJD has been reported in young adults with a shorter incubation period and usually fatal.

**cribriform** perforated like a sieve. *C. plate* part of the ethmoid bone. *See* ETHMOID.

**cricoid** ring-shaped. *C. cartilage* the ring-shaped cartilage at the lower end of the larynx.

**cri du chat syndrome** a hereditary congenital syndrome characterized by hypertelorism, microcephaly, severe mental deficiency, and a plaintive cat-like cry; due to the deletion of part of the short arm of chromosome 5.

**crisis** 1. a decisive point in acute disease; the turning point towards either recovery or death. *See* LYSIS. 2. a sudden paroxysmal intensification of symptoms in the course of a disease. 3. life crisis; a period of disorganization that occurs when a person meets an obstacle to an important life goal, such as the sudden death of a family member or a difficult family conflict. *Addisonian c., adrenal c.* symptoms of fatigue, nausea and vomiting and collapse accompanying an acute attack of adrenal failure. *Blast c.* a sudden, severe change in the course of chronic myelocytic leukaemia. The clinical picture resembles that

seen in acute myelogenous leukaemia, with an increase in the proportion of myeloblasts. *C. intervention* counselling or psychotherapy for patients in a life crisis that is directed at supporting the patient through the crisis and helping the patient to cope with the stressful event that precipitated it. *Identity c.* usually occurring during adolescence, manifested by a loss of the sense of the sameness and historical continuity of one's self, and inability to accept the role the individual perceives as being expected by society.

**criterion** the basis on which a decision is made, e.g. for drug dosage, treatment plans, research trials, etc.

**critical** 1. arising from a crisis. 2. implying serious risk or uncertainty as to outcome. *C. appraisal* an analysis of a research project using the parameters of research design, methodology, examination of results and relevance, e.g. relating the findings to practice. *C. care unit* a unit within a hospital that supports and treats patients with critical disorders or diseases of the vital physiological systems. May also be called intensive care unit. *See* INTENSIVE CARE UNIT. *C. path analysis* in project management tasks and actions are considered to be independent with the timing of each action crucial to the overall completion of the project. In clinical care a schedule or pathway of procedures, diagnostic tests for a patient is designed to ensure an efficient coordinated programme of treatment. *C. thinking* a purposeful, goal-directed approach based upon scientific evidence rather than assumption or memorization. Critical thinking is an organized approach to discovery that involves reflection and assimilation of information which enables the nurse or health care provider to arrive at an informed decision or to make a judgement.

**Crohn's disease** *B.B. Crohn, American physician, 1884–1983.* Regional ileitis. *See* ILEITIS.

**Crosby capsule** *W.H. Crosby, American physician, b. 1914.* A capsule attached to the end of a flexible tube which is swallowed by the patient. When the capsule reaches the small intestine, as seen on radiological examination, a biopsy of the intestinal mucosa may be taken.

**cross-matching** a test of the compatibility of donor blood to be transfused to a patient. *See* BLOOD GROUPS.

**cross-sectional study** a non-experimental research design that looks at data at one point in time, that is, in the immediate present.

**croup** a condition resulting from acute obstruction of the larynx caused by allergy, foreign body, infection or new growth; occurs chiefly in infants and children. There is spasmodic dyspnoea, a harsh cough and stridor.

**crown** that part of the tooth that appears above the gum.

**crowning** the stage in labour when the top of the infant's head becomes visible at the vulva.

**cruciate** resembling a cross. *C. ligament see* LIGAMENT.

**'crush' syndrome** the oedema, oliguria and other symptoms of acute renal failure that follow crushing of a part, especially a large muscle mass, causing the release of myoglobin into the circulation.

**crutch** appliance usually in the form of a light, tubular metal rod with hand grips and plastic loops for the forearms, to aid walking when the patient must not weight-bear (as in fractures of lower limbs) or when a lower limb is missing.

**cryaesthesia** abnormal sensitivity to cold.

**cryoanalgesia** the relief of pain by application of cold by cryoprobe to peripheral nerves.

**cryobank** a facility for freezing and preserving semen at low temperatures (usually –196.5 °C) for future use.

**cryoprecipitate** any precipitate that results from cooling. Of particular therapeutic value is the cryoprecipitate from fresh plasma, which is rich in factor VIII and is used to treat haemophilia.

**cryopreservation** maintenance of the viability of excised tissue or organs by storing at very low temperatures.

**cryosurgery** the use of extreme cold to destroy tissue.

**cryotherapy** therapeutic use of cold.

**cryptococcosis** infection caused by the yeast *Cryptococcus neoformans*, having a predilection for the brain and meninges but also invading the skin, lungs and other parts. It particularly affects persons immunocompromised by disease or therapy.

**cryptorchidism** failure of the testicles to descend into the scrotum; cryptorchism.

**CT** *see* COMPUTED AXIAL TOMOGRAPHY.

**Cu** symbol for *copper.*

**cubitus** 1. the forearm. 2. the elbow. *C. valgus* deformity of the elbow where the palm of the hand is abducted and thus faces outwards. *C. varus* deformity where there is adduction of the forearm.

**cue** something that gives a hint or idea of something else. A cue is a verbal or non-verbal signal in communication from one person to another. It is a remembered item which connects with further information or meaning.

**cued recall** retrieval of information from memory with the help of cues, perhaps using the first letter of the word or name to be remembered.

**culdoscope** an endoscope used in culdoscopy.

**culdoscopy** direct visual examination of the female viscera through an endoscope introduced into the pelvic cavity through the posterior vaginal fornix.

**culture** 1. the propagation of microorganisms or of living tissue cells in special media conducive to their growth. 2. a collective noun for the symbolic and acquired aspects of human society, including convention, custom and language. 3. a singular noun for the customs and features of an ethnic (racial, religious or social) group. *C. shock* A feeling of alienation often accompanied by feelings of depression and rejection that results from a radical change in culture, e.g. as a result of migration from one country to another.

**cumulative** adding to. *C. action* occurs when a dose of a slowly released drug is given too frequently and accumulates in the system leading to the development of toxic symptoms, e.g. with some barbiturates and digoxin.

**Cumulative Index to Nursing and Allied Health Literature.** abbreviated CINAHL. A computerized database of English language nursing and allied health literature published bi-monthly with a yearly cumulation.

**cupping** 1. the formation of a cup-shaped depression with the hand: (a) to produce a skin erythema, thereby improving local circulation; and (b) to loosen excessive secretions from air passages, and perhaps induce coughing. 2. the use of a cupping glass to stimulate skin blood flow.

**curative** anything which promotes healing by overcoming disease.

**curettage** [Fr.] the scraping of a surface with a curette for therapeutic purposes or to obtain biopsy material.

**curette** a spoon-shaped instrument used for the removal of unhealthy tissues by scraping.

**Curling's ulcer** an ulcer of the duodenum after severe burns of the body.

**cursor** on the computer screen, a blinking character that indicates where the next character will appear.

**curvature** the curving of a line, whether normal or abnormal. *Spinal c.* abnormal deviation of the vertebral column.

**Cushing's disease** *H.W. Cushing, American surgeon, 1869–1939.* A condition of oversecretion by the adrenal cortex due to an adenoma of the pituitary gland. Symptoms include obesity, abnormal distribution of hair and atrophy of the genital organs. A rare disorder.

**cushingoid** referring to symptoms resembling those of Cushing's disease, e.g. the side-effects of steroid therapy.

**cusp** a pointed or rounded projection, such as on the crown of a tooth, or a segment of a cardiac valve.

**cutaneous** pertaining to the skin.

**cutdown** an incision into a vein with insertion of a catheter for intravenous infusion. It is performed when an infusion cannot be started by venepuncture. Also used with hyperalimentation therapy when concentrated solutions need to be given into the superior vena cava.

**cuticle** the narrow band of epidermis extending from the nail wall on to the nail surface; also called eponychium.

**cyanocobalamin** vitamin $B_{12}$ (antianaemic factor) found in liver, eggs and fish. It combines with the intrinsic factor secreted in gastric juice for absorption and is essential for erythrocyte maturation. Administered by injection in the treatment of pernicious anaemia.

**cyanosis** a bluish appearance of the skin and mucous membranes, caused by imperfect oxygenation of the blood. It indicates circulatory failure and is common in respiratory diseases. It is also seen in 'blue babies'.

**cyberstalking** internet harassment, for example, repetitive unsolicited and/or inappropriate e-mails, including hate, obscene or threatening mail or live chat harassment. *See* BULLYING and HARASSMENT.

**cyclamate** a non-nutritive sweetener.

**cycle** a series of recurring events. *Cardiac c.* the events occurring between one heart beat and the next. *Menstrual c.* the changes that occur each month in the female reproductive system.

**cyclic** pertaining to or occurring in a cycle.

**cyclodialysis** an operation used in glaucoma to improve drainage from the anterior chamber of the eye at the corneoscleral junction.

**cyclodiathermy** a treatment for glaucoma without penetration of the eyeball. Diathermy is applied to the sclera to cause fibrosis around the ciliary body, so allowing the aqueous humour to drain.

**cycloplegia** paralysis of the ciliary muscle of the eye.

**cyclopropane** a gas used for general anaesthesia. It is not irritating to the respiratory tract but is highly inflammable and is therefore potentially dangerous.

**cyclothymia** the alteration of mood seen in manic-depressive psychosis.

**cyesis** pregnancy. *Pseudo-c.* signs and symptoms suggestive of pregnancy arising when no fertilization has taken place. 'Phantom pregnancy'.

**cyst** 1. a cavity or sac with epithelium, containing liquid or semi-solid matter. 2. a stage in the life cycle of certain protozoan parasites when they acquire tough protective coats. *Branchial c.* one formed in the neck from non-closure of the branchial cleft during development. *Chocolate c.* an ovarian cyst occurring in endometriosis. *Daughter c.* a small cyst that develops from a large one. *Dermoid c.* a congenital type containing skin, hair, teeth, etc. It is due to abnormal development of embryonic tissue. *Hydatid c.* the larval cyst stage of the tapeworm, usually found in the liver. *Meibomian c.* a swelling of a Meibomian gland caused by obstruction of its duct. *Multilocular c.* a cyst that is divided into compartments or locules. *Ovarian c.* a cyst of the ovary, usually non-malignant, but sometimes becoming very large and requiring surgical removal. *Retention c.* any cyst caused by blockage of a duct. *Sebaceous c.* a retention cyst caused by the blockage of a duct from a sebaceous gland so that the sebum collects. *Sublingual c.* a ranula. *Thyroglossal c.* one in the thyroglossal tract near the hyoid bone at the base of the tongue.

**cystathioninuria** a hereditary disorder of cystathionine metabolism, marked by increased concentrations in the urine. May be associated with learning difficulties.

**cysteine** a sulphur-containing amino acid formed by the ingestion of dietary proteins.

**cystic fibrosis** generalized hereditary disorder associated with accumulation of excessively thick and tenacious mucus and abnormal secretion of sweat and saliva; called also cystic fibrosis of the pancreas, and mucoviscidosis. The disease is inherited as a recessive trait and occurs particularly frequently in caucasians. The severity of cystic fibrosis varies widely. Although it is congenital, it may not manifest itself during the early weeks of life, or it may cause intestinal obstruction and perforation in the newborn. The chief cause of complications in cystic fibrosis is the extremely thick mucus predisposing to repeated infection. Therapeutic management is long term, initially centring on replacement of pancreatic enzymes, physiotherapy and antibiotics. Even with prompt and vigorous treatment permanent lung damage may occur. Lung or heart/lung transplants offer good results with an improved quality of life. Gene therapy is currently being developed. In those families with a history of the condition amniocentesis can be used to determine if a fetus is affected. Newborn babies can be screened for the disease as early diagnosis and treatment improves the long-term prognosis and life expectancy.

**cysticercosis** a disease caused by infestation with the cysticercus of *Taenia solium* (pork tapeworm). Has been eliminated from pig herds in the UK but may be found in immigrants or travellers who have ingested infected pork.

**cysticercus** the cystic or larval form of the tapeworm.

**cystine** an amino acid closely related to cysteine. Sometimes excreted in urine in the form of minute crystals (cystinuria).

**cystinosis** an inherited metabolic disorder in which cystine is deposited in the tissues.

**cystitis** inflammation of the urinary bladder.

**cystocele** a prolapse of the bladder into the vagina.

**cystodiathermy** the application of a high-frequency electric current to the bladder mucosa, usually for the removal of papillomas.

**cystography** radiography of the urinary bladder after the introduction of a radio-opaque contrast medium. *Micturating c.* radio-

graphic examination during the act of passing urine.

**cystoscope** an endoscope for examining the interior of the urinary bladder.

**cystostomy** the operation of making a temporary or permanent opening into the urinary bladder.

**cystotomy** incision of the urinary bladder for removal of calculi, etc. *Suprapubic c.* incision above the pubes.

**cystourethrography** radiography of the urinary bladder and urethra.

**cytogenetics** the study of cells during mitosis in order to examine the chromosomes and the relationship between chromosome abnormality and disease.

**cytology** the microscopic study of the form and functions of the cells of the body. *Exfoliative c.* an aid to the early diagnosis of malignant disease. Secretions or surface cells are examined for premalignant changes.

**cytolysin** a substance that causes cytolysis. *See* BACTERIOLYSIN and HAEMOLYSIN.

**cytolysis** the destruction of cells.

**cytomegalic inclusion disease** an infection due to cytomegalovirus. In the congenital form, there is hepatosplenomegaly with cirrhosis, and microcephaly with learning difficulties and developmental delay. Acquired disease may cause a clinical state similar to infectious mononucleosis.

**cytomegalovirus** a virus belonging to the herpes simplex group.

**cytopheresis** a technique to remove specific cellular components from the blood, e.g. white blood cells or platelets needed to treat a patient, or to remove abnormal constituents.

**cytoplasm** the protoplasmic part of the cell surrounding the nucleus.

**cytosine** one of the pyrimidine bases found in DEOXYRIBONUCLEIC

ACID (DNA). *C. arabinoside* an anti-metabolite used in the treatment of acute leukaemia. Cytarabine.

**cytotoxic** 1. having a deleterious effect upon cells. 2. an agent or drug that damages or destroys cells. Used to treat various forms of cancer and sometimes other conditions. The handling of cytotoxic drugs is a health and safety issue. Health care workers should follow local guidelines and policies regarding administration of these drugs.

**cytotoxin** a toxin having a specific toxic action on cells of special organs.

**D** symbol for *dioptre*.

**dacryolith** a calculus in a lacrimal duct.

**dacryoma** a benign tumour which arises from the lacrimal epithelium.

**dactyl** a finger or toe; a digit.

**dactylology** communication between individuals by signs made with the fingers and hands. Finger spelling.

**daltonism** colour-blindness; inability to distinguish red from green. *See* COLOUR VISION.

**dander** small scales from the hair or feathers of animals, which may be a cause of allergy in sensitive persons.

**dandruff** white scales shed from the scalp. If moist from serous exudate they have a greasy appearance.

**Darwinism** *C.R. Darwin, British naturalist, 1809–1882.* The theory of the evolution of species through natural selection.

**data** *sing.* datum; a collection of facts. *Continuous d.* data that have a continuous set of values, e.g. for variables such as height, weight and antibody titres in response to vaccination. *D. processing* the storage and analysis of data to produce statistical tabulations, often by computer. *D. Protection Act 1984* in the UK this Act gives people the right to know what information is held about them on computers, including health-related data. The Data Protection (Subject Access Modification) (Health) Order 1987 restricted access to health information which might cause serious physical or mental harm to an individual or reveal the identity of another person. The Act did not apply to manual records and in 1990 the Access to Health Records Act was passed to enable people to have access to any computerized or manual health-related records made after 1991. Patients and clients must apply to gain access to their records; the same exceptions to access as in the original Data Protection Act remain. *D. set* a collection of information made on a group and related to certain variables that are being investigated. *Discrete d.* data with a single value or characteristic, e.g. colour of hair.

**database** information collected, stored, reviewed and updated, and used for evaluation and audit; e.g. a patient care database, in which information is gained at the initial interview, forms part of the care plan and is available for the evaluation of treatment and care.

**day care** a specialized service for pre-school children, either as a substitute for or as an extension to family life. A similar service may be provided for the elderly needing care and support and to provide respite for family carers. *See* DAY CENTRE.

**day centre** a specialized facility that offers care, treatment and a respite service for the elderly or the mentally ill.

**day nursery** a centre for the care, during the daytime, of children up to the age of 5 years. Provided by the social services department or by voluntary agencies. Priority is given to children from 'at risk' families and to those with a handicap.

**day patient care** a service provided either in a specialized ward or in a hospital ward for treatment/ investigation/minor surgery. The patient is admitted and discharged on the same day.

**dB** symbol for *decibel*.

**D & C** dilatation and curettage.

**DDT** dichlorodiphenyltrichloroethane; dicophane. A powerful insecticide.

**deafness** complete or partial loss of hearing affecting about 10% of adults and more than 50% of people over 65 years of age. May be called 'hearing impairment' or 'hearing loss' especially when there is only partial loss of hearing. *Conduction or middle ear d.* deafness due to the sound wave failing to reach the cochlea. *Perceptive or nerve d.* deafness due to damage to the cochlea or auditory nerve.

**deamination** a process of hydrolysis, taking place in the liver, by which amino acids are broken down and urea is formed.

**death** the cessation of all physical and chemical processes that occur in all living organisms or their cellular components. *Brain d.* the diagnosis of clinical brain stem death is governed, in the UK, by a set of guidelines ratified by the Medical Royal Colleges and their Faculties. The testing procedure is performed twice by two different doctors to eliminate any observer error. The time interval between testing is not specified. For medicolegal purposes the time of death is that time when the second examination has been completed and the patient fulfils the criteria. Performance of the brain death criteria under the appropriate circumstances allows the patient a dignified death, reduces the agony of the relatives and releases scarce resources for other seriously ill patients. *Clinical d.* the absence of heart beat (no pulse can be felt) and cessation of breathing. *Cot d.* sudden infant death syndrome (SIDS). *D. certificate* certificate issued by the registrar for deaths after receipt of a preliminary certificate completed and signed by an attending doctor, indicating the date and probable cause of death. Only after issue of this certificate, indicating that the death has been registered, can the body be disposed of. *D. instinct* a concept, introduced by Freud, proposing a self-destructive drive opposed by the sexual instinct, which perpetually seeks a renewal of life. May manifest itself as a repetition compulsion with the aim of annihilating oneself. *D. rate* the number of deaths per stated number of persons (100 or 10 000 or 100 000) in a certain region in a certain period.

**debility** a condition of weakness and lack of physical tone.

**débridement** [Fr.] the removal of foreign substances and injured tissues from a traumatic wound. Part of the immediate treatment to promote healing.

**decalcification** removal of calcium salts, e.g. from bone in disorders of calcium metabolism.

**decapsulation** removal of a fibrous capsule.

**decay** 1. the gradual decomposition of dead organic matter. 2. the process or stage of ageing of living matter. *Radioactive d.* the process by which an unstable atom loses energy by the emission of gamma rays or beta or alpha particles and is transformed to a more stable atom.

**decerebrate** a person with brain damage whose neurological reactions are severely impaired and in whom cerebral functioning has ceased.

**decibel** *symbol* dB. A unit of intensity of sound, used particularly in estimating the degree of deafness.

**decidua** the thickened lining of the uterus for the reception of the fertilized ovum to protect the developing embryo. It is shed when pregnancy terminates.

**deciduous** falling off; subject to being shed, as deciduous teeth.

**decision-making** the act or process of choosing a preferred option or course of action from a set of alternatives. It forms the basis of almost all deliberate or voluntary behaviour. *D. rule* a formal or mechanical formula or principle for deciding on a course of action in response to input data. *D. theory* any theory that attempts to explain how decisions are reached. Most often applied to theories that use mathematical models to analyse human decision processes.

**decompensation** failure to compensate. In particular, failure of the heart to overcome disability or increased work load.

**decompression** return to normal environmental pressure after exposure to greatly increased pressure. *Cerebral d.* removal of a flap of the skull and incision of the dura mater for the purpose of relieving intracranial pressure. *D. sickness* a disorder characterized by joint pains, respiratory manifestations, skin lesions and neurological signs, occurring as a result of rapid reduction in air pressure. Aviators flying at high altitudes and persons breathing compressed air in caissons and diving apparatus are particularly susceptible to this disorder.

**decongestant** 1. reducing congestion or swelling. 2. an agent that reduces congestion or swelling, usually of the nasal membranes. Decongestants may be inhaled, taken as spray or nose drops, or used orally in liquid or tablet form.

**decontamination** the freeing of a person or an object of some contaminating substance such as nerve gas, infective or radioactive material, etc. Decontamination involves a combination of processes including cleaning, disinfection and sterilization. It is an important issue for public health in the prevention of hospital-acquired infection and minimizing the risk of the iatrogenic transmission of other organisms.

**decortication** an operation to strip the outer layer of an organ, e.g. the removal of the thickened pleura in the treatment of chronic empyema.

**decrudescence** diminution or abatement of the intensity of symptoms.

**decubitus** the position assumed when lying down. *D. ulcer* an ulcer due to interference with the local circulation from prolonged or severe pressure on the surface body tissue resulting in tissue anoxia and cell death; also called bedsore and pressure sore.

**decussation** a crossing, particularly of nerve fibres. A chiasma. *Pyramidal d.* the crossing of the pyramidal nerve fibres in the medulla oblongata.

**deep vein thrombosis** abbreviated DVT. A blood clot that forms in the deep veins of the lower leg; may be symptomless or can cause redness, swelling, tenderness and fever. The clot can travel and lodge in the heart or lungs (*see* PULMONARY EMBOLISM) resulting in sudden death. The so-called 'economy class syndrome' is the formation of a clot occurring during or just after a long journey in an aeroplane, where the lack of space restricts leg movements. Other risk factors are lower oxygen pressure and dehydration. The condition has also been reported in travellers after a long road journey without any breaks.

**defecation** elimination of waste and undigested food, as faeces, from the rectum.

**defence** behaviour directed to protection of the individual from injury. *Character d.* any character trait, e.g. a mannerism, attitude or affectation, which serves as a DEFENCE MECHANISM. *D. mechanism* in psychology, an unconscious mental process or coping pattern that lessens the anxiety associated with a situation or internal conflict and protects the person from mental discomfort. *Insanity d.* a legal concept that a person cannot be convicted of a crime if lacking criminal responsibility by reason of insanity at the time of commission of the crime.

**defervescence** the period of abatement of fever.

**defibrillation** the restoration of normal rhythm to the heart in ventricular or atrial fibrillation.

**defibrillator** an instrument by which normal rhythm is restored in ventricular or atrial fibrillation by the application of a high-voltage electric current.

**defibrination** the removal of fibrin from blood plasma to prevent clotting. Used in the preparation of sera.

**deficiency disease** a condition caused by dietary or metabolic deficiency, including all diseases due to an insufficient supply of essential nutrients.

**deficit** a deficiency or variation from that which is considered to be normal.

**defined daily dose** abbreviated DDD. The measure of the standard daily therapeutic dose of a drug. The World Health Organization publishes a list of DDs for various drugs.

**deglutition** the act of swallowing.

**dehiscence** splitting open, as of a wound.

**dehydration** excessive loss of fluid from the body by persistent vomiting, diarrhoea or sweating, or from the lack of intake. Severe dehydration is a serious condition that may lead to fatal shock, acidosis and the accumulation of waste products in the body, as in uraemia.

**déjà vu** [Fr.] an illusion that a new experience is a repetition of a previous experience.

**deleterious** harmful; injurious.

**delinquency** criminal or antisocial conduct, especially among juveniles.

**delirium** mental excitement. A common condition in high fever. It is marked by an irregular expenditure of nervous energy, incoherent talk and delusions. *D. tremens* an acute psychosis common in chronic alcoholism, usually following abstinence from alcohol. *Traumatic d.* a possible occurrence after severe head injury. There is much confusion and disorientation.

**delivery** childbirth; parturition.

**Delphi technique** a long-range forecasting technique in which qualitative value judgements are made about information. Judgements are made independently and anonymously, pooled and summarized before being fed back to the contributors for another round of opinion.

**deltoid** triangular. *D. muscle* the triangular muscle of the shoulder arising from the clavicle and scapula, with insertion into the humerus.

**delusion** a false idea or belief held by a person which cannot be corrected by reasoning. *D. of grandeur* erroneous belief in one's own greatness, wealth or position. *D. of* *persecution* paranoia. *Depressive d.* a sense of unworthiness or sinfulness.

**dementia** a global and progressive deterioration of the mental faculties which is irreversible and affects memory, intellect, judgement, personality and emotional control. Dementia is the result of an organic brain syndrome. The term 'brain failure' is gradually replacing the term dementia because it conveys the fact that brain failure is a process, while the term dementia simply suggests a state associated with nihilistic views on treatment and prognosis. *Arteriosclerotic d.* dementia due to insufficient blood supply to the brain caused by arteriosclerosis. *Presenile d.* occurring in people aged 40–60 years, it is due to early degeneration of small cerebral blood vessels. *See* ALZHEIMER'S DISEASE and CREUTZFELDT–JAKOB DISEASE. *Senile d.* dementia occurring in old age as the result of cerebral atrophy.

**demography** the statistical science dealing with populations, including matters of health, disease, births and mortality.

**De Morgan's spots** red or purplish raised spots in the skin consisting of a cluster of minute blood vessels. Found in middle-aged and older people, the spots becoming more numerous with increasing age. The spots may bleed if damaged but treatment is unnecessary. *See* AGE SPOTS.

**demulcent** an agent that soothes and allays irritation, especially of sensitive mucous membranes.

**demyelination** destruction of the medullary or myelin sheaths of nerve fibres, such as occurs in disseminated sclerosis. Demyelinization.

**dendrite** one of the protoplasmic filaments of a nerve cell by which impulses are transmitted from one neurone to another. Dendron.

**dendritic** 1. appertaining to a dendrite. 2. branching. *D. ulcer* a corneal ulcer caused by the virus of herpes simplex. It has a branching appearance as it spreads.

**denervation** severance or removal of the nerve supply to a part.

**dengue** a painful viral disease that occurs in tropical countries throughout the world. The virus that causes the disease, one of four types of a group B arbovirus, is carried by *Aedes* mosquitoes. Because of the intense pain in the bones, dengue is also known as breakbone fever.

**denial** a defence mechanism in which the existence of intolerable actions, ideas, changed circumstances, terminal illness, etc. is unconsciously denied.

**dental** relating to dentistry or to the teeth. *D. hygienist* a trained person carrying out dental procedures such as scaling of the teeth and oral cleansing, who works with the assistance of the dentist in providing preventative dental health care. *D. nurse* one who assists the dentist at the patient's side in passing instruments, preparing materials and generally assisting the dentist. *D. plaque* a sticky rough coating on the teeth formed by food deposits, bacteria and dead cells. It is the chief cause of dental decay if not removed regularly by good dental hygiene. *D. pulp* the tissue within the dental cavity containing nerves, blood and lymph vessels.

**dentine** the calcified substance forming the bulk of a tooth between the pulp and the enamel.

**dentist** a person qualified to practise dentistry.

**dentistry** the art and science of the teeth, mouth and associated tissues and bone. Dentistry also includes preventative dental care and education concerned with preserving the health of the teeth and gums as well as the supplying and fitting of dentures.

**dentition** the process of teething. *Primary d.* cutting of the temporary or milk teeth, beginning at the age of 6 or 7 months and continuing until the end of the second year. A full set consists of eight incisors, four canines and eight premolars: 20 teeth in all. Deciduous dentition. *Secondary d.* cutting of the permanent teeth, beginning in the sixth or seventh year, and being complete by the 12th to 15th year except for the posterior molars or 'wisdom teeth'. There are 32 permanent teeth: eight incisors, four canines, eight premolars or bicuspids and 12 molars. Permanent dentition. (*See* Figure.)

**dentoid** tooth-like.

**denture** a removable dental prosthesis, which may contain one artificial tooth, or several or a full set of teeth.

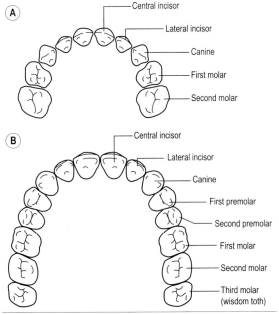

(A) PRIMARY DENTITION, (B) SECONDARY DENTITION

**deodorant** a substance that destroys or masks an offensive odour. *See* ANTIPERSPIRANT.

**deoxygenated** deprived of oxygen. *D. blood* that which has lost much of its oxygen in the tissues and is returning to the lungs for a fresh supply.

**deoxyribonucleic acid** abbreviated DNA. A nucleic acid of complex molecular structure occurring in cell nuclei as the basic structure of the genes. It is responsible for the control and passing on of hereditary characteristics, and is present in all body cells of every species, including unicellular organisms and DNA viruses. DNA molecules are linear polymers of small molecules called *nucleotides*, each of which consists of one molecule of the five-carbon sugar *deoxyribose*, bonded to a *phosphate* group and to one of the four *bases* twisted into a double helix. The four bases are two purines, *adenine* (A) and *guanine* (G), and two pyrimidines, *cytosine* (C) and *thymine* (T). The structure of DNA was described in 1953 by J.D. Watson and F.H.C. Crick.

**Department of Health** is the national headquarters of the NHS negotiating funding with the Treasury and the allocation of resources to the health services. It also provides strategic leadership to the NHS and social care organizations in England, setting their overall direction and establishing and monitoring standards. Its key objectives are: improving and maintaining health, with special attention to the needs of disadvantaged groups and areas; enhancing the quality and safety of all services for patients and users, providing faster access, more choice and control; improving the capacity, capability and efficiency of the health and social care systems; ensuring service modernization, IT investment and that new staff contracts provide value for money and quality; becoming more capable and efficient, with a reputation as an organization that is good to do business with and a good place to work. Similar government departments perform this role in Scotland, Wales and Northern Ireland. The Department makes reciprocal arrangements with other countries and represents the UK on health matters in the European Union, the World Health Organization and other international bodies.

**dependence** 1. addiction; the total psychophysical state of a user in which the usual or increasing quantities of the drug or activity (e.g. internet surfing or gambling) are required to prevent the onset of withdrawal symptoms. 2. the level of reliance a person has on others for carrying out the activities of daily living. *See* DEPENDENCY STUDIES.

**dependency** a state of relying on another for love, affection, mothering, comfort, security, food, warmth, shelter, protection, etc. *D. studies* the measurement of the need for care required by a patient based on the ability to carry out self-care. The main self-care activities measured are the ability to feed, the ability to carry out toilet requirements and the level of mobility, including dressing. *D. studies for staffing ratios* studies undertaken to determine the number of staff required to provide the appropriate skills to care for specific types and numbers of patient.

**depersonalization** a condition in which patients feel that their personality has changed so that they become onlookers observing their own actions. It may occur in almost any mental illness.

**depilatory** an agent that will remove hair.

**depressant** a drug that reduces functional activity of an organ. Anaesthetics, sedatives, tranquillizers and alcohol are depressants.

**depression** 1. a hollow or depressed area. 2. a lowering or decrease of functional activity. 3. in psychiatry, a morbid sadness, dejection or melancholy, distinguished from grief, which is realistic and proportionate to a personal loss. Profound depression may be symptomatic of a psychiatric disorder or it may constitute the principal manifestation of a neurosis or psychosis. *Endogenous d.* occurs sometimes without obvious cause in the course of manic-depressive psychosis. The mood change is associated with slowing of thought and action and feelings of guilt. *Recessive d.* occurs as a result of some event, such as illness, loss of money, bereavement.

**deprivation** loss or absence of parts, organs, powers, or things that are needed. *D. indices* national census variables that are used to assess the economic and social wellbeing within the population from whom the census has been taken. These include numbers of single parent families and overcrowded households, and levels of unemployment. *Emotional d.* deprivation of adequate and appropriate interpersonal or environmental experience in the early developmental years. *Maternal d. syndrome* a group of symptoms, including stunted emotional and physical development, arising in infants who have been deprived of care and love provided by a mother or mothering figure. Deprivation of maternal care during the first 3 years of life is thought to be particularly critical as this is the optimal period for the forming of social attachments. *Sensory d.* deprivation of the usual external stimuli and the opportunity for perception.

**Derbyshire neck** *see* GOITRE.

**derealization** loss of a sense of reality. Surroundings and events seem unreal.

**dereism** mental activity in which fantasy runs unhampered by logic and experience; describes autistic thinking.

**dermatitis** inflammation of the skin. *Contact d.* that arising from touching a substance to which the person is sensitive. *Ex-foliative d.* widespread scaling and itching of the skin, sometimes occurring as a reaction to treatment with certain drugs. *Industrial d., occupational d.* that caused by exposure to chemicals or other substances met with at work. *Sensitization d.* dermatitis due to an allergic reaction. *See* LATEX. *Traumatic d.* inflammation due to injury. *Varicose d.* dermatitis, usually of the lower portion of the leg, due to varicosities of the smaller veins. *X-ray d.* radiodermatitis; inflammatory reaction of the skin to radiotherapy.

**dermatoglyphics** study of the patterns of ridges of the skin of the fingers, palms, toes and soles. Of interest in anthropology and law enforcement as a means of establishing identity, and in medicine, both clinically and as a genetic indicator, particularly of chromosomal abnormalities.

**dermatographia** a condition in which urticarial weals occur on the skin if a blunt instrument or fingernail is lightly drawn over it.

**dermatology** the science of skin diseases.

**dermatomycosis** a fungal infection of the skin.

**dermatomyositis** a collagen disease producing inflammation of the voluntary muscles with necrosis of the muscle fibres.

**dermatosis** any skin disease, especially one which does not produce inflammation.

**dermis** the skin, especially the layer under the epidermis.

**dermoid** pertaining to the skin. *D. cyst see* CYST.

**desensitization** 1. the prevention or reduction of immediate hypersensitivity reactions by the administration of graded doses of allergen; hyposensitization. *See also* IMMUNOTHERAPY. 2. in behaviour therapy, the treatment of phobias and related disorders by intentionally exposing the patient, in imagination or in real life, to emotionally distressing stimuli.

**designer drugs** used to describe synthetic variants (drug analogues) of potent controlled drugs (including narcotics and stimulants) that are not themselves controlled. These substances currently circumvent existing drug legislation and many are relatively easy to synthesize from common industrial chemicals. Many designer drugs are extremely potent (some synthetic analogues of heroin are 1000 times as potent as heroin) and are consequently extremely dangerous.

**desquamation** peeling of the superficial layer of the skin, either in flakes or in powdery form.

**detachment** separation from or state of indifference to other people, one's surroundings or environment leading to social isolation. *D. of the retina* separation of the retina, or a part of it, from the choroid.

**detergent** a cleansing and antiseptic agent.

**deterioration** progressive impairment of function; worsening.

**detoxification** the process of neutralizing toxic substances; detoxication.

**detritus** debris; material that has disintegrated.

**detrusor** muscle of the urinary bladder, the action of which is to push down.

**detumescence** 1. the subsidence of a swelling. 2. the subsidence of an erect penis after ejaculation.

**development** the process of growth and differentiation. *Cognitive d.* the development of intelligence, conscious thought and problem-solving ability that begins in infancy. *Psychosexual d.* the development of the psychological aspects of sexuality from birth to maturity. *Psychosocial d.* the development of the personality, including the acquisition of social attitudes and skills, from infancy through to maturity.

**developmental** pertaining to development. *D. anomaly* absence, deformity or excess of body parts as the result of faulty development of the embryo. *D. milestones* significant behaviours used to mark the process of development (*see* AGE (ACHIEVEMENT)). Walking is a developmental milestone in locomotor development, conversation in cognitive development.

**deviance** generally any pattern of behaviour that violates prevailing standards of morality or behaviour within a society. The term is usually qualified to indicate the specific form of deviance.

**deviation** variation from the normal. In ophthalmology, lack of coordination of the two eyes. *Standard d.* in research, a method of grouping data on either side of the mean of a graph. In a normal distribution curve 68% of the data will be covered in one standard deviation above and below the mean. A measure of dispersion of scores around the mean value. It is the square root of variance.

**devitalized** devoid of vitality or life; dead.

**dextran** a plasma volume expander, formed of large glucose molecules, which, given intravenously, increases the osmotic pressure of blood.

**dextrocardia** location of the heart in the right side of the thorax.

**dextrose** an old chemical name for D-glucose, an important energy

| DIFFERENCES BETWEEN HYPERGLYCAEMIA AND HYPOGLYCAEMIA IN PATIENTS WITH DIABETES MELLITUS | | |
| --- | --- | --- |
| | Hyperglycaemia | Hypoglycaemia |
| Onset | Slow (2–3 days) | Rapid |
| History | Has not taken insulin/acute infection | Has taken insulin 1/2–4 hours previously, but has not eaten/has eaten but had unusual burst of energy |
| Patient reactions | Thirst Nausea Abdominal pain Constipation Vomiting | Irrational Bad-tempered Disorientated (may be mistaken for drunk) |
| Leads to | Ketoacidosis Drowsiness BP↓ Pulse weak and rapid Skin dry Tongue dry | Respirations normal No drowsiness BP normal Skin moist Tongue moist |
| Leads to | Coma | Coma |
| Needs | Insulin Restoration of fluid balance | Glucose |
| Avoided by | Recognition of early symptoms and taking appropriate action | |

source for all tissues and the sole energy source for the brain. Commonly used in intravenous infusion solutions and may also be used orally in rehydration solutions to replace electrolytes and fluids.

**diabetes** a disease characterized by excessive excretion of urine. *See* POLYURIA. Diabetes is a group of metabolic diseases characterized by hyperglycaemia resulting from defects in insulin secretion, insulin action or both. The chronic hyperglycaemia of diabetes is associated with long-term damage, dysfunction and failure of various organs, primarily the eyes, kidneys, nerves, heart and blood vessels (*see* Table). Because insulin is involved in the metabolism of carbohydrates, proteins and fats, diabetes is not limited to a disturbance of glucose metabolism. Polyuria, thirst and debility are common presenting symptoms. Type 1 diabetes (insulin-dependent diabetes mellitus, abbreviated IDDM) results from the destruction of the insulin-producing cells of the pancreas occurring most commonly in childhood or adolescence. Type 2 diabetes (non-insulin-dependent diabetes mellitus, abbreviated NIDDM) or maturity onset diabetes is due to an insufficiency of insulin and usually occurs after the age of 40 years. The goal of treatment is to maintain blood glucose and lipid levels within normal limits and to prevent complications. There is strong support for the concept that microvascular sequelae of the disease from retinopathy and kidney degeneration can be minimized by optimal control. In both types of diabetes treatment is aimed at promoting a sense of health and well-being. The diet must be controlled with adequate carbohydrate and the body weight stabilized. Type 1 is always treated with insulin. Type 2 may be treated with weight reduction, diet or the use of medications which promote the production of insulin by the pancreas. Insulin therapy has now been standardized at 100 units/ml. Combinations of soluble insulin with slower-acting preparations can be tailored to suit the individual patient in the 24-hour control of blood sugar. All insulin has to be given by injection, usually subcutaneously. Pump systems to deliver continuous insulin under the skin are available. Ongoing problems occur with reduced sensitivity of nerve endings causing patients to acquire infections, often on the feet, which may progress from a simple puncture-type wound to ulcer, which maybe become gangrenous leading to amputation if left untreated. *Brittle d.* the patient's diabetic condition is difficult to control because of alternating episodes of hyperglycaemia and hypoglycaemia. Also known as *unstable d.* or *labile d.* *D. insipidus* a disease resulting from insufficient secretion of the antidiuretic hormone by the pituitary gland, and which may follow injury, infection or be congenital, resulting in dehydration of the patient, polydipsia and polyuria.

**diabetic** 1. relating to diabetes. 2. a person affected with diabetes. *D. gangrene, d. retinopathy* and *d. cataract* are complications of diabetes mellitus.

**diabetogenic** inducing diabetes. Some drugs or physical conditions, such as pregnancy or disease, precipitate the symptoms of diabetes in those prone to the disease.

**diagnosis** determination of the nature of a disease. *Clinical d.* diagnosis made by the study of signs and symptoms. *Differential d.* the recognition of one disease among several presenting similar symptoms. *Nursing d.* a statement of a health care problem or the potential for one in the health status of the patient/client for which the nurse is competent to intervene and treat.

**dialysate** the material passing through the membrane in dialysis.

**dialyser** 1. the membrane used in dialysis. 2. the machine or 'artificial kidney' used to remove waste products from the blood in cases of renal failure.

**dialysis** the process by which crystalline substances will pass through a semipermeable membrane, whereas colloids will not. In medicine this process is usually employed to remove waste and toxic products from the blood in cases of renal insufficiency. *Peritoneal d.* use of the peritoneum as the semipermeable membrane. A dialysing solution is infused into the abdominal cavity and allowed to run out again when sufficient time has elapsed for dialysis to have occurred. Waste products are thus removed from the blood. *See* HAEMODIALYSIS.

**diameter** a straight line passing through the centre of a circle to opposite points on the circumference. *Cranial d's* measurement of the fetal head at term. If these are abnormal, delivery through the vagina may not be possible. *Pelvic d's* measurements between the bones and joints of the pelvis made in women to determine whether the fetus can pass through at the time of childbirth.

**diapedesis** the passage of white blood cells through the walls of blood capillaries.

**diaphoresis** perspiration; particularly profuse perspiration.

**diaphragm** 1. the muscular dome-shaped partition separating the thorax from the abdomen. 2. any separating membrane or structure. *Contraceptive d.* a rubber cap which occludes the cervix.

**diaphragmatic hernia** a protrusion of any or part of an abdominal organ through the diaphragm into the thoracic cavity.

**diaphysis** the shaft of a long bone.

**diarrhoea** rapid movement of faecal matter through the intestine resulting in poor absorption of water, nutritive elements and electrolytes, and producing abnormally frequent evacuation of watery stools. Commonest causes of diarrhoea include bacterial or viral infections, food sensitivity, laxatives, the use of antibiotics and dietary indiscretion. Other causes include irritable bowel syndrome and systemic diseases. Diarrhoea that persists for more than a week or is recurring requires medical investigation. *Tropical d.* sprue.

**diarthrosis** a freely moving articulation, e.g. ball and socket joint. A synovial joint.

**diastase** 1. an enzyme, formed during germination of seeds, which converts starch into sugar. 2. one of the pancreatic enzymes excreted in the urine and the saliva. *D. test* used to estimate the excretion of diastase and therefore pancreatic function.

**diastole** the phase of the cardiac cycle in which the heart relaxes between contractions; specifically, the period when the two ventricles are dilated by the blood flowing into them. *See* SYSTOLE.

**diathermy** production of heat in a body tissue by a high frequency electric current. *Medical d.* sufficient heat is used to warm the tissues but not to harm them. *Short-wave d.* used in physiotherapy to relieve pain or treat infection. *Surgical d.* of very high frequency; used to coagulate blood vessels or to dissect tissues. Cautery.

**DIC** disseminated intravascular coagulation.

**dichromatic** pertaining to colour-blindness when there is ability to see only two of the three primary colours. *See* COLOUR VISION DEFICIENCY.

**dicrotic** having a double beat. *D. pulse* a small wave of distension following the normal pulse beat; occurring at the closure of the aortic valve.

**diet** the customary amount and kind of food and drink taken by a person from day to day; more narrowly, a diet planned to meet the specific requirements of the individual, including or excluding certain foods. *Bland d.* one that is free from any irritating or stimulating foods. *Elimination d.* one for diagnosis of food allergy, based on omission of foods that might cause symptoms in the patient. *High-calorie d.* one that furnishes more calories than needed to maintain weight, often more than 3500–4000 kcal/day. *High-fibre d.* one relatively high in dietary fibre, which decreases bowel transit time and relieves constipation. *High-protein d.* one containing large amounts of protein, consisting largely of meats, fish, milk, peas, beans and nuts. *Hospital d.* a routine diet plan, provided in a hospital, that includes general, soft and liquid diets and modifications of them to suit the needs of specific patients. *Liquid d.* a diet limited to liquids or to foods that can be changed to a liquid state (*see also* LIQUID (DIET)). *Low-calorie d.* one containing fewer calories than needed to maintain weight, e.g. less than 1200 kcal/day for an adult. *Low-fat d.* one containing limited amounts of fat. *Low-residue d.* one with a minimum of cellulose and fibre and restriction of the connective tissue found in certain cuts of meat. It is prescribed for irritations of the intestinal tract, after surgery of the large intestine, in partial intestinal obstruction, or when limited bowel movements are desirable, as in colostomy patients. Also called low-fibre diet. *See* Appendix 1.

**dietary chaos syndrome** a syndrome in which patients believe that control of eating and body weight is the key to good health and wellbeing. A variety of approaches are used which include bulimia and periods of abstinence from food, the use of laxatives or prolonged chewing of food without swallowing. *See* ANOREXIA and BULIMIA.

**dietetics** the science of applying the principles of nutrition to the feeding of individuals or groups.

**dietary reference values** abbreviated (DRV). Published values (Department of Health) for most nutrients that provide for a range of intakes related to age, gender and activity required to maintain health. These values are based upon the nutritional requirements of groups living in the UK.

**dietitian** a person qualified in the principles of nutrition who applies these to the feeding of an individual or of a group of people usually in a shared setting, e.g. hospitals or residential homes. May also work in the commercial sector, e.g. food processing industry.

**differential** making a difference. *D. blood count see* BLOOD COUNT. *D. diagnosis see* DIAGNOSIS.

**differentiation** 1. the distinguishing of one thing from another. 2. the act or process of acquiring completely individual characteristics, such as occurs in the progressive diversification of cells and tissues in the embryo. 3. increase in morphological or chemical heterogeneity.

**diffuse** scattered or widespread, as opposed to localized.

**diffusion** 1. the spontaneous mixing of molecules of liquid or gas so that they become equally distributed. 2. dialysis.

**digestion** 1. the act or process of converting food into chemical substances that can be absorbed into the blood and utilized by the body tissues. 2. the subjection of a substance to prolonged heat and moisture, so as to disintegrate and soften it.

**digit** a finger or toe. *Accessory d., supernumerary d.* an additional digit occurring as a congenital abnormality.

**digital** coded in simple 'on–off' binary units such as in computers and the traditional view of the activation of neurones.

**digitalization** the administration of digitalis (digoxin) in a dosage schedule designed to produce and then maintain optimal therapeutic concentrations of its cardiotonic glycosides.

**dilatation, dilation** 1. the act of dilating or stretching. 2. the condition, as of an orifice or tubular structure, of being dilated or stretched beyond normal dimensions. *D. and curettage* expanding of the opening of the womb to permit scraping of the walls of the uterus; also called D & C. *D. of the heart* compensatory enlargement of the cavities of the heart, with thinning of the walls.

**dilator** 1. an instrument used for enlarging an opening or cavity such as the rectum, the male urethra or the cervix. 2. a muscle that causes dilatation. 3. a drug that causes dilatation, e.g. a vasodilator. *Hegar's d's* a series of dilators used to widen the cervical canal before examination of the uterus under anaesthesia.

**diluent** 1. diluting. 2. an agent that dilutes or renders less potent or irritant.

**dimethylphthalate** abbreviated DIMP. An insect repellent in liquid or ointment form that is effective for several hours when applied to the skin.

**Diogenes syndrome** gross self-neglect, usually in the elderly.

**dioptre** *symbol* D. The unit used in measuring lenses for spectacles. When parallel light enters a lens and focuses at a distance of 1 m, the refractive power of the lens is 1 dioptre, and from this basis abnormalities are calculated.

**diphtheria** a severe, notifiable, infectious disease, characterized by the formation of membranes in the throat and nose and rarely the skin (in an open wound), and toxic neurological and cardiac complications; caused by the bacillus *Corynebacterium diphtheriae*. Primary prevention is provided by the routine immunization of the population in childhood. *See* Appendix 9.

**Diphyllobothrium** a genus of large tapeworm. *D. latum*, the broad or fish tapeworm, grows up to 10 m long and may infest humans after the consumption of uncooked infected fish.

**diplegia** paralysis of similar parts on either side of the body.

**diplococcus** 1. any of the spherical, lanceolate or coffee-bean-shaped bacteria occurring, usually in pairs, as a result of incomplete separation after cell division in a single plane. 2. any organism of the genus *Diplococcus.*

**diploid** 1. having a pair of each chromosome characteristic of a species (in humans, 46). 2. a diploid individual or cell.

**diplopia** double vision, in which two images are seen in place of one, due to lack of coordination of the external muscles of the eye.

**dipsomania** a morbid craving for alcohol, which occurs in bouts.

**disability** any restriction or lack (resulting from an impairment) of ability to perform an activity in the manner or within the range considered normal for a human being. *Developmental d.* a substantial handicap of indefinite duration, with onset before the age of 18 years, and attributable to mental handicap, autism, cerebral palsy, epilepsy or other neuropathy.

**disaccharide** any of a class of sugars, e.g. maltose, lactose, each molecule of which yields two molecules of monosaccharide on hydrolysis. *D. intolerance* the inability to absorb disaccharides owing to an enzyme deficiency.

**disarticulation** separation; amputation at a joint.

**disc** a flattened circular structure. *Intervertebral d.* a fibrocartilaginous pad that separates the bodies of two adjacent vertebrae. *Optic d.* a white spot in the retina. It is the point of entrance of the optic nerve.

**discharge** 1. a setting free, or liberation; used for the release of a patient from hospital, clinic or therapy programme. 2. material or force set free. 3. an excretion or substance evacuated. *D. planning* the preparation required for the return of a patient to the usual life at home.

**disciplinary action** taken by the employer when a member of staff has made a serious error, acted unprofessionally or negligently or has been convicted of a criminal offence. The process follows an agreed disciplinary procedure. *See* Appendix 4.

**disclosing solution** a topically applied preparation which reveals plaque and other deposits on teeth by staining them. May also be given as a tablet to be chewed; any plaque is stained red.

**discography** radiographic examination after the injection of a radioopaque contrast medium into an intervertebral disc.

**discrete** composed of separate parts that do not become blended.

**disease** a definite pathological process having a characteristic set of signs and symptoms. It may affect the whole body or any of its parts, and its aetiology, pathology and prognosis may be known or unknown. (For separate diseases, *see* under individual names.)

**disengagement** the process by which an individual, usually elderly, gradually withdraws from the community and obligations towards friends and family. The effect of this process is to lead to social isolation for the individual with alienation and disregard from the community. This situation may be compounded by physiological deficits and handicaps. *D. theory* a psychosocial theory of ageing by which both society and the individual prepare for death by gradually reducing all social contacts which leads to poor relationships, egocentricity and sometimes depression.

**disimpaction** reduction of an impacted fracture.

**disinfect** to destroy microorganisms, but not usually bacterial spores, reducing the number of microorganisms to a level that is not harmful to health.

**disinfectant** an agent that destroys infection-producing organisms. Heat and certain other physical agents, such as steam, can be disinfectants, but in common usage the term is reserved for chemical substances such as glutaraldehyde, sodium hypochlorite or phenol. Disinfectants are usually applied to inanimate objects because they are too strong to be used on living tissues. Chemical disinfectants are not always effective against spore-forming bacteria.

**disinfection** the act of disinfecting. *Terminal d.* disinfection of a sick room and its contents at the termination of a disease.

**disinfestation** destruction of insects, rodents or pests present on the person or the clothes or in the surroundings, and which may transmit disease.

**dislocation** the displacement of a bone from its natural position upon another at a joint; luxation.

**dismemberment** the amputation of a limb or a part of it.

**disorientation** loss of proper bearings, or a state of mental confusion as to time, place or identity.

**displacement** removal to an abnormal location or position. *D. activity* in psychology, unconscious transference of an emotion from its original object on to a more acceptable substitute.

**disposition** a tendency to suffer from certain diseases.

**dissect** 1. to cut carefully in the study of anatomy. 2. during operation, to separate according to natural lines of structure.

**disseminated** widely scattered or dispersed. *D. intravascular coagulation* abbreviated DIC. Widespread formation of thromboses in the capillaries. It is a secondary complication of a diverse group of obstetric, surgical, haemolytic and neoplastic disorders.

**dissociation** separation. 1. the splitting up of molecules of matter into their component parts, e.g. by heat or electrolysis. 2. in psychology, the separation of ideas, emotions or experiences from the rest of the mind, giving rise to a lack of unity of which the patient is not aware.

**distal** situated away from the centre of the body or point of origin. The opposite of proximal.

**distension** enlargement. *Abdominal d.* enlargement of the abdomen by gas in the intestines or fluid in the abdominal cavity.

**distractibility** inability to focus or maintain attention on any one subject.

**distraction** 1. any thing that diverts a person's attention. 2. the location of joint surfaces caused by extension but without injury to the parts involved. 3. mental or emotional distress, anguish or confusion. *D. therapy* diverting the focus of attention on one activity, object or person to another. Used in the management of pain.

**distribution** 1. the sharing out or spreading of an agent, object or population within an area. 2. in research, the relative frequencies with which scores of a different size occur.

**diuresis** increased excretion of urine.

**diuretic** 1. increasing urine excretion or the amount of urine. 2. an agent that promotes urine secretion. Diuretic drugs are classified by chemical structure and pharmacological action, although a diuretic medication may contain drugs from one or more groups, e.g. loop diuretics, osmotic and potassium-sparing diuretics, and thiazides.

**diurnal** occurring during daytime or period of light. Diurnal animals have one period of rest and one of activity in 24 hours.

**diverticulitis** inflammation of a diverticulum. It is most common in the colon; lower abdominal pain with colic and constipation may occur. Intestinal obstruction or abscesses may develop as a result of collections of bacteria and irritating agents being trapped in small blind pouches formed in the intestinal walls.

**diverticulosis** the presence of diverticula in the colon without inflammation.

**diverticulum** a pouch or pocket in the lining of a hollow organ, as in the bladder, oesophagus or large intestine. *Meckel's d.* a small sac occurring in the ileum as a congenital abnormality.

**dizygotic, dizygous** pertaining to or derived from two separate zygotes (fertilized ova); said of non-identical twins.

**dizziness** a feeling of unsteadiness or haziness, accompanied by anxiety. *See* VERTIGO.

**DNA** deoxyribonucleic acid.

**Döderlein's bacillus** *A.S.G. Döderlein, German obstetrician and gynaecologist, 1860–1941.* A lactobacillus occurring normally in vaginal secretions.

**dolor** [L.] *pain.*

**domiciliary** within or at home. *D. midwifery* attending a woman in childbirth in her own home, by a midwife and possibly by the family doctor. *D. services* health and social services provided within the home of the patient/client.

**dominant** in genetics, capable of expression when carried by only one of a pair of homologous chromosomes. The opposite to recessive. *D. gene* one which will produce its characteristics when it is present in either a hetero- or homozygous state, i.e. it may be inherited from one parent only.

**'domino' booking** a plan of maternity care whereby a mother has her baby in a consultant unit, cared for by the community midwife. They return home following delivery after an interval of at least 6h. The name derives from *dom*iciliary midwife *in* and *out*.

**donor** 1. an organism that supplies living tissue to be used in another body, such as a person who furnishes blood for transfusion or an organ for transplantation. 2. a substance or compound that contributes part of itself to another substance (acceptor). **Universal d.** a person with group O blood; such blood is sometimes used in emergency transfusion. Transfusion of blood cells rather than whole blood is preferred.

**dopa** the precursor of dopamine and an intermediate product in the biosynthesis of noradrenaline and adrenaline. It is used in parkinson's disease and manganese poisoning. Also called L-dopa and levodopa.

**dopamine** a substance allied to noradrenaline and used in the treatment of cardiogenic shock. Also occurs naturally in the adrenal medulla and the brain, where it functions as a transmitter of nervous impulses.

**Doppler effect** the relationship of the apparent frequency of waves, as of sound, light and radio waves, to the relative motion of the source of the waves and the observer.

**Doppler ultrasound flowmeter** a device for measuring blood flow that transmits sound at a frequency of several megahertz along a blood vessel. Rapid pulsatile changes in flow as well as steady flow can be recorded; hence, it is helpful in assessing intermittent claudication, thrombus obstruction of deep veins and other abnormalities of blood flow in the major arteries and veins.

**dorsal** relating to the back or posterior part of an organ.

**dorsiflexion** bending backwards of the fingers or toes, i.e. upwards.

**dorsum** 1. the back. 2. the upper or posterior surface.

**dose** the amount of a drug taken at a given time or the amount of irradiation given to a patient. Drug dose can be expressed in terms of the weight of its active ingredient, the volume of liquid to be drunk or its effects upon the body tissues. The amount of radiation absorbed during a session of radiotheraphy is expressed in units called millisieverts. *See* RADIATION.

**dosimeter** one of various devices used to detect and measure exposure to radiation; worn by personnel near to radiation sources.

**double-blind trial** a test for the real effect of a new drug or treatment in clinical practice. Neither the patient nor the staff administering the treatment knows which of two apparently identical treatments is the new one being tested.

**douche** a stream of fluid directed to flush out a cavity of the body.

**doula** from the Greek word meaning 'woman who serves other women'; in maternity terms, one who provides emotional and practical support throughout pregnancy and labour. Doula birth companion training has been available in the UK since 1990, with a reduced training for qualified midwives, through the Birth and Bonding International organization.

**download** an action that is designed to transfer a file from a computer on the internet to your own computer by means of a modem and telephone line.

**Down's syndrome** *J.L.H. Down, British physician, 1828–1896.* A chromosomal abnormality, the commonest type having 47 instead of 46 chromosomes. The extra one is attached to the 21st pair, so that the condition is also called trisomy 21. This condition is associated with increasing maternal age. In the other form of Down's syndrome a translocation occurs, usually between chromosomes 14 and 21, as a structural rearrangement originating in the child, although the parents have normal chromosomes. Alternatively the translocations may occur as a result of a similar translocated chromosome in the parents; this increases the risk of the condition recurring in further pregnancies by 10%. The child exhibits certain features which include slanting eyes with specked iris, broad hands with a single palmar crease, short neck with loose skin and hypotonia. Other abnormalities may also occur, e.g. congenital heart disease. Learning difficulties are also present but the range of ability is wide.

**dracontiasis** a tropical disease caused by infestation with the guinea-worm; acquired by drinking contaminated water.

*Dracunculus* a genus of roundworms; includes the guinea-worm.

**drain** 1. to withdraw liquid generally. 2. any device by which a channel or open area may be established for exit of fluids or purulent material from a cavity, wound or infected area.

**drama-therapy** the therapeutic use of drama, in which clients are encouraged to act out their feelings in order to overcome problems.

**dream** mental activity that occurs during deep (*see* REM) sleep, usually in the form of vivid images, emotions and imagined events. Often rapidly forgotten on waking.

**dreaming** the activity of engaging in fantasies or speculation during quiescent waking periods. Also called daydreaming. Some research suggests that this activity helps to promote positive mental health for the individual concerned.

**dressing** material applied to cover a wound or a diseased surface of the body. *See* WOUND DRESSING.

**drive** in psychology, an urge or motivating force.

**droplet infection** infection due to inhalation of respiratory pathogens suspended in liquid particles exhaled from someone already infected.

**dropsy** an old-fashioned term used to describe excess fluid in the tissues (oedema).

**drug** 1. any medicinal substance. 2. a narcotic. 3. to administer a drug. *D. addiction* a state of periodic or chronic intoxication produced by the repeated consumption of a drug, characterized by: (a) an overwhelming desire or need (compulsion) to continue use of the drug and to obtain it by any means; (b) a tendency to increase the dosage; (c) a psychological and usually a physical dependence on its effects; and (d) a detrimental effect on the individual and on society. *D. idiosyncrasy* an individual response to a drug that is unique to that person and quite different from what is expected. *D. interaction* modification of the potency of one drug by another (or others) taken concurrently or sequentially. Some drug interactions are harmful and some may have therapeutic benefits. Present knowledge of drug interactions is limited. Drugs may also interact with various foods. In general, these interactions fall into three categories: (a) food malabsorption; (b) nutritional status; and (c) alteration of drug response by nutrients. In teaching patients self-care in the taking of prescribed medications, one should explain the need for meticulously following directions related to the intake of food and drink while the medication regimen is being followed. *D. misuse* the use of drugs for purposes other than those for which they are prescribed or recommended. The major groups of drugs and medicines generally considered to be most commonly misused are stimulants ('uppers'), depressants ('downers'), psychedelics and narcotics. **D. tolerance** a progressive reduction in the effect of a drug following repeated use. To achieve the desired effect increasingly larger doses of the medication are needed. **D. trial** the testing undertaken of any new drug before it becomes available for medical use.

**dry socket** infection of the soft tissues of a tooth socket, occurring 2 or 3 days after tooth extraction, often a lower molar. It is a painful condition requiring dental treatment with socket irrigation and local and/or systemic antibiotics.

**DSH** deliberate self-harm. *See* PARASUICIDE.

**Dubowitz score** a method used to assess gestational age in a low-birth-weight infant.

**Duchenne dystrophy** *G.B.A. Duchenne, French neurologist, 1806–1875.* Progressive muscular dystrophy occurring in childhood. *See* DYSTROPHY.

**duct** a tube or channel for the passage of fluid, particularly one conveying the secretion of a gland.

**ductless** without an excretory duct. **D. glands** ENDOCRINE glands.

**ductus** a duct. **D. arteriosus** a passage connecting the pulmonary artery and aorta in intrauterine life, which normally closes at birth. When it remains open it is called persistent ductus arteriosus. *See also* PATENT (DUCTUS ARTERIOSUS).

**dumping** the rapid evacuation of the contents of an organ. **D. syndrome** a feeling of fullness, weakness, sweating and dizziness which may occur after meals following a partial gastrectomy.

**duodenal** pertaining to the duodenum. **D. intubation** the use of a special tube which is passed via the mouth and stomach into the duodenum. Used for withdrawal of duodenal contents for pathological examination. **D. ulcer** a peptic ulcer occurring in the duodenum near the pylorus.

**duodenostomy** the formation of an artificial opening into the duodenum, through the abdominal wall, for purposes of feeding in cases of gastric disease.

**duodenum** the first 20–25 cm of the small intestine, from the pyloric opening of the stomach to the jejunum. The pancreatic and common bile ducts open into it.

**Dupuytren's contraction** or **contracture** *Baron G. Dupuytren, French surgeon, 1777–1835.* Contracture of the palmar fascia, causing permanent bending and fixation of one or more fingers (*see* Figure).

**dura mater** a strong fibrous membrane forming the outer covering of the brain and spinal cord.

**duty of care** a nurse, midwife or medical practitioner has an accepted duty to a patient or client irrespective of any contractual agreement existing between the parties. The law has developed a set of rules on the expected standard of care to assist in determining whether or not a professional has neglected their duty of care, based on the standards prevailing at the time of any case questioning the issue.

**duty of partnership** duty placed on NHS bodies and local government to develop joint local delivery plans involving other parts of the NHS, local voluntary organizations and businesses.

DUPUYTREN'S CONTRACTURE

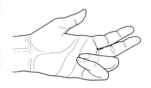

**dwarfism** the state of being short in stature. Arrest of growth and development, e.g. due to renal rickets, cretinism or deficient pituitary function.

**dysarthrosis** a deformed, dislocated or false joint.

**dyschondroplasia** a condition in which cartilage is deposited in the shaft of some bones. The affected bones become shortened and deformed.

**dyscrasia** a morbid condition, usually referring to an imbalance of component elements. *See also* BLOOD DYSCRASIA.

**dysdiadochokinesis** a sign of cerebellar disease in which the ability to perform rapid alternating movements, such as rotating the hands, is lost.

**dysentery** inflammation of the intestine, especially of the colon, with abdominal pain, tenesmus and frequent stools, often containing blood and mucus. The causative agent may be chemical irritants, bacteria, protozoa, viruses or parasitic worms. *Amoebic d.* common in tropical countries; caused by the protozoon *Entamoeba histolytica*. Spread is decreased in places with high standards of hygiene and sanitation. A notifiable disease in the UK. Also called amoebiasis. *Bacillary d.* the most common and acute form of the disease, caused by bacteria of the genus *Shigella*; *S. sonnei* is the most frequent cause in the UK. A notifiable disease. Also called shigellosis.

**dysfunction** impairment of function.

**dysgammaglobulinaemia** an immunological deficiency state marked by selective deficiencies of one or more, but not all, classes of immunoglobulin, resulting in heightened susceptibility to infectious diseases.

**dysgerminoma** a malignant tumour derived from germinal cells that have not been differentiated to either sex, occurring in either the ovary or the testicle.

**dyshidrosis** a disturbance of the sweat mechanism in which an itching vesicular rash may be present.

**dyskinesia** impairment of voluntary movement.

**dyslalia** impairment of speech, caused by a physical disorder.

**dyslexia** difficulty in reading or learning to read; accompanied by difficulty in writing and spelling correctly.

**dysmaturity** the condition of being small or immature for gestational age; said of fetuses that are the product of a pregnancy involving placental insufficiency or dysfunction. Also called small for dates, or light for gestational age.

**dysmenorrhoea** painful menstruation. *Primary (spasmodic) d.* painful menstruation occurring without apparent cause. The onset is usually shortly after puberty and occurs with each subsequent period. May be helped by hormonal therapy. *Secondary (congestive) d.* painful menstruation occurring in a woman who has previously had normal periods for some years. Often due to endometritis. The condition tends to worsen as the local congestion increases.

**dysostosis** abnormal development of bone.

**dyspareunia** painful or difficult coitus in women.

**dyspepsia** indigestion. There may be abdominal discomfort, flatulence, nausea and sometimes vomiting. *Nervous d.* dyspepsia in which anxiety and tension aggravate the symptoms.

**dysphagia** difficulty in swallowing.

**dysphasia** difficulty in speaking as the result of a brain lesion. There is a lack of coordination and an inability to arrange words in their correct order.

**dysplasia** abnormal development of tissue.

**dyspnoea** difficult or laboured breathing. *Expiratory d.* difficulty in expelling air. *Inspiratory d.* difficulty in taking in air.

**dyspraxia** partial loss of ability to perform coordinated movements.

**dysrhythmia** disturbance of a regularly occurring pattern. Often applied to an abnormality of rhythm of the brain waves, as shown in an electroencephalogram.

**dystaxia** difficulty in controlling voluntary movements.

**dystonia** a lack of tonicity in a tissue, often referring to the muscles.

**dystrophia** dystrophy. *D. myotonica* a rare hereditary disease of early adult life in which there is progressive muscle wasting and gonadal atrophy.

**dystrophy** a disorder of an organ or tissue caused by faulty nutrition of the affected part. Dystrophia. *Muscular d.* a group of hereditary diseases in which there is progressive muscular weakness and wasting.

**dysuria** difficult or painful micturition.

**ear** the organ of hearing and of equilibrium (*see* Figure). It consists of three parts: (a) the *external e.*, made up of the expanded portion, or pinna, and the auditory canal, separated from the middle ear by the drum, or tympanum; (b) the *middle e.*, an irregular cavity containing three small bones (incus, malleus and stapes) that link the tympanic membrane to the internal ear; it also communicates with the pharyngotym-panic tube and the mastoid cells; (c) the *internal e.*, which consists of a bony and a membranous labyrinth (the cochlea and semicircular canals).

**eating disorders** a general term for disturbed behaviour involving food, eating and body weight. *See* ANOREXIA, BULIMIA and DIETARY CHAOS SYNDROME.

**EB virus** Epstein–Barr virus.

**EBM** expressed breast milk. *See* EXPRESSION.

THE EAR

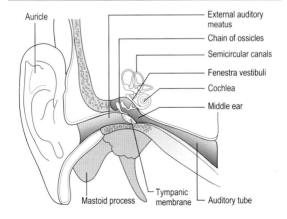

Auricle

External auditory meatus

Chain of ossicles

Semicircular canals

Fenestra vestibuli

Cochlea

Middle ear

Mastoid process

Tympanic membrane

Auditory tube

**Ebola haemorrhagic fever (EHF)** a severe and acute, often fatal, haemorrhagic viral disease, principally seen in central African countries caused by the Ebola virus, of the family *Filoviridae.* The incubation period ranges from 2 to 21 days and the patient presents with abrupt onset of high fever, weakness, muscle pain, headache and sore throat. This is quickly followed by more severe symptoms including vomiting, diarrhoea, rash, decreased kidney and liver functioning, and in some cases, both internal and external bleeding and death in up to 90% of cases. It occurs in sporadic outbreaks, frequently centred in health care settings in developing countries, where social and economic conditions often favour the spread of the virus. Ebola virus can be transmitted in several ways, the most significant being person-to-person through direct contact with body fluids (e.g. blood, semen, vaginal fluid) of an infected person. Transmission may occur through pregnancy and sexual activity. *See* MARBURG VIRUS DISEASE.

**ecchymosis** a bruise; an effusion of blood under the skin causing discoloration.

**eccrine** secreting externally. Applied particularly to the sweat glands, which are generally distributed over the body. *See* APOCRINE.

**ECG** electrocardiogram.

*Echinococcus* a genus of tapeworm. *E. granulosus* infests dogs and may also infect humans. The larval form develops into cysts (hydatids), which occur in the liver, lung, brain and other organs.

**echocardiography** a method of studying the movements of the heart by the use of ultrasound.

**echoencephalography** a method of brain investigation by ultrasonic echoes.

**echolalia** the pathological involuntary repetition of phrases or words spoken by another person.

**echopraxia** the automatic repetition of the movements of others.

**echovirus** a group of viruses (enteroviruses), the name of which was derived from the first letters of the description 'enteric cytopathogenic human orphan'. At the time of the isolation of the viruses the diseases they caused were not known, hence the term 'orphan'. It is now known that these viruses produce many types of human disease, especially aseptic meningitis, diarrhoea and respiratory diseases.

**eclampsia** a severe condition in which convulsions may occur as a result of an acute toxaemia of pregnancy.

**ecmnesia** forgetfulness of recent events with remembrance of more remote ones.

**ecology** the study of the relationship between living organisms and the environment.

**economy** the management of money or domestic affairs. *Token e.* in behaviour therapy, a programme of treatment in which the patient earns tokens, exchangeable for tangible rewards, by engaging in appropriate personal and social behaviour, and loses tokens for antisocial behaviour. *E. class syndrome See* DEEP VEIN THROMBOSIS.

**ecstasy** 1. a feeling of exaltation. It may be accompanied by sensory impairment and lack of activity but with an expression of rapture. 2. an illegal drug. It is widely used as an accompaniment to modern dance music. Has resulted in several fatalities in young people. Causes intense thirst leading to the drinking of large quantities of water resulting in fatal damage of the body's fluid balance, kidney failure and coma. Also known as 'MDMA', 'E' or 'ecky'.

**ECT**  electroconvulsive therapy.

**ectoderm**  the outer germinal layer of the developing embryo from which the skin and nervous system are derived.

**ectogenous**  produced outside an organism. *See* ENDOGENOUS.

**ectoparasite**  a parasite that spends all or part of its life on the external surface of its host, e.g. a louse.

**ectopia**  displacement or abnormal position of any part. *E. cordis* congenital malposition of the heart outside the thoracic cavity. *E. vesicae* a defect of the abdominal wall in which the bladder is exposed.

**ectopic**  1. pertaining to or characterized by ectopy. 2. located away from the normal position. 3. arising or produced at an abnormal site or in a tissue where it is not normally found. *E. pregnancy* pregnancy in which the fertilized ovum becomes implanted outside the uterus instead of in the wall of the uterus. Also called extrauterine pregnancy.

**ectopy**  displacement or malposition, especially if congenital.

**ectropion**  eversion of an eyelid, often due to contraction of the skin or to paralysis. It causes a persistent overflow of tears and hypertrophy of exposed conjunctiva.

**eczema**  1. a general term for any superficial inflammatory process involving primarily the epidermis, marked early by redness, itching, minute papules and vesicles, weeping, oozing and crusting, and later by scaling, lichenification and often pigmentation. 2. atopic dermatitis. Eczema is a common allergic reaction in children but it also occurs in adults. Childhood eczema often begins in infancy, the rash appearing on the face, neck and folds of elbows and knees. It may disappear by itself when an offending food is removed from the diet, or it may

become more extensive and in some instances cover the entire surface of the body. Severe eczema can be complicated by skin infections. The cause of eczema can be either exogenous (due to external or traumatic factors) or endogenous (due to internal or constitutional factors).

**edentulous**  without natural teeth.

**EEG**  electroencephalogram.

**effacement**  taking up of the cervix. The process by which the internal os dilates, so opening out the cervical canal and leaving only a circular orifice, the external os. This process precedes cervical dilatation, particularly in a primigravida, while both occur simultaneously in a multigravida during labour.

**effective**  1. the extent to which something succeeds. 2. a result produced by agent, action or force, e.g. resources to achieve desired outcomes. Cost effectiveness. *E. dose* The amount of a drug given to a patient to achieve the required treatment result.

**effector**  a motor or sensory nerve ending in a muscle, gland or organ.

**efferent**  conveying from the centre to the periphery. *See also* AFFERENT. *E. nerves* nerves coming from the brain to supply the muscles and glands.

**effleurage**  [Fr.] stroking movement in massage. In NATURAL CHILDBIRTH, a light circular stroke of the lower abdomen, done in rhythm to control breathing, to aid in relaxation of the abdominal muscles, and to increase concentration during a uterine contraction. The stroking is accomplished by moving the wrist only.

**effort syndrome**  a condition characterized by breathlessness, palpitations, chest pain and fatigue, caused by an abnormal anxiety; often found in soldiers but may also occur in other individuals.

**effusion**  the escape of blood, serum or other fluid into surrounding tissues or cavities.

**ego** in psychoanalytical theory, that part of the mind which the individual experiences as 'self'. The ego is concerned with satisfying the unconscious primitive demands of the 'id' in a socially acceptable form.

**egocentrism** a type of thinking in which a person has difficulty in seeing another's point of view. This self-centring is normal in young children but in adults may indicate delayed cognitive development.

**eidetic** having the ability to visualize exactly objects or events that have previously been seen. Having a photographic memory.

**ejaculation** 1. the act of ejecting semen, a reflex action that occurs as the result of sexual stimulation. 2. a sudden utterance or exclamation, which may be out of context.

**elastic** capable of stretching. *E. bandage* one that will stretch and will exert continuous pressure on the part bandaged. *E. stocking* a woven rubber stocking sometimes worn for varicose veins. *E. tissue* connective tissue containing yellow elastic fibres.

**elation** in psychiatry, a feeling of wellbeing or a state of excitement. It occurs to a marked degree in hypomania and to an intense degree in mania. *See* EUPHORIA.

**elbow** the joint between the upper arm and the forearm. It is formed by the humerus above and the radius and ulna below.

**elder abuse** *see* ABUSE.

**elective** usually pertaining to a surgical procedure that is performed by choice, as opposed to an emergency life-saving procedure. Timing of the procedure may also be arranged to be mutually convenient for the patient and surgeon.

**Electra complex** libidinous fixation of a daughter towards her father. The female version of the Oedipus complex.

**electrocardiogram** abbreviated ECG. A tracing made of the various phases of the heart's action by means of an electrocardiograph. The normal electrocardiogram is composed of a P wave, Q, R and S waves (known as the QRS COMPLEX, or QRS wave), and a T wave. The P wave occurs at the beginning of each contraction of the atria. The QRS wave occurs at the beginning of each contraction of the ventricles. The T wave seen in a normal electrocardiogram occurs as the ventricles recover electrically and prepare for the next contraction. There is a refractory period between these waves.

**electrocardiograph** a machine that records the electrical potential of the heart from electrodes on the chest and limbs.

**electrocautery** an instrument for the destruction of tissue by means of an electrically heated needle or wire loop.

**electrocoagulation** a method of coagulation using a high-frequency current. A form of surgical diathermy.

**electroconvulsive therapy** abbreviated ECT. Electroplexy. The passage of an electric current through the frontal lobes of the brain, which causes a convulsion. It is used in the treatment of severe depression. A general anaesthetic and muscle relaxant are given before treatment.

**electrocorticography** electroencephalography with the electrodes applied directly to the cortex of the brain during surgery to locate a small lesion, e.g. a scar.

**electrode** the terminal of a conducting system or cell of a battery, through which electricity enters or leaves the body; may be in the form of a plate or pad.

**electroencephalogram** abbreviated EEG. A tracing of the electrical activity of the brain. Abnormal rhythm is an aid to diagnosis in epilepsy and cerebral tumour.

**electroencephalograph** a machine for recording the electrical activity of the cortex of the brain. The electrodes are applied to the scalp.

**electrolysis** 1. chemical decomposition by means of electricity, e.g. an electric current passed through water decomposes it into oxygen and hydrogen. 2. the destruction of tissue by means of electricity, e.g. the removal of surplus hair.

**electrolyte** a compound which, when dissolved in a solution, will dissociate into ions. These ions are electrically charged particles and will thus conduct electricity. *E. balance* the maintenance of the correct balance between the different elements in the body tissues and fluids.

**electron** a negatively charged particle revolving round the nucleus of an atom. *E. microscope* a type of microscope employing a beam of electrons rather than a beam of light, which allows very small particles such as viruses to be identified.

**electronic health record** abbreviated EHR. Longitudinal record of a patient's health and health care which combines information from primary health care with periodic care from other institutions.

**electronic patient record** abbreviated EPR. Description of the care provided for a patient mainly by one organization, such as an acute hospital or Mental Health Trust.

**electrophoresis** a method of analysing the different proteins in blood serum by passing an electric current through the serum to separate the electrically charged particles. The particles gradually separate into bands as a result of the difference in rate of movement according to the electrical charge on the particles.

**electroplexy** electroconvulsive therapy.

**electroretinography** a method of examining the retina of the eye by means of electrodes and light stimulation for assessment of retinal damage.

**element** 1. any of the primary parts or constituents of a compound. 2. in chemistry, a simple substance that cannot be decomposed by ordinary chemical means; the basic 'stuff' of which all matter is composed.

**elephantiasis** a chronic disease of the lymphatics producing excessive thickening of the skin and swelling of the parts affected, usually the lower limbs. It may be due to filariasis in tropical and subtropical climates.

**elimination** the removal of waste matter, particularly from the body. Excretion.

**ELISA** abbreviation for enzyme-linked immunosorbent assay (also called enzyme immunoassay – EIA), a laboratory technique to identify the presence of an antibody or an antigen in a sample, such as blood or saliva. It is the principal technique used in testing for human immunodeficiency virus (HIV) infection. It is a highly accurate test, but positive results are always confirmed by additional testing.

**emaciation** excessive wasting of body tissues. Extreme thinness.

**e-mail** an electronic means of communication where messages are held on a server centrally prior to dispatch to the receiver's computer through a modem or network. *E. address* a series of characters that precisely identifies the location of an individual electronic mail box.

**emasculation** the removal of the penis or testicles; castration.

**embolectomy** surgical removal of an embolus, frequently arterial emboli that are cutting off the blood supply to the limbs.

**embolism** obstruction of a blood vessel by a travelling blood clot or particle of matter. *Air e.* the presence of gas or air bubbles, usually sucked into the large veins from a wound in the neck or chest. *Cerebral e.* obstruction of a vessel in the brain. *Coronary e.* the blockage of a coronary vessel with a clot. *Fat e.* globules of fat released into the blood from a fractured bone. *Infective e.* detached particles of infected blood clot from an area of inflammation which, obstructing small vessels, result in abscess formation, i.e. pyaemia. *Pulmonary e.* blocking of the pulmonary artery or one of its branches by a detached clot, usually due to thrombosis in the femoral or iliac veins. *Retinal e.* blockage, due to air or a blood clot, of the central retinal artery, resulting in loss of vision.

**embolus** a substance carried by the bloodstream until it causes obstruction by blocking a blood vessel. *See* EMBOLISM.

**embrocation** a liquid applied to the body by rubbing to treat strains. A liniment.

**embryo** the fertilized ovum in its earliest stages, i.e. until it shows human characteristics during the second month. After this it is termed a fetus.

**embryology** the study of the growth and development of the embryo from the unicellular stage until birth.

**emergency** a sudden crisis requiring urgent intervention. *E. planning* plan outlining how to deal with a serious incident, such as a major road accident, rail crash, bomb incident or chemical spill. Each level and part of the NHS has an emergency plan, which must relate to the emergency plans of other agencies, such as local authorities, police and fire services. *E. protection order* a court order whereby a child is arbitrarily removed from the care of the parents in the interests of the child's safety.

**emesis** vomiting.

**emic** perspectives that are shared and understood by members of a group, community or culture… 'the insiders'. These views may contrast to those of 'outsiders' (*see* ETIC). Used in ethnographic and qualitative research.

**emetic** an agent that can induce vomiting.

**eminence** a projection, usually rounded, from a surface, e.g. of a bone.

**emission** involuntary ejection (of semen).

**EMLA** a cream for local application to a skin site, containing a mixture of local anaesthetics. Particularly useful for children as it allows for painful tests and biopsies to be performed with minimal pain and discomfort.

**emollient** any substance used to soothe or soften the skin.

**emotion** feeling or affect; a state of arousal characterized by alteration of feeling tone and by physiological behavioural changes. The physical form of emotion may be outward and evident to others, as in crying, laughing, blushing or a variety of facial expressions; however, emotion is not always reflected in the appearance and actions even though psychic changes are taking place. Joy, grief, fear and anger are examples of emotions.

**emotional** 1. relating to the emotions. 2. arousing emotions or readily showing the emotions. *E. bias* situation in which emotional attitudes affect logical judgement. An emotional reaction. *E. deprivation* a lack of loving attention during a child's early years when there has been a failure to achieve a psychological and emotional tie between parent and child. This may lead to impulsive behaviour and an inability to sustain trusting relationships in later life. *See* BONDING. *E. disorders* characterized by swings in mood ranging from extreme excitement to one of depression. Emotional lability. *E. maturity* the achievement of maximum emotional control.

**empathy** the power of projecting oneself into the feelings of another person or into a situation.

**emphysema** the abnormal presence of air in tissues or cavities of the body. *Pulmonary e.* a chronic disease of the lungs. Distension of alveoli causes intervening walls to be broken down and bullae to form on the lung surface. It also causes distension of the bronchioles and eventual loss of elasticity so that inspired air cannot be expired, making breathing difficult. *Surgical e.* the presence of air or any other gas in the subcutaneous tissues, introduced through a wound and evidenced by crepitation on pressure.

**empirical** based on experience and not on scientific reasoning.

**empowerment** the capacity to empower, to give power or authority, e.g. to patients to take control over their own care and to work in partnership with care providers.

**empyema** a collection of pus in a cavity, most commonly referring to the pleural cavity.

**en face** [Fr.] a position in which the mother's face and that of her infant are on the same plane and approximately 20 cm apart; a position usually held during breastfeeding.

**enamel** the hard outer covering of the crown of a tooth.

**enarthrosis** a freely moving joint, e.g. ball and socket joint.

**encanthis** a small fleshy growth at the inner canthus of the eye, which may form an abscess.

**encapsulated** enclosed in a capsule.

**encephalin (enkephalin)** an opiate-like substance produced by the pituitary which has analgesic effects. This substance may also be produced synthetically. *See* ENDORPHIN.

**encephalitis** inflammation of the brain. There are many types of encephalitis, depending on the causative agent and the structures involved. The symptoms may be mild, with headache, general malaise and muscle ache similar to that associated with influenza. The more acute and serious symptoms may include fever, delirium, convulsions and coma, and in a significant number of patients result in death.

**encephalocele** herniation of the brain through the skull.

**encephalography** examination of the brain.

**encephalomalacia** softening of the brain.

**encephalomyelitis** inflammation of the brain and spinal cord.

**encephalomyelopathy** any disease condition of the brain and spinal cord.

**encephalopathy** cerebral dysfunction with diffuse disease or damage of the brain. Especially chronic degenerative conditions of toxic, nutritional or metabolic aetiology.

**encopresis** incontinence of faeces not due to organic defect or illness.

**endarterectomy** the surgical removal of the lining of an artery, usually because of narrowing of the vessel by atheromatous plaques. *Thrombo-e.* removal of a clot with the lining.

**endarteritis** inflammation of the innermost coat of an artery. *E. obliterans* a type that causes collapse and obstruction in small arteries.

**endemic** pertaining to a disease prevalent in a particular locality. *See* EPIDEMIC.

**endemiology** the study of all the factors pertaining to endemic disease.

**endocarditis** inflammation of the endocardium characterized by vegetations on the endocardium and heart valves. Due to infection by microorganisms, fungi or *Rickettsia*, or to rheumatic fever. Can affect all ages.

**endocardium** the membrane lining the heart.

**endocervicitis** inflammation of the mucous membrane lining the uterine cervix.

**endocrine** secreting within. Applied to those glands whose secretions (hormones) flow directly into the blood and not outwards through a duct. The chief endocrine glands are the thyroid, parathyroids, suprarenals and pituitary. The pancreas, stomach, liver, ovaries and testes also produce internal secretions. *See* EXOCRINE.

**endocrinology** the science of the endocrine glands and their secretions.

**endoderm** entoderm.

**endogenous** produced within the organism; *see* EXOGENOUS. *E. depression* one in which the disease derives from internal causes.

**endolymph** the fluid inside the membranous labyrinth of the ear.

**endometriosis** the presence of endometrium in an abnormal situation, e.g. in the ovaries, the intestines or the urinary bladder. The ectopic tissue undergoes the same hormonal changes as normal endometrium (*see* Figure on p. 137). As there is no outlet for bleeding when menstruation occurs, the woman suffers considerable pain.

**endometritis** inflammation of the endometrium.

**endometrium** the mucous membrane lining the uterus.

**endomyocarditis** inflammation of the lining membrane and muscles of the heart.

**endoparasite** a parasite that lives within the body of its host.

**endophthalmitis** inflammation of the ocular cavity and adjacent structures.

**endorphin** one of a group of opiate-like peptides produced naturally by the body at neural synapses at various points in the central nervous system, where they modulate the transmission of pain perceptions. Endorphins raise the pain threshold and produce sedation and euphoria; the effects are blocked by naloxone, a narcotic antagonist. Also known as enkephalins.

**endoscope** an lighted flexible or rigid instrument used for direct visual inspection of a hollow organ or cavity. May have a camera attached.

**endospore** *see* SPORE.

**endosteoma** a neoplasm in the medullary cavity of a bone.

**endosteum** the lining membrane of bone cavities.

**endothelioma** a malignant growth originating in the endothelium.

**endothelium** the membranous lining of serous, synovial and other internal surfaces.

**endotoxin** a poison produced by and retained within a bacterium, e.g. *Salmonella typhi*, which is released only after the destruction of the bacterial cell. *See* EXOTOXIN.

**endotracheal** within the trachea. *E. tube* an airway catheter which is inserted into the trachea when a patient requires ventilatory support. It also allows for the removal of secretions by suction.

**enema** 1. introduction of fluid into the rectum. 2. a solution introduced into the rectum to promote evacuation of faeces or as a means of administering nutrient or medicinal substances. 3. introduction of a radio-opaque material in a radiological examination of the colon (*barium e.*), or via a tube inserted into the jejunum in a radiological

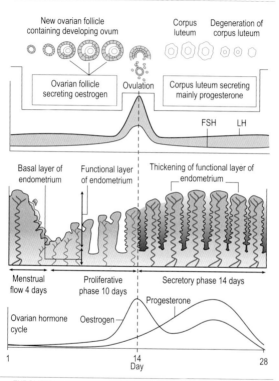

ENDOMETRIAL AND FOLLICULAR CHANGES DURING THE MENSTRUAL CYCLE

examination of the small bowel (*small bowel e.*).

**energy** the ability to do work or effect a physical change in status. Energy has many forms including light, heat and sound. Food through its breakdown within the body provides energy for human activity, strength, growth and vitality and this is measured in calories or joules. Carbohydrates provide 4 kcal/g and fats provide 9 kcal/g. *E. conservation* an occupational therapy technique that seeks to assist patients/clients in maximizing the use of limited physical energy to maintain quality of daily life. This approach is also used by nurses and other health care workers working with the elderly and physically disabled in the community. *E. requirements* the amount of energy that is required by a person for cell metabolism, growth and activity. This is influenced by age, gender, activity and health. *See* METABOLISM. A woman requires 2000Cal (500kJ) per day. A man requires 2500Cal (625kJ) per day. Excess energy foods are stored as fat. This fat provides a supplementary source of energy if the diet is inadequate.

**enervation** 1. general weakness and loss of strength. 2. removal of a nerve.

**engagement** the entry of the presenting part of the fetus, normally the head, into the true pelvis. Occurs in the last stage of pregnancy.

**enkephalin** either of two naturally occurring pentapeptides isolated from the brain, which have potent opiate-like effects and probably serve as neurotransmitters. They are classified as endorphins. *See* ENDORPHINS.

**enophthalmos** a condition in which the eyeball is abnormally sunken into its socket.

**ensiform** xiphoid; sword-shaped. *E. cartilage* the lowest portion of the sternum.

*Entamoeba* a genus of protozoa, some of which are parasitic in humans. *E. histolytica* the cause of amoebic dysentery.

**enteral** within the gastrointestinal tract. *e. diets* or *e. feeding* provides nutrition for those patients who are unable to ingest sufficient nutrients orally but who are able to utilize them in the body to provide for energy requirements and for healing. Feeding may be through nasogastric, gastrostomy or jejunostomy tubes by bolus, gravity or pump assisted. *See* PARENTERAL FEEDING.

**enteric** pertaining to the intestine. *E. coated* a special coating applied to tablets or capsules which prevents release and absorption of their contents until they reach the intestine.

**enteritis** inflammation of the small intestine.

**Enterobacteriaceae** a family of Gram-negative, rod-shaped bacteria, many of which are normally found in the human intestine.

**enterobiasis** infestation by threadworms.

*Enterobius* a genus of nematode worms. *E. vermicularis* the threadworm or pinworm, a small white worm parasitic in the upper part of the large intestine. Gravid females migrate to the anal region to deposit their eggs, sometimes causing severe itching. Infection and re-infection is frequent in children. Treatment is with an anthelmintic drug.

**enterococcus** any streptococcus of the human intestine. An example is *Streptococcus faecalis*, only harmful out of its normal habitat, when it may cause a urinary infection or endocarditis.

**enterocolitis** inflammation of both the large and the small intestine.

**enterokinase** an intestinal enzyme that converts trypsinogen into trypsin; enteropeptidase.

**enterostomy** the formation of an external opening into the small intestine. It may be (a) temporary, to relieve obstruction, or (b) permanent, in the form of an ileostomy in cases of total colectomy.

**enterotomy** any incision of the intestine.

**enterotoxin** a toxin that is produced by one of the many organisms that cause food poisoning. Such toxins frequently prove more resistant to destruction than the bacteria themselves.

**enterovirus** a virus that infects the gastrointestinal tract and then attacks the central nervous system. This subgroup includes Coxsackie, polio and echoviruses, and are now known, together with rhinoviruses, as picornaviruses.

**entoderm** the innermost of the three germ layers of the embryo along with the mesoderm (intermediate) and ectoderm (outer) layers. It gives rise to the lining of most of the respiratory tract and to the intestinal tract and its glands.

**entropion** inversion of an eyelid, so that the lashes rub against the eyeball.

**enucleation** removal of an organ or other mass intact from its supporting tissues, as of the eyeball from the orbit.

**enuresis** involuntary passing of urine, usually during sleep at night (bed-wetting).

**environment** the surroundings of an organism which influence its development and behaviour.

**environmental health** the concept that an individual's living and working environment has an impact upon health and well-being. Factors that can influence health include housing, food hygiene, refuse collection, infestation, and air and noise pollution, etc.

**enzyme** a protein that will catalyse a biological reaction. *See* CATALYST.

**enzyme-linked immunosorbent assay** *see* ELISA.

**eosin** a red dye used to stain biological specimens. A derivative of bromine and fluorescein.

**eosinophil** a cell having an affinity for eosin. A type of white blood cell containing eosin-staining granules.

**eosinophilia** excessive numbers of eosinophils present in the blood.

**ependyma** the membrane lining the cerebral ventricles and the central canal of the spinal cord.

**ependymoma** a neoplasm arising from the lining cells of the ventricles or central canal of the spinal cord. It gives rise to signs of hydrocephalus and is treated by surgery and radiotherapy.

**ephidrosis** profuse sweating; hyperhidrosis.

**epiblepharon** a congenital condition in which an excess of skin of the eyelid folds over the lid margin so that the eyelashes are pressed against the eyeball.

**epicanthus** a vertical fold of skin on either side of the nose, sometimes covering the inner canthus; a normal characteristic in persons of certain races, but anomalous in others.

**epicardium** the visceral layer of the pericardium.

**epicondyle** a protuberance on a long bone above its condyle.

**epicritic** pertaining to sensory nerve fibres in the skin which give the appreciation of touch and temperature.

**epidemic** the presence in a population of disease or infection in excess of that usually expected.

**epidemiology** the study of the distribution of diseases in populations. It includes the attack rate (incidence) and the numbers affected at any one time (prevalence).

**epidermis** the non-vascular outer layer or cuticle of the skin. It consists of layers of cells which protect the dermis.

**epidermoid** pertaining to certain tumours which have the appearance of epidermal tissue.

*Epidermophyton* a genus of fungi that attack skin and nails, but not hair. The cause of ringworm and athlete's foot.

**epididymis** [Gr.] an elongated, cord-like structure along the posterior border of the testis, whose coiled duct provides for the storage, transport and maturation of spermatozoa.

**epididymitis** inflammation of the epididymis.

**epididymo-orchitis** inflammation of the epididymis and the testis.

**epidural** outside the dura mater. *E. analgesia* also known as extradural or peridural anaesthesia. A form of pain relief for childbirth and chronic pain, obtained by the injection of a local analgesic into the epidural space in order to block the spinal nerves. It may be approached by two routes: (a) caudal, through the sacrococcygeal membrane covering the sacral hiatus; or (b) lumbar, through the intervertebral space and ligamentum flavum.

**epigastrium** that region of the abdomen situated over the stomach.

**epiglottis** a cartilaginous structure which covers the opening from the pharynx into the larynx during swallowing and prevents food from passing into the trachea.

**epilation** removal of hairs with their roots. It may be effected by pulling out the hairs or by electrolysis.

**epilatory** an agent that produces epilation.

**epilepsy** a group of conditions causing convulsive attacks due to disordered electrical activity of the brain cells. In a major attack of 'grand mal' the patient falls to the ground unconscious, following an aura or unpleasant sensation. There are first tonic and then clonic contractions, from which stage the patient passes into a deep sleep. A minor attack of 'petit mal' is a momentary loss of consciousness only. Both these types of epilepsy are idiopathic and are not caused by any damage to the brain. *Focal* or *Jacksonian e.* a symptom of a cerebral lesion. The convulsive movements are often localized and close observation of the onset and course of the attack may greatly

assist diagnosis. *Temporal lobe e.* characterized by hallucinations of sight, hearing, taste and smell, paroxysmal disorders of memory and automatism. Caused by temporal or parietal lobe disease.

**epileptiform** resembling an epileptic fit.

**epiloia** tuberous sclerosis. A congenital disorder with areas of hardening in the cerebral cortex and other organs, characterized clinically by mental handicap and epilepsy.

**epinephrine** adrenaline.

**epineurium** the sheath of tissue surrounding a nerve.

**epiphora** persistent overflow of tears, often due to obstruction in the lacrimal passages or to ectropion.

**epiphysis** the end of a long bone, developed separately from but attached by cartilage to the diaphysis (the shaft), with which it eventually unites. Growth in length takes place from the line of junction.

**episcleritis** inflammation of the outer coat of the eyeball. It is seen as a slightly raised bluish nodule under the conjunctiva.

**episiotomy** an incision made in the perineum when it will not stretch sufficiently during the second stage of labour.

**epispadias** a malformation in which there is an abnormal opening of the urethra on to the dorsal surface of the penis. *See* HYPOSPADIAS.

**epistaxis** bleeding from the nose.

**epithelioma** any tumour originating in the epithelium.

**epithelium** the surface layer of cells of the skin or lining tissues.

**epithelization** development of epithelium. The final stage in the healing of a surface wound. Epithelialization.

**Epstein–Barr virus** *M. A. Epstein, British pathologist, b. 1921; Y. Barr, Canadian pathologist, b. 1932.* A herpes virus that causes infectious mononucleosis. It has been isolated from cells cultured from Burkitt's lymphoma, and has been found in certain cases of nasopharyngeal cancer. Also called EB virus.

**Equality and Human Rights Commission** launched in 2007 the Commission is an independent statutory body established under the Equality Act 2006. This Commission took over responsibility for three former equality commissions: the Commission for Racial Equality, the Disability Rights Commission and the Equal Opportunities Commission. The Commission also has responsibility for other key areas of equality relating to age, gender reassignment, religion or belief, and sexual orientation as well as human rights.

**Equal Pay Act 1970** an Act, amended 2005, which came into force to eliminate discrimination between men and women with regard to their pay and conditions of employment.

**Erb's palsy** *W.H. Erb, German physician, 1840–1921.* Paralysis of the arm, often due to birth injury causing pressure on the brachial plexus or lower cervical nerve roots.

**erectile** having the power of becoming erect. *E. tissue* vascular tissue which, under stimulus, becomes congested and swollen, causing erection of that part. The penis consists largely of erectile tissue.

**erection** the enlarged and rigid state of the sexually aroused penis. Erection can also occur in the clitoris and the nipples of the female.

**erepsin** the enzyme of succus entericus, secreted by the intestinal glands, which splits peptones into amino acids.

**ergonomics** the scientific study of human beings in relation to their work and the effective use of human energy.

**ergosterol** a sterol occurring in animal and plant tissues which, on ultraviolet irradiation, becomes a potent antirachitic substance, vitamin $D_2$ (ergocalciferol).

**erogenous** arousing erotic feelings. *E. zones* areas of the body, stimulation of which produces erotic desire, e.g. the oral, anal and genital orifices and the nipples.

**erosion** the breaking down of tissue, usually by ulceration. *Cervical e.* a covering of columnar epithelium on the vaginal part of the uterine cervix, arising from erosion of the squamous epithelium, which normally covers it.

**erotic** pertaining to sexual love or lust.

**eroticism, erotism** a sexual instinct or desire; the expression of one's instinctual energy or drive, especially the sex drive.

**eructation** belching; the escape of gas from the stomach through the mouth.

**eruption** a breaking out, e.g. of a skin lesion, or the cutting of teeth.

**erysipelas** a febrile disease characterized by inflammation and redness of the skin and subcutaneous tissues, and caused by group A haemolytic streptococci.

**erysipeloid** an infective dermatitis or cellulitis due to infection with *Erysipelothrix insidiosa*; it usually begins in a wound (often the result of a prick by a fish bone) and remains localized, rarely becoming generalized and septicaemic.

**erythema** redness of the skin caused by congestion of the capillaries in its lower layers. It occurs with any skin injury, infection or inflammation. *E. induratum* a manifestation of vasculitis. *E. multiforme* an acute eruption of the skin, which may be due to an allergy or to drug sensitivity. *E. nodosum* a painful disease in which bright-red, tender nodes occur below the knee or on the forearm; it may be associated with tuberculosis.

**erythematous** characterized by erythema.

**erythrasma** a skin disease due to infection by *Coryne-bacterium minutissimum*, attacking the arm-pits or groins. It causes no irritation but is contagious.

**erythroblast** originally, any nucleated erythrocyte, but now more generally used to designate the nucleated precursor from which an erythrocyte develops.

**erythroblastosis** the presence of erythroblasts in the blood. *E. fetalis* a severe haemolytic anaemia with an excess of erythroblasts in the newly born. Due to rhesus incompatibility between the child's and the mother's blood.

**erythrocyanosis** swelling and blueness of the legs and thighs occurring mainly in young women and during cold weather.

**erythrocyte** a mature red blood cell. The cells contain haemoglobin and serve to transport oxygen. They are developed in the red bone marrow found in the cancellous tissue of all bones (*see* Figure). The haemopoietic factor vitamin B$_{12}$ is essential for the change from pro-erythroblast to normoblast, and iron, thyroxine and vitamin C are also necessary for its perfect structure. *E. sedimentation rate* abbreviated ESR. The rate at which the cells of citrated blood form a deposit in a graduated 200 mm tube (Westergren method). The normal is less than 10 mm of clear plasma in 1 hour. This is much increased in severe infection and acute rheumatism.

**erythrocythaemia** increase in numbers of red blood cells due to overactivity of the bone marrow; Vaquez' disease; polycythaemia vera.

**erythrocytopenia** erythropenia; deficiency in numbers of red blood cells.

**erythrocytosis** erythrocythaemia.

**erythroderma** abnormal redness of the skin, usually over a large area.

**erythropoiesis** the manufacture of red blood corpuscles.

**erythropoietin** a hormone, produced by the kidney, which stimulates the production of red blood cells in the bone marrow. *E. therapy* use of erythropoietin to promote new blood formation in the treatment of anaemia.

**erythropsia** a defect of vision in which all objects appear red. May occur after a cataract operation.

**eschar** a slough or scab which forms after the destruction of living tissue by gangrene, infection or burning.

*Escherichia* a genus of Enterobacteriaceae. *E. coli* an organism normally present in the intestines of humans and other vertebrates. Although not generally pathogenic, it may set up infections of the gallbladder, bile ducts,

---

ERYTHROCYTE DEVELOPMENT IN BONE MARROW

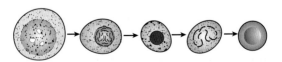

Proerythroblast    Erythroblast    Normoblast    Reticulocyte    Erythrocyte

and urinary and intestinal tracts. Strain O157, normally found in the gut of cattle, occasionally has been responsible for serious outbreaks of food poisoning in humans.

**esophoria** latent convergent strabismus. The eyes turn inwards only when one is covered up.

**esotropia** convergent strabismus. One or other eye turns inwards, resulting in double vision.

**ESP** extrasensory perception.

**ESR** erythrocyte sedimentation rate.

**ESRD** end-stage renal disease. *See* RENAL.

**essence** 1. an indispensable part of anything. 2. a volatile oil dissolved in alcohol.

**essential** indispensable. *E. amino acids* those amino acids that must be obtained in the diet and are necessary for the maintenance of tissue growth and repair. *See* AMINO ACID. *E. drugs* a concept developed by the World Health Organization as a scheme to extend the range of drugs to populations who have poor access because of the existing supply structure. A core drug list based on local health needs was developed. The World Health Organization perceives essential drug lists as an indication of those drugs needed to meet common national requirements in poorer countries. The lists are updated on a two-yearly basis with an emphasis on local ownership and the involvement of national policies in implementation. *E. fatty acids* unsaturated fatty acids that are necessary for body growth. *E. oils* specially prepared aromatic oils which are obtained from the different parts of plants including flowers, leaves, seeds, wood, roots and bark. Used in aromatherapy.

**ester** a compound formed by the combination of an acid and an alcohol, with the elimination of water.

**esterase** an enzyme that causes the hydrolysis of esters into acids and alcohol.

**ethanol** alcohol.

**ethanolamine** an intravenous sclerosing agent used to inject varicose veins.

**ether** a volatile inflammable liquid formerly used as a general anaesthetic agent.

**ethics** a code of moral principles. Each practitioner, upon entering a profession, is invested with the responsibility to adhere to the standards of ethical practice and conduct set by that profession. The Code of Professional Conduct for the Nurse, Midwife and Health Visitor, adopted by the NMC in 2000, provides guidance and advice for standards of practice and conduct that are essential for the ethical discharge of the practitioner's responsibility. *E. committee* a group of lay people with professional health care practitioners, nurses, doctors and other experts. They consider and discuss ethical issues within an NHS Trust and monitor research projects that involve the use of human subjects. *Nursing e. See* Appendix 4.

**ethmoid** a sieve-like bone separating the cavity of the nose from the cranium. The olfactory nerves pass through its perforations.

**ethnic** pertaining to a social group, members of which share cultural bonds or physical (racial) characteristics. *E. minority* a social grouping of people who share cultural or racial factors but who constitute a minority within the greater culture or society.

**ethnocentrism** the belief that one's own group, community, society or even way of doing things is superior to those of others, leading to mistrust or doubt about others' values and beliefs.

**ethnography** a qualitative research approach developed by anthropologists with the purpose of describing an aspect of a culture, but also aimed at learning about the culture or factor being studied.

**ethnology** the science dealing with the human races, their descent, relationship, etc.

**ethnomethodology** a sociological theory which concentrates on the case study using participant or non-participant observation.

**ethyl chloride** a volatile liquid used as a local anaesthetic. When sprayed on intact skin it causes local insensitivity, through freezing.

**ethylene oxide** a gas that is sporicidal and viricidal and capable of penetrating relatively inaccessible parts of an apparatus during sterilization. It is used for equipment which is too delicate to be sterilized by other methods.

**etic** the perspectives of a group, community or culture held by observers who are 'outsiders' or non-participants. *See* EMIC.

**etiolation** paleness of the skin due to lack of exposure to sunlight.

**etiology** *see* AETIOLOGY.

**eucalyptus oil** an oil derived from the leaves of the eucalyptus tree; it has mild antiseptic properties and is used in the treatment of nasal catarrh.

**eugenics** the study of measures that may be taken to improve future generations, both physically and mentally.

**eugeria** the state of a high quality of life in old age. Eugeria should be the normal state for the elderly but may be affected by physical or mental illness.

**eunuch** a castrated male.

**euphoria** an exaggerated feeling of wellbeing, often not justified by circumstances. Less extreme than ELATION.

**euplastic** capable of being transformed into healthy tissue. The term may be applied to a wound that is healing well.

**eurhythmics** gentle body exercises performed to music.

**European Union Nursing Directives** the EU directives seek to ensure that nurses and midwives from the member states of the EU receive similar educational programmes which meet defined standards to facilitate free movement of nursing personnel between the member states.

**European Medicines Evaluation Agency** authorizes the use of medicinal products in the European Union and works with national medicines regulatory bodies (*see also* MEDICINES AND HEALTHCARE PRODUCTS REGULATORY AGENCY).

**eustachian tube** *B. Eustachio, Italian anatomist, 1520–1574.* The pharyngotympanic tube.

**euthanasia** 1. an easy or good death. 2. the deliberate ending of life of a person suffering from an incurable disease; this can be voluntary or involuntary.

**euthyroid** having a normally functioning thyroid gland.

**evacuant** 1. promoting evacuation. 2. an agent that promotes evacuation.

**evacuation** 1. an emptying or removal, especially the removal of any material from the body by discharge through a natural or artificial passage. 2. material discharged from the body, especialy the discharge from the bowels.

**evacuator** an instrument that produces evacuation, e.g. one designed to wash out small particles of stone from the bladder after lithotripsy.

**evaluation** a critical appraisal or assessment; a judgement of the value, worth, character or effectiveness of that which is being assessed. In the health care field this includes assessment of the patient's position on the health/illness continuum, and of the effectiveness of patient care activities in bringing about a change in the patient's position. Accepted as the fourth phase of the nursing process.

**eventration** 1. the protrusion of the intestines through the abdominal wall. 2. removal of abdominal viscera.

**eversion** turning outwards. *E. of the eyelid* ectropion. The upper eyelid may be everted for examination of the eye or for the removal of a foreign body.

**evidence-based practice** systematically appraising clinical situations and then using up-to-date research findings as a basis for decisions by the nursing or other health-related professions, e.g. pharmacy or dentistry. An approach to clinical practice first developed at McMaster University (Canada) which is based on the following four principles: (a) clinical and other health care decisions should be *based on the best evidence* available from patients and populations as well as from the laboratory; (b) the patient's problem determines the nature and source of evidence to be sought, rather than habit, protocol or tradition; (c) identifying the best evidence calls for the integration of epidemiological and biostatistical ways of thinking with those derived from pathophysiology and clinical experience; (d) the conclusions of this search and critical appraisal of evidence are worthwhile only if they are translated into actions that affect patients.

**evisceration** removal of internal organs. *E. of the eye* removal of the contents of the eyeball, but not the sclera.

**evolution** the development of living organisms which change their characteristics during succeeding generations.

**evulsion** extraction by force.

**Ewing's tumour** *J. Ewing, American pathologist, 1866–1943.* A form of sarcoma usually affecting the shaft of a long bone in young adults.

**exacerbation** an increase in the severity of the symptoms of a disease.

**exanthem** an infectious disease characterized by a skin rash.

**exanthematous** pertaining to any disease associated with a skin eruption.

**excavation** scooping out. *Dental e.* the removal of decay from a tooth before inserting a filling.

**exception** in health care the justification for clinical variance made by a practitioner and usually peer-reviewed by others.

**excision** the cutting out of a part.

**excitation** the act of stimulating.

**excitement** a physiological and emotional response to a stimulus.

**excoriation** an abrasion of the skin.

**excrement** faecal matter; waste matter from the body.

**excrescence** abnormal outgrowth of tissue, e.g. a wart.

**excreta** the natural discharges of the excretory system: faeces, urine and sweat.

**excretion** the discharge of waste from the body.

**exercise** performance of physical exertion for improvement of health or correction of physical deformity. *Active e.* motion imparted to a part by voluntary contraction and relaxation of its controlling muscles. *Isometric e.* active exercise performed against stable resistance, without change in the length of the muscle. No movement occurs at any joints over which the muscle passes. *Passive e.* motion imparted to a segment of the body by another individual, or a machine or other outside force, or produced by voluntary effort of another segment of the patient's own body. *Range of movement (ROM) e's* exercises that move each joint through its full range of movement, that is, to the highest degree of movement of which each joint is normally capable.

**exfoliation** the splitting off from the surface of dead tissue in thin flaky layers.

**exhalation** 1. the giving off of a vapour. 2. the act of breathing out.

**exhibitionism** 1. showing off; a desire to attract attention. 2. exposing the genitals to persons of the opposite sex in socially unacceptable circumstances.

**exocrine** pertaining to those glands that discharge their secretion by means of a duct, e.g. salivary glands. *See* ENDOCRINE.

**exogenous** of external origin.

**exomphalos** 1. hernia of the abdominal viscera into the umbilical cord. 2. congenital umbilical hernia.

**exophthalmometer** an instrument for measuring the extent of protrusion of the eyeball.

**exophthalmos** abnormal protrusion of the eyeball which results in a marked stare. May be due to injury or disease and is often associated with thyrotoxicosis.

**exostosis** a bony outgrowth from the surface of a bone.

**exotoxin** a poison produced by a bacterial cell and released into the tissues surrounding it. *See* ENDOTOXIN.

**exotropia** divergent strabismus; the eyes turn outwards.

**expanded role** the opportunity for nurses, midwives and health visitors to undertake an expanded role in relation to patient care beyond that traditionally recognized. The professional framework for nurses, midwives and health visitors in relation to the expanded role is contained within the Nursing and Midwifery Council's code of Professional Conduct (*see* Appendix 5).

**expected date of delivery** abbreviated EDD. Used in midwifery and obstetrics to calculate the date of delivery of a baby. This is calculated by counting forwards 9 months and adding 7 days from the first day of the last normal menstrual period or counting back 3 months and adding 7 days.

**expected outcome** in a nursing care plan the rationale for a statement regarding a nursing intervention and what it is expected to achieve.

**expectorant** a remedy that promotes and facilitates expectoration.

**expectoration** sputum; secretions coughed up from the air passages. Its characteristics are a valuable aid in diagnosis and note should be taken of the quantity ejected, its colour and the amount of effort required. Frothiness denotes that it comes from an air-containing cavity; fluidity indicates oedema of the lung.

**experiental learning** learning from experiencing a situation. May also be facilitated with the use of role play or of a simulated situation and reflecting upon the experience.

**expiration** 1. the act of breathing out. 2. termination or death.

**exploration** the operation of surgically investigating any part of the body.

**expression** 1. the aspect or appearance of the face as determined by the physical or emotional state. 2. the act of squeezing out or evacuating by pressure, e.g. the removal of breast milk by hand or breast pump. 3. the manifestation of a heritable trait in an individual carrying the gene or genes that determine it.

**exsanguination** extensive blood loss due to internal or external haemorrhage.

**extended family** one that includes aunts, uncles, cousins and grandparents. *See* FAMILY.

**extension** 1. the straightening out of a flexed joint, such as the knee or elbow. 2. the application of traction to a fractured or dislocated limb by means of a weight.

**extensor** a muscle that extends or straightens a limb.

**exterior** on the outside.

**exteriorize** 1. to bring an organ or part of one to the outside of the body by surgery. 2. in psychiatry, to turn one's interests outwards.

**extra-** prefix denoting outside, additional or beyond.

**extracapsular** outside the capsule. May refer to a fracture occurring at the end of the bone but outside the joint capsule, or to cataract extraction.

**extracellular** outside the cell. *E. fluid* tissue fluid that surrounds the cells.

**extracorporeal membrane oxygenation** abbreviated ECMO. A life-support procedure, providing circulation and gas exchange outside the body using extrathoracic cannulation, for reversible profound respiratory and cardiac failure in infants and children. The procedure requires access to a central vein and a common carotid artery (for cardiac support) or a veno-venous approach (for respiratory support). Blood is circulated through the device by a roller pump with the infusion of oxygen via a semipermeable membrane which also allows for the removal of carbon dioxide. Body temperature is maintained by means of a heat exchanger, and access for the administration of drugs or blood sampling is possible through entry portals in the circuit. Intensive nursing, medical and physiotherapy care is required together with ventilation, continuous monitoring and regular assessment for pain and discomfort.

**extraction** 1. the process or act of pulling or drawing out. 2. the preparation of an extract. *Breech e.* extraction of an infant from the uterus in cases of breech presentation. *Vacuum e.* removal of the uterine contents by application of a vacuum. An alternative to the forceps method of delivering a baby.

**extrapyramidal** outside the pyramidal (cerebrospinal) tract. *E. system* the nerve tracts and pathways that are not within the pyramidal tracts.

**extrasensory** outside or beyond any of the known senses. *E. perception* abbreviated ESP. Appreciation of the thoughts of others or of current or future events without any normal means of communication.

**extrasystole** premature contraction of the atria or ventricles. *See* SYSTOLE.

**extrauterine** occurring outside the uterus. *E. pregnancy* ectopic gestation; development of a fetus outside the uterus.

**extravasation** effusion or escape of fluid from its normal course into surrounding tissues. *E. of blood* a bruise.

**extremity** distal part; a hand or foot.

**extrinsic** originating externally. *E. factor* a substance present in meat and other foodstuffs. Also called cyanocobalamin (vitamin $B_{12}$), it is necessary for the manufacture of red blood cells. The intrinsic factor produced in the stomach is necessary for the absorption of vitamin $B_{12}$. *E. muscle* a muscle originating away from the part that it controls, such as those controlling the movements of the eye.

**extroversion** turning inside out, e.g. of the uterus, as sometimes occurs after labour, or in psychol-

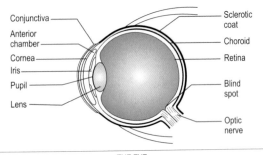

THE EYE

ogy the turning of thoughts to the external environment.

**extrovert** a person who is sociable, a good mixer, outgoing and interested in what is going on in the social enviroment. A personality type first described by Jung. *See* INTROVERT.

**extubation** removal of a tube used in intubation.

**exudation** the slow discharge of serous fluid through the walls of the blood cells and its deposition in or on the tissues.

**eye** the organ of sight. A globular structure with three coats. The nerve tissue of the retina receives impressions of images via the pupil and lens. From this the optic nerve conveys the impressions to the visual area of the cerebrum (*see* Figure). *E. contact* two people making direct contact in the vicinity of the other's eyes. Also called mutual gaze. Forms an important component of non-verbal communication in many cultures between people although the nurse will need to be sensitive to the cultural background of the person as some cultures consider direct eye contact inappropriate. *E. strain* fatigue of the eye(s) from overuse and tiredness; often associated with headaches. May be due to poor lighting or an uncorrected defect in focusing.

**eyelid** a protective covering of the eye, composed of muscle and dense connective tissue covered with skin, lined with conjunctiva and fringed with eyelashes. Eyelids contain the Meibomian glands.

**eyetooth** an upper canine tooth.

**F** symbol for *Fahrenheit* and *fluorine*.

**face** the front of the head from the forehead to the chin. *F. presentation* the appearance of the face of the fetus first at the cervix during labour.

**facet** a small flat area on the surface of a bone. *F. syndrome* a slight dislocation of the small facet joints of the vertebrae giving rise to pain and muscle spasm.

**facial** pertaining to the face or lower anterior portion of the head. *F. nerve* the seventh cranial nerve, which supplies the salivary glands and superficial face muscles. *F. paralysis see* PARALYSIS.

**facies** facial expression; it often gives some indication of the patient's condition. *Adenoid f.* the open mouth and vacant expression associated with mouth breathing and nasal obstruction. *Parkinson f.* fixed expression, due to paucity of movement of facial muscles, characteristic of Parkinsonism.

**faeces** waste matter excreted by the bowel, consisting of indigestible cellulose, food which has escaped digestion, bacteria (living and dead) and water.

**Fahrenheit scale** *G.D. Fahrenheit, German physicist, 1686–1736.* A scale of heat measurement. It registers the freezing point of water at 32°, the normal heat of the human body at 98.4°, and the boiling point of water at 212°. Symbol F. *See* CELSIUS.

**failure** inability to perform or to function properly. *F. to thrive* retardation of normal growth and development in an infant. Causes are numerous but malnutrition or difficulty in absorbing essential nutrients is a main factor, as well as those that are psychosocial in origin, e.g. maternal deprivation syndrome. *Heart f.* inability of the heart to maintain a circulation sufficient to meet the body's needs. *Kidney f., renal f.* inability of the kidney to excrete metabolites at normal plasma levels under normal loading, or inability to retain electrolytes when intake is normal; in the acute form, marked by uraemia and usually by oliguria, with hyperkalaemia and pulmonary oedema. *Respiratory f., ventilatory f.* a life-threatening condition in which respiratory function is inadequate to maintain the body's needs for oxygen supply and carbon dioxide removal while at rest.

**fainting** *see* SYNCOPE.

**faith healing** an attempt to cure disease or disability with the use of spiritual powers or by the influence of the personality of the healer.

**falciform** sickle-shaped. *F. ligament* a fold of peritoneum which separates the two main lobes of the liver and connects it with the anterior abdominal wall and the diaphragm.

**fall** moving downwards quickly and without control. The tendency

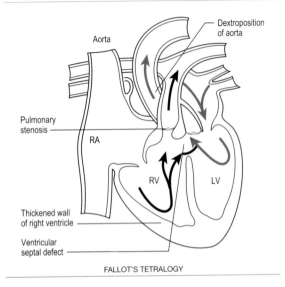

Aorta

Dextroposition of aorta

Pulmonary stenosis

RA

RV

LV

Thickened wall of right ventricle

Ventricular septal defect

FALLOT'S TETRALOGY

to fall to the ground increases with age when reflex actions are slower. Various conditions of the elderly, e.g. poor sight or walking disorders, increase the risk of falls as does the taking of sleeping pills or tranquillizer drugs. Broken bones are a common complication, most usually in women who are more prone to osteoporosis. A fall or the fear of falling can have an adverse psychological effect on an elderly person who may become reluctant to leave the home. Community care staff can provide practical advice and support to prevent or minimize further falls, e.g. ensuring that floor coverings and wiring are made safe, suitable footwear is worn, good lighting is available and hand rails are secure and safe.

**fallopian tube** *G. Fallopius, Italian anatomist, 1523–1563.* Uterine tube. One of a pair of tubes, about 10–14 cm long, arising out of the upper part of the uterus. The distal end of each tube is fimbriated and lies near an ovary. The tubes' function is to conduct the ova from the ovaries to the interior of the uterus. An oviduct.

**Fallot's tetralogy** *E.L.A. Fallot, French physician, 1850–1911.* A congenital cyanotic heart disease with four characteristic defects: (a) pulmonary stenosis; (b) interventricular defect of the septum; (c) overriding of the aorta, i.e. opening into both right and left ventricles;

(d) hypertrophy of the right ventricle. *See* Figure on p. 150.

**falx** a sickle-shaped structure. *F. cerebri* the fold of dura mater that separates the two cerebral hemispheres.

**familial** occurring in or affecting members of a family more than would be expected by chance.

**family** 1. a group of people who reside together and who may be related by blood or marriage, especially a husband, wife and their children. 2. a taxonomic category below an order and above a genus. *Blended f.* a family unit composed of a married couple and their offspring, including some from previous marriages. *Extended f.* a nuclear family and their close relatives, such as the children's grandparents, aunts and uncles. *Extended nuclear f.* a nuclear family who nevertheless make frequent social contacts with the extended family group despite geographical distance. *F. planning* the arrangement, spacing and limitation of the children in a family, depending upon the wishes and social circumstances of the parents. *F. centered care* a nursing approach to care and treatment of children which recognizes the needs of the family and their circumstances in the planning and delivery of services being provided for the child. *F. therapy* a therapeutic process whereby the psychotherapist uses family group therapy to resolve problems for one member of the family. *Nuclear f.* a couple and their children, by birth or adoption, who are living together and are more or less isolated from their extended family. *Single parent f.* a lone parent and offspring living together as a family unit.

**Fanconi's syndrome** F. Fanconi, Swiss paediatrician, 1892–1979. A rare inherited disorder of metabolism in which reabsorption of phosphate, amino acids and sugar by the renal tubules is impaired. The kidneys fail to produce acid urine, and resulting features are thirst, polyuria and rickets, leading to chronic renal failure.

**fang** the root of a tooth.

**fantasy** an imagined sequence of events or mental images that serves to satisfy unconscious wishes or to express unconscious conflicts.

**farmer's lung** a disease occurring in those in contact with mouldy hay. It is thought to be due to a hypersensitivity, with widespread reaction in the lung tissue. It causes excessive breathlessness.

**FAS** fetal alcohol syndrome.

**fascia** a sheath of connective tissue enclosing muscles or other organs.

**fasciculation** isolated fine muscle twitching which gives a flickering appearance.

**fasciculus** a small bundle of nerve or muscle fibres; a fascicle.

**fat** 1. the adipose or fatty tissue of the body. 2. neutral fat; a triglyceride which is an ester of fatty acids and glycerol. *F. soluble vitamins* those vitamins that are soluble in fat, i.e. vitamins A, D, E and K. *Wool-f.* lanolin. *See also* BROWN FAT.

**fatigue** a state of weariness which may range from mental disinclination for effort to profound exhaustion after great physical and mental effort. *Muscle f.* may occur during prolonged effort owing to oxygen lack and accumulation of waste products.

**fatty** containing or similar to fat. *F. acid see* ESSENTIAL. *F. degeneration* a degenerative change in tissue cells due to the invasion of fat and consequent weakening of the organ. The change occurs as a result of incorrect diet, shortage of oxygen in the tissues or excessive consumption of alcohol.

**fauces** the opening from the mouth into the pharynx. *Pillars of the f.* the two folds of muscle covered with mucous membrane that pass from the soft palate on either side of the fauces. One fold passes into the tongue, the other into the pharynx, and between them is situated the tonsil.

**favism** an acute haemolytic anaemia caused by ingestion of fava beans or inhalation of the pollen of the plant, usually occurring in certain individuals as a result of a genetic abnormality with a deficiency in an enzyme, glucose-6-phosphate dehydrogenase, in the erythrocytes. Called also fabism.

**favus** a type of ringworm infection rare in the UK, with formation of scabs, in appearance like a honeycomb. It usually affects the scalp and is due to a fungus infection (Trichophyton schoenleinii).

**Fe** symbol for iron.

**fear** a normal emotional response, in contrast to anxiety and phobia, to consciously recognized external sources of danger; it is manifested by alarm, apprehension or disquiet. *Obsessional f.* a recurring irrational fear that is not amenable to ordinary reassurance; a phobia.

**febrile** characterized by or relating to fever. *F. convulsion* a convulsion which occurs in early childhood and is associated with pyrexia.

**fecundation** fertilization.

**fecundity** the ability to produce offspring frequently. In demography, the physiological ability to reproduce, as opposed to fertility.

**feedback** a method of homostatic control where some of the output is returned as input for monitoring purposes. Feedback mechanisms are important in the regulation of such physiological processes as hormone and enzyme reactions. *F. treatment see* BIOFEEDBACK. *Negative f.* a rise in the output of a substance is detected and further output is thus inhibited. *Positive f.* a rise in output causes either a direct or indirect rise in the output of another substance.

**Felty's syndrome** *A.R. Felty, American physician, 1895–1963.* The triad of rheumatoid arthritis, splenomegaly and leukopenia. Often associated with anaemia, lymphadenopathy and vasculitic cutaneous ulceration.

**feminization** 1. the normal induction or development of female sexual characteristics. 2. the induction or development of female secondary sexual characteristics in the male. *Testicular f.* a condition in which the subject is phenotypically female, but lacks nuclear sex chromatin and is of XY chromosomal sex.

**femoral** pertaining to the femur. *F. artery* that of the thigh from groin to knee. *F. canal* the opening below the inguinal ligament through which the femoral artery passes from the abdomen to the thigh.

**femur** the thigh bone.

**fenestra** a window-like opening. *F. ovalis* the oval opening between the middle and the internal ear.

**ferritin** a complex formed of an iron and protein molecule; one of the forms in which iron is stored in the body.

**ferrous** containing iron. *F. fumarate, f. gluconate, f. succinate* and *f. sulphate* are iron salts which are given orally to treat iron-deficiency anaemia.

**ferrule** a rubber cap used on the end of walking sticks, frames and crutches to prevent slipping.

**fertilization** the impregnation of the female sex cell, the ovum, by a male sex cell, a spermatozoon. *In vitro f.* artificial fertilization of the ovum in laboratory conditions. The timing and conditions for implantation into a uterus have to be perfect if successful pregnancy is to ensue.

**fester** to become superficially inflamed and to suppurate.

**festination** an involuntary tendency to take short accelerating steps in walking; seen in conditions such as Parkinson's disease.

**fetal** pertaining to the fetus. *F. alcohol syndrome* abbreviated FAS. Physical and mental abnormalities due to excessive maternal alcohol intake during pregnancy. Abnormalities may include microcephaly, growth deficiencies, mental handicap, hyperactivity, heart murmurs and skeletal malformation. The exact amount of alcohol consumption that will produce fetal damage is unknown, but the periods of gestation during which the alcohol is most likely to result in fetal damage are 3–4.5 months after conception and during the last trimester. *F. assessment* determination of the wellbeing of the fetus. Assessment techniques and procedures include: (a) medical and family histories and physical examination of the mother; (b) ULTRASONOGRAPHY; (c) assessment of fetal activity using the Cardiff kick chart; (d) chemical assessment of placental function; (e) assays of amniotic fluid obtained by AMNIOCENTESIS; and (f) electronic and ultrasonic fetal heart rate monitoring. *F. distress* the clinical manifestation of fetal hypoxia which may be due to maternal or fetal causes. *F. position* a position resembling that of the fetus in the womb, sometimes adopted by a child or adult in a state of distress or depression.

**fetishism** a state in which an object is regarded with an irrational fear, or an erotic attraction which may be so strong that the object is necessary for achieving sexual excitement.

**fetor** an offensive smell.

**fetoscope** an endoscope for viewing the fetus in utero.

**fetus** the developing baby between the eighth week and the end of pregnancy.

**fever** 1. an abnormally high body temperature; pyrexia. 2. any disease characterized by marked increase of body temperature.

**fibre** a thread-like structure.

**fibreoptics** the transmission of light rays along flexible tubes by means of very fine glass or plastic fibres. Use is made of this in endoscopic instruments such as the gastroscope.

**fibrescope** an endoscope in which fibreoptics are used.

**fibrillation** a quivering, vibratory movement of muscle fibres. *Atrial f.* rapid contractions of the atrium causing irregular contraction of the ventricles in both rhythm and force. *Ventricular f.* fine rapid twitchings of the ventricles leading to circulatory arrest. Rapidly fatal unless it can be controlled.

**fibrin** an insoluble protein that is essential to clotting of blood, formed from fibrinogen by action of thrombin.

**fibrinogen** a soluble protein which is present in blood plasma and is converted into fibrin by the action of thrombin when the blood clots.

**fibrinolysin** a proteolytic enzyme that dissolves fibrin.

**fibrinolysis** the dissolution of fibrin by the action of fibrinolysin. The process by which clots are removed from the circulation after healing has taken place.

**fibrinopenia** a deficiency of fibrinogen in the blood. There is a tendency to bleed as the coagulation time is increased.

**fibroadenoma** a benign tumour of glandular and fibrous tissue. *See* ADENOMA.

**fibroangioma** a benign tumour containing both fibrous and vascular tissue.

**fibroblast** a connective tissue cell.

**fibrocartilage** cartilage with fibrous tissue in it.

**fibrochondritis** inflammation of fibrocartilage.

**fibrocystic** fibrous and cystic. *F. disease of the pancreas* an inherited disease affecting the mucus-secreting glands, the sweat glands and the pancreas. It is characterized by fatty stools and repeated lung infections. Mucoviscidosis; cystic fibrosis.

**fibroid** 1. having a fibrous structure. 2. a fibroma or a fibromyoma, usually one occurring in the uterus.

**fibroma** a benign tumour of connective tissue.

**fibromyoma** a tumour consisting of fibrous and muscle tissue; frequently found in or on the uterus.

**fibroplasia** the formation of fibrous tissue when a wound heals. *Retrolental f.* a condition characterized by the presence of fibrous tissue behind the lens, leading to detachment of the retina and blindness, attributed to use of excessively high concentrations of oxygen in the care of preterm infants.

**fibrosarcoma** a malignant tumour arising in fibrous tissue.

**fibrosis** fibrous tissue formation, such as occurs in scar tissue or as the result of inflammation. It is the cause of adhesions of the peritoneum or other serous membranes. *F. of the lung* condition that may precede bronchiectasis and emphysema.

**fibrositis** inflammation of fibrous tissue. The term is loosely applied to pain and stiffness, particularly of the back muscles, for which no other cause can be found.

**fibula** the slender bone from knee to ankle, on the outer side of the leg.

**field of vision** the area within view, as for the fixed eye or a camera, or in an operation.

**fight or flight response** activation of the sympathetic nervous system in response to danger or stress.

**filament** a small thread-like structure.

**Filaria** a genus of nematode worms which may be found in the connective tissues and lymphatics, having been transmitted to humans by mosquitoes. Found mainly in the tropics and subtropics.

**filariasis** an infection by filaria, particularly by Wuchereria bancrofti, resulting in blockage of the lymphatics, which causes swelling of the surrounding tissues. Elephantiasis may occur.

**filiform** thread-like. *F. papillae* the fine thread-like processes that cover the anterior two-thirds of the tongue.

**filter** a device for eliminating certain elements, such as (a) particles of certain size from a solution, or (b) rays of a certain wavelength from a stream of radiant energy.

**filtrate** the fluid that passes through a filter.

**filtration** 1. the removal of precipitate from a liquid by means of a filter. 2. the removal of rays of a certain wavelength from an electromagnetic beam. *F. angle* the angle of the anterior chamber of the eye through which the aqueous humour drains; blockage of this channel gives rise to glaucoma.

**fimbria** a fringe. *F. of the uterine tube* the thread-like projections that surround the pelvic opening of the uterine tube.

**finger** a digit of the hand. *Clubbed f.* one with enlargement of the terminal phalanx with constant osseous changes; occurs in many heart and lung diseases. *F. spelling* see SIGN LANGUAGE. *Hammer f., mallet f.* permanent flexion of the distal phalanx of a finger due to avulsion of the extensor tendon. *Trigger f.* temporary flexion of a finger which is overcome in a sudden jerk by active or passive extension of the finger. It is caused by thickening of the flexor tendon in a narrowed tendon sheath. *Webbed f's* fingers more or less united by strands of tissue; syndactyly.

**fingerprint** the impression left upon a surface of the ridged pattern of the skin of the fingertips. Loops, whorls, arches and combinations of these form distinct patterns for each human individual and not even identical twins have the same fingerprint pattern.

**first aid** emergency care and treatment of an injured person before complete medical and surgical treatment can be secured.

**fission** a form of asexual reproduction by dividing into two equal parts, as in bacteria. *Binary f.* the splitting in two of the nucleus and the protoplasm of a cell, as in protozoa. *Nuclear f.* the splitting of the nucleus of an atom, with the release of a great quantity of energy.

**fissure** a narrow slit or cleft. *Anal f.* a painful crack in the mucous membrane of the anus. *F. of Rolando* a furrow in the cortex of each cerebral hemisphere, dividing the sensory from the motor area; the central sulcus.

**fistula** an abnormal passage between two epithelial surfaces, usually connecting the cavity of one organ with another or a cavity with the surface of the body. *Anal f.* the result of an ischiorectal abscess where the channel is from the anus to the skin. *Biliary f.* a leakage of bile to the exterior, following operation on the gallbladder or ducts. *Blind f.* one which is open at only one end. *Faecal f.* one in which the channel is from the intestine through the wound caused by an operation on the intestines when sepsis is present. *Rectovaginal f.* fistula from the rectum to the vagina which may result from a severe perineal tear during childbirth. *Tracheo-oesophageal f.* an opening from the trachea into the oesophagus; a congenital deformity. *Vesicovaginal f.* an opening from the bladder to the vagina, either from error during operation or from ulceration, as may occur in carcinoma of the cervix.

**fit** a commonly used term for paroxysmal motor discharges leading to sudden convulsive movements, as in epilepsy, eclampsia and hysteria.

**fitness** associated with a sense of wellbeing, and the ability to undertake sustained physical exertion without undue breathlessness. Fitness needs to be maintained on a regular basis by the person taking regular physical exertion or exercise.

**fixation** 1. the process of rendering something immovable, such as a joint or a fractured bone. 2. in psychology, a term used to describe a failure to progress wholly or in part through the normal stages of psychological development to a fully developed personality. 3. in optics, directing the sight straight at an object.

**flaccid** soft, flabby. *F. paralysis see* PARALYSIS.

**flail** exhibiting abnormal or pathological mobility. *F. chest* a loss of stability of the chest wall due to multiple rib fractures or detachment of the sternum from the ribs as a result of a severe crushing chest injury. The loose chest segment moves in a direction that is the reverse of normal. *F. joint* an unusually movable joint.

**flap** a mass of tissue, used for grafting in plastic surgery, which is left attached to its blood supply and used to repair defects either adjacent to it or at some distance from it.

**flare** the response of the skin to an allergic or hypersensitivity reaction. Reddening of the skin that spreads outwards.

**flatfoot** a condition due to absence or sinking of the medial longitudinal arch of the foot, caused by weakening of the ligaments and tendons.

**flatulence** excessive formation of gases in the stomach or intestine.

**flatulent** suffering from flatulence. *F. distension* swelling due to gas in the stomach or intestines. It is a common complication after abdominal operations and is caused by intestinal stasis.

**flatus** gas in the stomach or intestine.

**flea** a small, wingless blood-sucking insect parasite. The common human flea, *Pulex irritans*, rarely transmits disease. Cat and dog fleas, *Ctenocephalides*, are also relatively harmless. The rat fleas *Xenopsylla* and *Nosopsyllus* are the vectors of bubonic plague.

**flexion** bending; moving a joint so that the two or more bones forming it draw towards each other. *Plantar f.* bending the fingers or toes downwards.

**Flexner's bacillus** S. Flexner, American bacteriologist, 1863–1946. One of the group of pathogenic bacteria which cause bacillary dysentery; *Shigella flexneri*.

**flexor** any muscle causing flexion of a limb or other part of the body.

**flexure** a bend or curve.

**flight of ideas** the rapid movement of ideas and speech from one fragmentary topic to another that occurs in mania.

**floaters** wisps or strands within the eye that are visible to the patient. Usually caused by detachment and collapse of the vitreous humour and the normal ageing process.

**flooding** 1. excessive loss of blood from the uterus. 2. a form of desensitization for the treatment of phobias and related disorders. The patient is repeatedly exposed, in imagination or real life, to emotionally distressing aversive stimuli of high intensity. Also called implosion.

**florid** having a flushed facial appearance.

**flowmeter** an instrument used to measure the flow of liquids or gases.

**fluctuation** a wave-like motion felt on palpation of the abdomen.

**fluid** 1. a liquid or gas; any liquid of the body. 2. composed of molecules which freely change their relative positions without separation of the mass. *Amniotic f.* the fluid within the amnion that bathes the developing fetus and protects it from mechanical injury. *Body f's* the fluids within the body, composed of water, electrolytes and non-electrolytes. The volume and distribution of body fluids vary with age, sex and amount of adipose tissue (*see* Figure on p. 157). *Cerebrospinal f.* the fluid contained within the ventricles of the brain, the subarachnoid space and the central canal of the spinal cord. *Extracellular f.* fluid outside the cell, constituting one third of the total body fluid *F. chart* a chart kept by nurses recording the daily intake and output of fluids for a patient. The amount of intake and output is usually totalled every 24 hours. The chart provides a crude indicator for the patient's fluid balance status. *Interstitial f.* the extracellular fluid bathing most tissues, excluding the fluid within the lymph and blood vessels. *Intracellular f.* fluid within the cell, constituting two thirds of the total body fluid.

**fluid balance** a state in which the volume of body water and its solutes (electrolytes and non-electrolytes) is within normal limits and there is normal distribution of fluids within the intracellular and extracellular compartments. The total volume of body fluids should be about 60% of the body weight.

**fluke** one of a group of parasitic flatworms (Trematoda). Different varieties may affect the blood, the intestines, the liver or the lungs.

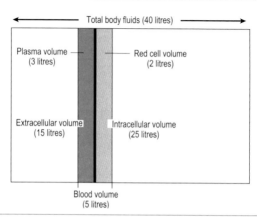

TOTAL BODY FLUIDS

**fluorescein** a dye used to detect corneal ulceration. When it is dropped on the eye the ulcer stains green.

**fluorescence** the property of reflecting back light waves, usually of a lower frequency than those absorbed so that invisible light (e.g. ultraviolet) may become visible.

**fluorescent** capable of producing fluorescence. *F. screen* a screen that becomes fluorescent when exposed to X-rays. *F. treponemal antibody test* a serological test for syphilis; the first to become positive after infection.

**fluoridation** the adding of fluorine to water, in those areas where it is lacking, in order to reduce the incidence of dental caries. Fluorine may also be added to tooth paste as a caries preventative.

**fluorine** *symbol* F.

**fluoroscope** an instrument for the study of moving internal organs and contrast medium using X-rays.

**flush** a redness of the face and neck. *Hectic f.* one occurring in conditions such as septic poisoning and pulmonary tuberculosis. *Hot f.* one occurring during the menopause, accompanied by a feeling of heat.

**flutter** an irregularity of the heart beat.

**focus** 1. the point of convergence of light or sound waves. 2. the local seat of a disease. *F. group* small group led by a leader, with the aim of generating data on a designated topic through discussion and interaction. A research technique.

**focusing** the ability of the eye to alter its lens power to focus correctly at different distances.

**folic acid** one of the VITAMINS of the B complex. Folic acid is involved in the synthesis of amino acids and DNA; its deficiency causes megaloblastic anaemia. Green vegetables, liver and yeast are major sources. *F. a. antagonist* any antimetabolite cytotoxic drug that inhibits the action of the folic acid enzyme.

**folie à deux** [Fr.] the occurrence of identical psychoses simultaneously in two closely associated persons.

**follicle** a very small sac or gland. *Hair f.* the sheath in which a hair grows. *F.-stimulating hormone* abbreviated FSH. A hormone, produced by the anterior pituitary gland, which controls the maturation of the GRAAFIAN FOLLICLES in the ovary.

**follicular** pertaining to a follicle. *F. conjunctivitis* inflammation occurring in the lower conjunctival fornix. *F. tonsillitis* tonsillitis arising from infection of the tonsillar follicles.

**folliculosis** an abnormal increase in the number of lymph follicles. *Conjunctival f.* a benign non-inflammatory overgrowth of follicles of the conjunctiva of the eyelids.

**fomentation** treatment by warm, moist applications; also, the substance thus applied.

**fomites** inanimate objects or material on which disease-producing agents may be conveyed.

**fontanelle** a soft membranous space between the cranial bones of an infant (*see* Figure). *Anterior f.* that between the parietal and frontal bones, which closes at about the age of 18 months. Rickets causes delay in this process. *Posterior f.* the junction of the occipital and parietal bones, at the sagittal suture, which closes within 3 months of birth.

**food** anything which, when taken into the body, serves to nourish or build up the tissues or to supply body heat. *F. additives see* ADDITIVES. *F. allergy* sensitivity to one or more of the components of a normal diet, e.g. peanuts, cow's milk or eggs. The reaction to the allergen usually occurs within a short period of ingesting the trigger

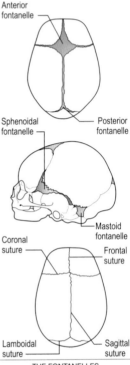

THE FONTANELLES

food and includes lip swelling, vomiting, abdominal distension and diarrhoea. Serious allergies can cause anaphylactic shock requiring a self-administered injection of adrenalin. The only effective treatment is total avoidance of the offending food. *See* ANAPHYLAXIS. *F. intolerance* an adverse reaction to a food or to a specific food ingredient that occurs each time the substance is ingested that is not due to food poisoning or involves the immune system. The specific cause of food intolerance may be difficult to trace, others more recognizable, e.g. lactose intolerance is due to a genetic deficiency of the enzyme lactase needed for the digestion of lactose in milk. *F. poisoning* a group of notifiable acute illnesses caused by ingestion of contaminated food. It may result from toxaemia from foods, such as those inherently poisonous or those contaminated by poisons, foods containing poisons formed by bacteria, or food-borne infections. Food poisoning usually causes inflammation of the gastrointestinal tract (gastroenteritis). This may occur quite suddenly, soon after the food has been eaten. The symptoms are acute, and include tenderness, pain or cramps in the abdomen, nausea, vomiting, diarrhoea, weakness and dizziness. *See* BOTULISM.

**Food Standards Agency** organization charged with protecting health in relation to food, with powers to act throughout the food chain to develop policies. Advises consumers, ministers and the food industry on all aspects of food safety and standards.

**foot** the terminal part of the lower limb. *Athlete's f.* ringworm of the foot; tinea pedis. *F. drop* inability to keep the foot at the correct angle owing to paralysis of the flexors of the ankle. *F. presentation* the presentation of one or both legs instead of the head during labour.

**foramen** an opening or hole, especially in a bone. *F. magnum* the hole in the occipital bone through which the spinal cord passes. *F. ovale* the hole between the left and right atria in the fetus. *Obturator f.* the large hole in the innominate

bone. *Optic f.* the opening in the posterior part of the orbit through which the optic nerve and the ophthalmic artery pass.

**forceps** surgical instruments used for lifting or compressing an object. *Artery f. (Spencer Wells f.)* compress bleeding points during an operation. *Cheatle f.* long forceps for lifting utensils. *Obstetric f.* various patterns are used in difficult labour to facilitate delivery. *Vulsellum f.* have claw-like ends for exerting traction.

**forensic** pertaining to or applied in legal proceedings. *F. medicine* the branch that is concerned with the law and has a bearing on legal problems. It includes the investigation of unexplained death or injury. *F. psychiatry* the consideration of current mental health laws and their relationship to mental health care and the consideration of issues such as diminished responsibility and fitness to stand trial. Mental health nurses work closely with the justice system and courts for offenders with mental health problems.

**foreskin** the prepuce.

**forgetfulness** the inability to remember or recall events, appointments, objects, etc. that make for daily life. Failure to retrieve memories may occur as a normal result of inattention although it is a common difficulty that develops with increasing age. In the elderly worsening forgetfulness may be associated with the development of dementia.

**formaldehyde** a gaseous compound with strongly disinfectant properties. It is used in solution for disinfection of excreta and utensils and also in the preparation of toxoids from toxins.

**formula** 1. an expression, using numbers or symbols, of the composition of, or of directions for preparing, a compound, such as a medicine; or of a procedure to follow to obtain a desired result; or of a single concept. 2. a mixture for feeding an infant, composed of milk and/or other ingredients.

**formulary** a prescriber's handbook of drugs. *See* BRITISH NATIONAL FORMULARY.

**fornix** an arch. *Conjunctival f.* the reflection of the conjunctiva from the eyelids on to the eyeball. *F. cerebri* an arched structure at the back and base of the brain. *F. of the vagina* the recesses at the top of the vagina in front (anterior f.), back (posterior f.) and sides (lateral f.) of the cervix uteri.

**fossa** a small depression or pit. Usually applied to fossae in bones. *Cubital f.* the triangular depression at the front of the elbow. *Iliac f.* the depression on the inner surface of the iliac bone. *Pituitary f.* the depression in the sphenoid bone. *See* SELLA TURCICA.

**foster children** children under the care of foster parents.

**foster parents** persons who undertake for reward the care of children who are not related to them within the meaning of the Children Act (1989).

**Fothergill's operation** *W.E. Fothergill, British gynaecologist, 1865–1926.* Amputation of the cervix, with anterior and posterior colporrhaphy for prolapse of the uterus.

**Foundation NHS Trusts** Foundation Trusts are subject to the same standards, performance ratings and systems of inspection as other NHS organizations, although they are free from the direction of the Secretary of State for Health. They have greater autonomy in the management of the organizational finances and are accountable to the Independent Regulator and inspected by the Commission for Healthcare Audit and Inspection. Members of the local community and staff directly elect represen-tatives to serve on the Board of Governors.

**fourchette** [Fr.] the fold of membrane at the perineal end of the vulva.

**fovea** a fossa; a small depression, particularly that of the retina which contains a large number of cones, giving form and colour, and is therefore the area of most accurate vision.

**fracture** 1. to break a part, especially a bone. 2. a break in the continuity of bone. The signs and symptoms are pain, swelling, deformity, shortening of the limb, loss of power, abnormal mobility, and crepitus. Fractures are generally caused by trauma, by either a direct or an indirect force on the bone. Fractures may also be caused by muscle spasm or by disease that results in decalcification of the bone. The different types and classification of fractures are shown in the Figure on p. 161. *March f.* a hairline crack in the long bone of the foot caused by repeated trauma associated with long marches and with jogging. *Pathological f.* one due to weakening of the bone structure by pathological processes, such as neoplasia, osteomalacia or osteomyelitis. *Pott's f.* a fracture dislocation of the ankle involving the lower end of the fibula and sometimes the internal malleolus of the tibia. *Spontaneous f.* one that occurs as a result of little or no violence, usually of a bone weakened by disease.

**frame** a rigid supporting structure or a structure for immobilizing a part. *Braun f.* a metal frame used to elevate the lower limb in fractures of the tibia and fibula. *Quadriplegic standing f.* a device for supporting in the upright position a patient whose four limbs are paralysed. *Stryker f.* one consisting of canvas stretched on anterior and posterior

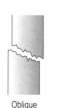
Oblique

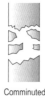
Comminuted

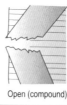
Open (compound)

Greenstick

FRACTURES OF BONE

frames, on which the patient can be rotated around the longitudinal axis. *Walking f.* a walking aid with three or four legs.

**freckle** a brown pigmented spot on the skin. *Hutchinson's melanotic f.* a non-invasive malignant melanoma which occurs mainly on the faces of middle-aged women.

**free association** in psychoanalysis a spontaneous mental process whereby words used in a non-logical chain suggest ideas, thoughts or feelings without selection or repression.

**Freedom of Information Act** all NHS organizations are required to have a publication scheme which sets out the type of information that it publishes or intends to publish, the form in which the information is published and details of any changes. NHS organizations must answer requests for information within the terms of the individual right of access given by the Act. This applies to all types of recorded information held by the organization regardless of its date, although the Act does include some specific exemptions.

**Frei's test** *W.S. Frei, German dermatologist, 1885–1943.* An intradermal test to aid the diagnosis of lymphogranuloma venereum.

**Freiberg's disease** *A.H. Freiberg, American surgeon, 1868–1940.*
Osteochondritis of the second metatarsal bone, in which there is pain on walking and standing.

**frenotomy** the cutting of the frenulum of the tongue to cure tongue-tie.

**frenulum** frenum; a fold of mucous membrane which limits the movement of an organ. *F. of the tongue* the fold under the tongue.

**Freudian** *S. Freud, Austrian psychiatrist, 1856–1939.* Relating to the theories of Freud, who was the originator of psychoanalysis and the psychoanalytical theory of the cause of neurosis.

**friable** easily crumbled or torn.

**friction** the act of rubbing one object against another. *F. massage* a circular or transverse pressure applied by fingertip or thumb to a localized area. Used for the relief of pain. *F. murmur* the grating sound heard in auscultation when two rough surfaces rub together, as in dry pleurisy.

**Friedländer's bacillus** *K. Friedländer, German pathologist, 1847–1887.* The cause of a rare form of pneumonia. *Klebsiella friedländeri.*

**Friedreich's ataxia** or **disease** *N. Friedreich, German physician, 1825–1882.* A rare form of hereditary ataxia.

**frigidity** an absence of normal sexual desire; usually refers to women.

**Frölich's syndrome** *A. Frölich, Austrian neurologist, 1871–1953.* A group of symptoms associated with disease of the pituitary body: increased adiposity, atrophy of the genital organs, and development of feminine characteristics.

**frontal** 1. relating to the forehead. 2. relating to the front or anterior aspect of a structure.

**frostbite** impairment of circulation, chiefly affecting the fingers, the toes, the nose and the ears, due to exposure to severe cold. The first stage is represented by chilblains. Advanced cases show thrombosis and dry gangrene.

**frottage** [Fr.] 1. a rubbing movement in massage. 2. sexual gratification by rubbing against another person's body.

**frozen shoulder** a stiff and painful shoulder; capsulitis. Treatment may include stretching under anaesthesia, combined with exercises and pain relief. The cause is unknown.

**frozen watchfulness** the state of a young child who is unresponsive to its surroundings, but is clearly aware of them. The state of frozen watchfulness is usually a marker of child abuse.

**fructose** fruit sugar, a monosaccharide.

**FSH** follicle-stimulating hormone.

**fugue** a period of altered awareness during which a person may wander for hours or days and perform purposive actions although memory for the period may be lost. It may follow an epileptic fit or occur in hysteria or schizophrenia.

**fulguration** the destruction by diathermy of papillomata (warts), particularly inside the urinary bladder.

**fulminating** sudden in onset and rapid in course.

**fumigation** disinfection by exposure to the fumes of a vaporized germicide.

**function** 1. the natural action or intended purpose of a person,

organ or structure. 2. to perform special work or an action.

**fundus** the base of an organ or the part farthest removed from the opening. *F. of the eye* the posterior part of the inside of the eye as shown by the ophthalmoscope. *F. of the stomach* that part above the cardiac orifice. *F. of the uterus* the top of the uterus; that part farthest from the cervix.

**fungate** to grow rapidly and produce fungus-like growths. Often occurs in the late stages of malignant tumours.

**fungicide** a preparation that destroys fungal infection.

**fungiform** shaped like a fungus or mushroom.

**fungus** a low form of vegetable life which includes mushrooms and moulds. Some varieties cause disease, such as actinomycosis and ringworm.

**funnel chest** a developmental deformity in which there is a depression in the sternum and an inward curvature of the ribs and costal cartilages.

**furor** a state of intense excitement during which violent acts may be performed. This may occur after an epileptic fit.

**furuncle** a boil.

**furunculosis** a staphylococcal infection represented by many, or crops of, boils.

**furunculus** a furuncle. *F. orientalis* a protozoal infection, mainly of the tropics, which causes a chronic ulceration. Cutaneous leishmaniasis.

**fusiform** shaped like a spindle.

**fusion** 1. the union between two adjacent structures. 2. the coordination of separate images of the same object in the two eyes into one image.

*Fusobacterium* a genus of anaerobic Gram-negative bacteria found as normal flora in the mouth and large bowel, and often in necrotic tissue, probably as secondary invaders.

**g** symbol for *gram*.

**G** symbol for *guanine*.

**Ga** symbol for *gallium*.

**gag** 1. an instrument placed between the teeth to keep the mouth open. 2. the reflex action that occurs when the back of the throat is stimulated.

**gait** manner of walking. *Ataxic g.* the foot is raised high, descends suddenly, and the whole sole strikes the ground. *Cerebellar g.* a staggering walk indicative of cerebellar disease. *Four-point g.* a method which may be adopted when using sticks or crutches, which allows maximum stability. *Spastic g.* stiff, shuffling walk, the legs being kept together.

**galactorrhoea** 1. an excessive flow of milk. 2. secretion of milk after breast feeding has ceased.

**galactosaemia** an inborn error of metabolism in which there is inability to convert galactose to glucose. The disorder becomes manifest soon after birth and is characterized by feeding problems, vomiting, diarrhoea, abdominal distension, enlargement of the liver and mental handicap. Treatment consists of exclusion from the diet of milk and all foods containing galactose or lactose.

**galactose** a monosaccharide derived from lactose. D-Galactose is found in lactose or milk sugar and cerebrosides of the brain. *G. tolerance test* a laboratory test to determine the liver's ability to convert the sugar galactose into glycogen.

**gallbladder** the sac under the lower surface of the liver, which acts as a reservoir for bile.

**gallium** *symbol* Ga. A radioisotope used in detecting some soft-tissue disorders.

**gallop rhythm** heart rhythm that may occur when there is ventricular overload.

**gallstone** a concretion formed in the gallbladder or bile ducts. Gallstones vary in size and may be multiple and faceted. *G. colic see* BILIARY (COLIC).

**gamete** a sex cell which combines with another to form a zygote, from which a complete organism develops. A spermatozoon or an ovum.

**gamete intrafallopian transfer** abbreviated GIFT. A technique for assisting conception. The woman must have at least one patent fallopian tube. Oocytes and spermatozoa are mixed in the laboratory and introduced into a fallopian tube, and the fertilized egg may then become embedded in the uterus.

**gametocyte** a cell that is undergoing gametogenesis.

**gametogenesis** the production of the gametes by the gonads.

**gamma** the third letter in the Greek alphabet. *G. camera* an apparatus for depicting a part of the body into which radioactive isotopes emitting gamma rays have been introduced. *G. encephalography* a method of localizing a brain tumour by using radioactive isotopes emitting gamma rays. *G.-globulin* a class of plasma proteins composed almost entirely of IgG, an IMMUNOGLOBULIN protein that contains most antibody activity. *G. rays* electromagnetic rays, of shorter wavelength and with greater penetration than X-rays, which are given off by certain radioactive substances and which are used in radiotherapy. Also used in the sterilization of articles that would be destroyed by the heat and moisture required in autoclaving.

**ganglion** 1. a collection of nerve cells and fibres, forming an independent nerve centre, as is found in the sympathetic nervous system. 2. a cystic swelling on a tendon.

**ganglionectomy** excision of a ganglion.

**gangrene** death of body tissue, generally in considerable mass, due either to loss of blood supply or to the effects of certain infections. *Dry g.* occurs gradually and results from slow reduction of the blood flow in the arteries. There is no subsequent bacterial decomposition; the tissues become dry and shrivelled. It occurs only in the extremities, and can occur with ARTERIOSCLEROSIS and DIABETES (MELLITUS). *Gas g.* results from dirty lacerated wounds infected by anaerobic bacteria, especially species of *Clostridium*. It is an acute, severe, painful condition in which muscles and subcutaneous tissues become filled with gas and a serosanguineous exudate. *Moist g.* caused by sudden stoppage of blood, resulting from burning by heat or acid, severe freezing, physical accident that destroys the tissue, or a clot or other embolism. At first, tissue affected by moist

gangrene has the colour of a bad bruise, and is swollen and often blistered. The gangrene is likely to spread with great speed. Toxins are formed in the affected tissues and absorbed.

**Ganser's syndrome (state)** *S.J.M. Ganser, German psychiatrist, 1853–1931.* Amnesia, disturbance of consciousness and hallucinations, associated with senseless answers to questions, and absurd acts. Usually a transient response to a troublesome situation, e.g. prisoners on remand (prison psychosis).

**gargle** 1. a solution for rinsing the mouth and throat. 2. to rinse the mouth and throat by holding a solution in the open mouth and agitating it by expulsion of air from the lungs.

**gargoylism** *see* HURLER'S SYNDROME.

**gas** molecules of a substance very loosely combined; a vapour. *G. and air analgesia* an authorized form of analgesia using nitrous oxide and air, by which the pains of labour are lessened without affecting uterine contractions. *Laughing g.* nitrous oxide. *Marsh g.* methane. *Sternutatory g.* one that causes sneezing. *Tear g.* one that is irritating to the eyes and causes excessive lacrimation.

**Gasser's ganglion** *J.L. Gasser, Austrian anatomist, 1723–1765.* The trigeminal ganglion. The ganglion of the sensory root of the fifth cranial nerve.

**gastrectomy** excision of part or whole of the stomach. *Billroth g.* removal of most of the lesser curvature and pyloric portion and joining of the duodenum to the refashioned stomach. This cuts down the production of secretin and acid. *Partial g.* removal of a part, usually the distal portion, of the stomach. Commonly performed in the surgical treatment of peptic ulcer. *Polya g.* removal of the first part of the duodenum and the greater part of the stomach, and anastomosis of the stomach to the jejunum. The blind portion of the duodenum supplies the bile and pancreatic and duodenal secretions.

**gastric** pertaining to the stomach. *G. analysis* analysis of the stomach contents by microscopy and tests to determine the amount of acid present. *G. bypass* surgical creation of a small gastric pouch that empties directly into the jejunum through a gastrojejunostomy, thereby causing food to bypass the duodenum; performed for the treatment of gross OBESITY. *G. flu* a popular term for what may be any of several disorders of the stomach and intestinal tract. The symptoms are nausea, diarrhoea, abdominal cramps and fever. *G. juice* the clear fluid secreted by the glands of the stomach to assist digestion. It contains an enzyme called pepsin, which acts upon proteins in the presence of weak hydrochloric acid. *G. lavage* a treatment for some types of poisoning where the stomach contents are washed out through a stomach tube. *G. ulcer* ulceration of the gastric mucosa, associated with hyperacidity and often precipitated by *Helicobacter pylori* organisms. The condition is often aggravated by stress.

**gastrin** a hormone, secreted by the walls of the stomach, which excites continued secretion of digestive juice while food is in the stomach.

**gastritis** inflammation of the lining of the stomach.

**gastro-oesophagostomy** a surgical anastomosis between the stomach and the oesophagus.

**gastrocnemius** the principal muscle of the calf of the leg. It flexes both the ankle and the knee.

**gastrocolic** pertaining to the stomach and colon. *G. reflex* after a meal, increased peristalsis causes the colon to empty into the rectum. This gives rise to a desire to defecate.

**gastroduodenostomy** a surgical anastomosis between the stomach and the duodenum.

**gastroenteritis** inflammation of the stomach and intestines causing episodes of nausea, vomiting, appetite loss, fever, abdominal pain and diarrhoea. A mild episode usually only lasts a few days but a severe one may cause dehydration, shock and collapse especially in children and the elderly. The illness maybe caused by any one of a number of organisms: bacteria, bacterial toxins, viruses and other organisms in food and water.

**gastroenterology** the study of diseases of the gastrointestinal tract.

**gastroenterostomy** a surgical anastomosis between the stomach and small intestine.

**gastroileac** pertaining to the stomach and ileum. *G. reflex* food entering the stomach sets up powerful peristalsis in the ileum and opening of the ileocaecal valve.

**gastrointestinal** pertaining to the stomach and intestine. *G. tract* the alimentary tract.

**gastrojejunostomy** a surgical anastomosis between the stomach and the jejunum.

**gastroscope** an endoscope especially designed for passage into the stomach to permit examination of its interior. The gastroscope is a hollow, cylindrical tube, fitted with special lenses and lights, which acts by reflecting light and creating a mirror effect, making it possible to 'go around corners', and facilitating visualization of the curvature of the stomach.

**gastrostomy** the creation of an opening into the stomach. This procedure is done to provide for the administration of food and liquids when stricture of the oesophagus or other conditions make swallowing impossible. *See* ARTIFICIAL (FEEDING).

**gastrotomy** a surgical incision of the stomach.

**gastrula** an early stage in the development of the fertilized ovum.

**gate control theory of pain** theory proposing that a neural mechanism in the dorsal horns of the spinal cord acts like a gate which can increase or decrease the flow of nerve impulses from peripheral fibres to the central nervous system. It is the position of the gate that determines how much information is transmitted to the brain and therefore on the amount of pain generated. Influences such as anxiety and anticipation cause the gate to open and therefore increase the level of pain experienced, whereas other factors may cause the gate to close, thereby reducing the pain.

**gatekeepers** the individuals or groups in an organization who regulate access to goods and services, e.g. the general practitioner's receptionist.

**gateway drug** generic name for alcohol, cocaine or cannabis referring to their supposed roles as conduits leading on to the taking of harder drugs.

**Gaucher's disease** *P.C.E. Gaucher, French physician, 1854–1918.* A rare familial disease in which fat is deposited in the reticuloendothelial cells, causing an enlarged spleen and anaemia.

**gauze** a thin open-meshed material used for dressing wounds.

**gavage** [Fr.] forced feeding; the giving of fluids and nourishment by oesophageal or other type of tube directly into the stomach.

**gay** popular term for a homosexual, usually male. *G. bowel syndrome* the damaging effects of male homosexual practices on the lower bowel; also includes anal fissures, anal fistulas, haemorrhoids and ulcers.

**Geiger counter** *H. Geiger, German physicist, 1882–1945.* An instrument for detecting and registering radioactivity. The apparatus is sensitive to the rays emitted.

**gelatin** an albuminoid, obtained from connective tissue or bone. Used in pharmacy for suppositories and capsules, and in bacteriology as a culture medium. In absorbable film and sponge, it is used in surgical procedures.

**gender** the perceived differences between the two sexes that generates social differentiation, inequality, discrimination and prejudice. Gender is a social identity and distinct from 'sex' which relates to the biological differences between men and women. *G. identity* the concept or inner feeling that a person has of being male and masculine or female and feminine. Differentiation of gender identity begins in infancy, continuing through childhood, and reinforced in adolescence. This includes parental attitudes and expectations as well as psychological and social pressures. *G. identity disorder* a psychiatric label for those disorders marked by a sense of inappropriateness and attendant discomfort concerning one's sexual anatomy and sex role. This category usually includes transvestism, transsexualism and gender identity disorders in childhood.

**gene** one of the biological units of heredity, self-reproducing and located at a definite position (locus) on a particular chromosome. *Dominant g.* one that is capable of transmitting its characteristics irrespective of the genes from the other parent. *G. therapy* the use of 'healthy' genes to cure or treat a hereditary disease.

*Recessive g.* one that can pass on its characteristics only if it is present with a similar recessive gene from the other parent. *See* MENDEL'S THEORY.

**General Household Survey (GHS)** started in 1971, now under the auspices of the Office for National Statistics; initially for use by all government departments but also provides a secondary data source for the social sciences. It is a continuous survey and includes five main areas of investigation: family data, employment, housing, education and health.

**General Medical Council** abbreviated GMC. The regulating body of all medical practitioners within the UK; the medical equivalent of the Nursing and Midwifery Council. It licenses doctors to practise and is charged with: (a) keeping the register of practising doctors up to date; (b) fostering good medical practice; (c) promoting high standards in medical education; and (d) dealing firmly and fairly with doctors whose fitness for practice is in doubt.

**general practitioner** abbreviated GP. The role of the general practitioner or primary care physician in the UK is unique. Besides being the first point of contact for most patients, GPs must offer the first treatment or referral for all problems which are presented to them. In addition, GPs give personal and continuing care to their patients and families, often over the course of many years.

**General Social Care Council** abbreviated GSCC. An independent regulatory body which safeguards public protection by promoting and monitoring high standards of conduct, practice and training for social care workers. The council regulates the workforce with a code of practice for all social care workers and their employers and maintaining a register of social care workers.

**generic** 1. pertaining to a genus. 2. non-proprietary, relating to a drug name not protected by a trademark, usually descriptive of the drug's chemical structure.

**genetic** 1. pertaining to reproduction or to birth or origin. 2. inherited. *G. code* the arrangement of genetic material stored in the DNA molecule of the chromosome. *G. counselling* supportive service for prospective parents who can receive advice as to the likelihood of their children being born with a genetically transmitted disorder. *G. engineering* the alteration of a genome of an organism to change its heritable characteristics. In practice this technique currently is used to mass produce a variety of drugs and vaccines used in medical treatment, e.g. growth hormone and human insulin. Further development offers enormous scope for the advancement of medicine in the treatment of disease and genetic disorders. *G. screening* tests used to screen individuals whose genotypes are associated with specific diseases. These individuals may develop the disease itself or pass it on to their offspring.

**genetics** the study of heredity and natural development.

**genitalia** the organs of reproduction.

**genitourinary** referring to both the reproductive organs and the urinary tract.

**genotype** the genetic characteristics of an individual either over the genome as a whole or at one particular locus.

**genupectoral** relating to the knee and chest. *G. position* the knee–chest position. *See* POSITION.

**geriatrics** the branch of medicine covering old age and the disorders arising from it.

**germ** 1. a microbe. 2. that from which something may develop; a seed.

**German measles** *See* RUBELLA.

**germicide** an agent capable of destroying pathogenic microorganisms.

**germinoma** a neoplasm of the testis or ovum.

**gerontology** the study of the changes associated with old age and the ageing processes. Includes both mind and body and involves many disciplines, e.g. psychology, sociology, pharmacology, biology and social care.

**Gessells developmental chart** *A. Gessell, American psychologist, 1880–1961*. A chart that shows the expected motor, social and psychological development of children.

**gestaltism** a theory of holism in psychology which claims that ideas come as a whole and are not subdivisible.

**gestation** the period of development of the young in mammals, from the time of fertilization of the ovum to birth. *See also* PREGNANCY. *Ectopic g.* fetal development in some part other than the uterus, usually the uterine tube. *G. period* the duration of pregnancy; in the human female about 280 days when measured from the first day of the last menstrual period. *See also* EXPECTED DATE OF DELIVERY.

**Ghon focus** *A. Ghon, Czechoslovakian pathologist, 1866–1936*. The primary lesion of pulmonary tuberculosis, as seen on chest radiograph, after it has healed by fibrosis and calcification.

**giardiasis** *A. Giard, French biologist, 1846–1908*. An infection with *Giardia lamblia*, a pear-shaped protozoon that causes a persistent protracted diarrhoea, often resulting in intestinal malabsorption.

**gigantism** abnormal growth of the body, often due to overactivity of the anterior lobe of the pituitary gland.

**Gilles de la Tourette's syndrome (disease)** *G.E.A.B. Gilles de la Tourette, French neurologist, 1857–1904*. Multiple tics, especially of the face and upper part of the body, often associated with involuntary obscene utterances. The condition usually has its onset in childhood and often becomes chronic. The cause is unknown.

**gingiva** the gum; connective tissue surrounding the necks of the teeth.

**gingivectomy** the surgical removal of the gum margins to get rid of pockets and improve the shape of the gums.

**gingivitis** inflammation of the gums.

**ginko** extract from the maidenhair tree, used by herbalists and naturopaths and claimed to be helpful in circulatory disorders, reduced circulation in the brain, senility, depression and premenstrual syndrome.

**ginseng** extract of the root of plants of genus *Panax*, used widely in Chinese medicine; reputed to have the power to cure many diseases and to have properties to improve sexual health and impotence.

**gland** an organ composed of specialized cells which secrete fluid prepared from the blood, either for use in the body, or for excretion as waste material. *Ductless (endocrine) g.* one that produces an internal secretion but has no canal (duct) to carry the secretion away, e.g. the thyroid gland. *Exocrine g.* one that discharges its secretion through a duct, e.g. the parotid gland. *Lymph g. see* LYMPH (NODES). *Mucous g.* one that secretes mucus.

**glanders** a disease of horses communicable to humans, and caused by the glanders bacillus, *Pseudomonas mallei*.

**glandular** pertaining to a gland. *G. fever see* MONONUCLEOSIS, INFECTIOUS.

**glans** [L.] *acom.* An acorn-shaped body, such as the rounded end of the penis or the clitoris.

**Glasgow Coma Scale** a standardized system for quickly evaluating the level of consciousness in the critically ill. Measures include: eye opening according to four criteria, verbal response against five criteria, and motor response using six criteria. Scores of 7 or less qualify as 'coma'. Coma is defined as no response and no eye opening.

**glass test** a simple test for meningitis that involves pressing a clear glass against a rash. If the rash remains visible it may indicate purpura, which occurs in meningitis. *See* MENINGITIS.

**glaucoma** raised intraocular pressure. *Closed-angle g.* one that occurs when there is a mechanical defect in the drainage angle; may be primary or secondary. It may be acute, when there is pain and blurring of vision, or chronic, when there may be no pain, but a gradual loss of vision. *Open-angle g.* chronic primary glaucoma in which the angle remains open but drainage becomes gradually diminished; tends to run in families. *Primary g.* one that occurs without any previous disease. It is a common cause of blindness, partial or complete, in the elderly. *Secondary g.* one that occurs when some ocular disease is complicated by an increase in intraocular pressure.

**gleet** chronic gonococcal urethritis marked by a transparent mucous discharge.

**glenoid** resembling a hollow. *G. cavity* the socket of the shoulder joint.

**glia** neuroglia; the connective tissue of the brain and spinal cord.

**glioblastoma** a malignant glioma arising in the cerebral hemispheres.

**glioma** a malignant tumour composed of neuroglial cells affecting the brain and spinal cord; seldom metastasizes.

**globulins** a protein group, forming constituents of the blood (*serum g.*) and cerebrospinal fluid.

**globus** a ball or globe. *G. hystericus* a symptom of hysteria when a patient feels unable to swallow because there is a lump in the throat. *G. pallidus* the pale medial part of the lentiform nucleus of the brain.

**glomerulitis** inflammation of the glomeruli of the kidney.

**glomerulonephritis** a bilateral, non-infectious inflammation of the kidneys. The cause is unknown but the condition is associated with immunological disturbance. It may be acute, presenting rapidly but reversibly, or it may be chronic, presenting slowly and irreversibly.

**glomerulosclerosis** degenerative changes in the glomerular capillaries of the renal tubule, leading to renal failure.

**glomerulus** the tuft of capillaries within the nephron, which filters urine from the blood.

**glossal** relating to the tongue.

**glossitis** inflammation of the tongue.

**glossolalia** 'speaking in tongues'; unintelligible speech. The patient speaks in an imaginary language.

**glossopharyngeal** pertaining to the tongue and pharynx. *G. nerve* the ninth cranial nerve.

**glossoplegia** paralysis of the tongue.

**glottis** the space between the vocal cords. The term is sometimes used for that part of the larynx which is associated with voice production.

**glucagon** a polypeptide produced by the pancreas. It aids glycogen breakdown in the liver and raises the blood sugar level.

**glucocorticoid** any corticoid substance that raises the concentration of liver glycogen and blood sugar,

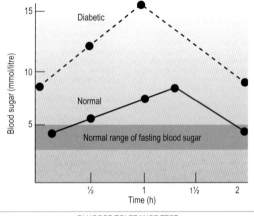

GLUCOSE TOLERANCE TEST

i.e. cortisol (hydrocortisone), cortisone and corticosterone.

**gluconeogenesis** the production of glucose from the non-nitrogen portion of the amino acids after deamination. It occurs in the liver and kidneys.

**glucose** dextrose or grape-sugar; a simple sugar, a monosaccharide in certain foodstuffs, especially fruit, and in normal blood; the chief source of energy for living organisms. *See also* DEXTROSE. *G.-6-phosphate dehydrogenase* a red-cell enzyme. Inherited deficiency causes a tendency to haemolytic anaemia. *See* FAVISM. *G. tolerance test* test in which a quantity of glucose is given and the concentration of glucose in the blood is estimated at intervals afterwards (*see* Figure). Used mainly when diabetes mellitus is suspected.

**glue ear** the accumulation of sticky material in the middle ear resulting in impaired hearing, most common in young schoolchildren.

**glue sniffing** solvent abuse.

**glutamic acid** one of the 22 amino acids formed by the digestion of dietary protein.

**glutamic–oxaloacetic transaminase** an enzyme found in cardiac muscle and the liver. Raised serum levels (SGOT) may indicate an acute myocardial infarction or the presence of liver disease.

**glutamic–pyruvic transaminase** an enzyme found in the liver. Measurement of serum levels (SGPT) is used in the study and diagnosis of liver diseases.

**glutaraldehyde** a disinfectant active against all viruses, fungi, vegetative bacteria and spores. Used in aqueous solution for sterilization of non-heat-resistant equipment.

**gluteal** relating to the buttocks. *G. muscles* three muscles that form the fleshy part of the buttocks.

**gluten** a sticky protein found in wheat and other cereals, e.g. rye and barley. Gluten consists of two proteins: gliadin and glutenin. Some people are sensitive to gluten, which causes in them intestinal malabsorption (gluten-induced enteropathy). *G.-induced enteropathy see* COELIAC DISEASE.

**glycaemic index** GI the classification of carbohydrate foods based on their overall effects on blood glucose levels. Carbohydrates are ranked 1 to 100. Foods with a low GI factor, e.g. wholegrain cereals, raise blood glucose levels a little and are absorbed more slowly and evenly, whereas those with a high GI factor, e.g. refined flours and sugars, raise blood glucose sharply and considerably. Low level GI diets have been shown to improve blood glucose and lipid levels in people with type 1 and type 2 diabetes.

**glycerin** a colourless syrupy substance obtained from fats and fixed oils. It has a hygroscopic action. As an emollient it is an ingredient of many skin preparations. *G. suppository* one composed of glycerin and gelatin, used as an evacuant. *G. of thymol* an antiseptic mouthwash and gargle.

**glycine** a non-essential amino acid.

**glycogen** the form in which carbohydrate is stored in the liver and muscles. Animal starch. *G. storage disease* inherited disease in which there is a deficiency in the synthesis of glycogen. This accumulates in the liver, causing enlargement.

**glycogenesis** the process of glycogen formation from the blood glucose.

**glycogenolysis** the breakdown of glycogen in the body so that it may be utilized.

**glycosuria** an excess of glucose in the urine, a symptom of diabetes mellitus. *Renal g.* sugar in the urine, in an otherwise healthy person, due to an inherited inability to reabsorb glucose normally.

**gnathic** pertaining to the jaw.

**goal** a statement of what a nursing intervention is expected to achieve in either the short or longer term. May also be referred to as an outcome. *See* NURSING.

**goblet cell** a goblet-shaped cell, found in the intestinal epithelium, which produces mucus.

**goitre** enlargement of the thyroid gland, causing a swelling in the front part of the neck. Simple endemic goitre, sometimes referred to as Derbyshire neck, is usually caused by lack of iodine in the diet. *Colloid g.* an enlarged but soft thyroid gland with no signs of hyperthyroidism. *Exophthalmic g.* hyperthyroidism with marked protrusion of the eyeballs (exophthalmos). Graves' disease. *Intrathoracic g.* enlargement of the gland mainly in the thorax, so the swelling may not be easily visible. *Sporadic g.* a simple non-toxic enlargement. *Substernal g.* enlargement of the gland under the sternum so that swelling in the neck may not be apparent. *Toxic g.* signs of excess of thyroxine in the blood, where the gland has not been previously enlarged. The patient complains of weight loss and is generally nervous. Exophthalmos may be present.

**gold** *symbol* Au. A metallic element used in treating rheumatoid arthritis. *Radioactive g.* an isotope that gives off beta and gamma rays. Used, in the form of small grains or seeds, in the treatment of some malignant conditions.

**Golgi apparatus** *C. Golgi, Italian histologist, 1844–1926.* Specialized structures seen near the nucleus of a cell during microscopic examination.

**Golgi's organ** the sensory end-organs in muscle tendons that are sensitive to stretch.

**gonad** a reproductive gland; the testicle or ovary.

**gonadotrophic** having influence on the gonads. *G. hormone* gonadotrophin.

**gonadotrophin** any hormone having a stimulating effect on the gonads. Two such hormones are secreted by the anterior pituitary: follicle-stimulating hormone (FSH) and luteinizing hormone (LH), both of which are active, but with differing effects, in the two sexes. *Chorionic g.* a gonad-stimulating hormone produced by cytotrophoblastic cells of the placenta; used in the treatment of underdevelopment of the gonads and to induce ovulation in infertile women.

**gonioscope** an apparatus for examining the angle of the anterior chamber of the eye.

**goniotomy** an operation for glaucoma; it consists in opening Schlemm's canal under direct vision.

**gonococcus** *Neisseria gonorrhoeae*, a diplococcus which causes gonorrhoea.

**gonorrhoea** a common venereal disease caused by *Neisseria gonorrhoeae* infecting the genital tract of either sex, causing a discharge and pain on micturition, although the disease is often asymptomatic in females. Spread by the bloodstream, it may give rise to iritis or arthritis. Scar tissue formation may bring about urethral stricture or infertility owing to occlusion of the uterine tubes. The eyes of babies may be infected at birth during passage through the birth canal of an infected mother. The condition is called OPHTHALMIA (NEONATORUM) (notifiable disease). In the past it was a major cause of blindness in babies.

**gonorrhoeal** relating to gonorrhoea. *G. arthritis* intractable infection of joints, causing great pain and disability.

**goose-flesh** the reaction of the skin to cold and fear. The blood vessels and hair follicles in the skin contract causing the hair to stand up giving the impression of plucked poultry skin. Also known as goose pimples.

**gout** a form of arthritis with an excess of uric acid in the blood. It is characterized by painful inflammation and swelling of the smaller joints, especially those of the big toe and thumb. Inflammation is accompanied by the deposit of urates around the joints.

**Graafian follicle** *R. de Graaf, Dutch physician and anatomist, 1641–1673.* A follicle which is formed in the ovary and contains an ovum. A follicle matures during each menstrual cycle, ruptures and releases the ovum (ovulation), which is then picked up by the fimbriated end of the uterine tube.

**graft** 1. any tissue or organ for implantation or transplantation. 2. to implant or transplant such tissue. *Autogenous g.* a graft taken from and given to the same individual. *Bone g.* a portion of bone transplanted to repair another bone. *Corneal g.* a portion of cornea, usually from a recently dead person, used to repair a diseased cornea. *Homologous g.* tissue obtained from the body of another animal of the same species but with a genotype differing from that of the recipient; a homograft or allograft. *Pedicle g.* a skin graft, one end of which remains attached to its original site until the grafting has become established.

**graft-versus-host disease (reaction)** abbreviated GVH disease. A condition that occurs when immunologically competent cells or their precursors are transplanted into an immunologically incompetent recipient (host) that is not histocompatible with the donor.

Characteristic signs include skin lesions, ulceration, alopecia, painful joints and haemolytic anaemia. GVH disease is a frequent complication of bone marrow transplants. Human leukocyte antigen (HLA) matching of the donor and recipient reduces the possibility of GVH disease.

**gram** *symbol* g. The fundamental SI unit of weight, equal to one thousandth of a kilogram.

**Gram's stain** *H. Gram, Danish physician, 1853–1938.* A method of staining bacteria which is used to classify them into Gram-negative and Gram-positive.

**grand mal** [Fr.] major epilepsy. *See* EPILEPSY.

**grande multipara** a woman who has borne four or more children. Increasing parity can lead to an increased risk of problems in pregnancy, labour and the puerperium.

**granular** containing small particles. *G. casts* the degenerated cells from the lining of renal tubules excreted in the urine in certain kidney disorders.

**granulation** 1. the division of a hard solid substance into small particles. 2. the growth of new tissue by which ulcers and wounds heal when the edges are not in apposition. It consists of new capillaries and fibroblasts which fill in the space and later form fibrous tissue. The resulting scar is often unsightly.

**granulocyte** any cell containing granules in its cytoplasm, especially polymorphonuclear leukocytes which contain neutrophilic, basophilic and eosinophilic granules in their cytoplasm.

**granulocytopenia** a marked reduction in the number of granulocytes in the blood. The condition may precede agranulocytosis.

**granuloma** a tumour composed of granulation tissue, usually due to chronic infection or invasion by a foreign body.

**granulomatosis** an infection producing granulomata. *Lipoid g.* xanthomatosis; Hand–Schüller–Christian disease. *Malignant g.* lymphadenoma; Hodgkin's disease.

**gravel** small 'sandy' calculi formed in the kidneys and bladder, and sometimes excreted with the urine. They can also form in the gallbladder where they can accumulate or cause low-grade cholecystitis.

**Graves' disease** *R.J. Graves, Irish physician, 1796–1853.* Exophthalmic goitre; thyrotoxicosis.

**gravid** pregnant.

**gravity** weight. *Specific g.* the weight of a substance compared with that of an equal volume of water.

**gray** *symbol* Gy. The SI unit used to denote the absorbed dose in radiation therapy.

**grey-scale display** a method to show the texture of tissue on ultrasound display. The amplitude of each echo is represented by varying shades of grey. A bright white outline is seen from specular surfaces, a mottled grey from various tissue areas, and black from collections of fluid, such as the bladder and amniotic sac.

**grid** a chart with horizontal and vertical lines on which curves may be plotted.

**grief** *see* BEREAVEMENT.

**groin** the junction of the upper thigh with the abdomen. The groins slope outwards and upwards from the pubic region.

**grounded theory** a qualitative research approach which emphasizes the process of theory generation from systematically collected and stored data, the concept being that the theory remains 'grounded in' the data, demonstrating the fit between the theory and the supporting empirical evidence.

**group practice** medical or midwifery practice carried out by a team of general practitioners or midwives (often independent midwives) working together.

**group therapy** a form of psychotherapy in which a group of 4–12 patients meets regularly with the therapist in order to discuss and share problems, anxieties and fears in a psychotherapeutic setting. The group also provides emotional support for self-revelation and a structured environment for trying out new ways of relating to people.

**growing pains** recurrent quasirheumatic limb pains peculiar to early youth, once believed to be caused by the growing process. It is now recognized that growth does not cause pain and that these pains can be a symptom of many different disorders.

**growth** 1. the progressive development of a living thing, especially the process by which the body reaches its point of complete physical development. 2. an abnormal formation of tissue, such as a tumour. *G. hormone* a substance that stimulates growth, especially a secretion of the anterior lobe of the pituitary gland that directly influences protein, carbohydrate and lipid metabolism, and controls the rate of skeletal and visceral growth. *See* CREUTZFELDT–JAKOB DISEASE.

**guanine** a purine base, one of the constituents of all nucleic acids.

**guardian *ad litem*** a person usually from the local authority social service department, who is appointed by a court to look after the interests of a child before its full Adoption Order is granted. Meanwhile the prospective adoptive parents have continuous possession of the child, and are visited and interviewed by the guardian *ad litem* to ensure that the home will be satisfactory.

**guardian Caldicott** a named member of an NHS Trust who is responsible for agreeing and reviewing internal protocols governing the protection and use of patient identified information by staff within the health care system. This nominated person is also responsible for ensuring that these protocols meet the requirements of relevant national guidance and/or policies and that all systems in place are regularly monitored. *See* CALDICOTT GUARDIAN.

**guided imagery** a complementary therapy that uses pleasant mental images of events, feelings or sensations as a distraction method in coping with pain.

**Guillain–Barré syndrome** *G. Guillain, French neurologist, 1876–1961; A. Barré, French neurologist, 1880–1967.* Acute infective polyneuritis. After an infection, usually respiratory, there is a general weakness or paralysis which frequently affects the respiratory muscles as well as the peripheral ones.

**guilt** feelings of self-blame and reproach causing distress to the individual who believes that they have contravened accepted cultural, moral and ethical standards of behaviour. A deep, lasting and sometimes seemingly inappropriate sense of guilt is often a feature of psychiatric disorder.

**guinea-worm** a nematode worm, *Dracunculus medinensis*, which burrows into human tissues, particularly into the legs or feet.

**Gulf War syndrome** experienced by military personnel during the Gulf War and later wars as a variety of symptoms including chronic fatigue, muscle and joint pains, headaches, memory loss, depression and irritability. Possibly due to chemical exposure (e.g. to insecticides or nerve gas) or the interaction of multiple vaccinations and drugs given to protect personnel from the perceived threat of chemical or biological warfare combined with prolonged fatigue and stress.

**gumboil** the opening on the gum of an abscess at the root of a tooth.

**gumma** a soft, degenerating tumour characteristic of the tertiary stage of syphilis. It may occur in any organ or tissue.

**gustatory** relating to taste.

**Guthrie test** 1. a sensitive screening test. 2. test performed on a small amount of blood, usually taken from the heel stab and carried out on a neonate between the 6th and 14th days of life to diagnose PHENYLKETONURIA.

**gut** the intestine.

**gutta** a drop. *G. percha* the juice of a tropical tree which, when dried, forms an elastic semisolid substance. Used in dentistry as a root filler.

**GVH disease** graft-versus-host disease.

**Gy** symbol for *gray.*

**gynaecologist** one who specializes in the diseases of the female genital tract.

**gynaecology** the science of those diseases that are peculiar to the female genital tract.

**gynaecomastia** excessive growth of the male breast.

**gypsum** plaster of Paris (calcium sulphate).

**gyrus** a convolution, as of the cerebral cortex.

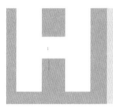

**H** symbol for *hydrogen*.

**habit** automatic response to a specific situation acquired as a result of repetition and learning. *Drug h.* drug addiction. *H. forming* drugs that may lead to physiological addiction. *H. retraining* technique used by nurses to retrain patients in the process for control of micturition. The patient is encouraged to void at set times according to an agreed baseline chart but may use the lavatory at other times. *H. training* a method used in psychiatric nursing whereby deteriorated patients can be rehabilitated and taught personal hygiene by constant repetition and encouragement.

**habilitation** the process of assisting a patient towards achieving the maximum social and physical independence of their potential. The patient/client is usually someone handicapped from birth who is learning and not relearning a skill.

**habituation** gradual adaptation to a stimulus or to the environment. The acquisition of a habit, e.g. a condition resulting from the repeated consumption of a drug, but with little or no tendency to increase the dose; there may be psychic but no physical dependence on the drug.

**haemangioma** a benign tumour formed by dilated blood vessels. *Strawberry h.* a birthmark, which may become very large, but frequently disappears in a few years.

**haemarthrosis** an effusion of blood into a joint.

**haematemesis** vomiting of blood. If it has been in the stomach for some time and become partially digested by gastric juice, it is of a dark colour and contains particles resembling coffee grounds.

**haematin** the iron-containing part of haemoglobin.

**haematocele** a swelling produced by effusion of blood, e.g. in the sheath surrounding a testicle or a broad ligament.

**haematocolpos** an accumulation of blood or menstrual fluid in the vagina.

**haematocrit** the volume of red cells in the blood. Usually expressed as a percentage of the total blood volume.

**haematology** the science dealing with the nature, functions and diseases of blood.

**haematoma** a swelling containing clotted blood.

**haematomyelia** an effusion of blood into the spinal cord.

**haematuria** the presence of blood in the urine, due to injury or disease of any of the urinary organs.

**haemochromatosis** a condition in which there is high absorption and deposition of iron leading to a high serum level, pigmentation of the skin and liver failure. Bronze diabetes.

**haemoconcentration** a loss of circulating fluid from the blood resulting in an increase in the proportion of red blood cells to plasma. The viscosity of the blood is increased.

**haemodialysis** the removal of waste material from the blood of a patient with acute or chronic renal failure by means of a dialyser or artificial kidney. The apparatus is coupled to an artery and dialysis is achieved by the blood and rinsing fluid (DIALYSATE) passing through a semipermeable membrane. Blood is returned through a vein.

**haemoglobin (Hb)** the complex protein molecule contained within the red blood cells which gives them their colour and by which oxygen is transported.

**haemoglobinopathy** any one of a group of hereditary disorders, including sickle-cell anaemia and thalassaemia, in which there is an abnormality in the production of haemoglobin.

**haemolysin** a substance that destroys red blood cells.

**haemolysis** the disintegration of red blood cells. Excessive haemolysis, which may produce anaemia, may be caused by injection with viruses or bacteria, drugs, chemicals and incompatible blood transfusions.

**haemolytic** having the power to destroy red blood cells. **H. disease of the newborn** a condition associated with rhesus incompatibility. *See* RHESUS FACTOR.

**haemophilia** a condition characterized by impaired coagulability of the blood, and a strong tendency to bleed. Over 80% of all patients with haemophilia have haemophilia A (classic haemophilia), which is characterized by a deficiency of clotting factor VIII. Haemophilia B (Christmas disease), which affects about 15% of all haemophiliac patients, results from a deficiency of factor IX. Inherited as an X-linked recessive trait, it is

transmitted by females only, to their male offspring. In order to avoid the debilitating and crippling effects of haemophilia, treatment must raise the level of the deficient clotting factor and maintain it in order to stop local bleeding. The patient must learn to avoid trauma and to obtain prompt treatment for bleeding episodes. Before surgery or dental treatment the patient must be given an infusion of the appropriate clotting factor.

*Haemophilus* a genus of Gramnegative rod-like bacteria. *H. ducreyi* the cause of soft chancre. *H. influenzae* a species once thought to be the cause of epidemic influenza; it produces a highly fatal form of meningitis, especially in infants. *H. pertussis* the cause of whooping cough; Bordet–Gengou bacillus.

**haemophthalmia** bleeding into the vitreous of the eye, usually the result of trauma; haemophthalmos.

**haemopneumothorax** the presence of blood and air in the pleural cavity, usually the result of injury.

**haemopoiesis** the formation of red blood cells, which normally takes place in the bone marrow and continues throughout life. **Extramedullary h.** the formation of blood cells other than in the bone marrow, e.g. in the liver or spleen.

**haemopoietic** relating to blood cell formation. **H. factors** those necessary for the development of red blood cells, e.g. vitamin $B_{12}$ and folic acid.

**haemoptysis** the coughing up of blood from the lungs or bronchi. Being aerated, it is bright-red and frothy.

**haemorrhage** an escape of blood from a ruptured blood vessel, externally or internally. Arterial haemorrhage involves bright-red blood which escapes in rhythmic spurts, corresponding to the beats of the heart. Venous haemorrhage involves dark-red blood which escapes in an even flow. Haemorrhage may also be: primary, at the time of operation or injury; reactionary or recurrent, occurring later when the blood pressure rises and a ligature slips or a vessel opens up; secondary, may be several days after injury, and usually due to sepsis. Special types are as follows. *Antepartum h.* that which occurs before labour starts. *See* PLACENTA (PRAEVIA). *Cerebral h.* an episode of bleeding into the cerebrum; one of the three main forms of STROKE. *Concealed h.* collection of the blood in a cavity of the body. *Intracranial h.* bleeding within the cranium, which may be extradural, subdural, subarachnoid or cerebral. *Intradural h.* bleeding beneath the dura mater. It may be due to injury and causes signs of compression. The cerebrospinal fluid will be bloodstained. *Postpartum h.* that which occurs within 12–24 hours of delivery, from the genital tract, and which either measures 500 ml or more, or which adversely affects the woman's condition. Secondary postpartum haemorrhage is excessive bleeding more than 24 hours after delivery.

**haemorrhagic** pertaining to or characterized by haemorrhage. *H. disease of the newborn* a self-limited haemorrhagic disorder of the first days of life, caused by deficiency of vitamin K-dependent blood clotting factors II, VII, IX and X. It should be prevented by the prophylactic administration of vitamin K to all newborn babies. *Viral h. fevers* a group of notifiable virus diseases of diverse aetiology but with similar characteristics of fever, headache, myalgia, prostration and haemorrhagic symptoms. They include dengue haemorrhagic fever, Marburg disease, Ebola virus disease, Lassa fever and yellow fever.

**haemorrhoid** a 'pile' or locally dilated rectal vein. Piles may be either external or internal to the anal sphincter. Pain is caused on defecation, and bleeding may occur.

**haemorrhoidectomy** the surgical removal of haemorrhoids.

**haemosiderosis** iron deposits in the tissues resulting from excessive haemolysis of red blood cells.

**haemostasis** the arrest of bleeding or the slowing up of blood flow in a vessel.

**haemostatic** a drug or remedy for arresting haemorrhage; a styptic.

**haemothorax** blood in the thoracic cavity, e.g. from injury to soft tissues as a result of fracture of a rib.

**HCAI** a health care associated infection.

**hair** a delicate keratinized epidermal filament growing out of the skin. The root of the hair is enclosed beneath the skin in a tubular follicle. Erect hair has a minimal role in thermoregulation of the body. If the body is too cold arrector pili muscles contract in the skin, pulling the hairs upright and trapping an insulating layer of air. *See* GOOSE-FLESH. *H. analysis* used as an adjunct to other tests in preconception care of women to assess nutritional status and detect the concentration of up to 18 metals. High levels of some metals such as lead may be associated with congenital abnormalities. Deficiencies of substances such as zinc can be treated with dietary advice and/or supplements. (*see* Figure on p. 179). *H. ball see* BEZOAR.

**half-life** 1. the time it takes for a substance to decay to one-half of its original value. 2. in pharmacology, the time it takes for the level of a drug to decrease to one-half in the blood. This is used to determine the dosing level required for therapeutic treatment.

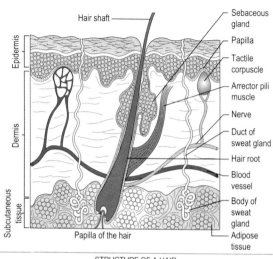

STRUCTURE OF A HAIR

**Halal** meat from an animal that has been killed according to Islamic law and is therefore lawful to be eaten by Muslims.

**halitosis** foul-smelling breath.

**hallucination** a sensory impression (sight, touch, sound, smell or taste) that has no basis in external stimulation. Hallucinations can have psychological causes, as in mental illness, or they can result from drugs, alcohol, or organic illnesses, such as brain tumour or senility. People subjected to sensory deprivation or overwhelming physical stress sometimes suffer from temporary hallucinations.

**hallucinations rating scale** abbreviated HRS. A scale that uses 11 items to determine auditory hallucinations in patients. It also assesses the way in which the hallucinations are experienced and controlled by the patient.

**hallucinogen** an agent that causes hallucinations, e.g. LSD and cannabis.

**hallux** the big toe. *H. valgus* a deformity in which the big toe is bent towards the other toes (*see* Figure on p. 180). *H. varus* a deformity in which the big toe is bent outwards away from the other toes.

**halo** a circular structure, such as a luminous circle seen surrounding an object or light. *Glaucomatous h., h. glaucomatosus* a narrow light zone surrounding the optic disc in glaucoma.

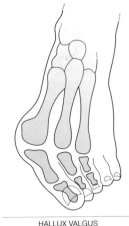

HALLUX VALGUS

**halo effect** a beneficial effect noted after a health care intervention, visit or research project. The halo effect cannot be attributed to the content of the interview, visit or project but is the outcome of indefinable factors as a result of the intervention.

**halo splint** an orthopaedic device used to immobilize the head and neck to assist in the healing of cervical injuries and postoperatively after cervical surgery.

**halogen** any of the five non-metallic elements chlorine, iodine, bromine, astatine and fluorine.

**hamartoma** a benign nodule which is an overgrowth of mature tissue.

**hammer** the malleus. **H.-toe** a deformity in which the first phalanx is bent upwards, with plantar flexion of the second and third phalanx.

**hamstring** the flexors of the knee joint that are situated at the back of the thigh.

**hand** the terminal part of the arm below the wrist. *Claw h.* a paralytic condition in which the hand is flexed and the fingers contracted, caused by injury to nerves or muscles. *Cleft h.* a congenital deformity in which the cleft between the third and fourth fingers extends into the palm. *H., foot and mouth disease* a mild infectious disease in children, caused by Coxsackie virus, which results in vesicle formation on all three sites. Not the same as foot and mouth disease. *H. washing see* Appendix 12.

**hand–arm vibration syndrome** pain and numbness with blanching in the hand and arm due to the use of vibrating tools, usually in the workplace. The syndrome tends to develop slowly over time and gangrene may develop. Exposure to cold tends to aggravate the condition.

**Hand–Schüller–Christian disease** *A. Hand, American paediatrician, 1868–1949; A. Schüller, Austrian neurologist, 1874–1958; H.A. Christian, American physician, 1876–1951.* A disease of the reticuloendothelial system in which granulomata containing cholesterol are formed, chiefly in the skull.

**hand washing** *See* Appendix 12.

**handicap** a disadvantage for a given individual, resulting from an impairment or a disability that limits or prevents the fulfilment of a role (depending on age, sex, and social and cultural factors) for that individual.

**Hansen's disease** *G.H.A. Hansen, Norwegian physician, 1841–1912.* Leprosy, caused by Hansen's bacillus, *Mycobacterium leprae. See* LEPROSY.

**haploid** having one set of chromosomes after division instead of two.

**harassment** any repetitive physical or verbal conduct that causes another person alarm or distress, including physically threatening, humiliating, offensive or derogatory acts or utterances. Harassment is unlawful and examples include bullying, workplace violence, sexual harassment, racial, age or gender discrimination and cyberstalking. Harassment can occur in health care settings and this may take many forms, but an example is when a consultant, manager or senior professional repeatedly makes derisory or critical comments to another member of staff in front of patients or colleagues leading that person losing confidence and feeling powerless in the workplace.

**hard drugs** an imprecise term used in relation to drugs that are highly addictive, e.g. heroin or cocaine, and therefore prone to misuse.

**Harrison's groove** or **sulcus** *E. Harrison, British physician, 1789–1838.* A horizontal groove along the lower border of the thorax corresponding to the costal insertion of the diaphragm; seen in rickets.

**Hartmann's solution** a saline solution containing sodium lactate used intravenously in treating acidosis.

**Hartnup disease** a hereditary defect in amino acid metabolism which may cause learning difficulties (named after the first person found to suffer from it).

**Hashimoto's disease** *H. Hashimoto, Japanese surgeon, 1881–1934.* A lymphoadenoid goitre caused by the formation of antibodies to thyroglobulin. It is an autoimmune condition giving rise to hypothyroidism.

**hashish** Indian hemp. *See* CANNABIS.

**haustration** a haustrum, or the process of forming one.

**haustrum** any one of the pouches formed by the sacculations of the colon.

**Haversian canal** *C. Havers, British physician and anatomist, 1650–1702.* One of the minute canals that permeate compact bone, containing blood and lymph vessels to maintain its nutrition. *See* BONE.

**Hawthorne effect** the term given to the usual beneficial effect of a study on the persons participating in the study. It was named after an industrial management study in the USA, where the effect was first identified.

**hay fever** an atopic ALLERGY characterized by sneezing, itching and watery eyes, running nose and a burning sensation of the palate and throat. It is a localized anaphylactic reaction to an extrinsic allergen, most commonly pollens and the spores of moulds. When the allergen comes in contact with mast-cell-bound IgE immunoglobulin in the tissues of the conjunctiva, nasal mucosa and bronchial tree, the cells release mediators of ANAPHYLAXIS and produce the characteristic symptoms of hay fever. *See* ATOPY.

**HCG** human chorionic gonadotrophin. *See* GONADOTROPHIN.

**HCl** hydrochloric acid.

**He** symbol for *helium*.

**head** the anterior or superior part of a structure or organism, in vertebrates containing the brain and the organs of special sense. **H. injury** traumatic injury to the head resulting from a fall or violent blow. Such an injury may be open or closed and may involve a brain CONCUSSION, skull fracture, or contusions of the brain. All head injuries are potentially dangerous because there may be a slow leakage of blood from damaged blood vessels into the brain, or the formation of a blood clot which gradually increases pressure against brain tissue. Long-term effects of head injury may include chronic headache, disturbances in mental and motor function, and a host of other symptoms that may or may not be psychogenic. Organic brain damage and post-traumatic epilepsy resulting from scar formation are possible sequels to head injury. *H. lice see* PEDICULUS.

**headache** a pain or ache in the head. A symptom rather than a disorder. It accompanies many diseases and conditions, including emotional distress. *See also* MIGRAINE.

**Heaf test** *F.G.R. Heaf, British physician, 1894–1973.* A form of tuberculin testing. A drop of tuberculin solution on the skin is injected by means of a number of very short needles mounted on a spring-loaded device (Heaf's gun).

**healing** the process of return to normal function after a period of disease or injury. *H. by first intention* union of the edges of a clean incised wound without visible granulations, and leaving only a faint linear scar. *H. by second intention* union of the edges of an open wound by the formation of granulations from the bottom and sides. *H. by third intention* union of a wound that is closed surgically several days after the injury.

**health** the World Health Organization (WHO) states that 'Health is a state of complete physical, mental and social wellbeing and not merely the absence of disease or infirmity.' *H. assessment* an evaluation made by a health care professional of an individual's health status, which takes account of the health history and lifestyle together with the findings of a physical examination. *H. centre* primary health care organization for providing ambulatory health care and coordinating the efforts of all health agencies, commonly focused around the general practitioner's services. *H. culture* a system that attempts to explain and treat health problems and illness and to maintain health. Part of the wider culture to which people belong, it may be a traditional or a biomedical system. *H. education officer* an officer appointed to make health education resources available to the community. *H. promotion* A programme to effect health improvements in individuals, communities or populations through a strategy of surveillance planned on a community basis. Programmes include offering screening systems, immunization and health education. Supported by the World Health Organization as a process of orientating communities to move health services from a treatment approach to one of prevention. *H. services* the term is usually employed to connote the system or programme by which health care is made available to the population and financed by government or private enterprise, or both. *H. statistics* summated data on any aspect of the health of populations; for example, mortality, morbidity, use of health services, treatment outcome, costs of health care. *Holistic h.* a system of preventive medicine that takes into account the whole individual, and that person's own responsibility for wellbeing, with the total influences (social, psychological, environmental) that affect health, including nutrition, exercise and mental relaxation. *Public h.* the field of medicine that is concerned with safeguarding and improving the health of the community as a whole.

**Health and Safety at Work Act 1974** comprehensive legislation that came into force in 1975. It deals with the welfare, health and safety of all employers and employees, except domestic workers in a private house. *See* Appendix 10.

**Health and Safety Commission** organization responsible for the administration of the Health and Safety at Work Act 1974. Its mission is to ensure that risks to people's health and safety from work activities are properly controlled. The Commission reviews health and safety legislation and makes proposals for changes.

**Health and Safety Executive** a corporate entity which advises and assists the Health and Safety Commission in its functions. The executive has specific statutory responsibilities, including the enforcement of health and safety law. The executive's staff includes inspectors, policy advisers, lawyers, technologists, scientific officers, and nursing and medical experts.

**health care assistant** abbreviated HCA. A support worker in the clinical area who works with the supervision of registered practitioner who is responsible for the quality of care delivered by the HCA. A HCA may be registered at level 1, 2 or 3 of the National Council for Vocational Qualifications (NCVQ) having completed the approved courses.

**health care-associated infection** (HCAI; sometimes abbreviated as HAI); also known as nosocomial infections. An infection acquired during an episode of health care in either acute (hospital) or non-acute settings, usually as a result of a clinical intervention, such as urinary catheterization or the insertion of a vascular access device.

**health care system** an organized plan of health services. The term is usually employed to denote the system or programme by which health care is made available to the population and financed by government or private enterprise or both.

**health education** various methods of education aimed at the prevention of disease. All nurses, midwives and health visitors have particular responsibilities and opportunities to promote good health.

**Health Improvement Programme** abbreviated HImP. A local strategy for improving health within a community, which is updated each year. Developed and led by a health authority, it must result in coordinated and shared strategy involving the health authority, Foundation Trusts, local NHS Trusts, local authorities, primary care groups, dentists, voluntary and partner organizations with local people. It is designed to cover the main health needs and health care requirements of the local people within the defined area, together with the investment required in local health services to meet these needs. Also includes the health targets set by central government from 'Our Healthier Nation', etc.

**Health of the Nation Outcome Scale** abbreviated HoNOS. A scale of 12 items that assess risk behaviours, deterioration and/or improvement with health and social functioning. Used in mental health care.

**Health Professions Council (HPC)** is a UK independent body created in 2001 to protect the public by setting and maintaining standards for those health care professionals which it regulates. It currently regulates thirteen professions which include: arts therapists; biomedical scientists; chiropodists/podiatrists; clinical scientists; dieticians; occupational therapists; operating department practitioners; orthoptists; paramedics; physiotherapists; prosthetists/orthotists; radiographers; speech and language therapists. *See* Appendix 5.

**Health Protection Agency** abbreviated HPA. Agency established in 2003 as the national organization for England and Wales. It is dedicated to protecting people's health and reducing the impact of infectious diseases, chemical, radiation and poison hazards. It brings together the expertise of health and scientific professionals working in public health departments, communicable diseases, infection control, laboratories and universities working with poisonous, chemical and radiation hazards and those concerned with emergency planning.

**Health Service Commissioner (Health Service Ombudsman UK)** appointed to protect the interests of patients in relation to the administration and provision of health care delivered in the NHS. The Commissioner is responsible to Parliament and can investigate complaints and allegations of maladministration by a health authority, NHS Trusts and the clinical practice of medical practitioners. See OMBUDSMAN.

**health visitor** a registered nurse who may also be a midwife and who has completed a university course in social and preventative medicine leading to a health visiting qualification. The main area of responsibility of health visitors is health education and preventative care of mothers and children under 5 years old, although some specialize in school health and preventative care of the elderly.

**hearing** the reception of sound waves and their transmission onwards to the brain in the form of nerve impulses. *H. aid* an apparatus, usually electronic, to amplify sounds before they reach the inner ear. *H. therapy* the support and rehabilitation of people with hearing difficulties, tinnitus or vertigo. It includes the teaching of lip reading, the use of hearing aids and providing tinnitus retraining therapy.

**heart** a hollow, muscular organ which pumps the blood throughout the body, situated behind the sternum slightly towards the left side

HEART

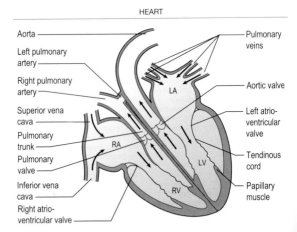

Aorta
Left pulmonary artery
Right pulmonary artery
Superior vena cava
Pulmonary trunk
Pulmonary valve
Inferior vena cava
Right atrio-ventricular valve

Pulmonary veins
Aortic valve
Left atrio-ventricular valve
Tendinous cord
Papillary muscle

LA
RA
LV
RV

of the thorax (*see* Figure on p. 184). *H. attack* myocardial infarction. *H. block* impairment of conduction in heart excitation; often applied specifically to atrioventricular heart block. *H. failure* may be acute, as in coronary thrombosis, or chronic. *H.–lung machine* an apparatus used to perform the functions of both the heart and the lungs during heart surgery. *H. murmur* an abnormal sound heard in the heart, frequently caused by disease of the valves. Occurs when the blood flow through the heart exceeds a certain velocity. *H. rate* the number of heart beats per minute. The normal resting heart rate is 60–100 beats per minute, and should be monitored for rate, strength and rhythm. *H. sounds* the normal heart sounds correspond to the closure of the four valves of the heart:- First heart sound = 'LUB' sound corresponding to the closure of the mitral and tricuspid valves. Second heart sound = 'DUP' sound with closure of the aortic and pulmonary valves. *Maximum h. rate* used in sports medicine to assess an individual's heart during exercise. It is equal to 220 minus the age of the person.

**heartburn** indigestion marked by a burning sensation in the oesophagus, often with regurgitation of acid fluid.

**heat** warmth. A form of energy, which may cause an increase in temperature or a change of state, e.g. the conversion of water into steam. *H. exhaustion* a rapid pulse, anorexia, dizziness, and cramps in arms, legs or abdomen, sometimes followed by sudden collapse, caused by loss of body fluids and salts under very hot conditions. *Prickly h.* miliaria; heat rash. Acute itching caused by blocking of the ducts of the sweat glands following profuse sweating. *H. stroke* a severe life-threatening condition resulting from prolonged exposure to heat. *See* SUNSTROKE.

**hebephrenia** a form of schizophrenia characterized by thought disorder and emotional incongruity. Delusions and hallucinations are common.

**Heberden's nodes** *W. Heberden, British physician, 1710–1801.* Bony or cartilaginous outgrowths causing deformity of the terminal finger joints in osteoarthritis.

**hebetude** emotional dullness. A common symptom in dementia and schizophrenia.

**hectic** occurring regularly. *H. fever* a regularly occurring increase in temperature; it is frequently observed in pulmonary tuberculosis. *H. flush* a redness of the face accompanying a sudden rise in temperature.

**hedonism** excessive devotion to pleasure.

**Heimlich manoeuvre** now referred to as abdominal thrust. *See* Appendix 2.

*Helicobacter* a genus of spiral and flagellated Gram-negative bacteria. *H. pylori* a species found in the stomach. May cause damage to the prostaglandins protecting the mucosal cells in the stomach wall, leading to progressive gastritis and ulceration.

**heliotherapy** treatment of disease by exposure of the body to sunlight.

**helium** *symbol* He. An inert gas sometimes used in conjunction with oxygen to facilitate respiration in obstructional types of dyspnoea and for decompressing deep-sea divers.

**helix** 1. a spiral twist. Used to describe the configuration of certain molecules, e.g. deoxyribonucleic acid (DNA). 2. the outer rim of the auricle of the ear.

**Hellin's law** one in about 89 pregnancies ends in the birth of twins;

one in 89², or 7921, in the birth of triplets; one in 89³, or 704 969, in the birth of quadruplets. Infertility treatments have raised the rate of multiple pregnancies.

**helminthiasis** an infestation with worms.

**hemeralopia** day blindness. The vision is poor in a bright light but is comparatively good when the light is dim. *See* NYCTALOPIA.

**hemianopia** partial blindness, in which the patient can see only half of the normal field of vision. It arises from disorders of the optic tract and of the occipital lobe.

**hemicolectomy** the removal of the ascending and part of the transverse colon with an ileotransverse colostomy (*see* Figure).

**hemiparesis** paralysis on one side of the body; hemiplegia.

**hemiplegia** paralysis of one half of the body, usually due to cerebral disease or injury. The lesion is on the side of the brain opposite to the side paralysed.

**hemisphere** a half sphere. In anatomy, one of the two halves of the cerebrum or cerebellum.

**Henle's loop** *F.G.J. Henle, German anatomist, 1809–1885.* The U-shaped loop of the uriniferous tubule of the kidney.

**Henoch's purpura** *E.H. Henoch, German paediatrician, 1820–1910.* Allergic PURPURA.

**heparin** an anticoagulant formed in the liver and circulated in the blood. Injected intravenously it prevents the conversion of prothrombin into thrombin, and is used in the treatment of thrombosis.

**hepatectomy** excision of a part or the whole of the liver.

**hepatic** relating to the liver. *H. flexure* the angle of the colon that is situated under the liver.

**hepaticojejunostomy** the anastomosis of the hepatic duct to the jejunum, usually created after extensive excision for carcinoma of the pancreas.

**hepaticostomy** a surgical opening into the hepatic duct.

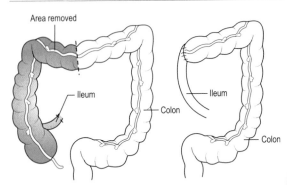

HEMICOLECTOMY     TRANSVERSE ILEOCOLOSTOMY

Area removed

Ileum

Ileum

Colon

Colon

**hepatitis** inflammation of the liver. *Amoebic h.* inflammation that may arise during amoebic dysentery and lead to liver abscesses. *Anicteric h.* viral hepatitis without jaundice, tending to occur chiefly in infants and young children; symptoms include mild anorexia and gastrointestinal disturbances, slight fever, and enlargement and tenderness of the liver. *Fulminant h.* (acute hepatitis with coma) an acute fulminating form of hepatitis resulting from extensive hepatic necrosis. It may be due to: (a) toxic liver injury, as in carbon tetrachloride poisoning or paracetamol overdose; (b) a hypersensitivity reaction to a drug, such as halothane; or (c) viral hepatitis. Death is usually caused by acute yellow atrophy of the liver. *Viral h.* an acute, notifiable, infectious hepatitis caused by one of several different viruses that infect human liver cells, e.g. hepatitis A virus (HAV), hepatitis B virus (HBV), hepatitis C virus (HCV) and hepatitis E virus (HEV).

**hepatization** the alteration of lung tissue into a solid mass resembling liver, which occurs in acute lobar pneumonia.

**hepatogenous** arising in the liver. Applied to jaundice in which the disease arises in the parenchymal cells of the liver.

**hepatolenticular** pertaining to the liver and the lentiform nucleus. *H. degeneration* Wilson's disease; a progressive condition, usually occurring between the ages of 10 and 25 years. There are tremors of the head and limbs, pigmentation of the cornea and sometimes defective twilight vision.

**hepatoma** a primary malignant tumour arising in the liver cells.

**hepatomegaly** an enlargement of the liver.

**hepatosplenomegaly** enlargement of the liver and spleen, such as may be found in kala-azar.

**hepatotoxic** applied to drugs and substances that cause destruction of liver cells, e.g. alcohol.

**herbal medicine** a form of complementary or alternative medicine in which plants are used for their therapeutic properties.

**herd immunity** the immunity of a population. When there is a high enough number of persons in a population immune to a particular infection, the infection fails to spread because of the absence of enough susceptibles. For example, in measles this could probably be achieved by vaccination of 90–95% of the population.

**hereditary** derived from ancestry; inherited.

**heredity** the transmission of both physical and mental characteristics to the offspring from the parents. Recessive characteristics may miss one or two generations and reappear later.

**hermaphrodite** an individual whose gonads contain both testicular and ovarian tissue. These may be combined or there may be a testis on one side and an ovary on the other. The external genitalia may be indeterminate or of either sex. *Pseudo-h.* one whose gonads are histologically of one sex but in whom the genitalia have the appearance of the opposite sex. *True h.* one who possesses both male and female gonads.

**hermeneutics** the study of meanings in social behaviour and experience. Denotes the art, skill or theory of interpreting human behaviour, speech and writings in terms of intentions and meanings.

**hermetic** airtight. A wound dressing may be sealed to ensure that the wound is not exposed to air.

**hernia** a protrusion of any part of the internal organs through

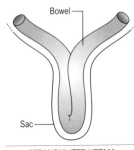

STRANGULATED HERNIA

the structures enclosing them. *Cerebral h.* a protrusion of brain through the skull. *Diaphragmatic h.* and *hiatus h.* a protrusion of a part of the stomach through the oesophageal opening in the diaphragm. *Femoral h.* a loop of intestine protruding into the femoral canal. More common in females. *Hiatus h. see* DIAPHRAGMATIC H. *Incisional h.* a hernia occurring at the site of an old wound. *Inguinal h.* protrusion of the intestine through the inguinal canal. This may be congenital or acquired, and is commoner in males. A rupture. *Irreducible h.* a hernia that cannot be replaced by manipulation. *Reducible h.* a hernia that can be returned to its normal position by manipulative measures. *Strangulated h.* a hernia of the bowel in which the neck of the sac containing the bowel is so constricted that the venous circulation is impeded, and gangrene will result if not treated promptly (*see* Figure). *Umbilical h.* protrusion of bowel through the umbilical ring. This may be congenital or acquired. *Vaginal h.* rectocele or cystocele.

**hernioplasty** a plastic repair of the abdominal wall performed after reduction of a hernia.

**herniorrhaphy** removal of a hernial sac and repair of the abdominal wall.

**herniotomy** an operation to removal a hernial sac.

**heroin** a diacetate of morphine used as an analgesic and abused illicitly for its euphoriant effects. The drug readily induces physical dependence and may be sniffed, smoked ('chasing the dragon') or injected subcutaneously or intravenously ('shooting up' or 'mainlining'). Street names for heroin include 'smack', 'H' and 'horse'. *H. baby* a baby that has received regular heroin (morphine) via the placenta before birth and who shows signs of withdrawal after birth. Withdrawal symptoms may persist for 1–4 weeks and include vomiting, diarrhoea, sweating, breathing difficulties and hyperactivity.

**herpes** an inflammatory skin eruption showing small vesicles caused by a herpes virus. *H. simplex* a viral infection which gives rise to localized vesicles in the skin and mucous membranes and is characterized by latency and subsequent recurrence. It is caused by herpes simplex viruses types 1 and 2. Type 1 infection is common in children and is often symptomless. Type 2 infection is common in older age groups and is associated with sexual activity. Recurrent attacks may occur. Lesions appear on the cervix, vulva and surrounding skin in women and on the penis in men. In homosexual men rectal lesions are common. To prevent neonatal herpes, Caesarean is recommended for women presenting with clinical genital tract herpes within two weeks of delivery. *Congenital h. simplex* a serious neonatal condition with a generalized vesicular rash, causing encephalitis and death. *H. zoster* a local manifestation of reactivation of infection of the varicella zoster virus, the causative agent of chickenpox, characterized by a vesicular rash in the area of distribution of a sensory nerve. Called also shingles.

**herpes virus** one of a group of DNA-containing viruses. They include the causative agents of herpes simplex, herpes zoster, chickenpox, cytomegalic inclusion disease and infective mononucleosis.

**heterochromia** a difference in colour in the irises of the two eyes or in different parts of one iris. It may be congenital or secondary resulting from inflammation.

**heterosexual** 1. pertaining to, characteristic of or directed towards the opposite sex. 2. a person with erotic interests directed towards the opposite sex.

**heterotropia** a marked deviation of the eyes; strabismus or squint.

**heterozygous** possessing dissimilar alternative genes for an inherited characteristic, one gene coming from each parent. One gene is dominant and the other is recessive. *See* HOMOZYGOUS.

**hexachlorophane** a detergent and germicidal compound commonly incorporated in soaps and dermatological agents. Topical preparations have been associated with severe neurotoxicity and should not be used on children under 2 years old except on medical advice.

**Hg** *symbol for* mercury.

**hiatus** a space or opening. *H. hernia* a protrusion of a part of the stomach through the oesophageal opening in the diaphragm.

**Hib** an injectable vaccine which protects against *Haemophilus influenzae* type B which causes severe respiratory and ear infections and meningitis. Offered to infants at ages of 2, 3 and 4 months.

**hiccup** hiccough; a spasmodic contraction of the diaphragm causing an abrupt inspiratory sound.

**hidrosis** the excretion of sweat.

**high-altitude sickness** the condition resulting from difficulty in adjusting to diminished oxygen pressure at high altitudes. It may take the form of mountain sickness, high-altitude pulmonary oedema or cerebral oedema.

**high dependency unit** abbreviated HDU. For those patients who do not need intensive care in the clinical situation but reguire a greater degree of specialist monitoring and observation than in a general ward, nursing and medical care is provided in the high dependency unit.

**higher education institutions** abbreviated HEI. Universities and colleges which provide academic programmes to diploma and degree level, including programmes of midwifery and nursing.

**highly active antiretroviral therapy** abbreviated HAART. A treatment regimen that incorporates a combination of different antiviral drugs for human immunodeficiency viral infection. Sometimes also called ART, antiretroviral therapy.

**hilum** hilus; a recess in an organ by which blood vessels, nerves and ducts enter and leave it.

**hindbrain** that part of the brain consisting of the medulla oblongata, the pons and the cerebellum.

**hip** 1. the region of the body at the articulation of the femur and the innominate bone at the base of the lower trunk. These bones meet at the hip joint. Called also *coxa*. 2. loosely, the hip joint. *Total h. replacement* replacement of the femoral head and acetabulum with prostheses that are cemented into the bone; called also *total h. arthroplasty*. The procedure is done to replace a severely damaged arthritic hip joint.

**hippus** alternate contraction and dilatation of the pupils. This occurs in various diseases of the nervous system, e.g. multiple sclerosis.

**Hirschsprung's disease** *H. Hirschsprung, Danish physician, 1831–1916.* See MEGACOLON.

**hirsute** hairy.

**hirsutism** excessive hairiness.

**hirudin** the active principle in the secretion of the leech and certain snake venoms that prevents clotting of blood.

*Hirudo* a genus of leeches. *H. medicinalis* the medical leech.

**histamine** an enzyme that causes local vasodilatation and increased permeability of the blood vessel walls. Readily released from body tissues, it is a factor in allergy response, greatly increases gastric secretion of hydrochloric acid and increases the heart rate.

**histidine** one of the ten essential amino acids formed by the digestion of dietary protein. Histamine is derived from it.

**histiocyte** a stationary macrophage of connective tissue. Derived from the reticuloendothelial cells, it acts as a scavenger, removing bacteria from the blood and tissues.

**histiocytosis** a group of diseases of bone in which granulomata containing histiocytes and eosinophil cells appear. See LETTERER–SIWE DISEASE and HAND–SCHÜLLER–CHRISTIAN DISEASE.

**histocompatibility** the ability of cells to be accepted and to function in a new situation. Tissue typing reveals this and ensures a higher success rate in organ and tissue transplantation.

**histogram** a bar-chart. Statistical values are expressed as blocks on a graph.

**histology** the science dealing with the minute structure, composition and function of tissues.

**histolysis** the disintegration of tissues.

**histoplasmosis** infection caused by inhalation of the spores of a yeast-like fungus, *Histoplasma capsulatum*. Usually symptomless, the infection may progress and produce a condition resembling tuberculosis.

**HIV** human immunodeficiency virus.

**HIV disease** the entire spectrum of cellular and clinical disease from initial infection and asymptomatic disease to early and late symptomatic disease (AIDS) and death, caused by human immunodeficiency virus (HIV) infection. See HUMAN IMMUNODEFICIENCY VIRUS.

**hives** urticaria.

**Hodgkin's disease** *T. Hodgkin, British physician, 1798–1866.* Lymphadenoma, a malignant condition of the reticuloendothelial cells. There is progressive enlargement of lymph nodes and lymph tissue all over the body. Treated by radiotherapy and cytotoxic drugs. This disease has a good prognosis.

**holism** a philosophy in which the person is considered as a functioning whole rather than as a composite of several systems. May be spelt wholism.

**holistic** pertaining to holism. *H. health care* a comprehensive approach to health care that implies body–mind–spirit consideration in all actions and interventions for the patient, while recognizing the concept of the uniqueness of the individual and the influence of external and internal environmental factors on health.

**Homans' sign** *J. Homans, American surgeon, 1877–1954.* Pain elicited in the calf when the foot is dorsiflexed. Indicative of venous thrombosis.

**home** the place where a person lives. *H. assessment* made by an occupational therapist to assess the home environment for a patient, in order to determine the need for any adaptations appropriate to the patient's needs to maintain independent living at home. *H. birth* the delivery of a baby in the mother's home. Women can choose to deliver their babies and receive care from a community or independent midwife and general practitioner. *H. carers* members of community care teams organized by local authority social services who provide care in the home for older and/or disabled people as part of an agreed care package. Formerly called home helps. *H. help service* a branch of the social services department, which provides domestic and housekeeping assistance to those in need. It is on either a short-term or long-term basis, and payment is according to means. *H. page* the first page of an internet website.

**homeopathy** a system of medicine promulgated by C.F.S. Hahnemann (*German physician, 1755–1843*) and based upon the principle that 'like cures like'. Remedies are given which can produce in the patient the symptoms of the disease to be cured, but they are administered in minute doses.

**homeostasis** a tendency of biological systems to maintain stability while continually adjusting to conditions that are optimal for survival.

**homicide** the killing of a human being. *Culpable h.* covers murder (malice aforethought), manslaughter (without malice aforethought), causing death by reckless driving, and infanticide. *Non-culpable h.* covers justifiable homicide (e.g. lawful execution) and excusable homicide (misadventure or accident).

**homogeneous** uniform in character. Similar in nature and characteristics.

**homogenize** to make homogeneous. To reduce to the same consistency.

**homogenous** derived from the same source.

**homograft** a tissue or organ transplanted from one individual to another of the same species. An allograft.

**homolateral** on the same side; ipsilateral.

**homologous** 1. in anatomy, having the same embryological origin although performing a different function. 2. in chemistry, possessing a similar structure. *H. chromosomes* those that pair during meiosis and contain an identical arrangement of genes in the DNA pattern.

**homologue** a part or organ which has the same relative position or structure as another one.

**homoplasty** surgical replacement of defective tissues with a homograft.

**homosexual** 1. of the same sex. 2. a person who is sexually attracted to a person of the same sex.

**homosexuality** sexual and emotional orientation towards persons of the same sex.

**homozygous** possessing an identical pair of genes for an inherited characteristic. *See* HETEROZYGOUS.

**hookworm** *see* ANCYLOSTOMA.

**hordeolum** a stye; inflammation of the sebaceous glands of the eyelashes.

**hormone** a chemical substance that is generated in one organ and carried by the blood to another, in which it excites activity. *H. replacement therapy* abbreviated as HRT. The giving of prepared hormones as a substitute for those hormones that the body no longer produces or that have been lost as a result of surgery. A combination of oestrogenic hormones is commonly given to women for the relief of menopausal symptoms and the prevention of osteoporosis.

**Horner's syndrome** *J.F. Horner, Swiss ophthalmologist, 1831–1886.* A condition in which there is a lesion on the path of sympathetic nerve fibres in the cervical region. The symptoms include enophthalmos, ptosis, a contracted pupil and a decrease in sweating.

**Horton's syndrome** *B.T. Horton, American physician, 1895–1980.* Severe headache caused by the release of histamine in the body.

**hospice** the concept of a hospice is that of a caring community of professional and non-professional people, together with the family. Emphasis is on dealing with emotional and spiritual problems as well as the medical problems of the terminally ill. Of primary concern is control of pain and other symptoms, keeping the patient at home for as long as possible or desirable, and making the remaining days as comfortable and meaningful as possible. After the patient dies, family members are given support throughout their period of bereavement.

**hospital** an institution for the care, diagnosis and treatment of the sick and injured. *H.-acquired infection see* (HOSPITAL-ACQUIRED) INFECTION. **H. Information System (HIS)** a computerized network of hospitals, laboratories, Primary Care Trusts and other health care facilities spread throughout Europe to meet and collate data relating to the social and health care needs in each area. May also be used to describe the system within an individual NHS Trust or unit.

**host** the animal, plant or tissue on which a parasite lives and multiplies. *Definitive* or *final h.* one that harbours the parasite during its adult sexual stage. *Intermediate h.* one that shelters the parasite during a non-reproductive period.

**hourglass contraction** a contraction near the middle of a hollow organ, such as the stomach or uterus, producing an outline resembling an hourglass shape.

**housemaid's knee** prepatellar bursitis; inflammation of the prepatellar bursa, which becomes distended with serous fluid.

**HRT** hormone replacement therapy.

**human chorionic gonadotrophin** *see* GONADOTROPHIN.

**Human Fertilization and Embryology Act 1990** an amended version of the 1967 Abortion Act. Termination of pregnancy must be performed before 24 weeks of pregnancy by a registered medical practitioner, agreed with a second doctor that the woman or her family would suffer physical, mental or social trauma if the pregnancy were to continue, or if the baby is at risk of gross physical or mental abnormality. Termination of pregnancy may be performed at any time if there is serious risk to the mother's life if the pregnancy were to continue. *See* ABORTION.

**Human Fertilization and Embryology Authority** non-departmental body that licenses and monitors NHS and private fertility clinics. It is also charged with ensuring that research is carried out responsibly.

**human immunodeficiency virus** abbreviated HIV. A lentivirus that belongs to a group of viruses known as retroviruses and causes AIDS in humans. There are two main types of HIV: HIV-1, the predominant AIDS-causing virus in the world, and HIV-2, also an AIDS-causing virus that is found more commonly in countries on the west coast of Africa. HIV is transmitted sexually, parenterally, from mother to child (during pregnancy, at time of birth, or in the postnatal period from breast feeding) and more rarely, iatrogenically. Most people become infected sexually through unprotected penetrative vaginal or anal sexual intercourse. Unprotected means that the male insertive partner has not worn a good-quality, intact rubber latex condom. Parenteral transmission is usually associated with injecting drug users sharing contaminated injection equipment. Blood tests to identify HIV infection detect antibodies to the virus and may not be positive for 8–12 weeks following primary infection. Because it is not possible to detect all HIV-infected patients, all health care workers in direct patient contact should practise universal infection control precautions. *See* UNIVERSAL PRECAUTIONS.

**Human Rights Act 1998** incorporates into domestic law the European Convention on Human Rights. The intention is to embed values of fairness, respect for human dignity and inclusiveness in the public services. The law prohibits any public authority acting in a way that is incompatible with a Convention right, acknowledging the principles and values of fairness together with respect for human dignity as core concepts covered by the Act.

**humidity** the degree of moisture in the air. *H. therapy* the therapeutic use of water to prevent or correct a moisture deficit in the respiratory tract. The principal reasons for employing humidity therapy are: (a) to prevent drying and irritation of the respiratory mucosa; (b) to facilitate ventilation and diffusion of oxygen and other therapeutic gases being administered; and (c) to aid in the removal of thick and viscous secretions that obstruct the air passages. Another important use of water aerosol therapy is to aid in obtaining an induced sputum specimen.

**humour** any fluid of the body, such as lymph or blood. *Aqueous h.* the

fluid filling the anterior chamber of the eye. *Vitreous h.* the jelly-like substance that fills the chamber of the eye between the lens and the retina.

**humour and laughter therapy** an amusing intervention used by a health care professional or patient and designed to benefit the patient.

**Huntington's disease** *G.S. Huntington, American physician, 1851–1927.* A rare, degenerative inherited disorder of the brain in which there is progressive chorea and mental deterioration (dementia).

**Hurler's syndrome** *G. Hurler, Austrian paediatrician, 1889–1965.* An inherited disorder in which learning difficulties are caused by excess mucopolysaccharides being stored in the brain and reticuloendothelial system. Formerly known as gargoylism.

**Hutchinson's teeth** *Sir J. Hutchinson, British surgeon, 1828–1913.* Typical notching of the borders of the permanent incisor teeth occurring in congenital syphilis.

**hyaline** resembling glass. *H. degeneration* a form of deterioration that occurs in tumours and is due to deficiency of blood supply. It precedes cystic degeneration. *H. membrane disease see* RESPIRATORY (DISTRESS SYNDROME OF NEWBORN).

**hyaluronidase** an enzyme that facilitates the absorption of fluids in subcutaneous tissues.

**hydatid** a cystic swelling containing the embryo of *Echinococcus granulosus*. It may be found in any organ of the body, e.g. in the liver. 'Daughter cysts' are produced from the original. Infection is from contaminated foods, e.g. salads. *H. disease* the result of the presence of hydatids in the lungs, liver or brain.

**hydatidiform** resembling a hydatid cyst. *H. mole see* MOLE.

**hydraemia** a modification of the blood in which there is an excess of plasma in relation to the cells.

A degree of hydraemia is physiological in pregnancy.

**hydramnios** an excessive amount of amniotic fluid in the uterus during pregnancy. It is associated with maternal diabetes, congenital abnormalities especially of the central nervous system and with uniovular twins. Sometimes used synonymously with polyhydramnios.

**hydrarthrosis** a collection of fluid in a joint.

**hydrate** a compound of an element with water, to combine with water.

**hydroa** a childhood hypersensitivity of the skin to sunlight, resulting in the formation of a vesicular eruption on the exposed parts, with intense irritation.

**hydrocarbon** a compound of hydrogen and carbon. Fats are of this type.

**hydrocele** a swelling caused by accumulation of fluid, especially in the tunica vaginalis surrounding the testicle.

**hydrocephalus** 'water on the brain'. Enlargement of the skull due to an abnormal collection of cerebrospinal fluid around the brain or in the ventricles. It may be either congenital or acquired from infection, trauma or tumour. The most effective treatment is surgical correction employing a shunting technique.

**hydrochloric acid** HCl, a colourless compound of hydrogen and chlorine. It is present, in 0.2% solution, in gastric juice and aids digestion.

**hydrocolloid dressings** absorbent dressings with a soft spongy consistency that are applied to wounds that are subject to pressure, for example those in the sacral area or on heels. They relieve pain from the site, rehydrate and encourage debridement and healing.

**hydrogel dressings** wound dressings that rehydrate dry necrotic tissue, reduce pain and promote healing.

**hydrogen** *symbol* H. A combustible gas, present in nearly all organic compounds, which, in combination with oxygen, forms water. **H. ion concentration** the amount of hydrogen in a liquid, which is responsible for its acidity. The degree of acidity is expressed in pH values: the higher the hydrogen ion concentration, the greater the acidity, and the lower the pH value. The concentration in the blood is of importance in acidosis. **H. peroxide** $H_2O_2$, a strong disinfectant cleansing and bleaching liquid used, diluted in water, for cleansing wounds.

**hydrolysis** the process of splitting up into smaller molecules by uniting with water.

**hydrometer** an instrument for estimating the specific gravity of fluids, e.g. a urinometer.

**hydronephrosis** an accumulation of urine in the pelvis of the kidney, resulting in atrophy of the kidney structure, due to an obstruction to the flow of urine from the kidney. The condition may be: (a) congenital, due to malformation of the kidney or ureter; or (b) acquired, due to an obstruction of the ureter by tumour or stone, or to back pressure from stricture of the urethra or an enlarged prostate gland.

**hydropathy** the treatment of disease by the use of water internally and externally; hydrotherapy.

**hydropericarditis** inflammation of the pericardium resulting in serous fluid in the pericardial sac.

**hydroperitoneum** *see* ASCITES.

**hydrophobia** 1. rabies. 2. irrational fear of water.

**hydropneumothorax** the presence of fluid and air in the pleural space.

**hydrops** [L.] abnormal accumulation of serous fluid in the tissues or in a body cavity; also called dropsy. *Fetal h., h. fetalis* gross oedema of the entire body of the newborn infant, occurring in haemolytic disease of the newborn.

**hydrotherapy** the treatment of disease by means of water, e.g. douching or bathing.

**hydrothorax** fluid in the pleural cavity due to serous effusion, as in cardiac, renal and other diseases.

**hydroureter** an accumulation of urine in a ureter.

**hygiene** 1. the science of health and its preservation. 2. a condition of practice, such as cleanliness, that is conducive to preservation of health. *Communal h.* the maintenance of the health of the community by the provision of a pure water supply, efficient sanitation, good housekeeping, etc. *Industrial h.* (occupational health) care of the health of workers in an industry. *Mental h.* the science dealing with development of healthy mental and emotional reactions and habits. *Oral h.* the proper care of the mouth and teeth. *Personal h.* individual measures taken to preserve one's own cleanliness and wellbeing.

**hygroma** a swelling caused by fluid. *Cystic h.* a cystic lymphangioma of the neck. *Subdural h.* a collection of clear fluid in the subdural space.

**hygrometer** an instrument for measuring the water vapour in the air.

**hygroscopic** readily absorbing moisture. An example is glycerin, which is used in suppositories as a means of aiding evacuation by moistening the faeces.

**hymen** a fold of mucous membrane partially closing the entrance to the vagina. *Imperforate h.* a membrane which completely occludes the vaginal orifice.

**hyoid** shaped like a U. *H. bone* a U-shaped bone above the thyroid cartilage, to which the tongue is attached.

**hyperacidity** excessive acidity. *Gastric h.* hyperchlorhydria.

**hyperactive** exhibiting hyperactivity; hyperkinetic.

**hyperactivity** abnormally increased activity. Developmental hyperactivity of children (hyperkinesia) is characterized by very restless, impulsive behaviour. These children are usually aged between 2 and 4 years, inattentive and have a poor concentration span. Other features that may be associated with hyperactivity include aggression, anxiety, poor eating and sleeping patterns, and social and learning difficulties. Persistent hyperactivity is know as attention deficit hyperactivity disorder which may require assessment and treatment. *See* ATTENTION DEFICIT SYNDROME.

**hyperaemia** excess of blood in any part.

**hyperaesthesia** excessive sensitiveness to touch or to other sensations, e.g. taste or smell.

**hyperalimentation** a programme of parenteral administration of all nutrients for patients with gastrointestinal dysfunction; also called total parenteral alimentation (TPA) and total parenteral nutrition (TPN). Although the term hyperalimentation is commonly used to designate total or supplementary nutrition by intravenous feedings, it is not technically correct inasmuch as the procedure does not involve an abnormally increased or excessive amount of feeding. *See* NUTRITION (PARENTERAL). *See* Appendix 1.

**hyperasthenia** extreme weakness.

**hyperbaric** at a greater pressure than normal; applied to gases under greater than atmospheric pressure. *H. oxygenation* exposure to oxygen under conditions of greatly increased pressure. The patient is placed in a sealed enclosure, called a hyperbaric chamber. Compressed air is introduced;

at the same time the patient is given pure oxygen through a face mask. Patients suffering from tetanus and gas gangrene, infections caused by bacteria that are resistant to antibiotics but vulnerable to oxygen, are helped by hyperbaric oxygenation. The technique is also useful in radiotherapy for cancer. When full of oxygen, cancer cells seem more vulnerable to radiation. Carbon monoxide poisoning can be treated by hyperbaric oxygenation. Carbon monoxide molecules, displacing the oxygen in the erythrocytes, usually cause asphyxiation, but hyperbaric oxygenation can often keep the patient alive until the carbon monoxide has been eliminated from the body's system.

**hyperbilirubinaemia** an excess of bilirubin in the blood.

**hypercalcaemia** an excess of calcium in the blood. May rarely be caused by overadministration of vitamin D, hyperparathyroidism, thyrotoxicosis, prolonged immobility, breakdown of bone by malignant disease, or impaired renal function.

**hypercalciuria** a high level of calcium in the urine leading to renal stone formation.

**hypercapnia** an increased amount of carbon dioxide in the blood, causing overstimulation of the respiratory centre. Hypercarbia.

**hypercatabolism** an excessive rate of catabolism leading to wasting or destruction of a part or tissue.

**hyperchloraemia** an excess of chloride in the blood.

**hyperchlorhydria** an excess of hydrochloric acid in the gastric juice.

**hypercholesteraemia, hypercholesterolaemia** excess of cholesterol in the blood. Predisposes to atheroma and gallstones.

**hyperemesis** excessive vomiting. *H. gravidarum* an uncommon,

serious complication of pregnancy, characterized by severe and persistent vomiting, the aetiology of which is not fully understood.

**hyperextension** the forcible extension of a limb beyond the normal. It is used to correct orthopaedic deformities.

**hyperflexion** the forcible bending of a joint beyond the normal.

**hypergalactia, hypergalactosis** excessive secretion of milk.

**hyperglycaemia** excess of sugar in the blood (normal 2.5–4.7 mmol/litre when fasting); a sign of diabetes mellitus. *See* HYPOGLYCAEMIA; Table on p. 117.

**hyperhidrosis** excessive perspiration; hyperidrosis.

**hyperkalaemia** an excess of potassium in the blood. If untreated, this will lead to cardiac arrest.

**hyperkeratosis** hypertrophy of the horny layers of the skin.

**hyperkinesis** a condition in which there is excessive motor activity. *See* HYPERACTIVITY.

**hyperlipaemia** an excess of fat or lipids in the blood.

**hypermastia** 1. the presence of one or more supernumerary breasts. 2. overdevelopment of one or both breasts.

**hypermetropia** hyperopia; long-sightedness. The light rays entering the eye converge beyond the retina. Clear vision can be obtained by the wearing of spectacles or contact lenses.

**hypermotility** excessive movement. *Gastric h.* increased muscle action of the stomach wall, associated with increased secretion of hydrochloric acid.

**hypernatraemia** an excess of sodium in the blood, usually diagnosed when the plasma sodium is above 150 mmol/litre. It is the result of loss of water and electrolytes from the body caused by diarrhoea, polyuria, excessive sweating or inadequate fluid intake.

**hyperostosis** a thickening of bone; a bony outgrowth; exostosis.

**hyperparathyroidism** excessive activity of the parathyroid glands, causing drainage of calcium from the bones, with consequent fragility and liability to spontaneous fracture.

**hyperphasia** excessive talkativeness.

**hyperpituitarism** overactivity of the pituitary gland.

**hyperplasia** excessive formation of normal cells in a tissue or organ, which increases in size.

**hyperpnoea** overbreathing; hyperventilation; an abnormal increase in the rate and depth of breathing.

**hyperprolactinaemia** increased levels of prolactin in the blood; in women, it is associated with infertility and may lead to galactorrhoea. In men it may cause impotence and loss of libido.

**hyperpyrexia** an excessively high body temperature, i.e. over 41°C.

**hypersensitivity** abnormal sensitivity, especially to a particular antigen. The reactions include allergies (such as asthma) and anaphylaxis. *Contact h.* produced by contact of the skin with a chemical substance having the properties of an antigen or hapten; it includes contact dermatitis (*see* CONTACT). *Delayed h.* a slowly developing increase in cell-mediated immune response (involving T lymphocytes) to a specific antigen, as occurs in graft rejection, autoimmune disease, etc. *Immediate h.* antibody-mediated hypersensitivity characterized by lesions resulting from release of histamine and other mediators of hypersensitivity from reagin-sensitized mast cells, causing increased vascular permeability, oedema and smooth muscle contraction; it includes anaphylaxis and atopy.

**hypersplenism** overactivity of an enlarged spleen resulting in the destruction of blood cells and platelets.

**hypertelorism** abnormally increased distance between two organs or parts. *Ocular h., orbital h.* increase in the interocular distance, often associated with craniofacial dysostosis and sometimes with mental handicap.

**hypertension** persistently high BLOOD PRESSURE. In adults, it is generally agreed that a blood pressure is abnormally high when the resting, supine arterial systolic pressure is equal to or greater than 140 mmHg and the diastolic pressure is equal to or greater than 90 mmHg. A diagnosis of hypertension should be based on a series of readings rather than a single measurement and which will vary with age. Hypertension is very common and usually symptomless but may cause headaches and visual disturbances when severe. Its incidence is highest in men, the middle-aged and the elderly. Associated factors are smoking, high-salt diet, obesity, a family history, lack of exercise and a high degree of stress. Lifestyle changes are recommended, e.g. losing weight, giving up smoking, adopting a low-salt diet. Antihypertensive drugs may be needed to maintain blood pressure readings within reasonable levels. *Essential h.* high blood pressure without demonstrable change in kidneys, blood vessels or heart.

**hyperthermia** an exceedingly high body temperature. *Malignant h.* a serious condition, sometimes arising during general anaesthesia.

**hyperthyroidism** excessive activity of the thyroid gland. *See* THYROTOXICOSIS.

**hypertonic** 1. showing excessive tone or tension, as in a blood vessel or muscle. 2. describing a solution that has greater osmotic pressure than normal physiological tissue fluid. *See* HYPOTONIC.

**hypertrichosis** excessive growth of hair on any part of the body.

**hypertrophy** an increase in the size of a tissue or a structure caused by an increase in the size of the cells that compose it (as opposed to an increase in the number of cells). *See* HYPERPLASIA.

**hyperuricaemia** an excess of uric acid in the blood. *See* GOUT.

**hyperventilation** 1. increase of air in the lungs above the normal amount. 2. abnormally prolonged and deep breathing, usually associated with acute anxiety or emotional tension Hyperpnoea. Also occurs in uncontrolled diabetes mellitus, kidney failure and in some lung disorders. Symptoms occur as a result of an abnormal loss of carbon dioxide from the blood and include faintness, tetany and a tense feeling of not being able to take a full breath.

**hypervitaminosis** a condition caused by the intake of an excessive quantity of vitamins.

**hypervolaemia** abnormal increase in the volume of circulating fluid (plasma) in the body.

**hyphaema** haemorrhage into the anterior chamber of the eye.

**hypnosis** an artificially induced passive state in which there is increased amenability and responsiveness to suggestions and commands. In hypnosis, a drowsy phase is followed by a sleep. It may also be used to produce painless childbirth and tooth extraction.

**hypnotherapy** treatment by hypnosis or by the induction of prolonged sleep.

**hypnotic** an agent that causes sleep; a soporific.

**hypnotism** the practice of hypnosis.

**hypocalcaemia** a deficiency of calcium in the blood.

**hypocapnia** a deficiency of carbon dioxide in the blood.

**hypochloraemia** a deficiency of chloride in the blood.

**hypochlorhydria** a lower than normal amount of hydrochloric acid in the gastric juice.

**hypochlorite** any salt of hypochlorous acid used in solution to yield chlorine, a disinfecting and germicidal agent.

**hypochondria** a morbid preoccupation or anxiety about one's health. The sufferer feels that first one part of the body and then another part is the seat of some serious disease.

**hypochondriac** one affected by hypochondria. *H. region* the hypochondrium.

**hypochondrium** the upper region of the abdomen on each side of the epigastrium.

**hypodermic** beneath the skin; applied to subcutaneous injections and to the syringes used for such injections.

**hypofibrinogenaemia** a lack of fibrinogen in the blood. This may occur in severe trauma or haemorrhage or as an inherited condition.

**hypogammaglobulinaemia** a deficiency of gamma-globulin in the blood, rendering the person susceptible to infection.

**hypogastrium** the lower middle area of the abdomen, immediately below the umbilical region.

**hypoglossal** under the tongue. *H. nerve* the 12th cranial nerve.

**hypoglycaemia** a condition in which the blood sugar level is less than normal. Usually arising in diabetic patients as a result of insulin overdosage, delay in eating or a rapid combustion of carbohydrate. *See* HYPERGLYCAEMIA; Table on p. 117.

**hypokalaemia** a low potassium level in the blood. This is likely to be present in dehydration and with the repeated use of diuretics.

**hypomania** a degree of elation, excitement and activity higher than normal but less severe than that present in mania.

**hypometropia** myopia; short-sightedness.

**hypomotility** deficient power of movement in any part.

**hyponatraemia** a deficiency of sodium in the blood.

**hypoparathyroidism** a lack of parathyroid secretion, leading to a low blood calcium and tetany.

**hypophysis** an outgrowth. *H. cerebri* the pituitary gland.

**hypopituitarism** deficiency of secretion from the anterior lobe of the pituitary gland, causing excessive deposition of fat in children. *See* FRÖLICH'S SYNDROME. Dwarfism may result. In adults asthenia, drowsiness and adiposity may occur, together with an impairment of sexual activity and premature senility.

**hypoplasia** imperfect development of a part or organ.

**hypopnoea** shallow breathing.

**hypoproteinaemia** a deficiency of serum proteins in the blood.

**hypoprothrombinaemia** a deficiency of prothrombin in the blood, leading to a tendency to bleed. *See* HAEMOPHILIA.

**hyposecretion** a deficiency in secretion from any glandular structure or secreting cells.

**hyposensitivity** a lack of sensitivity, especially to a particular allergen with which the patient may have been exposed over a period.

**hypospadias** a developmental anomaly in the male in which the urethra opens on the underside of the penis or on the perineum.

**hypostasis** 1. a sediment or deposit. 2. congestion of blood in a part, due to slowing of the circulation.

**hypostatic** relating to hypostasis. *H. pneumonia see* PNEUMONIA.

**hypotension** abnormally low arterial blood pressure; hypopiesis.

*Controlled* or *induced h.* an artificially produced lowering of the blood pressure so that an operation field is rendered practically bloodless. *Orthostatic* or *postural h.* temporary hypotension when the patient stands up, producing giddiness and sometimes a faint.

**hypotensive** producing a reduction in tension, especially pertaining to a drug that lowers the blood pressure.

**hypothalamus** in the brain a portion of greymatter lying beneath the thalamus at the base of the cerebrum, and forming the floor and part of the lateral wall of the third ventricle. It influences peripheral autonomic mechanisms, endocrine activity and many somatic functions, e.g. a general regulation of water balance, body temperature, sleep, thirst and hunger, and the development of secondary sexual characteristics. It plays an important role in the regulation of protein, fat and carbohydrate metabolism, body fluid volume and electrolyte content, and internal secretion of endocrine hormones.

**hypothermia** 1. a severe reduction in the core body temperature to below 35°C. The condition usually arises gradually and may prove fatal if untreated. It is most common among babies and elderly people. 2. artificial cooling of the body to reduce the oxygen requirements of the tissues. Generalized lowering of the body temperature is used in three main situations: (a) to control fever, as in malignant hyperthermia; (b) to enable certain cardiac and neurological operations to be carried out; and (c) to protect the brain from raised intracranial pressure in patients with head injuries or following drowning.

**hypothesis** a supposition that appears to explain a group of phenomena and is assumed as a basis of reasoning and experimentation. A starting point for further investigations from known facts.

**hypothrombinaemia** a diminished amount of thrombin in the blood, with a consequent tendency to bleed.

**hypothyroidism** an insufficiency of thyroid secretion. In children it may produce cretinism. In adults it leads to myxoedema.

**hypotonia** 1. deficient muscle tone. 2. deficient tension in the eyeball.

**hypotonic** describing a solution that has a lower osmotic pressure than another one. *See* HYPERTONIC.

**hypoventilation** hypopnoea; shallow breathing, usually at a very slow rate. It may cause a build-up of carbon dioxide in the blood.

**hypovolaemia** a reduction in the circulating blood volume due to external loss of body fluids or to loss from the blood into the tissues, as in shock.

**hypoxaemia** an insufficient oxygen content in the blood.

**hypoxia** a diminished amount of oxygen in the tissues. *Anaemic h.* low oxygen content due to deficiency of haemoglobin in the blood.

**hysterectomy** removal of the uterus. *Abdominal h.* removal via an abdominal incision. *Subtotal h.* removal of the body of the uterus only. *Total h.* removal of the body and cervix.

*Vaginal h.* removal through the vagina. *Wertheim's h.* additional excision of the parametrium, upper vagina and lymph glands. Radical abdominal hysterectomy.

**hysteria** a psychoneurosis in which the individual converts anxiety created by emotional conflict into physical symptoms, e.g. tics, mutism or paralysis of an arm or leg, that have no organic basis; formerly called conversion reaction or conversion hysteria. The term hysteria is also used to describe a state of tension or excitement in which there is a temporary loss of control over the emotions.

**hysterical** relating to hysteria.

**hystero-oöphorectomy** excision of the uterus and the ovaries.

**hysterosalpingography** radiographic examination of the uterus and uterine tubes after the injection of a radio-opaque dye. Uterosalpingography.

**hysterosalpingostomy or an anastomis** the operation of forming an anastomosis, or opening, between the distal portion of the uterine tube and the uterus in an effort to overcome infertility when the medial portion is occluded or excised.

**hysterotomy** incision of the uterus, usually in order to remove a fetus in mid-pregnancy when it is too late to perform a therapeutic abortion.

**I** symbol for *iodine*.

**iatrogenesis** additional patient problems, complications or disease brought about by the activities of physicians, surgeons or other health care professionals, including new infections, unwanted effects of drug therapy and psychological distress.

**ice** water in a solid state, at or below freezing point. *Dry i.* carbon dioxide snow. *I. bag* a rubber or plastic bag half-filled with pieces of ice and applied near or to a part to relieve pain or swelling.

**ichthyosis** a congenital abnormality of the skin in which there is dryness and roughness, the horny layer is thickened and large scales appear.

**ICM** International Confederation of Midwives.

**ICN** infection control nurse (*see* INFECTION); International Council of Nurses.

**ICP** intracranial pressure.

**ICSH** interstitial cell stimulating hormone.

**icterus** jaundice. *I. gravis* a fatal form of jaundice occurring in pregnancy. Acute yellow atrophy. *I. gravis neonatorum* haemolytic disease of the newborn. *See* RHESUS FACTOR.

**ICU** intensive care unit.

**id** that part of the personality, containing the instinctive drives, which leads to gratification of primitive needs and which exists in the unconscious.

**idea** a mental impression or conception. *Autochthonous i.* a strange idea that comes into the mind in some unaccountable way, but is not a hallucination. *Compulsive i.* an idea that persists despite reason and will and that drives one to action, usually inappropriate. *Dominant i.* a morbid or other impression that controls or colours every action and thought. *Fixed i.* a persistent morbid impression or belief that cannot be changed by reason. *I. of reference* the incorrect idea that the words and actions of others refer to oneself, or the projection of the causes of one's own imaginary difficulties upon someone else.

**identical** exactly alike. *I. twins* twins of the same sex developing from a single fertilized ovum.

**identification** a mental mechanism by which an individual adopts the attitudes and ideas of another, often admired, person.

**identity** part of the 'self concept' of being distinguishable and separate from others. *I. crisis* one in which the individual loses the sense of self-distinctiveness and role in society. Occurs most commonly in the transition from one phase of life to the next, e.g. during adolescence.

**ideology** 1. the science of the development of ideas. 2. the body of ideas characteristic of an individual or of a social unit.

**ideomotion** the association of ideas and muscle action, as in involuntary acts.

**idiopathic** self-originated; applied to a condition the cause of which is not known.

**idiosyncrasy** 1. a habit or quality of body or mind peculiar to any individual. 2. an abnormal susceptibility to an agent (e.g. a drug) that is peculiar to the individual.

**Ig** immunoglobulin of any of the five classes: IgA, IgD, IgE, IgG and IgM.

**ileal** referring to the ileum. *I. conduit* a surgical procedure in which the ureters are transplanted into the ileum, an isolated loop of which is then brought to the surface of the abdomen in order to allow the urine to drain into a bag.

**ileitis** inflammation of the ileum. *Regional i.* Crohn's disease. A chronic condition of the terminal portion of the ileum in which granulation and oedema may give rise to obstruction.

**ileocolitis** inflammation of the ileum and colon.

**ileocolostomy** the making of a permanent opening between the ileum and some part of the colon.

**ileoproctostomy** surgical anastomosis between the ileum and the rectum; ileorectal anastomosis.

**ileorectal** referring to the ileum and rectum. *I. anastomosis* ileoproctostomy.

**ileosigmoidostomy** an operation carried out when most of the colon has to be removed and an anastomosis is made between the ileum and the sigmoid colon.

**ileostomy** an artificial opening (stoma) created from the ileum and brought to the surface of the abdomen for the purpose of evacuation. Ileostomy is an inevitable part of proctocolectomy. An ileostomy may be temporary or permanent. *I. bags* disposable bags to collect the liquid faecal matter discharged from an ileostomy. The bags can be adhesive or worn on a belt.

**ileum** the last part of the small intestine, terminating at the caecum.

**ileus** intestinal obstruction, especially failure of peristalsis. The condition frequently accompanies peritonitis and usually results from disturbances in neural stimulation of the bowel. The principal symptoms of ileus are abdominal pain and distension, vomiting (the vomitus may contain faecal material) and constipation. If the intestinal obstruction is not relieved, the patient becomes extremely ill with SHOCK and DEHYDRATION.

**iliac** pertaining to the ilium. *I. artery* the right and left arteries form the terminal branches of the abdominal aorta and supply blood to the pelvic region and the lower limbs. *I. crest* the crest of the hip bone. *I. fossa* the depression on the concave surface of the iliac bone. *I. vein* the right and left veins join to form the inferior vena cava and drain the blood from the lower limbs and pelvis.

**ilium** the haunch bone; the upper part of the hip bone.

**illness** a condition marked by pronounced deviation from the normal healthy state; sickness. *I. behaviour* the way in which ill individuals regard the structure and function of their own body, interpret symptoms and seek treatment for their condition.

**illusion** a mistaken perception due to a misinterpretation of a sensory stimulus; believing something to be what it is not.

**image** 1. the mental recall of a former precept. 2. the optical picture transferred to the brain cells by the optic nerve.

**imaging** diagnostic techniques that are used to produce images of organs or tissues within the body.

These may be plain X-rays to view dense structures such as bone, or contrast X-rays used to view internal organs, e.g. barium X-rays to examine the oesophagus, stomach and small intestine. Newer techniques include ultrasonography. Computerized tomography (CT) uses X-rays and a scanner, and is particularly useful in examination of the head, chest and abdomen; other techniques include radionuclide scans and magnetic resonance and positron emission tomography (*see* MAGNETIC RESONANCE IMAGING and RADIONUCLIDE). Some of these techniques use computers to process the data and produce the image.

**imago** [L.] 1. in psychoanalysis, a childhood memory or fantasy of a loved person that persists in adult life. 2. the adult or definitive form of an insect.

**imbalance** lack of balance, e.g. of endocrine secretions, between water and electrolytes, or of muscles.

**immature** unripe; not fully developed, as in a cataract when only a part of the lens is opaque.

**immiscible** incapable of being mixed, e.g. oil and water.

**immobilize** to render incapable of being moved, as by a plaster of Paris cast.

**immune** protected against a particular infection or allergy. *I. response* the (in general) helpful events that follow activation of the immune system, including T lymphocyte activity (cell-mediated responses) and B lymphocyte activity (humoral responses). Immune responses are involved in protecting persons from disease following infection and are also involved in the rejection of transplanted organs and tissues that the body recognizes as foreign, or non-self.

**immunity** the resistance possessed by the body to infectious diseases, foreign tissues, foreign non-toxic substances and other ANTIGENS. The opposite of susceptibility. Immunological responses in humans can be divided into two broad categories: humoral immunity, which takes place in the body fluids and is concerned with antibody and complement activities; and cell-mediated or cellular immunity, which involves a variety of activities designed to destroy or at least contain cells that are recognized by the body as alien and harmful. Both types of response are instigated by lymphocytes that originate in the bone marrow as stem cells and later are converted into mature cells having specific properties and functions. The two kinds of lymphocyte that are important to the establishment of immunity are T lymphocytes (T cells), which kill cells infected with viruses and other intracellular parasites, and B lymphocytes (B cells). B lymphocytes mature into plasma cells that are primarily responsible for forming antibodies, thereby providing humoral immunity. Cellular immunity is dependent upon T lymphocytes and is primarily concerned with a delayed type of immune response as occurs in the rejection of transplanted organs, defence against some slowly developing bacterial diseases, allergic reactions and certain autoimmune diseases.

**immunization** the act of creating immunity by artificial means. *I. schedule* a standard schedule for immunization against infectious diseases (*see* Appendix 9).

**immunoassay** a quantitative estimate of the proteins contained in the blood serum.

**immunodeficiency** a deficiency of the immune response, either that mediated by humoral antibody or by immune lymphoid cells. *I. disorders* acquired or congenital conditions in which the body's immune system fails to protect against infection, foreign material and some forms of cancer.

**immunoglobulin** *See* ANTIBODY.

**immunology** the study of immunity and the body's defence mechanisms.

**immunosuppression** inhibition of the formation of antibodies to antigens that may be present; used in transplantation procedures to prevent rejection of the transplanted organ or tissue.

**immunosuppressive** 1. pertaining to or inducing immunosuppression. 2. an agent that induces immunosuppression.

**immunotherapy** 1. treatment by immunization. Sometimes used in the treatment of some cancers and chronic disorders, e.g. rheumatoid arthritis. 2. the establishing of passive immunity.

**immunotransfusion** transfusion of blood from a donor previously rendered immune to the disease affecting the patient.

**impaction** a state of being wedged. *Dental i.* the condition in which a tooth, usually a molar, is unable to erupt through the gum because it is lodged in position by bone or the other teeth. *Faecal i.* a collection of putty-like or hardened faeces in the rectum or sigmoid colon.

**impairment** any loss or abnormality of psychological, physiological or anatomical structure or function.

**impalpable** incapable of being felt by manual examination. May apply to an organ or a tumour.

**imperforate** without an opening. *I. anus* a congenital defect in which this opening is closed. *I. hymen* complete closure of the vaginal opening by the hymen.

**impermeable** not permitting the passage of fluid or molecules.

**impetigo** an acute contagious inflammation of the skin marked by pustules and scabs; of streptococcal or staphylococcal origin. It occurs mainly on the face and limbs, particularly those of children.

**implant** any substance grafted into the tissues; may be living cells or inert materials. *Hormone i.* a hormonal pellet which may be implanted subcutaneously. *Intraocular lens i.* a plastic lens which may be implanted in the eye after lens extraction. *Plastic i.* a silicone implant which may be used in plastic surgery, e.g. to reshape the breast.

**implantation** the act of planting or setting in. 1. the embedding of the fertilized ovum in the wall of the uterus. 2. the placing of a drug within the tissues. 3. the surgical introduction of healthy tissue to replace tissue that has been damaged.

**implementation** the third phase of the nursing process signifying the giving of care in relation to defined nursing interventions and goals. During implementation the nursing care plan is tested for effectiveness and accuracy. Data gathering continues and plans may change on the basis of new information obtained. The implementation phase concludes with the recording of the activities performed and the response of the patient. *See* ASSESSMENT and EVALUATION.

**implosion** in behaviour therapy, a form of desensitization used in the treatment of phobias and related disorders. *See* FLOODING.

**impotence** inability in a man to carry out sexual intercourse from either psychological or physical causes.

**impregnation** insemination; rendering pregnant.

**impression** an imitation of a person or thing. In dentistry, a mould made of a toothless jaw or of the teeth and surrounding tissues, used in the construction of dentures and dental braces.

**impulse** 1. a sudden pushing force. 2. a sudden uncontrollable act. 3. nerve impulse. *Cardiac i.* movement of the chest wall caused by the heart beat. *Nerve i.* the electrochemical process propagated along nerve fibres.

**IMV** intermittent mandatory ventilation.

**inaccessibility** a state of unresponsiveness characteristic of certain psychiatric patients, e.g. schizophrenics.

**inarticulate** 1. without joints. 2. unable to speak intelligibly.

**incarcerated** held fast. Applied to (a) a hernia that is immovable, and therefore only curable by operation, and (b) a pregnant uterus held under the sacral brim.

**incest** sexual intercourse between close blood relatives, e.g. brothers and sisters; marriage between them is legally or culturally prohibited. Some form of incest taboo is found in all known societies, although the relationships prohibited vary.

**incidence** the number of particular new events which occur in a population in a given period of time. For example, the number of new cases of a disease, such as measles, expressed per 1000 of population per year.

**Incident Report** a report the completion of which is required by NHS Trusts and other health care facilities following any accident or untoward incident involving a patient, visitor or member of staff. These incidents may be clinical, e.g. cardiac arrest or the incorrect administration of a medication, but can also include such issues as the loss of a patient's belongings. Also known as a Critical Incident Report.

**incipient** beginning to exist.

**incision** 1. in surgery, a cut into soft tissue. 2. the act of cutting.

**incisor** one of the four front teeth in the centre of each jaw.

**inclusion** something that is enclosed or the act of enclosing. *I. bodies* particles that are temporarily enclosed in the cytoplasm of a cell. For example, in trachoma virus particles can be seen in the conjunctival epithelial cells.

**incoherent** 1. unconnected; inconsistent. 2. uttering speech that is disconnected and rambling.

**incompatibility** the state of two or more substances being antagonistic, or destroying the efficiency of each other. Applied to mixtures of drugs, and to blood. *See* BLOOD GROUPS.

**incompetence** inefficiency. *Aortic i.* failure of the aortic valves to regulate the flow of blood. *Mitral i.* failure of the mitral valve to close properly.

**incontinence** inability to control natural functions or discharges. *Faecal i.* inability to control the movements of the bowels. *Overflow i.* that from an overfull bladder, most common in elderly men with urinary obstruction. *Paralytic i.* loss of control of anal and urethral sphincters due to injury to nerve centres. *Stress i.* that which is due to a defect in the urethral sphincters and is liable to occur when intra-abdominal pressure is increased, as in coughing or lifting heavy weights; most common in women with weak pelvic muscles. *Urinary i.* inability to control the outflow of urine.

**incoordination** inability to adjust various muscle movements harmoniously.

**increment** an increase or addition.

**incremental** to build up as in the contractions of labour or to add in stages.

**incrustation** the formation of a crust or scab on a wound.

**incubation** the development and growth of microorganisms and animal embryos. *I. period* the period between the date of infection and the appearance of symptoms of an infectious disease.

**incubator** 1. a warmed servo-controlled Perspex box for nursing ill and preterm babies. 2. an apparatus used to develop bacteria at a uniform temperature suitable to their growth.

**incus** the small anvil-shaped bone of the middle ear. The second auditory ossicle.

**independent nursing practice** any nursing intervention for which the nurse alone is responsible. Such interventions are based upon the nurse's assessment, care planning, goal setting and evaluation, without instruction from other health care providers.

**indicator** 1. the index finger, or the extensor muscle of the index finger. 2. any substance that indicates the appearance or disappearance of a chemical by a colour change or attainment of a certain pH.

**indigenous** occurring naturally in a certain locality.

**indigestion** *see* DYSPEPSIA.

**indolent** slow-growing. Reluctant to heal. Largely painless. *I. ulcer* a chronic ulcer of the skin or mucous membrane.

**induction** the act of initiating something. *Electromagnetic i.* the production of an electric current in a body because of its nearness to an electrified (or magnetized) body. *I. of abortion* the intentional bringing about of an abortion. *I. of anaesthesia* the start of the administration of a general anaesthetic. *I. of labour* the artificial starting of the process of childbirth.

**induration** the abnormal hardening of a tissue or organ.

**industrial** referring to industry. *I. or occupational diseases* those

that are caused by the nature of the work. *Prescribed i. diseases* those for which sickness benefit is payable, including those that are notifiable under the Factories Act 1961.

**inebriation** the condition of being intoxicated by alcohol; drunkenness.

**inert** having no action. *I. gas* a gas which does not react with other elements, e.g. neon.

**inertia** sluggishness; inability to move except when stimulated by an external force. *Uterine i.* lack of muscle contraction during the first and second stages of labour.

**infant** a child under 1 year of age. Educationally, a child under 7 years of age. *Floppy i., floppy i. syndrome* a congenital myopathy of infants, marked clinically by myotonia and muscle weakness. *I. feeding* the supplying of nutrition to an infant. Breast milk is the ideal food for the baby and if breast feeding is established satisfactorily for the first few months it can aid physical and emotional development. Where it is not possible an infant food formula can be given. *I. mortality rate* the number of deaths of children under 1 year of age per 1000 live births in any one year. *Premature i.* one born before the state of maturity. *See* PRETERM INFANT.

**infanticide** the killing of a child during the first year of its life when she may be psychologically disturbed. Occurs in association with some psychiatric disorders, e.g. depressive illness.

**infantile** concerning an infant; childish. *I. paralysis* poliomyelitis.

**infantilism** persistence of the characteristics of childhood into adult life, marked by underdevelopment of the reproductive organs, and often short stature.

**infarct** the wedge-shaped area of necrosis in an organ produced by the blocking of a blood vessel, usually due to an embolus. *Red i.* a haemorrhage infarct. Red blood cells infiltrate the area. *White i.* an anaemic infarct. The area is suddenly deprived of blood and is pale.

**infarction** the formation of an infarct. *Myocardial i.* an infarct of the heart muscle following a coronary thrombosis. *Pulmonary i.* an infarct resulting from obstruction of a branch of the pulmonary artery by embolism or thrombosis.

**infection** 1. invasion and multiplication of microorganisms in body tissues, especially that causing local cellular injury due to competitive metabolism, toxins, intracellular replication or antigen–antibody response. 2. an infectious disease. *Aerobic i.* infection caused by an aerobe. *Airborne i.* infection by inhalation of organisms suspended in air on water droplets, droplet nuclei or dust particles. *Anaerobic i.* infection caused by an ANAEROBE. *Cross i.* infection transmitted between patients infected with different pathogenic microorganisms. *Droplet i.* infection due to inhalation of respiratory pathogens suspended on liquid particles exhaled by someone already infected. *Health care-associated infections* those acquired during episodes of health care, usually but not exclusively in hospitals. A prevalence survey in 2006 found that 8.2% of patients in hospitals in England had acquired a healthcare-associated infection. The most common causative agents are *Escherichia coli, Proteus, Pseudomonas* and *Klebsiella* among the Gram-negative organisms, and *Staphylococcus* and *Enterococcus* among the Gram-positive organisms. *See also* INFECTION (CONTROL). *I. control* the utilization of procedures and techniques in the surveillance, investigation and compilation of statistical data in

order to reduce the spread of infection, particularly hospital-acquired infections. Practitioners in infection control are frequently nurses who are employed by NHS Trusts and other health care facilities. They have titles such as Director of Infection Prevention and Control (DIPC), Consultants in Infection Prevention and Control and Infection Prevention and Control Practitioners/Nurses, and they function as liaison between staff, nurses, doctors, department heads, infection control commitees and the health authority. Such practitioners also assume some responsibility for teaching patients and their families, as well as employees. *Mixed i.* infection with more than one kind of organism at the same time. *Opportunistic i.* an infection with a microorganism that does not usually cause disease but may do so when the patient's resistance to infection is lowered, e.g. after surgery. *Secondary i.* infection by a pathogen superimposed upon an infection by a pathogen of another kind. *Sexually transmitted i.* an infection transmitted by sexual intercourse or by intimate contact with the genitals, mouth and rectum. *See* SEXUALLY TRANSMITTED INFECTION. *Subclinical i.* infection associated with no detectable symptoms but caused by microorganisms capable of producing easily recognizable diseases, such as poliomyelitis or mumps; it is detected by the production of antibody, or by delayed hypersensitivity exhibited in a skin test reaction to such antigens as tuberculoprotein.

**infectious** caused by or capable of being communicated by infection (*see* Table on p. 208). *I. disease* disease resulting from multiplication of microorganisms in the body. Most are communicable, but not all. *See also* COMMUNICABLE

| INFECTIOUS DISEASES | | | |
|---|---|---|---|
| Disease | Incubation period (days) | Period of infectivity | |
| Chickenpox (varicella) | 10–20 | 2–3 days before until 10 days after onset of rash | Notifiable in Scotland and N. Ireland |
| Diphtheria | 2–7 | Until culture of three consecutive nose swabs proves negative | Notifiable UK |
| Enteric fevers Typhoid Paratyphoid | 6–21 | Until at least 1 month after onset of disease and six consecutive negative stools | Notifiable UK |
| Measles (morbilli) | 6–12 | 4 days before until 4 days after onset of rash | Notifiable UK |
| Mumps (parotitis) | 12–28 | 2 days before onset until resolution of symptoms | Notifiable UK |
| Pertussis (whooping cough) | 7–14 | 7 days before until 3 weeks after onset of cough | Notifiable UK |
| Rubella (German measles) | 14–21 | During incubation period until 2 days after resolution of symptoms | Notifiable UK |

DISEASE. *I. mononucleosis* glandular fever. An acute virus infection, characterized by sore throat and glandular enlargement, caused by the Epstein–Barr (EB) virus. A common infection worldwide, particularly prevalent in older children and young adults in Western countries. The source of infection is human and spread is by oropharyngeal secretions: for example, during kissing. The incubation period is 4–6 weeks and infectivity after the disease may be prolonged.

**infective** infectious, capable of producing infection; pertaining to or characterized by the presence of pathogens.

**inferior** lower. *I. vena cava* the lower large vein.

**inferiority** lesser rank, stature, position or ability. *I. complex see* COMPLEX.

**infertility** inability of a woman to conceive or of a man to bring about conception.

**infestation** the presence of animal parasites, e.g. mites, ticks or worms, in or on the body, in clothing or in a house.

**infibulation** an extensive form of female circumcision performed in some cultures in which the clitoris and labia are removed and the vaginal entrance narrowed. *See* CIRCUMCISION.

**infiltration** the entrance and diffusion of some substance not usually found there, either fluid or solid, into tissues or cells. *I. analgesia* the injection into tissues of a local analgesic solution.

**inflammation** a localized protective response elicited by injury or destruction of tissues, which serves to destroy, dilute or wall off both the injurious agent and the injured tissue. The cardinal signs are heat, swelling, pain and redness (*see* Figure). *Acute i.* sudden onset of inflammation, with marked and progressive symptoms. *Catarrhal i.* inflammation in which mucous surfaces are attacked, with stimulation of exudation. *Chronic i.* inflammation that develops slowly. Granulation tissue forms and tends to localize the infection. *Diffuse i.* extensive inflammation, as in nephritis and cellulitis. *Suppurative i.* one marked by pus formation. *Traumatic i.* that which follows an injury.

**inflammatory bowel disease** abbreviated IBD. Collective term for a group of chronic disorders affecting the small and/or large intestines that results in pain, bleeding and diarrhoea. *See* CROHN'S DISEASE.

**influenza** an acute viral infection of the respiratory tract, occurring in isolated cases, epidemics and pandemics. Also called 'flu.' Transmission is by droplet inhalation and the period of infectivity lasts from 1 day before the onset of symptoms until up to 7 days later. In the UK, most cases occur between December and May, with the peak incidence being in February. There is fever, headache, pain in the back and limbs, anorexia and sometimes nausea and vomiting. The fever subsides in 2–3 days, leaving a feeling of lassitude. There is no specific drug cure for influenza, but an influenza vaccine is available, the formulation of which is changed annually to include recently circulating strains of viruses on recommendation of the World Health Organization. Annual vaccination is advised for persons with chronic heart, lung or renal disease, those with diabetes, and patients on immunosuppressive therapy. It should also be advised for people over 65 years old and residents of residential and nursing homes.

**informal patient** a patient who has entered hospital voluntarily, i.e. without any statutory requirements for detention.

INFLAMMATION

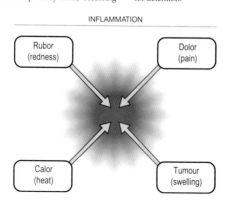

**informatics** discipline that integrates science, computer science and information science in systematizing, identifying, collecting, processing and managing data. *Nursing i.* the way in which nurses, managers, researchers and practitioners use information systems in their work, enabling technology to develop a body of readily available knowledge to support the practice of nursing and the delivery of health care.

**informed choice** in order to make decisions about their own health care and treatment mentally competent patients need to be given information regarding their own condition that is accurate, non-judgemental and valid, in language that is jargon free and understandable. This enables the patient to make an informed choice from the treatment options. In some situations an interpreter may be required.

**informed consent** *see* CONSENT.

**infrared** rays of a lower wavelength than those in the visible spectrum. They can produce radiant heat which is used in the treatment of rheumatic conditions. *See* ULTRAVIOLET RAYS.

**infusion** 1. the process of extracting the soluble principles of substances (especially drugs) by soaking in water. 2. the solution thus produced. 3. the slow therapeutic introduction by gravity of fluid other than blood into a vein.

**ingestion** the taking in of food and drugs by mouth.

**inguinal** relating to the groin. *I. canal* the channel through the abdominal wall, above Poupart's ligament, through which the spermatic cord and vessels pass to the testis in the male, and which contains the round ligament of the uterus in the female. *I. ligament* Poupart's ligament; that connecting the anterior superior spine of the ilium to the tubercle of the pubis.

**inhalation** 1. the drawing of air or other substances into the lungs. 2. any drug or solution of drugs, administered (as by means of nebulizers or aerosols) by the nasal or oral respiratory route.

**inhaler** an apparatus used for administering an inhalation.

**inherent** a characteristic that is innate or natural and essentially a part of the person.

**inheritance** the acquisition of qualities and characteristics from parents and ancestors.

**inhibition** arrest or restraint of a process. In psychiatry, the unconscious restraining of an instinctual drive.

**injection** 1. the forcing of a liquid into a part, as into the subcutaneous tissues, the vascular tree or an organ (*see* Figure on p. 211). 2. a substance so forced or administered; in pharmacy, a solution of a medicament suitable for injection. 3. prominence of small blood vessels on the surface of an organ or tissue, frequently indicating the vascular phase of an inflammatory response. *Depot i.* the giving of a medication by injection, usually intramuscularly, that can be absorbed slowly over a period of time. Many drugs and hormones are given in this way. *Hypodermic i.* that made just below the skin; a subcutaneous injection. *Intramuscular i.* that made into a muscle. *Intrathecal i.* that made into the subarachnoid space of the spinal cord. *Intravenous i.* that made into a vein. *Subcutaneous i.* that made into the subcutaneous tissues; a hypodermic injection.

**inlay** material inserted to replace a defect in a tissue: for example, a bone graft or a filling cast in metal to fit a hole in a tooth.

**innate** inborn; present in the individual at birth.

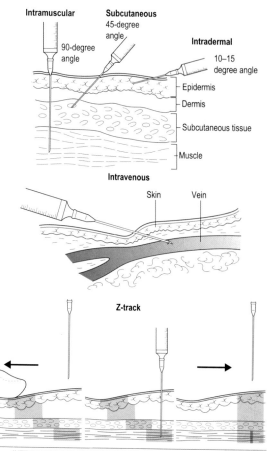

INTRAMUSCULAR, SUBCUTANEOUS, INTRADERMAL AND Z-TRACK
INTRAVENOUS INJECTIONS

**innervation** nerve supply to a part.

**innocent** as applied to a tumour, benign or non-malignant.

**innocuous** harmless.

**innominate** unnamed. *I. artery* a branch of the aorta, now termed the brachiocephalic trunk. *I. bone* the hip bone, formed by the union of the ilium, ischium and pubis.

**inoculation** 1. introduction of pathogenic microorganisms, injected material, serum or other substances into tissues of living organisms or into culture media. 2. introduction of a disease agent (usually a live infectious agent) into a healthy individual to produce a mild form of the disease, followed by IMMUNITY.

**inorganic** of neither animal nor vegetable origin.

**inotropic** affecting the force or energy of muscular contractions, particularly the heart muscle. Beta-blocking drugs are said to be inotropic.

**inquest** a legal inquiry held by a coroner, with or without a jury, into the cause of sudden or unexpected death.

**insanity** a legal term for mental illness, roughly equivalent to PSYCHOSIS and implying inability to be responsible for one's acts.

**insecticide** one of a large group of chemical compounds that kill insect pests.

**insemination** 1. fertilization of an ovum by a spermatozoon. 2. introduction of semen into the vagina. *Artificial i.* insemination by means other than sexual intercourse. The semen can be either the husband's (AIH) or some other donor's (AID).

**insensible** 1. unable to perceive with the senses. 2. unconscious. 3. imperceptible to the senses.

**insertion** 1. the act of implanting. 2. something that is implanted. 3. the attachment of a muscle to the bone that it moves.

**insidious** approaching by stealth. A term applied to any disease that develops imperceptibly.

**insight** mental awareness. The capacity of individuals to estimate a situation or their own behaviour or the connection between their present attitudes and past experiences. In psychiatry, a recognition by patients that they are ill. Insight in this connection may be complete, partial or absent, and may alter during the course of the illness.

**in situ** [L.] *in the original position.*

**insoluble** not capable of being dissolved in a liquid.

**insomnia** inability to sleep.

**inspiration** the act of drawing in the breath.

**inspissated** thickened, through evaporation or absorption of fluid.

**instillation** the act of pouring a liquid into a cavity drop by drop, e.g. into the eye.

**instinct** a complex of unlearned responses characteristic of a species. *Death i.* in psychoanalysis, the latent instinctive impulse towards death; the drive to reduce tensions by reaching the ultimate tensionless state of death. *Herd i.* the instinct or urge to be one of a group and to conform to its standards of conduct and opinion.

**institutionalization** a condition of apathy and withdrawal occurring in residents of long-stay institutions, prisons, etc., as a result of rigid routines and lack of independence. The person may resist leaving because the routine has become predictable and familiar, making minimal demands.

**insufficiency** inadequacy. Used to describe the failure of function of an organ, such as the heart, stomach, liver or muscles.

**insufflation** the act of blowing air, gas or powder into a cavity of the body.

**insulin** a protein hormone formed in the beta cells of the pancreatic islets of Langerhans. The major fuel-regulating hormone, it is secreted into the blood in response to a rise in concentration of blood glucose or amino acids. A deficiency results in diabetes mellitus. Various types of commercially prepared insulin are available. There are three main groups: rapid-acting, intermediate-acting and long-acting. Diabetic patients react differently in the rate at which they absorb and utilize insulin; therefore the duration of action varies from patient to patient. Insulin is measured in units. The concentration used is 100 units/ml. This strength allows for accurate measurement of dosage and reduces the possibility of error in calculating an individual dose. *I. pump* a device consisting of a syringe filled with a predetermined amount of short-acting insulin, a plastic cannula and a needle, and a pump that periodically delivers the desired amount of insulin.

**insulin dependent diabetes mellitus** type 1 diabetes mellitus.

**insulinoma** a benign adenoma of the islet cells of the pancreas, causing hypoglycaemia.

**insult** any trauma, irritation, poisoning or injury to the body.

**integrated therapy** a combination of complementary therapies with orthodox medicine to facilitate healing and promote the wellbeing of the patient. A biopsychosocial approach to care.

**integument** 1. the skin. 2. a layer of tissue covering a part or organ of the body.

**intellect** the mind, thinking faculty, reasoning or understanding.

**intelligence** 1. the capacity to understand. 2. general mental ability. *I. quotient* abbreviated IQ. The ratio of the mental age to the chronological age expressed as a percentage. *I. test* a test designed to measure the level of intelligence, usually expressed as an IQ.

**Intensive Care Unit** abbreviated ICU. A hospital unit in which are concentrated special equipment and specially trained personnel for the care of seriously ill patients requiring immediate and continuous monitoring and treatment. Also called critical care unit (CCU), intensive therapy unit (ITU). *Neonatal ICU* abbreviated NICU. An intensive care unit that is designated solely for small, preterm neonates and those neonates requiring surgery or other specialized care. *Paediatric ICU* abbreviated PICU. A unit providing intensive care solely for seriously ill children.

**intention** a process of healing.

**intercellular** between the cells of a structure. May be applied to the connective tissue or to fluid bathing the cells.

**intercostal** between the ribs. *I. muscles* muscles situated between the ribs and controlling their movements during inspiration and expiration.

**intercourse** 1. social exchange. 2. sexual intercourse or coitus.

**intercurrent** occurring at the same time. Describes a disease occurring during the course of another disease in the same person.

**interdisciplinary** joint working between professional disciplines: nursing, social work, clergy, medical staff, physiotherapy and other allied health professions.

**interferon** a protein, produced by cells infected by a virus, which has an inhibitory effect on the multiplication of the invading viruses, thus preventing uninfected cells from becoming infected and hastening recovery from viral disease. Human interferon preparations, products of genetic engineering, are used in the treatment of some cancers and hepatitis B and C.

**interlobular** between lobules. *I. veins* branches of the portal vein in the liver.

**intermediate care** the purpose of services designed to assist the transition for a patient or client from medical and social dependence to day-to-day independence. A range of services have the potential to fulfil this function as people move from hospital to home, where the objectives of care are not primarily medical, the patient's discharge destination is anticipated, and a clinical outcome of recovery (or restoration of health) is desired. Specifically excluded are services such as convalescence or hotel beds that do not have therapeutic input (King's Fund definition).

**intermenstrual** occurring between two menstrual periods.

**intermission** a temporary interruption, particularly of a feverish condition.

**intermittent** occurring at intervals. *I. claudication* see CLAUDICATION. *I. fever* one in which the temperature drops to normal or lower, at times. *I. mandatory ventilation* abbreviated IMV. A type of mechanical ventilation in which the VENTILATOR is set to deliver a prescribed tidal volume at specified intervals, and a high-flow gas system permits the patient to breathe spontaneously between cycles. *I. peritoneal dialysis* see DIALYSIS. *I. pneumatic compression hose* a stocking worn to prevent deep vein thrombosis of upper and lower leg. *I. positive airway ventilation* abbreviated IPAV; also known as intermittent positive pressure ventilation, abbreviated IPPV. A method of assisted ventilation in which oxygen or air is used under pressure to inflate the lungs when the patient is unable to breathe spontaneously.

**internal** situated on the inside. *I. haemorrhage* one occurring in a cavity or into the tissues. *I. secretion* one in which the hormones pass directly into the bloodstream from the secreting gland.

**International Classification of Diseases** abbreviated ICD. A publication of the World Health Organization produced approximately every 10 years listing all known disease categories.

**International Council of Nurses** abbreviated ICN. Founded in 1899 to represent worldwide international nurses' associations as a corporate organization.

**internet** a global computer network with millions of connected computers. By connecting to this network, it is possible to access a wide range of information including health-related information and provide for the transmission of electronic mail. NHSNet links all NHS Trusts and can exchange information with other health care organizations and agencies. *I. addiction syndrome* first described in 1994 and characterized by excessive or pathological 'internet surfing' which may lead to financial hardship, sleep deprivation, isolation and even job or relationship loss due to the excessive hours spent on the internet. *See* DEPENDENCE.

**interphase** the period between two cell divisions during which the chromosomes are not easily visible.

**intersex** 1. a congenital abnormality in which anatomical features of both sexes are evident. 2. a person displaying intersexuality.

**intersexuality** an intermingling of the characters of each sex, including physical form, reproductive tissue and sexual behaviour, in one individual, as a result of some flaw in embryonic development.

**interstitial** situated within the tissue spaces or between the tissues. *I. cell stimulating hormone* abbreviated ICSH. Luteinizing hormone.

*I. fluid* the fluid in which body cells are bathed. It acts as an intermediary between the cells and the blood. Extracellular fluid. *I. keratitis* see KERATITIS. *I. nephritis* chronic nephritis associated with fibrosis and hypertension.

**intertrigo** an irritating, eczematous skin eruption caused by the chafing of two moist skin surfaces.

**intervention** in health care, any act carried out to prevent harm to patients or to improve, promote or enhance their physical, mental or spiritual wellbeing.

**intervertebral** between the vertebrae. *I. disc* the pad of fibrocartilage between the bodies of the vertebrae. Protrusion of the contents of the disc may give rise to sciatica by exerting pressure on the nerve roots.

**interviewing** process involving a semi-structured meeting and conversational style that allows the interviewer to probe for information and is widely used in everyday situations. This technique is also used at the initial stage of patient assessment in developing a nursing care plan. Interviews are used as a method of data collection involving face-to-face or telephone questioning by the researcher; most often used in qualitative research.

**intestinal** referring to the intestine.

**intestine** that part of the alimentary canal that extends from the stomach to the anus. *Small i.* the first 6 m from the pylorus to the caecum, consisting of the duodenum, the jejunum and the ileum. *Large i.* the final 2 m, consisting of the caecum, the ascending, transverse and descending colon, and the rectum.

**intima** the innermost coat of an artery or vein.

**intolerance** lack of power to endure. Applied to the effect of some drugs on individuals, e.g. iodine and quinine. See IDIOSYNCRASY.

**intoxication** 1. poisoning by drugs or harmful substances. 2. the condition produced by excessive use of alcohol.

**intra-abdominal** within the abdomen.

**intra-articular** within a joint capsule. *I-a. injection* injection into a joint capsule, applicable to hydrocortisone, for example.

**intracapsular** within a capsule, usually of a joint. *I. extraction* the removal of the whole lens with its capsule in the treatment of cataract.

**intracellular** within a cell. *I. fluid* the water and its dissolved salts found within the cells.

**intracerebral** within the brain substance. *I. haemorrhage* an escape of blood in the cerebrum, most often arising from the middle cerebral artery or from an aneurysm.

**intracranial** within the skull. *I. abscess* one arising within the brain or meninges. *I. aneurysm* dilatation of one of the cerebral vessels. It may be congenital or acquired. *I. pressure* abbreviated ICP. The pressure exerted by the cerebrospinal fluid within the subarachnoid space and ventricles of the brain.

**intractable** not able to be relieved, controlled or cured.

**intradermal** between the layers of the skin.

**intradural** within the dura mater. *I. haemorrhage* see HAEMORRHAGE.

**intragastric** within the stomach.

**intrahepatic** within the liver. Referring to a condition of the liver cells or connective tissue.

**intralobular** within a lobule. *I. veins* veins that collect blood from within the lobules of the liver.

**intramedullary** 1. within the medulla oblongata. 2. within the bone marrow. *I. nail* a metal pin used for the internal fixation of fractures.

**intramuscular** within muscle tissue.

**intranet** A computer network designed to meet the internal needs of a single organization, e.g. the NHS.

It is not necessarily open to the internet and is not accessible by individuals from outside the organization.

**intraocular** within the eyeball.

**intraorbital** within the orbit of the eye.

**intraosseous** within a bone. *I. infusion* the process of supplying fluid into the narrow cavity of a bone in a life-threatening situation.

**intraperitoneal** within the peritoneal cavity.

**intrathecal** within the meninges of the spinal cord, usually in the subarachnoid space.

**intratracheal** endotracheal; within the trachea. *I. anaesthesia* inhalation anaesthesia. *See* ANAESTHESIA.

**intrauterine** within the uterus. *I. contraceptive device* abbreviated IUCD. A contraceptive device introduced into the uterine cavity. *I. growth retardation* associated with a poor blood supply to the placenta, or maternal disease. Other factors include infection during pregnancy, maternal smoking or drug addiction. The infant at birth is 'small for dates' and falls below the tenth percentile of appropriate gestational age for infants. *I. insemination* abbreviated IUI. Following the induction of ovulation fresh sperm are introduced into the uterus with ultrasound supervision; allows fertilization to take place naturally in the uterine tubes. *See* IN VITRO FERTILIZATION. *I. life* fetal development in the uterus.

**intravenous** within a vein. *I. flow rate* the rate at which fluids, medications and blood products flow into the bloodstream during intravenous infusion. The flow rate is usually ordered by the doctor as total volume (ml) per total hours or, in the case of drugs, total dose per total hours. *I. infusion* the therapeutic introduction of a fluid, such as saline, into a vein. The infusion works by gravity, in that the container of fluid is higher than the blood vessel into which the fluid is being introduced. *I. urography* radiographic examination of the urinary tract after the injection of a radio-opaque contrast medium into a vein.

**intraventricular** within a ventricle; may apply to a cerebral or a cardiac ventricle.

**intrinsic** particular to or contained within an organ. *I. factor* a glycoprotein, contained in the gastric juices, which is necessary for the absorption of extrinsic factor (vitamin $B_{12}$).

**introitus** [L.] an opening or entrance into a hollow organ or cavity. *I. vaginae* the vulva.

**introjection** a mental process by which individuals take into themselves the personal characteristics of another person, usually those of someone much loved or admired.

**introspection** a subjective study of the mind and its processes, in which individuals study their own reactions.

**introversion** 1. a turning inwards within itself of a hollow organ. 2. preoccupation with oneself, with reduction of interest in the outside world.

**introvert** a person whose interests are turned inwards upon the self. *See* EXTROVERT.

**intubation** the introduction of a tube into a part of the body, particularly into the air passages to allow air to enter the lungs.

**intussusception** prolapse of one part of the intestine into the lumen of an immediately adjacent part (*see* Figure on p. 217), causing OBSTRUCTION (INTESTINAL).

**inunction** 1. rubbing an oily or fatty preparation containing a medicinal ingredient into the skin, with absorption of the drug. 2. any preparation so applied.

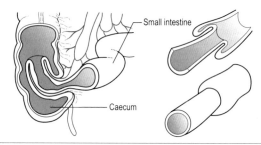

EXAMPLE OF INTUSSUSCEPTION

**invagination** 1. the folding inwards of a part, thus forming a pouch. 2. intussusception.

**invasion** 1. the entry of bacteria into the body. 2. the entrance of parasites into the body of a host.

**invasive** 1. having the quality of invasiveness. 2. involving puncture or incision of the skin or insertion of an instrument or foreign material into the body; said of diagnostic techniques.

**invasiveness** 1. the ability of microorganisms to enter the body and spread in the tissues. 2. the ability to infiltrate and actively destroy surrounding tissue, a property of malignant tumours.

**inversion** a turning upside down or inside out. **Sexual i.** homosexuality. **Uterine i.** the condition of the uterus after parturition when a part of its upper segment protrudes through the cervix.

**investigations** procedures performed to establish a diagnosis, to monitor a person's health, disease or the effectiveness of treatment. They are classified as non-invasive where there is no direct entry into the body, e.g. recording body weight, or invasive, e.g. endoscopy or blood sampling.

**in vitro** the occurrence of a phenomenon in laboratory experiments (literally 'within a glass', e.g. a test tube) and not necessarily reflecting what happens within the human body. For example, a drug may exhibit certain characteristics in vitro that may or may not occur inside the body. *See* IN VIVO. *I. v. fertilization* a technique used to treat infertility for women who have blocked uterine tubes. The woman is given hormone therapy which promotes the maturity of more than one egg at the same time. These eggs are harvested by laparoscopy and fertilized with sperm in the laboratory until a blastocyte is formed. Usually two or more of the fertilized eggs are implanted into the woman's uterus; if these become safely embedded pregnancy continues normally.

**in vivo** occurrence of a phenomenon or effect within the living body as opposed to in vitro.

**involucrum** new bone which forms a sheath around necrosed bone, as in chronic osteomyelitis.

**involuntary** independent of the will. *See* VOLUNTARY. *I. muscle* one that acts without conscious control: for instance, the heart and stomach muscles.

**involution** 1. turning inwards; describes the contraction of the uterus after labour. The process whereby the uterus returns to its normal size. 2. the progressive degeneration occurring naturally with advancing age, resulting in shrivelling of organs or tissues.

**iodine** *symbol* I. A non-metallic element with a distinctive odour, obtained from seaweed. Iodine is essential in nutrition, being especially prevalent in the colloid of the THYROID (GLAND). It is used in the treatment of HYPOTHYROIDISM and as a topical antiseptic. It is a frequent cause of poisoning. Iodine is opaque to X-rays and can be combined with other compounds for use as contrast media in diagnostic radiology.

**ion** an atom or group of atoms having a positive (cation) or negative (anion) electric charge by virtue of having gained or lost one or more electrons. Substances forming ions are electrolytes (*see* ELECTROLYTE). *See* HYDROGEN.

**ionization** the breaking up of molecules into electrically charged particles or ions when an electric current is passed through an electrolytic solution.

**ionizing radiation** *see* RADIATION.

**iontophoresis** the introduction through the skin of therapeutic ions by ionization.

**IPAV** intermittent positive airway ventilation.

**IPPV** intermittent positive pressure ventilation.

**ipsilateral** occurring on the same side. Applied particularly to paralysis or other symptoms occurring on the same side as the cerebral lesion causing them.

**IQ** **intelligence quotient.** *See* INTELLIGENCE.

**IRDS** infant respiratory distress syndrome. *See* RESPIRATORY.

**iridectomy** excision of a part of the iris, usually for the treatment of glaucoma.

**iridium** *symbol* Ir. A radioactive metal, often used in the form of wires or hairpins to treat superficial malignancies, e.g. those of the tongue, cheek or breast.

**iridocele** herniation of a part of the iris through a corneal wound.

**iridocyclitis** inflammation of the iris and ciliary body.

**iridodonesis** trembling of the iris due to lack of support from the lens in dislocation of the lens or after a cataract extraction.

**iridoptosis** prolapse of the iris.

**iris** the coloured part of the eye, made of two layers of muscle, the contraction of which alters the size of the pupil and so controls the amount of light entering the eye. *I. bombé* a bulging forwards of the iris due to pressure of the aqueous humour when its passage into the anterior chamber is obstructed.

**iritis** inflammation of the iris, causing pain, photophobia, contraction of the pupil and discoloration of the iris. *See* UVEITIS.

**iron** *symbol* Fe. A metallic element, present in the body in small quantities and essential to life. A deficiency may produce anaemia.

**irradiation** the treatment of disease by electromagnetic radiation.

**irreducible** incapable of being replaced in a normal position. Applied to a fracture or a hernia.

**irrigation** the washing out of a cavity or wound with a stream of lotion or water.

**irritable** reacting excessively to a stimulus. *I. bowel syndrome* (IBS) mucous colitis; spastic colon. The patient complains of disordered bowel function with abdominal pain, but no organic disease can be found.

**irritant** an agent causing stimulation or excitation.

**irritation** 1. a condition of undue nervous excitement resulting from abnormal sensitiveness. 2. itching of the skin. *Cerebral i.* a stage of excitement present in many brain conditions and typical of the recovery stage of concussion.

**ischaemia** a deficiency in the blood supply to a part of the body. *Myocardial i.* ischaemia of the heart muscles, which causes angina pectoris.

**ischiorectal** concerning the ischium and the rectum *I. abscess* a collection of pus in the ischiorectal connective tissue. An anal fistula may result.

**ischium** the lower posterior bone of the pelvic girdle.

**Ishihara colour charts** *S. Ishihara, Japanese ophthalmologist, 1879–1963.* Patterns of dots of the primary colours on similar backgrounds which make numbers or patterns. The numbers or patterns can be seen by a normal-sighted person, but one who is colour-blind will only be able to identify some of them, depending on the type of colour-blindness.

**islet of Langerhans** *P. Langerhans, German pathologist, 1847–1888.* One of a group of cells in the pancreas that produce insulin and glucagon; islet of the pancreas.

**isograft** a tissue graft from one identical twin to another.

**isoimmunization** the development of antibodies against an antigen derived from an individual of the same species, e.g. a rhesus-negative woman may immunize herself against her fetus, if it is rhesus-positive, by forming specific ANTIBODY.

**isolation** the separation of a person with an infectious disease from those non-infected. *I. period* quarantine; the length of time during which a patient with an infectious fever is considered capable of infecting others by contact.

**isoleucine** one of the ten essential amino acids that are vital for health in the adult.

**isometric** having equal dimensions. *I. exercises* the contraction and relaxation of muscles without producing movement; used to maintain muscle tone after a fracture.

**isotonic** having uniform tension. *I. solution* a solution of the same osmotic pressure as the fluid with which it is compared. Normal saline (0.9% solution of salt in water) is isotonic with blood plasma.

**isotope** one of the several forms of an element with the same atomic number but different atomic weights. *Radioactive i.* an unstable isotope which decays and emits alpha, beta or gamma rays. May be used in the diagnosis and treatment of malignant disease.

**isthmus** a narrow connection between two larger bodies or parts, e.g. the band of tissue between the two lobes of the thyroid gland.

**itch** a skin eruption with irritation. *Baker's i.* eczema of the hands due to the proteins of flour. *Barber's i.* sycosis; tinea barbae. *Dhobi i.* TINEA (CRURIS). The name is derived from the belief in India that the spread of infection was due to washermen (dhobis) wearing their clients' clothes. *I. mite* the cause of scabies, *Sarcoptes scabiei.* *Washerwomen's i.* dermatitis of the hands due to the constant use of detergents.

**itching** an intense irritating sensation of the skin that causes the sufferer to scratch the part affected. Generalized itching may occur as a result of excessive bathing and using irritant detergent soaps and foams. Itching is common in the elderly who often have a dry skin, and also commonly occurs in pregnancy. Some people experience general itching as a result of taking certain drugs.

**ITP** idiopathic thrombocytopenic purpura.

**ITU** intensive therapy unit.

**IUCD** intrauterine contraceptive device.

**IVF** in vitro fertilization. *See* FERTILIZATION.

**IVP** intravenous pyelography (*see* UROGRAPHY).

**IVU** intravenous urography (*see* UROGRAPHY).

**J** symbol for *joule*.

**Jacksonian epilepsy** *J.H. Jackson, British neurologist, 1835–1911.* Focal motor EPILEPSY.

**Jacquemier's sign** *J.M. Jacquemier, French obstetrician, 1806–1879.* Blueness of the lining of the vagina seen from the early weeks of pregnancy.

**jargon** the terminology used and generally understood only by those who have knowledge of that speciality, e.g. medical jargon, legal jargon.

**Jarman index** a system for weighting a general medical practice population to indicate the health needs of the population served according to local social factors and conditions.

**jaundice** icterus; a yellow discoloration of the skin and conjunctivae, due to the presence of bile pigment in the blood. It may be one of the following types: (a) *Haemolytic j.* due to excessive destruction of red blood cells, causing increase of bilirubin in the blood. The liver is not involved. *Acholuric j.* is of this type. It is characterized by increased fragility of the red blood cells. (b) *Hepatocellular j.* the liver cells are damaged by either infection or drugs. (c) *Obstructive j.* the bile is prevented from reaching the duodenum owing to obstruction by a gallstone, a growth or a stricture of the common bile duct. (d) *Physiological j.* (icterus neonatorum) occurs within the first few days of life, and is caused by the breakdown of the excessive number of red blood cells present in the newborn.

**jaw** a bone of the face in which the teeth are embedded. *Lower j.* the mandible. *Upper j.* the two maxillae.

**jealousy** intense concern for the loss of affection or attention of another person; may also be exhibited as being envious of someone else's achievements or advantages. *Morbid j.* preoccupation with the potential sexual infidelity of one's partner. Morbid jealousy is usually caused by a personality disorder but may also occur in those suffering from organic brain disease or alcohol dependency.

**jejunal biopsy** removal of a small piece of the jejunum for histological and enzyme examination. Used to confirm Crohn's disease, coeliac disease and other malabsorption syndromes. The biopsy is taken using a a flexible endoscope passed down through the mouth into the jejunum.

**jejunoileostomy** the making of an anastomosis between the jejunum and the ileum.

**jejunostomy** the making of an opening into the jejunum through the abdominal wall.

**jejunum** the portion of the small intestine from the duodenum to the ileum; about 2.4 m in length.

**jelly** a soft, coherent, resilient substance; generally, a colloidal semisolid mass. *Contraceptive j.* a non-greasy jelly used in the vagina for prevention of conception (*see* CONTRACEPTION). *Petroleum j.* a purified mixture of semisolid hydrocarbons obtained from petroleum (also called petrolatum). *Wharton's j.* the soft, jelly-like intracellular substance of the umbilical cord, which insulates the vein and arteries, preventing occlusion and fetal hypoxia.

**jerk** a sudden muscular contraction. *Knee j.* a kicking movement produced by tapping the tendon below the patella. Used with other jerks, such as the ankle jerk, to test the nervous reflexes.

**jet lag** the lack of balance that occurs between local time and the person's biological rhythms that results from air travel over a long distance, especially in an easterly direction and to a lesser extent westwards. Sleep, memory and concentration are disturbed and there is a persistent feeling of tiredness usually lasting 2–3 days as the body adjusts to the time change.

**jigger** a sand flea, found in the tropics, which burrows into the soles of the feet and causes severe irritation.

**jogger's heel** a painful condition of the heel caused by repeatedly striking the heel against the ground or road surface when running or jogging.

**jogger's nipple** soreness of the nipple(s) caused by friction of clothing against them; occurs in runners and athletes. Prevention is by applying petroleum jelly before running.

**jogging** running at a slow even pace. A popular form of street exercise.

**joint** an articulation; the point of junction of two or more bones, particularly one which permits movement of the individual bones relative to each other.

**Joint Planning** a statutory obligation placed upon local authorities and health authorities to collaborate in planning care provision for their areas (NHS Act 1977). A need was identified for these authorities to work closely together in the development and provision of services for client groups.

**joule** *symbol* J. The SI unit of energy.

**judgement** the ability of an individual to estimate a situation, to arrive at reasonable conclusions and to decide on a course of action.

**judicial review** a legal process by which individuals or organizations can challenge government or public body decisions. Any person or organization with sufficient interest and concern regarding a decision that has been made, e.g. by a health sector organization, can apply for a review to the Lord Chancellor's Office. This relates to the legal process in England and Wales only.

**jugular** relating to the neck. J. *veins* several veins in the neck which drain the blood from the head.

**Jungian theory** *C.G. Jung, Swiss psychologist and psychiatrist, 1875–1961.* The concept that certain ideas from past experiences are present in the unconscious and controlled by the way in which the person views the world. Jung called these shared ideas the 'collective unconscious' as an entity common to all human beings. Jung considered that each person also had a 'personal unconscious' containing personal life experiences. Jung separated individuals into personality types: the externally sensitive type who directs energy outwards, and the introvert whose energies are inwardly directed. The goal of Jungian psychotherapy is to permit the individual to become what they essentially are, i.e. to encourage individual development.

**junk food** convenience or fastfood high in monosodium glutamate.

**jurisprudence** the science of law. Medical jurisprudence is another name for forensic medicine.

**juvenile** relating to young people.

**juvenile chronic arthritis** a rare form inflammatory arthritis affecting children, most often girls, between the ages of 2 and 4 years or at puberty; usually affects four or more joints. Management is based around the relief of pain, suppression of the inflammatory process and the prevention of deformity. Formerly known as Still's disease.

**juxta-articular** near a joint.

**juxtaglomerular** near to a glomerulus of the kidney. *J. cells* specialized cells found in the kidney which appear to play an important part in the control of aldosterone release.

**juxtaposition** an adjacent, or side by side position.

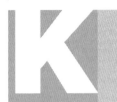

**K** symbol for *potassium*.

**kala-azar** visceral leishmaniasis. A tropical disease caused by the protozoan parasite *Leishmania donovani* which is carried by the sandfly. Symptoms include enlargement of the liver and spleen, anaemia and wasting. The disease is often fatal.

**kangaroo care** the use of skin-to-skin contact between the premature but stable infant and parent or caregiver. The infant in nappy and cap rests on the mother's or father's exposed chest either in a sling or blanket; vital signs can be kept monitored. The skin contact has a soothing effect, calming and warming the infant while promoting bonding between parent and baby.

**Kaposi's sarcoma** *M.K. Kaposi, Austrian dermatologist, 1837–1902.* A multifocal, metastasizing, malignant reticulosis with angiosarcoma-like features, involving chiefly the skin. Kaposi's sarcoma is a major feature of this disease, characterized by the development of bluish-red cutaneous nodules usually on the lower extremities, most often on the toes or feet, increasing in size and number and spreading to more proximal sites especially on the face and nose.

**Kaposi's spots** a serious complication of infantile eczema occurring on exposure to herpes simplex virus infection. More commonly known as Kaposi's varicelliform eruption.

**karyotype** 1. the chromosomal constitution and arrangement of a cell of an individual. 2. the pattern that is seen when human chromosomes are photographed during metaphase. The pictures are then enlarged and paired according to the length of their short arm.

**Kawasaki disease** a rare, acute inflammatory disorder of young children. Cause and mode of transmission not known but may be a sequela of a viral infection. Symptoms include fever, rash, sore throat and cervical lymphadenopathy and in some children cardiac complications. Occurs mainly in Japan and the USA. Also called mucocutaneous lymph node syndrome.

**kcal** kilocalorie.

**Kegel exercises** *Dr Arnold H. Kegel, a US gynaecologist 1894–1981.* Specific exercises to strengthen the pelvic–vaginal muscles as a means of controlling stress incontinence in women.

**Keller's operation** *W.L. Keller, American surgeon, 1874–1959.* An operation for correcting hallux valgus.

**keloid** hard, raised scar tissue in the skin, common in people with dark skins. A type occurs in a healed wound due to overgrowth of fibrous tissue, causing the scar to be raised above the skin level.

**Kennedy Report** a report entitled 'Learning from Bristol: the report of the public enquiry into children's heart surgery at the Bristol Royal Infirmary 1984–1995' (published 2001) which has resulted in a change of culture in the NHS. The intention is that patients are able to be active partners in their care.

**Kennedy's syndrome** *F. Kennedy, American neurologist, 1884–1952.* Ipsilateral optic atrophy caused by a frontal lobe tumour which involves one of the optic nerves.

**keratectomy** excision of a portion of the cornea.

**keratic** 1. horny. 2. relating to the cornea. *K. precipitates* inflammatory exudates adhering to the back of the cornea; a sign of iritis and cyclitis.

**keratin** an albuminoid substance which forms the principal constituent of all horny tissues.

**keratinize** to make or become horny.

**keratitis** inflammation of the cornea. The causes may be physical (trauma, exposure to dust, vapours or ultraviolet light) or due to infectious conditions such as corneal and dendritic ulcers. *Interstitial k.* deep chronic keratitis, usually arising in congenital syphilis. *Striate k.* inflammation that appears in lines due to the folding over of the cornea after injury or operation, particularly one for cataract.

**keratocele** descemetocele; protrusion of Descemet's membrane through the base of a corneal ulcer. A horny growth of the skin.

**keratoconjunctivitis** inflammation of both the cornea and the conjunctiva of the eye.

**keratoiritis** inflammation of both the cornea and iris.

**keratomalacia** ulceration and softening of the cornea due to a deficiency of vitamin A.

**keratometer** ophthalmometer. An instrument by which the amount of corneal astigmatism can be measured accurately.

**keratophakia** keratoplasty in which a slice of donor's cornea is shaped to a desired curvature and inserted between layers of the recipient's cornea to change its curvature and to correct hypermetropia.

**keratoplasty** a plastic operation on the cornea, including corneal grafting.

**keratoscope** an instrument for examining the eye to detect keratoconus. Placido's disc.

**keratosis** a skin disease marked by excessive growth of the epidermis or horny tissue.

**keratotomy** incision of the cornea.

**kerion** a complication of ringworm of the scalp, with formation of pustules.

**kernicterus** a condition in the newborn marked by severe neural symptoms, associated with high levels of bilirubin in the blood; it is commonly a sequela of icterus gravis neonatorum and may result in learning disabilities.

**Kernig's sign** *V.M. Kernig, Russian physician, 1840–1917.* A sign of meningitis. When the thigh is supported at right angles to the trunk, the patient is unable to straighten the leg at the knee joint.

**ketogenic** forming or capable of being converted into ketone bodies.

**ketone** an organic compound containing the carbonyl group (CO) attached to two hydrocarbon groups. Ketones are produced by the metabolization of fats.

**ketonuria** the presence of ketones in urine; acetonuria.

**ketosis** the condition in which ketones are formed in excess in the body and accumulate in the blood. Severe acidosis may occur.

**ketosteroid** a steroid hormone which contains a ketone group attached to a carbon atom. *17-k's* are excreted in the urine and formed from the adrenal corticosteroids, testosterone and, to a lesser extent, oestrogens.

**key worker** a person (commonly a social worker) designated as coordinator for action where several people are involved in the care of a person or family. The key worker is also responsible for calling a case conference.

**kick chart** a method of fetal assessment carried out by the mother. The number of kicks or movements felt during the day is counted and noted. If fewer than 10 kicks are felt in a 12 hour daytime period on two consecutive occasions, the mother is advised to contact her midwife or doctor immediately. This is a subjective assessment, and is usually combined with other tests of fetal wellbeing. Also known as a movement chart.

**kidney** one of two organs situated in the lumbar region, which purify the blood and secrete urine. The kidney secretes renin and renal erythropoietic factor. *Artificial k.* the apparatus used to remove retained waste products from the blood when kidney function is impaired. *Granular k.* the small fibrosed kidney of chronic nephritis. *Horseshoe k.* a congenital defect producing a fusion of the two kidneys into a horseshoe shape. *K. failure* the condition in which renal function is severely impaired and the organs are unable to maintain the fluid and electrolyte balance of the body. *K. transplant* the surgical implantation of a kidney taken from a live donor or from one who has recently died. Used in the treatment of renal failure. *Polycystic k.* a congenital bilateral condition of multiple cysts replacing kidney tissue.

**kilocalorie** *symbol* kcal. One thousand calories, a unit of food energy.

**kilojoule** *symbol* kJ. One thousand joules, a unit of food energy (1 kcal = 4.184 kJ).

**Kimmelstiel–Wilson syndrome** *P. Kimmelstiel, German pathologist, 1900–1970; C. Wilson, British physician, b. 1906.* A degenerative complication of DIABETES (MELLITUS), with albuminuria, oedema, hypertension, renal insufficiency and retinopathy; may lead to kidney failure. Called also intercapillary glomerulosclerosis.

**kinaesthesia** the combined sensations by which position, weight and muscular position are perceived.

**kinanaesthesia** an inability to perceive the sensation of movements of parts of the body.

**kinase** an enzyme activator; *see* ENTEROKINASE and THROMBOKINASE.

**kineplasty** plastic amputation; amputation in which the stump is so formed as to be utilized for producing motion of the prosthesis.

**kinetic** producing or pertaining to motion.

**King's Fund** King Edward's Hospital Fund for London was founded in 1897 for the support, by the giving of grants, of voluntary hospitals in London. Since the inception of the National Health Service in 1948, it has been concerned with the funding of experimental schemes, particularly relating to the management of services. *K. F. bed* a bed fitted with jointed springs which may be adjusted to various positions, developed as the result of research undertaken on behalf of and funded by the King's Fund. *K. F. audit programme* an audit process used in health care settings, developed by the King's Fund.

**kinin** a polypeptide which occurs naturally and is a powerful vasodilator.

**kinship** relationship. *K. studies* in anthropology, the study of kin (relatives) and their patterns of marriage, descent, inheritance, habitation, social values health beliefs and economics.

**Kirschner wire** *M. Kirschner, German surgeon, 1879–1942.* A thin wire that may be passed through a bone to apply skeletal traction.

**kiss of life** the expired air method of artificial respiration, by either mouth-to-nose or mouth-to-mouth breathing. *See* Appendix 2.

**kJ** symbol for *kilojoule*.

**Klebs–Löffler bacillus** *T.A.E. Klebs, German bacteriologist, 1834–1913; F.A.J. Löffler, German bacteriologist, 1852–1915.* Former name for *Corynebacterium diphtheriae*, the causative agent of diphtheria.

**Klebsiella** a genus of Gram-negative bacteria (family Enterobacteriaceae).

**Kleihauer test** a microscopic test to detect fetal cells in the maternal circulation, usually done immediately after delivery so that, if the mother is rhesus-negative and the fetus rhesus-positive, anti-D immunoglobulin may be given to prevent isoimmunization.

**kleptomania** an irresistible urge to steal when there is often no need and no particular desire for the objects. Often associated with depression.

**Klinefelter's syndrome** *H.F. Klinefelter, American physician, b. 1912.* A congenital chromosome abnormality in which each cell has three sex chromosomes, XXY, rather than the usual XX or XY, making a total of 47 (normal is 46). Affected men have female breast development and small testes and are infertile.

**knee** the joint between the femur and the tibia. ***K.cap*** the patella. ***Housemaid's k.*** prepatellar bursitis. ***K. jerk*** an upward jerk of the leg obtained by striking the patellar tendon when the knee is passively flexed. ***Knock-k.*** a condition in which the knees turn inwards towards each other; genu valgum.

**kneecap** the patella.

**Koch's bacillus** *R. Koch, German bacteriologist, 1843–1910.* Former name for *Mycobacterium tuberculosis*, the causative organism of tuberculosis.

**Köhler's disease** *A. Köhler, German physician and radiologist, 1874–1947.*

Osteochondritis of the navicular bone of the foot, occurring in children.

**koilonychia** the development of brittle, spoon-shaped nails which may occur in iron-deficiency anaemia.

**Koplik's spots** *H. Koplik, American paediatrician, 1858–1927.* Small white spots that sometimes appear on the mucous membranes inside the mouth in measles on the second day of onset, before the general rash.

**Korotkoff's method** *N.S. Korotkoff, Russian physician, 1874–1920.* A method of finding the systolic and diastolic blood pressure by listening to the sounds produced in an artery while the pressure in a previously inflated cuff is gradually reduced.

**Korsakoff's syndrome** or **psychosis** *S.S. Korsakoff, Russian neurologist, 1854–1900.* A chronic condition in which there is impaired memory, particularly for recent events, and the patient is disorientated for time and place. It may be present in psychosis of infective, toxic or metabolic origin, or in chronic alcoholism.

**kosher** food that is prepared and cooked in accordance with Jewish dietary laws it is eaten by practising Jews.

**kraurosis** dryness and shrinking of a part of the body. ***K. vulvae*** a degenerative condition of the vulva. May be treated by giving oestrogen preparations.

**Krebs cycle** *Sir H.A. Krebs, German–British biochemist, 1900–1981.* A series of reactions during which the aerobic oxidation of pyruvic acid takes place. This is part of carbohydrate metabolism. ***K. urea c.*** the way in which urea is formed in the liver.

**Küntscher nail** *G. Küntscher, German orthopaedic surgeon, 1902–1972.* An intramedullary nail used in treating fractures of long bones, especially the shaft of the femur.

**Kupffer's cells** *K.W. von Kupffer, German anatomist, 1829–1902.* Phagocytic reticuloendothelial cells of the liver which form bile from haemoglobin released by disintegrated erythrocytes.

**Kveim test** *M.A. Kveim, Norwegian physician, 1892–1966.* A test for sarcoidosis in which antigen from the lymph nodes or spleen of a sarcoidosis patient is injected intradermally.

**kwashiorkor** a condition of protein malnutrition occurring in children in underprivileged populations. Fatty infiltration of the liver arises and may cause cirrhosis.

**kymograph** an instrument for recording variations or undulations, arterial or other.

**kyphoscoliosis** an abnormal curvature of the spine in which there is forward and sideways displacement.

**kyphosis** posterior curvature of the spine; humpback.

**l** symbol for *litre*.

**label** 1. a classifying name given to a person or object. When a label is given to someone there is a tendency for that person to be perceived by others and often by themselves as having the characteristics implied by the label, and being nothing more than that and therefore undervalued. *See* STIGMA. 2. a means of providing data when attached to an item, e.g. drugs, food or surgical dressings.

**labial** pertaining to the lips or labia.

**labile** unstable. Applied to those chemicals that are subject to change or readily altered by heat.

**lability** instability. *L. of mood* the tendency to sudden changes of mood of short duration.

**labium** a lip. *L. majus pudendi* the large fold of flesh surrounding the vulva. *L. minus pudendi* the lesser fold within the labium majus.

**labour** parturition or childbirth, which takes place in three stages: (a) dilatation of the cervix uteri; (b) passage of the child through the birth canal; and (c) expulsion of the placenta. *Induced l.* labour brought on by artificial means before term, as in cases of contracted pelvis, or if overdue. *Obstructed l.* labour in which there is a mechanical hindrance. *Precipitate l.* labour in which the baby is delivered extremely rapidly. *Premature l.* labour which occurs after the 24th week of pregnancy and before fullterm. *Spontaneous l.* that which occurs without being artificially induced or accelerated. *Spurious l.* ineffective labour pains which sometimes precede true labour pains.

**labyrinth** the structures forming the internal ear, i.e. the cochlea and semicircular canals. *Bony l.* the bony canals of the internal ear. *Membranous l.* the soft structure inside the bony canals.

**labyrinthectomy** excision of the labyrinth.

**labyrinthitis** inflammation of the labyrinth, causing vertigo.

**laceration** a wound with torn and ragged edges.

**lacrimal** relating to tears. *L. apparatus* the structures secreting the tears and draining the fluid from the conjunctival sac (*see* Figure on p. 230). *L. gland* a gland that secretes tears, which drain through two small openings in the eyelids (*l. puncta*) into a pair of ducts (*l. canaliculi*) into the sac and finally into the nasal cavity through the nasolacrimal duct. Situated in the outer and upper corner of the orbit.

**lacrimation** an excessive secretion of tears.

**lacrimator** a substance that causes excessive secretion of tears, e.g. tear gas.

**lactagogue** any agent that promotes the secretion or flow of milk; galactagogue.

**lactalbumin** an albumin of milk.

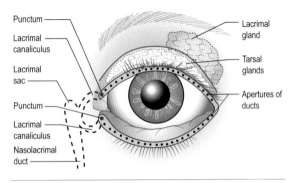

Punctum
Lacrimal canaliculus
Lacrimal sac
Punctum
Lacrimal canaliculus
Nasolacrimal duct
Lacrimal gland
Tarsal glands
Apertures of ducts

LACRIMAL APPARATUS

**lactase** an enzyme, produced in the small intestine, which converts lactose into glucose and galactose.

**lactate** 1. any substance given to promote lactation. 2. any salt of lactic acid. 3. to secrete milk. *L. dehydrogenase* abbreviated LD, LDH. An enzyme that catalyses the interconversion of lactate and pyruvate. Widespread in tissues and particularly abundant in kidney, skeletal muscle, liver and myocardium. It has five isoenzymes denoted $LD_1$ to $LD_5$. The 'flipped' pattern, in which the serum $LD_1$ level is greater than the $LD_2$ level, is indicative of an acute myocardial infarction. This pattern occurs within 12–24 hours after the attack.

**lactation** 1. the period during which the infant is nourished from the breast. 2. the process of milk secretion by the mammary glands.

**lacteal** 1. consisting of milk. 2. a lymphatic duct in the small intestine which absorbs chyle.

**lactic** pertaining to milk. *L. acid* an acid formed by the fermentation of lactose or milk sugar. It is produced naturally in the body as a result of glucose metabolism. An excess of the acid accumulating in the muscles may cause cramp.

**lactiferous** conveying or secreting milk.

*Lactobacillus* a genus of Grampositive, rod-shaped bacteria, many of which produce fermentation.

**lactoferrin** an iron-binding protein found in neutrophils and bodily secretions (milk, tears, saliva, bile, etc.), having bactericidal activity and acting as an inhibitor of colony formation by granulocytes and macrophages.

**lactogenic** stimulating the production of milk. *See* LUTEOTROPHIN.

**lactose** milk sugar consisting of glucose and galactose. *L. intolerance* the ingestion of milk containing lactose results in the patient experiencing severe abdominal colic and diarrhoea due to a deficiency of the lactose-splitting enzyme (betagalactosidase) in the lining of the small intestine.

**lactovegetarian** 1. a person who subsists on a diet of milk or milk products and vegetables. 2. pertaining to such a diet.

**lactulose** a synthetic disaccharide which is used as a laxative.

**lacuna** a small cavity or depression in any part of the body.

**Laënnec's disease** *R.T.H. Laënnec, French physician, 1781–1826.* The most common type of cirrhosis of the liver, frequently attributable to high alcohol consumption.

**laevulose** fruit sugar; fructose.

**laking** haemolysis of the red blood cells. The cells swell and burst and the haemoglobin is released.

**lallation** a babbling, infantile form of speech.

**Lamaze method** *F. Lamaze, French obstetrician, 1890–1957.* A method of preparing for natural childbirth developed by Fernand Lamaze, and based on the technique of training the mind and body for the purpose of modifying perception of pain during labour and delivery. *See* CHILDBIRTH (NATURAL).

**lambdoid** shaped like the Greek letter lambda, i.e. Λ or λ. **L. suture** the junction of the occipital bone with the parietals.

**lambliasis** giardiasis.

**lamella** 1. a thin layer, membrane or plate, as of bone. 2. a thin medicated disc of gelatin used in applying drugs to the eye. The gelatin dissolves and the drugs are absorbed.

**lamina** a bony plate or layer.

**laminectomy** excision of the posterior arch of a vertebra, sometimes performed to relieve pressure on the spinal cord or nerves.

**Lancefield's groups** *R.C. Lancefield, American bacteriologist, 1895–1981.* Divisions of B-haemolytic streptococci, which are classified on the basis of serological action into groups A–R. Most human infections are due to group A.

**Landry's paralysis** *J.B.G. Landry, French physician, 1826–1865.* Guillain–Barré syndrome; acute ascending polyneuritis.

**Landsteiner's classification** *K. Landsteiner, Austrian biologist, 1868–1943.* A system of blood groups; the ABO system, consisting of groups A, B, AB and O. *See* BLOOD GROUPS.

**language** the means of human communication consisting of the use of the spoken or written word in a structured way. Gestures of hands, head and even the body may be involved, although this is reflected differently from one setting to another, e.g. from a formal presentation to the greeting a friend. Cultural background too plays a part in the use or absence of gestures. **L. disorders** problems affecting the ability to communicate and/or comprehend the spoken and/or written word. *See* SPEECH.

**lanugo** the fine hair that covers the body of the fetus and newly born infants, especially those who are premature. Also called down.

**laparoscopy** viewing of the abdominal cavity by passing an endoscope through the abdominal wall.

**laparotomy** incision of the abdominal wall for exploratory purposes.

**laryngeal** pertaining to the larynx.

**laryngectomy** excision of the larynx.

**laryngismus** a spasmodic contraction of the larynx. **L. stridulus** a crowing sound on inspiration, following a period of apnoea, due to spasmodic closure of the glottis. It occurs in children, particularly those suffering from rickets. *See* CROUP.

**laryngitis** inflammation of the larynx causing hoarseness or loss of voice due to acute infection or irritation by gases.

**laryngopharynx** the lower portion of the pharynx connecting with the larynx.

**laryngoscope** an endoscopic instrument for examining the larynx or for aiding the insertion of endotracheal tubes or the bronchoscope.

**laryngospasm** a reflex, prolonged contraction of the laryngeal muscles that is liable to occur on insertion or withdrawal of an endotracheal tube.

**laryngostenosis** contraction or stricture of the larynx.

**laryngostomy** the making of an opening into the larynx to provide an artificial air passage.

**laryngotomy** an incision into the larynx to make a temporary opening in an emergency when the larynx is obstructed. Tracheostomy.

**laryngotracheal** referring to both the larynx and trachea.

**laryngotracheitis** inflammation of both the larynx and trachea.

**laryngotracheobronchitis** an acute viral infection of the respiratory tract which occurs particularly in young children.

**larynx** [Gr.] the muscular and cartilaginous structure, lined with mucous membrane, situated at the top of the trachea and below the root of the tongue and the hyoid bone. The larynx contains the vocal cords and is the source of the sound heard in speech. Also called the voice box.

**laser** *light amplification by stimulated emission of radiation.* An apparatus producing an extremely concentrated beam of light that can be used to cut metals. When used in the treatment of neoplasms, detached retina, diabetic retinopathy and macular degeneration, and some skin conditions, eye protection must be worn by the operator.

**Lassa fever** a West African viral haemorrhagic fever with insidious onset and an incubation period of 6–21 days. It is a zoonosis, the reservoir of infection of which is the multimammate rat. Devastating outbreaks of person-to-person transmission have occurred in hospitals in West Africa by direct contact with blood, urine or semen from infected patients. It can also be contracted by the airborne route. In the UK prevention is dependent on the early detection of cases and their isolation, and strict precautions to protect health care staff caring for febrile patients from Africa from inoculation or other accidents.

**lassitude** a feeling of extreme weakness and apathy.

**latent** temporarily concealed; not manifest. *L. heat* the heat absorbed by a substance during a change in state, e.g. from water into steam. When condensation occurs this heat is released. *L. period* 1. the incubation period of an infectious disease. 2. the time between the application of a nerve stimulus and the reaction.

**lateral** situated at the side; therefore, away from the centre.

**lateroversion** a turning to one side, such as may occur of the uterus.

**latex** a milky fluid derived from tapping the rubber tree *Hevea brasiliensis* found mainly in Thailand, Indonesia and Malaysia. It comprises an aqueous suspension of globules of rubber hydrocarbon coated with proteins. *L. allergy* a reaction to latex proteins, varying in severity. It is a significant occupational health problem for health care workers. Latex is a component of many medical supplies, e.g. various tubes, materials and gloves. Latex gloves have been frequently implicated due either to the latex or to the proteins used in the powders that lubricate the gloves for ease of use.

**lavage** the washing out of a cavity. *Colonic l.* the washing out of the colon. *Gastric l.* the washing out of the stomach.

**laxatives** a group of drugs used to treat constipation or to evacuate the bowel before surgery on the large bowel. May be used orally, in suppositories or in enemas. There are different categories of laxative based upon their method of working: (a) bulk forming, e.g. methyl cellulose, that increase volume, encouraging the passage of a softer and bulkier stool; (b) stimulant laxatives that cause the intestinal wall to contract and speed up the elimination of faeces, e.g. senna or bisacodyl; (c) softeners, e.g. liquid paraffin, that lubricate and facilitate the passage of faeces; (d) osmotic laxatives primarily used in enemas that increase the fluid in the bowel by osmosis, e.g. magnesium sulphate or lactulose. Laxatives may also be given in a combined form of softener and stimulant.

**LE** lupus erythematosus. *LE cell* a mature neutrophilic polymorphonuclear leukocyte that has phagocytized a large, spherical inclusion derived from another neutrophil; a characteristic of lupus erythematosus, but also found in analogous connective tissue disorders.

**lead** *symbol* Pb. A metallic element, many of the compounds of which are highly poisonous. *L. poisoning* a condition that usually occurs in children as the result of excessive lead in the atmosphere, or from chewing objects covered with paint containing lead. The symptoms and signs include malaise, diarrhoea and vomiting, and sometimes encephalitis. There is often pallor and a blue line around the gums. The use of lead in paints is now controlled by legislation and safety regulations.

**learning** knowledge or skills gained, or behaviour modified through being taught or from study. Learning occurs as a result of using intelligence, memory, insight and understanding. *L. curve* a person's rate of progress in gaining experience or new skills which can be represented as a graph. *L. difficulties* problems with learning arise as a result of a range of mental and physical problems. *L. disability* the preferred term to the one formely used of 'mental handicap'. Essentially disorders are characterized by substantial deficits in scholastic or academic skills.

**lecithin** one of a group of phospholipids that are found in the cell tissues and are concerned in the metabolism of fat.

**leech** *Hirudo medicinalis*, an aquatic worm which sucks blood and secretes hirudin (an anticoagulant) in its saliva. Historically used to withdraw blood from patients. May now be used following some forms of surgery, e.g. plastic or microsurgery, to restore the patency of collapsed or blocked blood vessels. Leeches are also occasionally used to drain a haematoma from a wound.

**leg** the lower limb, from knee to ankle. *Barbados l.* elephantiasis. *Bow-l.* genu varum. *Scissor l.* condition in which the patient is crosslegged, such as occurs in cerebral diplegia. *White l.* phlegmasia alba dolens. Acute oedema in a leg due to lymphatic blockage. Rarely occurs now but was most commonly seen in women after childbirth.

**Legionella pneumophila** a species of Gram-negative, non-acid-fast, rod-shaped bacteria which require both cysteine and iron for growth; the causative agent of LEGIONNAIRES' DISEASE and PONTIAC FEVER.

**legionellosis** a disease caused by infection with *Legionella* species, such as *L. pneumophila*. A notifiable disease in Scotland.

**legionnaires' disease** a pulmonary form of legionellosis, resulting from infection with *Legionella* *pneumophila*. It is contagious and may be fatal. Symptoms include fever, confusion, pain in the muscles and across the chest, a dry cough and a partial loss of kidney function. It is associated with an infected water supply in public buildings such as hotels, hospitals and large office blocks, a cause of both community and hospital acquired infection. The infective organism is spread by droplets; there is no person to person spread.

**leiomyoma** a benign smooth muscle tumour (fibroid) most commonly found in the uterus.

**leiomyosarcoma** a malignant muscle tumour.

*Leishmania* a genus of parasitic flagellated protozoa which infect the blood of humans and are the cause of leishmaniasis.

**leishmaniasis** a group of diseases caused by one of the protozoan *Leishmania* parasites. See KALA-AZAR.

**lens** 1. a piece of glass or other material shaped to transmit light rays in a particular direction. 2. the transparent crystalline body situated behind the pupil of the eye. It serves as a refractive medium for rays of light. **Contact l.** a thin sheet of glass or plastic moulded to fit directly over the cornea. Worn instead of spectacles.

**lentigo** a brownish or yellowish spot on the skin. A freckle. *L. maligna* Hutchinson's melanotic freckle. See FRECKLE.

*Lentivirus* from Latin *lentus* (slow) + virus. A group of retroviruses that cause disease in animals and humans, including HIV-1 and HIV-2 (*see* HUMAN IMMUNODEFICIENCY VIRUS). These viruses are associated with slowly progressive diseases.

**leontiasis** an osseous deformity of the face which produces a lion-like appearance. It occurs sometimes in leprosy and rarely in osteitis deformans.

**lepidosis** any scaly eruption of the skin.

**leprosy** Hansen's disease. A chronic infection of the skin, mucous membrane and nerves with *Mycobacterium leprae*. It is predominantly a disease of warm climates which is transmitted by prolonged contact. There is an insidious onset of symptoms, mainly involving the skin and nerves, after an incubation period of between 1 and 30 years. The disease can be classified into three types: (a) lepromatous, which is a steadily progressive form, often resulting in paralysis, disfigurement and deformity; this form is often complicated by tuberculosis; (b) tuberculoid, which is often self-limiting and generally runs a more benign course; and (c) indeterminate, in which there are skin symptoms representative of both lepromatous and tuberculoid forms. Leprosy is now treated with a range of antimicrobial drugs.

**leptomeningitis** inflammation of the pia mater and arachnoid membranes of the brain and spinal cord.

*Leptospira* a genus of spirochaetes. *L. icterohaemorrhagiae* the cause of spirochaetal jaundice (Weil's disease).

**leptospirosis** any of a group of notifiable infectious diseases due to serotypes of *Leptospira*. The best known is Weil's disease, or leptospiral jaundice; others are mud fever, autumn fever and swineherd's disease. The aetiological agent is a spiral organism that is common in water. Initially the symptoms include fever, rigors, vomiting, headache and often jaundice. Diagnosis may be difficult because the symptoms resemble those of several other diseases. Jaundice is a key symptom. Sanitation measures can reduce the spread of the disease in both humans and animals.

**lesbianism** sexual and emotional orientation of one woman to another; female homosexuality.

**Lesch–Nyhan syndrome** *M. Lesch, American physician, b. 1939; W.L. Nyhan Jr, American physician, b. 1926.* A hereditary disorder of purine metabolism transmitted as an X-linked recessive trait with physical and mental handicap, compulsive self-mutilation of fingers and lips by biting, spasticity, cerebral palsy and impaired renal function.

**lesion** any pathological or traumatic discontinuity of tissue or loss of function of a part. Lesion is a broad term, including wounds, sores, ulcers, tumours, cataracts and any other tissue damage. Lesions range from the skin sores associated with eczema to the changes in lung tissue that occur in tuberculosis.

**lethargy** a condition of drowsiness or stupor that cannot be overcome by the will.

**Letterer–Siwe disease** *E. Letterer, German physician, 1895–1982; S.A. Siwe, German physician, 1897–1966.* Reticuloendotheliosis of early childhood, marked by a haemorrhagic tendency, eczematoid skin eruption, hepatosplenomegaly with lymph node involvement, and progressive anaemia.

**leucine** a naturally occurring essential amino acid, vital for growth in infants and for nitrogen equilibrium in adults.

**leuco-** for words beginning thus, see *leuco-*.

**leukaemia** a progressive, malignant disease of the blood-forming organs, marked by abnormal proliferation and development of leukocytes and their precursors in the blood and bone marrow. It is accompanied by a reduced number of erythrocytes and blood platelets, resulting in anaemia and increased susceptibility to infection and haemorrhage. Other typical symptoms include fever, excessive bruising, breathlessness, pain in the joints and bones and swelling of the lymph nodes, spleen and liver. Leukaemia is classified clinically on the basis of (a) the duration and character of the disease (acute or chronic), and (b) the cell line involved, i.e. myeloid (myelocytic, myeloblastic, granulocytic) or lymphoid (lymphatic, lymphoblastic, lymphocytic). A widely used classification of acute leukaemia based on cell type is the French American British (FAB) classification. The incidence of the disease is growing and the increase is only partially explained by increased efficiency of detection. Treatment options may include a combination of: chemotherapy, radiotherapy, steroid therapy, bone marrow or stem cell transplant. Antibiotics are commonly required.

**leukocyte** a white blood corpuscle. There are three types: (a) granular (polymorphonuclear cells) formed in bone marrow, consisting of neutrophils, eosinophils and basophils; (b) lymphocytes (formed in the lymph glands); and (c) monocytes (*see* Figure and Table on p. 236).

**leukocytolysis** destruction of white blood cells.

**leukocytosis** an increase in the number of leukocytes in the blood. Often a response to infection.

**leukoderma** an absence of pigment in patches or bands, producing abnormal whiteness of the skin. Vitiligo.

**leukodystrophy** a degenerative disorder of the brain which starts during the first few months of life and leads to mental, visual and motor deterioration.

**leukonychia** white patches on the nails due to air underneath.

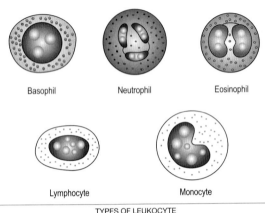

Basophil    Neutrophil    Eosinophil

Lymphocyte    Monocyte

TYPES OF LEUKOCYTE

| NORMAL LEUKOCYTE COUNT | |
|---|---|
| Cell type | No. cells/litre |
| Neutrophils | $3.5–7.5 \times 10^9$ |
| Eosinophils | $0.04–0.4 \times 10^9$ |
| Basophils | $0.01–0.1 \times 10^9$ |
| Lymphocytes | $1.5–4.0 \times 10^9$ |
| Monocytes | $0.2–0.8 \times 10^9$ |

**leukopenia** a decreased number of white cells, usually granulocytes, in the blood.

**leukophoresis** withdrawal of blood for the selective removal of leukocytes. The remaining blood is retransfused.

**leukoplakia** a chronic inflammation, characterized by white thickened patches on the mucous membranes, particularly on the tongue, gums and inside of the cheeks. *L. vulvae* thickening of the mucous membrane of the labia with the appearance of scattered white patches.

**leukopoiesis** the formation of white blood cells. Leukocytopoiesis.

**leukorrhoea** a viscid, whitish discharge from the vagina.

**levator** a muscle that raises a structure or organ of the body.

**levels of care** the six divisions of the HEALTH CARE SYSTEM; preventive care, primary care, secondary or acute care, tertiary care, restorative care and continuing care.

**LH** luteinizing hormone.

**Li** symbol for *lithium*.

**liaison** communication and contact between groups, units and/or agencies and organizations. *L. health visitor* nurse appointed to facilitate communications between the hospital and the community services for the benefit of the patient's care at home after discharge from the inpatient unit.

**libido** 1. the vital force or impulse which brings about purposeful action. 2. sexual drive in Freudian psychoanalysis, the motive force of all human beings.

**lichen** a group of inflammatory infections of the skin in which the tions. *L. planus* raised flat patches of dull, reddish-purple colour, with a smooth or scaly surface.

**lichenification** the stage of an eruption when it resembles lichen.

**lid** eyelid. *Granular l.* trachoma. *L. lag* jerky movement of the upper lid when it is being lowered. A sign of exophthalmic goitre (thyrotoxicosis).

**lie** a position or direction. *L. of fetus* the position of the fetus in the uterus. The normal lie is longitudinal.

**life event** a sociological term used to describe major events in a person's life, e.g. leaving home for the first time, getting married, moving house, changing a job.

**life expectancy** the average length of life based upon prevailing mortality trends. It is influenced by health status and illness record, but also by social factors: education, occupation, ethnicity and environmental factors such as sanitation and quality of housing. Currently demographic differences are widening, with life expectancy in the north of England and Scotland being significantly less than in the south.

**life long learning** a process of personal, social and professional development throughout the life span of the individual.

**life support system** the equipment and technology used to maintain the life of a patient who is not otherwise able to survive.

**lifestyle** the pattern of daily living that an individual develops. On the initial assessment of a person entering the healthcare services this is considered in relation to the delivery of care by healthcare workers in order that the aims and objectives for care can be individualized.

**lift assessment** the choice of the most appropriate lift method to

use when moving a patient, as from bed to chair. Factors that need to be taken into account include: whether the patient is conscious or unconscious; if there is a visual, hearing or cognitive impairment present; the presence of equipment, e.g. urinary drainage, IV lines or monitors; the body weight of the person.

No particular method of lifting is suggested as correct or appropriate in all situations. Rather, that safe lifting or manual handling practices should be used at all times. Lifting devices are the first option when implementing manual handling activities. *See also* MANUAL HANDLING.

**ligament** 1. a band of fibrous tissue connecting bones forming a joint. 2. a layer or layers of peritoneum connecting one abdominal organ to another or to the abdominal wall. *Annular l.* the ring-like band that fixes the head of the radius to the ulna. *Cruciate l.* crossed ligaments within the knee joint. *Inguinal l.* that between the pubic bone and anterior iliac crest. *Round l.* for example, one of the two anterior ligaments of the uterus, passing through the inguinal canal and ending in the labia majora. There are also round ligaments of the femur and of the liver.

**ligation** the application of a ligature.

**ligature** a thread of silk, catgut or other material used for tying round a blood vessel to stop it bleeding.

**light** electromagnetic waves which stimulate the retina of the eye. *L. adaptation* the changes that take place in the eye when the intensity of the light increases or decreases. *L. coagulation* a method of treating retinal detachment by directing a beam of strong light from a carbon arc through the pupil to the affected area.

**lightening** the relief experienced in pregnancy, 2–3 weeks before labour, when the uterus sinks into the pelvis and ceases to press on the diaphragm.

**limbus** an edge or border. *Corneal l.* the border where the cornea joins the sclera.

**liminal** pertaining to the threshold of perception.

**linctus** a thick syrup given to soothe and allay coughing.

**linea** [L.] *a line.* **L. alba** the tendinous area in the centre of the abdominal wall into which the transversalis and part of the oblique muscles are inserted. **L. albicantes** white streaks that appear on the abdomen when it is distended by pregnancy or a tumour. **L. aspera** the rough ridge on the back of the femur on which muscles are inserted. **L. nigra** the pigmented line that often appears in pregnancy on the abdomen between the umbilicus and the pubis.

**linear** pertaining to a line. **L. accelerator** a megavoltage machine for accelerating electrons so that powerful X-rays are given off for use in the treatment of deep-seated tumours.

**lingual** pertaining to the tongue.

**lingula** a tongue-like structure, such as the projection of lung tissue from the left upper lobe.

**liniment** a liquid to be applied externally by rubbing on to the skin.

**lip** 1. the upper or lower fleshy margin of the mouth. 2. any lip-like part; labium. *Cleft l.* congenital fissure of the upper lip.

**lip reading** understanding of speech through observation of the speaker's lip movements; called also speech reading.

**lipaemia** the presence of excess fat in the blood. Sometimes a feature of diabetes. **L. retinalis** condition in which the retinal blood vessels appear to be filled with milk owing to the presence of an excess of fat in the blood.

**lipase** fat-splitting enzyme; any enzyme that catalyses the splitting of fats into glycerol and fatty acids. Measurement of the serum lipase level is an important diagnostic test for acute and chronic pancreatitis.

**lipid** one of a group of fatty substances that are insoluble in water but soluble in alcohol or chloroform. They form an important part of the diet and are normally present in the body tissues providing a source of energy and insulation. Lipids are also an important constituent of some cell structures. **L. disorders** metabolic disorders that result in abnormal amounts of lipids in the body leading to hyperlipidaemia; this can cause atherosclerosis and pancreatitis. There are also some rare hereditary disorders. **L. lowering drugs** a group of drugs used in treating hyperlipidaemia to prevent or slow the progression of coronary heart disease and severe atherosclerosis.

**lipolysis** the breakdown of fats by the action of bile salts and enzymes to a fine emulsion and fatty acids.

**lipoma** a benign tumour composed of fatty tissue, arising in any part of the body, and developing in connective tissue. *Diffuse l.* a tumour of fat in an irregular mass, without a capsule, occurring above the pelvis.

**lipoprotein** one of a group of fatty proteins present in blood plasma.

**liposarcoma** a malignant tumour of the fat cells.

**liposuction** the removal by suction of excess fat in the body through a small skin incision. Most commonly used cosmetically as a means of contour reduction or reshaping. Also called lipectomy.

**liquid** 1. a substance that flows readily in its natural state. 2. flowing readily, neither solid nor gaseous. **L. diet** a diet limited to the intake of liquids or foods that can be changed to a liquid state. A liquid diet may be restricted to clear liquids or it may be a full liquid diet.

**liquor** a watery fluid; a solution. **L. amnii** the fluid in which the fetus floats; amniotic fluid.

**Listeria** Baron J. Lister, British surgeon, 1827–1912. A genus of Gram-negative bacteria which produce upper respiratory disease, septicaemia and encephalitic disease in humans. They can be transmitted by the consumption of infected, unpasteurized dairy produce, or by direct contact with infected animals or contaminated soil. Newborn infants, pregnant women, the elderly and the immunosuppressed are more susceptible to infection.

**listeriosis** infection with organisms of the genus Listeria.

**lithiasis** the formation of calculi. **Conjunctival l.** the formation of small white chalky areas on the inner surface of the eyelids.

**lithosis** pneumoconiosis resulting from inhalation of particles of silica, etc., into the lungs.

**lithotripsy** the crushing of calculi in the bladder; lithotrity.

**litmus paper** a blotting paper impregnated with blue pigment obtained from lichen and used for testing the reaction of fluids. **Blue l.** turned red by an acid. **Red l.** turned blue by an alkali.

**litre** symbol l. The SI unit of capacity. One cubic decimetre.

**liver** the large gland situated in the right upper area of the abdominal cavity. It is essential to life. Its chief functions are: (a) formation of bile; (b) production of plasma proteins except gamma-globulins; (c) storage of carbohydrates as glycogen, iron and vitamins A, D, E and K; (d) regulation of metabolism of fat, protein and carbohydrate;

(e) detoxication of drugs and other substances; (f) the formation and destruction of erythrocytes; (g) production of prothrombin and fibrinogen; (h) heat production; and (i) phagocytic action on bacteria. **Cirrhotic l.** fibrotic changes which occur in the liver as the result of degeneration of the liver cells, often as a result of alcoholism. **L. biopsy** the taking of a small core of liver tissue through a liver biopsy needle under a local anaesthetic. Allows for microscopic examination to aid diagnosis of a wide range of disorders of the liver. **L. function tests** blood tests used to assess liver function including: alanine aminotransferase, alkaline phosphatase, aspartate aminotransferase, gamma-glutamyltransferase, serum bilirubin and serum proteins. **L. transplant** the transplantation of a liver from a suitable donor in the treatment of liver failure.

**livid** descriptive of the bluish-grey discoloration of the skin produced by congestion of blood.

**living will** a statement signed by a person requesting and indicating what should be done in the event of becoming totally incapacitated or terminally ill. It enables the writer, while still alive, to refuse resuscitation or other measures to maintain life.

**LOA** left occipitoanterior. Refers to a possible position of the fetus in the uterus.

**loading dose** in pharmaco-therapeutics, the administration of a drug in larger doses than the body can eliminate in order to bring the concentration of the drug within the body to an effective level. After this, the daily dose is gradually reduced.

**lobar** relating to a lobe.

**lobe** a section of an organ, separated from neighbouring parts by fissures. The liver, lungs and brain are divided into lobes.

**lobectomy** removal of a lobe, e.g. of the lung.

**lobular** relating to a lobule.

**lobule** a small lobe, particularly one making up a larger lobe.

**local authority** the local government.

**local supervising authority** abbreviated LSA. Currently, the Strategic Health Authorities within England are designated as the LSAs. The Health Inspectorate Wales is the designated authority in Wales, in Scotland and Northern Ireland the Health Boards are the designated authorities. The functions of the LSAs are specified in the Nursing & Midwifery Order 2001, with the statutory duties further specified in the Midwives rules and standards Nursing Midwifery Council (NMC) 2004. The LSAs are accountable to the NMC for ensuring that these duties are carried out. The role of the LSA Midwifery Officer is to ensure that the supervision of midwifery is carried out to a satisfactory standard for all midwives practising within their geographical boundaries. This officer has a leadership role in providing expert advice on professional matters and is responsible for the appointment of the Supervisors of Midwives (who must be practising midwives) within the area who provide midwives with a local framework of on-going support and supervision.

**localize** 1. to limit the spread, e.g. of disease or infection, to a certain area. 2. to determine the site of a lesion.

**lochia** the discharge of blood and tissue debris from the uterus after childbirth, lasting for 2–3 weeks. Initially lochia is bright red and gradually becomes paler.

**lockjaw** tetanus.

**locomotor** pertaining to movement from one place to another. *L. ataxia* tabes dorsalis. *See* ATAXIA.

**loculated** divided into small locules or cavities.

**loculus** a small cystic cavity, one of a number.

**locum tenens** [L.] *holding the place.* A person, usually a doctor, who substitutes for another over a period of time; usually referred to as a locum.

**locus of control** the ideas and beliefs that people have about the way in which they can control external events in their lives. Those with an internal locus of control tend to expect that any change or reinforcement is the result of their own efforts or behaviour and will want to be actively involved in any health care measures. Those with an external locus of control see themselves as being dependent upon luck, fate or the actions of 'powerful others' and are therefore fatalistic about any health care provision or treatment.

**log roll** a nursing technique used to turn a reclining patient from one side to the other. The patient lies on the back with arms folded across the chest, and legs extended. The nurses manipulate the underlying drawsheet so that the patient is rolled on to one side or the other.

**logorrhoea** excessive and often unintelligible volubility.

**loiasis** infestation of the conjunctiva and eyelids with a parasite worm, *Loa loa*. A tropical condition.

**loin** the area of the back between the thorax and the pelvis.

**long sight** hypermetropia.

**longitudinal study** an investigation that involves making observations of the same group at sequential time intervals. Longitudinal studies are valuable as a means of studying human development or change and may also be used to observe change

**loosening** in psychiatry, a disorder of thinking in which associations of ideas become so shortened, fragmented and disturbed as to lack logical relationship.

**LOP** left occipitoposterior. Refers to a possible position of the fetus in the uterus.

**lordosis** a form of spinal curvature in which there is an abnormal forward curve of the lumbar spine.

**lotion** a medicinal solution for external application to the body. Lotions usually have a soothing or antiseptic effect. *Calamine l.* a soothing mixture containing calamine and zinc oxide. *Evaporating l.* a dilute alcoholic solution applied to bruises. *Lead l.* a weak solution of lead acetate used for sprains and bruises where the skin is unbroken.

**louse** a general term covering a number of small insects that are parasitic to humans and to other mammals and birds. Three varieties are parasitic to humans: (a) *Pediculus capitis*, the head louse; (b) *Pediculus corporis*, the body louse; and (c) *Phthirus pubis*, which infects the coarse hair on the body and also the eyebrows. Diseases known to be transmitted by lice are typhus fever, relapsing fever and trench fever.

**lozenge** a medicated tablet with a sugar basis, used to treat mouth and throat conditions.

**LSA** local supervising authority.

**LSD** *see* LYSERGIDE.

**lubb-dupp** representation of the sounds heard through the stethoscope when listening to the normal heart: *lubb* when the atrioventricular valves shut, and *dupp* when the semilunar valves meet each other.

**lucid** clear, particularly of the mind. *L. interval* period of clear thinking that may occur in cerebral injury between two periods of unconsciousness or as a sane interval in a mental disorder.

**lumbago** pain in the lower part of the back. It may be caused by muscular strain or by a prolapsed intervertebral disc ('slipped disc').

**lumbar** pertaining to the loins. *L. puncture* insertion of a trocar and cannula into the spinal canal in the lower back and withdrawal of cerebrospinal fluid for diagnostic and sometimes treatment purposes.

**lumbosacral** relating to both the lumbar vertebrae and the sacrum. *L. support* a corset aimed at both supporting and restricting movement in that region. *L. vertebra* one of the five vertebrae in the lower back lying between the thoracic vertebrae and the sacrum.

**lumen** the space inside a tube.

**lumpectomy** the surgical excision of only the local lesion (benign or malignant) of the breast.

**Lund and Browder chart** a chart used for the calculation of the surface area of a burn. At birth the size and area of the head is large compared with the adult, and the legs and thighs constitute a much smaller proportion of the total body surface. On admission to a burns unit or ward the area of the body burned is mapped on to the Lund and Browder chart and the area of the burn affecting each portion of the body surface is calculated.

**lung** one of a pair of conical organs of the respiratory system, consisting of an arrangement of air tubes terminating in air vesicles (alveoli) and filling almost the whole of the thorax. The alveoli are the sites of gaseous exchange in the lungs. Atmospheric oxygen is absorbed and carbon dioxide from the pulmonary capillaries is released and excreted in expiration from the lungs. The right lung has three lobes and the left lung two. They are connected with the air by means of the bronchi and trachea.

**lupus** a chronic skin disease having many manifestations. *L. erythematosus* abbreviated LE. An inflammatory disease, affecting both the internal organs and the skin, which finally produces a round plaque-like area of hyperkeratosis. It is thought to be due to an autoimmune reaction to sunlight, infection or other unknown cause. *L. vulgaris* a tuberculous disease of the skin producing brownish nodules, frequently on the nose or cheek, and severe scarring.

**luteinizing hormone** abbreviated LH. One of three hormones produced by the anterior pituitary gland which control the activity of the gonads.

**luteotrophin** an anterior pituitary hormone which stimulates the formation of the corpus luteum and the production of milk. Prolactin.

**luxation** the dislocation of a joint. *L. of the lens* displacement of the lens of the eye into the anterior chamber or posteriorly into the vitreous humour.

**Lyme disease** a zoonosis transmitted by ticks and characterized by a rash (erythema chronicum migrans), arthritis and aseptic meningitis, caused by the spirochaete *Borrelia burgdorferi*.

**lymph** the fluid from the blood which has transuded through capillary walls to supply nutriment to tissue cells. It is collected by lymph vessels which ultimately return it to the blood. *L. nodes* or *glands* structures placed along the course of lymph vessels, through which the lymph passes and is filtered of foreign substances, e.g. bacteria. These nodes also make lymphocytes. *Plastic l.* an inflammatory exudate which tends to cause adhesion between structures and so limit the spread of infection. *Vaccine l.* a lymph preparation obtained from calves or other animals and used for vaccination.

**lymphadenectomy** excision of a lymph gland or nodes.

**lymphadenitis** inflammation of a lymph gland.

**lymphadenopathy** any disease condition of the lymph nodes.

**lymphangiectasis** dilatation of the lymph vessels due to some obstruction of the lymph flow. It may be congenital.

**lymphangiography** radiographic examination of lymph vessels after the insertion of a radio-opaque contrast medium.

**lymphangioma** a swelling composed of dilated lymph vessels.

**lymphangitis** inflammation of lymph vessels, manifested by red lines on the skin over them. It occurs in cases of severe infection through the skin.

**lymphatic** referring to lymph. *L. system* the system of vessels and glands through which the lymph is returned to the circulation. The vessels end in the thoracic duct and the right lymphatic duct.

**lymphoblast** an early developmental cell that will mature into a lymphocyte.

**lymphocyte** a white blood cell formed in the lymphoid tissue. Lymphocytes produce immune bodies to overcome and protect against infection.

**lymphocythaemia** an excessive number of lymphocytes in the blood. Lymphocytosis.

**lymphocytopenia** absence or scarcity of lymphocytes in the blood. Lymphopenia.

**lymphoedema** a condition in which the intercellular spaces contain an abnormal amount of lymph due to obstruction of the lymph drainage.

**lymphogranuloma** Hodgkin's disease. *L. venereum* a sexually transmitted disease, caused by a virus; primarily a tropical condition.

**lymphoma** lymphadenoma. Used to denote any malignant condition of the lymphoid tissue. Generally these diseases are classified as either Hodgkin's or non-Hodgkin's lymphomas. *Burkitt's l.* a type of lymphoma found predominantly in East Africa and affecting the jaws of children.

**lymphopoiesis** the production of lymphocytes. Occurs chiefly in the bone marrow, lymph nodes, thymus, spleen and gut wall.

**lymphosarcoma** a term formerly used to denote a malignant lymphoma (with the exception of Hodgkin's disease).

**lyophilization** a method of preserving biological substances in a stable state by freeze-drying. It may be used for plasma, sera, bacteria, viruses and tissues.

**lysin** a specific antibody present in the blood that can destroy cells. *See* BACTERIOLYSIN.

**lysine** an essential amino acid formed by the digestion of dietary protein. It is vital for normal health.

**lysis** 1. the gradual decline of a disease, especially of a fever. The temperature falls gradually, as in typhoid. *See* CRISIS. 2. the destruction of cells.

**lysosome** a particle, found in the cytoplasm of cells, which causes the breakdown of metabolic substances and foreign particles (e.g. bacteria) within the cell.

**lysozyme** an enzyme present in tears, nasal mucus and saliva that can kill most bacteria coming into contact with it.

**m** symbol for *metre* and *misce* (mix).

**M** symbol for *molar*.

**McBurney's point** *C. McBurney, American surgeon, 1845–1913*. The spot midway between the anterior iliac spine and the umbilicus where pain is felt on pressure if the appendix is inflamed.

**maceration** softening of a solid by soaking it in liquid. **Neonatal m.** the natural softening of a dead fetus in the uterus.

**Mackenrodt's ligaments** *A.K. Mackenrodt, German gynaecologist, 1859–1925*. The transverse or cardinal ligaments that support the uterus in the pelvic cavity.

**Macmillan nurses** qualified nurses who have also received special training in the management of pain relief, palliative care and the provision of emotional support to cancer patients and their families. This nursing service is provided either in the patient's home through the Macmillan home visiting service, in hospital or in a hospice. Supported by the Macmillan Cancer Relief charity founded to improve the quality of life for people with cancer and their families.

**macrocyte** an abnormally large red corpuscle found in the blood in some forms of anaemia.

**macrocythaemia** the presence of abnormally large red cells in the blood. Macrocytosis.

**macronutrient** an essential nutrient that has a large minimal daily requirement (greater than 100 mg); calcium, phosphorus, magnesium, potassium, sodium and chloride are macronutrients.

**macrophage** a large reticuloendothelial cell which has the power to ingest cell debris and bacteria. It is present in connective tissue, especially when there is inflammation.

**macroscopic** discernible with the naked eye. The opposite of microscopic.

**macrostomia** an abnormal development of the mouth in which the mandibular and maxillary processes do not fuse and the mouth is excessively wide.

**macula** a spot or discoloured area of the skin, not raised above the surface; a macule. **M. corneae** a small area of opacity in the cornea, seen through an ophthalmoscope as a deeper red. **M. degeneration** the loss of retinal pigment cells and damage to the macula. Occurs with ageing and results in the loss of colour vision and progressive visual impairment. **M. lutea** the yellow central area of the retina, where vision is clearest.

**maculopapular** displaying both maculae and papules. **M. eruption** a rash comprised of both maculae and papules, as in measles.

**Madura foot** mycetoma of the foot.

**maduromycosis** a chronic disease caused by *Madurella mycetoma*. The most common form is Madura foot.

**magnesium** *symbol* Mg. A bluish-white metallic element. It occurs widely in mineral sources and is present in some of the body tissues. *M. carbonate* and *m. hydroxide* neutralizing antacids used in hyperacidity. *M. sulphate* a saline purgative. Epsom salts. *M. trisilicate* an antacid powder taken after food for dyspepsia and peptic ulceration.

**magnetic resonance imaging (MRI)** an imaging technique based on the NUCLEAR MAGNETIC RESONANCE properties of the hydrogen nucleus. Cross-sectional images in any plane of the body for examination may be obtained. MRI is without hazard to the patient.

**maintenance order** a court decision that requires a person to give a regular payment to someone for whom they have responsibility, e.g. a father of a child.

**Makaton** one of the sign languages.

**mal** [Fr.] *disease*. *Grand m., petit m.* forms of epilepsy. *M. de mer* seasickness.

**malabsorption** inability of the small intestine to absorb certain substances. It may be the cause of a deficiency disease due to the lack of an essential factor.

**malacia** softening of tissues. *See also* KERATOMALACIA and OSTEOMALACIA.

**maladaptation** the inability to make normal adjustments in personal relationships and in society which may result in stress, ill health and abnormal behaviour.

**maladjustment** in psychiatry, a failure to adjust to the environment.

**malaise** a feeling of general discomfort and illness.

**malalignment** displacement, especially of the teeth from their normal relation to the line of the dental arch.

**malaria** a serious, notifiable infectious illness characterized by periodic chills, fever, sweating and splenomegaly. Serious and often fatal complications may arise in falciparum malaria. It is endemic in parts of Africa, Asia and Central and South America, and is estimated to occur at the rate of 100 million cases each year throughout the world. Treatment is with antimalarial drugs although drug resistance has occurred. Many of the antimalarial drugs have side-effects and emphasis should be placed upon prevention in malarial areas, e.g. covering up the skin, use of insect repellents and chemoprophylactic drugs. Epidemics usually occur in areas where mosquitoes persist in large numbers. The disease is caused by a parasite of the genus *Plasmodium* introduced into the blood by mosquitoes of the genus *Anopheles*. The attacks are periodic, every 48–72 hours according to the type of plasmodium. For *P. vivax* it lasts 48 hours, *P. malariae* 72 hours, and *P. falciparum* 36–48 hours. *Airport m.* a term sometimes used to describe malaria occurring at or near an airport, in a country normally free of the disease, and spread by infected mosquitoes brought in on an aeroplane from an endemic area. Control measures include disinsectization of aircraft where appropriate.

**malformation** deformity; a structural defect.

**malignant** tending to become progressively worse and to result in death; having the properties of anaplasia, invasiveness and metastasis; said of tumours.

**malingering** wilful, deliberate and fraudulent feigning or exaggeration of the symptoms of illness or injury to attain a consciously desired end.

**malleolus** one of the two protuberances on either side of the ankle joint. *Lateral m.* that on the outer surface at the lower end of the fibula. *Medial m.* that on the inner surface at the lower end of the tibia.

**malleus** the hammer-shaped bone in the middle ear.

**malnutrition** the condition in which nutrition is defective in quantity or quality.

**malocclusion** an abnormality of dental development which causes overlapping of the bite.

**Malpighian body** M. *Malpighi, Italian anatomist, physician and physiologist, 1628–1694.* The glomerulus and Bowman's capsule of the kidney.

**malposition** an abnormal position of any part of the body.

**malpractice** failure to maintain accepted standards and cause harm. Professional misconduct.

**malpresentation** any abnormal position of the fetus at birth that renders delivery difficult or impossible.

**Malta fever** brucellosis; undulant fever.

**maltase** a sugar-splitting enzyme which converts maltose to glucose. Present in pancreatic and intestinal juice.

**maltose** the sugar formed by the action of digestive enzymes on starch.

**malunion** faulty repair of a fracture.

**mammary** relating to the breasts.

**mammography** radiographic or infrared examination of the breast to detect abnormalities.

**mammoplasty** a plastic operation to reduce the size of abnormally large, pendulous breasts or augment the size of very small breasts.

**mammothermography** an examination of the breast that depends on the more active cells producing heat that can be shown on a thermograph; it may indicate abnormalities of the breast tissue.

**mandible** the lower jawbone.

**mania** a disordered mental state of extreme excitement, especially the manic type of manic-depressive psychosis. Also used as a word termination to denote obsessive preoccupation with something, as in kleptomania.

**manic** pertaining to mania. *M.-depressive psychosis* a mental illness characterized by mania or endogenous depression. The attacks may alternate between mania and depression or the patient may just have recurrent attacks of mania or depression. A bipolar disorder: *See* BIPOLAR.

**manipulation** use of the hands to produce a desired movement, such as in reducing a fracture or a hernia. Its use is important in orthopaedics, physiotherapy, osteopathy and in chiropractice.

**mannitol** a sugar alcohol occurring widely in nature; an osmotic diuretic used for forced diuresis.

**manometer** an instrument for measuring the pressure of liquids or gases.

**Mantoux test** C. *Mantoux, French physician, 1877–1947.* A tuberculin skin test in which a solution of purified protein derivative (PPD)-tuberculin is injected intradermally into either the anterior or posterior surface of the forearm. The test is read 48–72 hours after injection. It is considered positive when the induration at the site of injection is more than 10 mm in diameter.

**manual** involving the use of the hands. *M. evacuation of the bowel* a nursing technique used to evacuate the bowel following use of faecal softening agents (*see* LAXATIVES) in a severely constipated patient. This procedure is less commonly used now due to the possibility of causing rectal trauma and distress to the patient. *M. expression of urine* pressure is placed upon the abdomen by using the hands at regular intervals to encourage the patient to void when the bladder is paralysed. *M. handling* technically the moving, lifting or supporting of a load. In the work environment this is now subject to regulations and guidelines to reduce the risk of back injuries for nurses and health care workers; these regulations are enforced by the Health and Safety Executive. *M. handling equipment* any piece of equipment that facilitates the transfer of persons or objects, e.g. monkey poles, slide sheets, transfer boards (Patslides), mechanical lifters or hoists. *M. handling risk* following an initial assessment, any hazard or risk that has the potential to cause harm or illness to the patient during the manoeuvre.

**manubrium** the upper part of the sternum to which the clavicle is attached.

**MAOI** monoamine oxidase.

**maple syrup urine disease** an inborn error of metabolism in which there is an excess in the urine of certain amino acids; the urine smells like maple syrup. There are learning difficulties, spasticity and convulsions.

**marasmus** severe and chronic malnutrition producing a gradual wasting of the tissues, owing to insufficient or unassimilated food, occurring especially in infants.

**Marburg virus disease** a severe and acute, often-fatal, haemorrhagic viral disease, similar to Ebola virus disease, principally seen in central African countries caused by the Marburg virus, of the family *Filoviridae*. The incubation period ranges from 5 to 10 days and patients present with abrupt onset of high fever, weakness, muscle pain, headache and sore throat. This is quickly followed by more severe symptoms including vomiting, diarrhoea, rash, decreased kidney and liver functioning, and in some cases, both internal and external bleeding and death

in up to 90% of cases. It occurs in sporadic outbreaks, frequently centred in health care settings in developing countries, where social and economic conditions often favour the spread of the virus. Marburg virus can be transmitted in several ways, the most significant being person-to-person through direct contact with body fluids (e.g. blood, semen, vaginal fluid) of an infected person. *See* EBOLA VIRUS DISEASE.

**Marfan's syndrome** *B.J.A. Marfan, French paediatrician, 1858–1942.* A hereditary disorder in which there is excessive height with very long digits, a high arched palate, hypertonus and dislocation of the lens of the eyes; heart disease commonly occurs.

**marijuana** *Cannabis indica;* Indian hemp. *See* CANNABIS.

**marrow** the substance contained in the middle of long bones and in the cancellous tissue of all bones. *M. puncture* investigatory procedure in which marrow cells are aspirated from the sternum or iliac crest. *Red m.* that found in all cancellous tissue at birth. Blood cells are made in it. *Yellow m.* the fatty substance contained in the centre of long bones in later life.

**masculinization** the development in a woman of male secondary sexual characteristics.

**mask** 1. A covering for the mouth and nose and sometimes for the whole face, designed to protect the wearer or patient in preventing the inhalation of pathogenic organisms or toxic substances. Masks are also used in the administration of oxygen and other aerosol medications. 2. A facial expression characteristic of a certain disorder or condition. *Aerosol m.* used with a nebulizer that humidifies the inspired air or oxygen. *Parkinson's m.* an unblinking, fixed facial expression characteristic of patients with Parkinson's disease. **M. of pregnancy.** A brownish patchy discolouration on the face and neck occuring during pregnancy in some women and disappears after delivery. **Venturi m.** *see* VENTURI MASK.

**Maslow's hierarchy of needs** *A.H. Maslow, American psychologist, 1908–1970.* A hierarchical ranking, in ascending order of importance, concerning human needs and the aim of realizing one's full potential. Physiological needs for oxygen, nutrition, shelter, sleep, etc., are the most basic and need to be met first before one is able to deal in successive order with the need for safety, security, love and belonging, self-esteem and ultimately the need for self-actualization (*see* Figure).

MASLOW'S HIERARCHY OF NEEDS

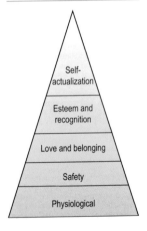

**masochism** a sexual perversion in which pleasure is derived from suffering mental or physical pain.

**mass** 1. The quantity of material in an object or body. Can be measured in terms of the force that is needed to accelerate it. 2. A lump of undefined shape. **M. number** the total mass of protons and neutrons in an atom.

**massage** the application of diverse manual techniques of touch, stroking, rubbing, kneading and manipulating the body to stimulate circulation and to promote a sense of wellbeing. Used in physiotherapy and as a complementary therapy. **External cardiac m.** the application of rhythmic pressure to the lower sternum to cause expulsion of blood from the ventricles and restart circulation in cases of cardiac arrest.

**masseter** the muscle of the cheek chiefly concerned in mastication.

**mast cell** a large connective tissue cell found in many body tissues, including the heart, liver and lungs. Mast cells contain granules which release heparin, serotinin and histamine in response to inflammation or allergy.

**mastalgia** pain in the breast.

**mastectomy** amputation of the breast. **Radical m.** removal of the breast, axillary lymph glands and the pectoral muscle.

**mastication** the act of chewing food.

**mastitis** inflammation of the breast, usually due to bacterial infection.

**mastoid** breast- or nipple-shaped. **M. antrum** the cavity in the mastoid process which communicates with the middle ear, and contains air. **M. cells** hollow spaces in the mastoid bone. **M. operation** drainage of mastoid cells when infection spreads from the middle ear. **M. process** the breast-shaped prominence on the temporal bone which projects downwards behind the ear and into which the sternocleido-mastoid muscle is inserted.

**mastoidectomy** removal of diseased bone and drainage of the mastoid antrum in severe purulent mastoiditis.

**mastoiditis** inflammation of the mastoid antrum and cells.

**masturbation** the production of sexual excitement by friction of the genitals.

**materia medica** the science of the source and preparation of drugs used in medicine.

**maternal** pertaining to the mother. *M. mortality rate* the number of deaths in childbirth per 1000 births.

**matrix** 1. that tissue in which cells are embedded. 2. in research, a matrix is an arrangement of data, which may consist of numbers or text in rows and columns. Matrices are used as part of overall data management, for accessing important data, retaining data for analysis throughout (and after) a research study.

**matter** substance. *Grey m.* a collection of nerve cells or non-medullated nerve fibres. *White m.* medullated nerve fibres massed together, as in the brain.

**maturation** ripening or developing.

**maxilla** one of the pair of bones forming the upper jaw and carrying the upper teeth.

**maxillary** pertaining to the upper jawbones.

**maxillofacial** pertaining to the maxilla and the face.

**MCHC** mean corpuscular haemoglobin concentration.

**MCV** mean corpuscular volume.

**ME** myalgic encephalomyelitis. *See* CHRONIC FATIGUE SYNDROME.

**measles** morbilli; rubeola. An acute, infectious, statutorily notifiable disease of childhood caused by a virus spread by droplets. Endemic and worldwide in distribution. Onset is catarrhal before the rash appears on the fourth day. Koplik's spots are diagnostic earlier. Secondary infection may give rise to the serious complication of otitis media or bronchopneumonia. Vaccination provides a high degree of immunity and may be offered with protection against mumps and rubella (MMR). *German m. see* RUBELLA.

**measles, mumps and rubella vaccine** abbreviated MMR. An injectable vaccine offered to children aged 12–15 months. *See* Appendix 9.

**meatus** an opening or passage. *Auditory m.* the opening leading into the auditory canal. *Urethral m.* the opening of the urethra to the exterior.

**mechanism of labour** the sequence of movements whereby the fetus adapts itself to pass through the maternal passages during the process of birth.

**Meckel's diverticulum** *J.F. Meckel, German anatomist and surgeon, 1781–1833.* The remains of a passage which, in the embryo, connected the yolk sac and intestine, evident as an enclosed sac or tube in the region of the ileum.

**meconium** the first intestinal discharges of a newly born child. Dark green and consisting of epithelial cells, mucus and bile. *M. ileus* intestinal obstruction due to blockage of the bowel by a plug of meconium in a neonate with cystic fibrosis.

**median** 1. placed in the centre. 2. in a series of values, the value middle in position.

**mediastinum** the space in the middle of the thorax, between the two pleurae.

**medical** pertaining to medicine. *M. audit* an evaluative process applied to the quality of clinical practice, often by peer review of routine or specially collected records of individual cases. Judgements are frequently made on the appropriateness of the processes carried out during the management of the case, in light of the outcome. Deaths are frequently the subject of medical audit, two established examples being the Confidential Enquiry into Maternal Deaths (carried out at national level), and local reviews of perinatal deaths. *See* AUDIT. *M. certificate see* MEDICAL STATEMENT below. *M. device* a product used for or by a patient or service user (excluding drugs) for: (a) diagnosis, prevention, monitoring, treatment or alleviation of disease; (b) alleviation of, or compensation for, an injury or impairment; (c) investigation, replacement or modification of the anatomy or of a physiological process. *M. jurisprudence* medical science as applied to aid the law, e.g. in the case of death by poisoning, violence, etc. Forensic medicine. *See* FORENSIC. *M. laboratory scientific officer* abbreviated MLSO. An allied health professional skilled in the theory and practice of clinical laboratory procedures. *M. model* the traditional approach to the diagnosis and treatment of disease in the Western world. The medical practitioner, using a problem-solving approach, focuses on the disease process and the deficits identified in the body organs and tissues. *M. social worker* a professionally qualified worker who looks after the patients' socioeconomic and welfare needs. *M. statement* advises how long a patient should refrain from work. When the patient is claiming sickness benefit, the statement must be sent to the local social security office. *M. statistics* that branch of statistics concerned with data relating to health and health services. Traditionally these include the use of routine data relating to death, illness and use of hospitals, clinics, etc. The term is also often used to encompass statistics derived from aspects of medical research, such as the conduct of trials of new drugs or procedures.

**medicalization** 1. the extension of medical authority into areas previously regarded as being nonmedical, where the lay or a popular approach prevailed, e.g. pregnancy and childbirth. 2. the tendency to view undesirable conduct as illness and therefore requiring medical intervention.

**medicament** any medicinal substance used in treatment.

**medicated** impregnated with a medicinal substance.

**medication** 1. a substance administered to a patient for therapeutic purposes. 2. the treatment of a patient by means of drugs.

**medicinal** 1. having therapeutic qualities. 2. pertaining to a medicine.

**medicine** 1. any drug or remedy. 2. the art and science of the diagnosis and treatment of disease and the maintenance of health. 3. the non-surgical treatment of disease. *Public Health m.* that specialty which deals with all aspects of medical care in the community, including notification and control of infectious diseases, preschool and school health care, and factors affecting the health of the population as a whole. *Emergency m.* that specialty which deals with the acutely ill or injured who require immediate medical treatment. *Forensic m.* the application of medical knowledge to questions of law; medical jurisprudence. Also called legal medicine. *Group m.* the practice of medicine by a group of doctors, usually representing various specialties, who are associated together for the cooperative diagnosis, treatment and prevention of disease. *Legal m.* forensic medicine.

*Nuclear m.* that branch of medicine concerned with the use of radionuclides in the diagnosis and treatment of disease. *Physical m.* that branch of medicine using physical agents in the diagnosis and treatment of disease. It includes the use of heat, cold, light, water, electricity, manipulation, massage, exercise and mechanical devices. *Preventive m.* the science aimed at preventing disease. *Proprietary m.* any chemical, drug or similar preparation used in the treatment of diseases, if such article is protected against free competition as to name, product, composition or process of manufacture by secrecy, patent, trademark or copyright, or by other means. *Psychosomatic m.* the study of the interrelations between bodily processes and emotional life. *Space m.* that branch of aviation medicine concerned with conditions to be encountered in space. *Sports m.* the field of medicine concerned with injuries sustained in athletic endeavours, including their prevention, diagnosis and treatment.

**Medicines and Healthcare products Regulatory Agency** abbreviated MHRA. Responsible for the regulation of medicines and health care products. Its primary objective is to protect public health by taking all possible steps to ensure that medicines, health care products and medical equipment are safe for those who use them.

**meditation** an altered state achieved by concentrating on an object, word or idea. *Transcendental m.* an exercise in contemplative relaxation that promotes a feeling of wellbeing and calmness. It also induces changes in physiological functions, e.g. lowering of the metabolic rate, decreased cardiac output and reduced oxygen consumption, and is used in various complementary therapies.

**medium** in bacteriology, a preparation for the culture of microorganisms. *Contrast m.* a substance used in radiography to make visible structures that could not otherwise be seen.

**MEDLARS** *Medical Literature Analysis and Retrieval System.* A computerized system of the National Library of Medicine at the National Institutes of Health, Bethesda USA from which the *Index Medicus* is produced. This is available in the UK in the larger academic libraries.

**Medline** an electronic database providing abstracts of thousands of biomedical studies.

**medulla** 1. bone marrow. 2. the innermost part of an organ, particularly the kidneys, lymph glands and suprarenal glands. *M. oblongata* that portion of the spinal cord that is contained inside the cranium. In it are the nerve centres that govern respiration, the action of the heart, etc.

**medullary** pertaining to the marrow or a medulla. *M. cavity* the hollow in the centre of long bones.

**medullated** having a myelin covering. *M. nerve fibre* one enclosed in a myelin sheath.

**medulloblastoma** a rapidly growing tumour of neuroepithelial origin occurring in childhood and appearing near the fourth ventricle of the brain. The tumour is highly radiosensitive.

**megacolon** extreme dilatation and hypertrophy of the large intestine. When the condition is congenital it is known as Hirschsprung's disease.

**megakaryocyte** a large cell of the bone marrow, responsible for blood platelet formation.

**megaloblast** an abnormally large nucleated cell from which mature red blood cells are derived.

**megalocephaly** 1. abnormal largeness of the head. 2. leontiasis ossea.

**megalomania** delusions of grandeur or self-importance.

**megaureter** dilatation of the ureter.

**Meibomian cyst** *H. Meibom, German anatomist, 1638–1700.* A small swelling of the Meibomian gland caused by obstruction of its duct. If untreated, it may become infected. A chalazion.

**Meibomian glands** Small sebaceous glands situated beneath the conjunctiva of the eyelid; tarsal glands.

**meibomianitis** a bilateral chronic inflammation of the Meibomian glands.

**meiosis** 1. a stage of reduction cell division when the chromosomes of a gamete are halved in number ready for union at fertilization. 2. contraction of the pupil of the eye; miosis.

**melaena** darkening of the faeces by blood pigments.

**melancholia** a state of extreme DEPRESSION.

**melanin** a dark pigment found in the hair, the choroid of the eye, the skin and in melanotic tumours.

**melanism** a condition marked by an abnormal deposit of dark pigment in the skin or other tissue. Melanosis.

**melanocyte** a cell of the skin pigment melanin. *M.-stimulating hormone* abbreviated MSH. Hormone produced in the pituitary gland which stimulates the formation of melanin.

**melanoderma** a patchy pigmentation of the skin.

**melanoma** a malignant tumour arising in any pigment-containing tissues, especially the skin and more rarely the eye. The incidence of melanoma is rising worldwide amongst light skinned people due to increased exposure to sunlight. Preventative measures should be taken such as limiting exposure to sunlight especially between 11:00 hours and 14:00 hours. Protective clothing should also be worn with the use of an effective sunscreen for children and adults. *Amelanotic m.* an unpigmented malignant melanoma.

**melanuria** the presence of black pigment in the urine. Occurs in melanotic sarcoma and porphyria.

**membrane** a thin elastic tissue covering the surface of certain organs and lining the cavities of the body. *Basement m.* the interface between epithelial cells and the underlying connective tissue. *Mucous m.* a membrane that secretes mucus and lines all cavities connected directly or indirectly with the skin. *Serous m.* membrane lining the abdominal cavity and thorax and covering most of the organs within.

**memory** the mental faculty that enables one to register, retain and recall previously experienced sensations, impressions, information and ideas. The ability of the brain to retain and to use knowledge gained from past experience is essential to the process of learning. Short-term memory involves the registration of received information but this is lost quickly unless the information is repeated constantly. Important information that needs to be retained is stored in long-term memory and can be recalled. Memory provides a person with a life history which is central to the concept of the 'individual self'. The exact way in which the brain remembers is not completely understood; it is believed that a portion of the temporal lobe of the brain acts as a memory centre, drawing on memories stored in other parts of the brain. *M. disturbances* any disorder of the memory functions whether of registration, retention, recall or recognition. The disorders are varied in character and in causation. The most common problem is difficulty in recall, i.e. short-term memory, that develops with age. More severe loss of memory may be an early symptom of dementia. *Procedural m.* that part of memory that stores information needed to do routine tasks that involve a sequence of steps, e.g. switching on a computer.

**menarche** the first appearance of menstruation.

**Mendel's theory** *G.J. Mendel, Abbot of Brünn, 1822–1884.* The theory that the characters of sexually reproducing organisms are handed on to the offspring in fixed ratios and without blending.

**Menière's disease** or **syndrome** *P. Menière, French physician, 1799–1862.* A disease of the inner ear causing attacks of vertigo and tinnitus with progressive deafness.

**meninges** the membranes covering the brain and spinal cord. There are three: the dura mater (outer), arachnoid mater (middle) and pia mater (inner).

**meningioma** a slow-growing, usually benign tumour developing from the arachnoid and pia mater.

**meningism** a condition in which there are signs of cerebral irritation similar to meningitis but where no causative organism can be isolated.

**meningitis** inflammation of the meninges due to organisms such as bacteria, viruses and fungi. Meningitis causes fever, intense headache, intolerance to light and sound with rigidity of muscles especially those in the neck (*see* KERNIG'S SIGN). Convulsions with severe vomiting and delirium may also occur in the more severely ill patient. A petechial rash that does not disappear when pressure is applied (*see* GLASS TEST) may also occur in patients with meningococcal septicaemia. Therapy involves the use of appropriate antimicrobial drugs, together with intensive care interventions if required,

combined with skilled nursing care and support. Meningitis is a notifiable disease, and its causal organism, if known, should also be stated. *Meningococcal m.* cerebrospinal fever. An epidemic form with a rapid onset caused by *Neisseria meningitidis* infection. *Tuberculous m.* inflammation of tuberculous origin.

**meningocele** a protrusion of the meninges through the skull or spinal column, appearing as a cyst filled with cerebrospinal fluid. *See* SPINA (BIFIDA).

**meningococcus** *Neisseria meningitidis.* A diplococcus, the microorganism of cerebrospinal meningitis.

**meningoencephalitis** inflammation of the brain and meninges.

**meningomyelocele** a protrusion of the spinal cord and meninges through a defect in the vertebral column. Myelomeningocele. *See* SPINA (BIFIDA).

**meniscectomy** surgical removal of a semilunar cartilage from the knee joint.

**meniscus** 1. the convex or concave surface of a liquid as observed in its container. 2. a lens having one convex and one concave surface. 3. a semilunar cartilage of the knee joint.

**menopause** the span of time during which the menstrual cycle wanes and gradually stops; also called change of life and climacteric. It is the period when ovaries stop functioning and therefore menstruation and childbearing cease. Usually occurs between the 45th and 50th years of life. There may be an associated hormonal imbalance which causes symptoms such as night sweats, hot flushes, diminished libido and extreme lethargy. *Artificial m.* an induced cessation of menstruation by surgery or by irradiation.

**menorrhagia** an excessive flow of the menses; menorrhoea.

**menses** the discharge from the uterus during menstruation.

**menstrual** relating to the menses. *M. cycle* the monthly cycle commencing with the first day of menstruation, when the endometrium is shed, proceeding through a process of repair and hypertrophy till the next period. It is governed by the anterior pituitary gland and the ovarian hormones, oestrogen and progesterone (*see* Figure on p. 137).

**menstruation** the monthly discharge of blood and endometrium from the uterus, starting at the age of puberty and lasting until the menopause. *Anovular m., anovulatory m.* periodic uterine bleeding without preceding ovulation. *Vicarious m.* discharge of blood at the time of menstruation from some organ other than the uterus, e.g. epistaxis, which is not uncommon.

**mental** 1. pertaining to the mind. 2. pertaining to the chin. *M. age* a measurement based on testing a person's intellectual development usually compared to standardized data for a chronological age. For example, a 13-year-old child with learning difficulties may have a mental age of 5. *Mental Capacity Act 2005* governs decision-making on behalf of adults who have lost mental capacity or where the incapacitating condition has been present since birth. *M. disorder* a temporary or permanent change in an individual's mental state which makes the person unable to function in daily life as well as they would normally do. Mental illness or disorder is defined in the English Mental Health Act as 'mental illness, arrested or incomplete development of mind, psychopathic disorder and any other disorder or disability of mind'. *M. handicap* a former term for learning disability. *See* LEARNING DISABILITY. *M. health* a state of wellbeing characterized by the absence of mental or behaviour disorder whereby the person has made a satisfactory adjustment as an individual, and to the community, in relation to emotional, personal, social and spiritual aspects of their life. *M. Health Act Commission* abbreviated MHAC. A special health authority with the responsibility for the care and welfare of individuals detained under the provisions of the Mental Health Act. *M. Health Acts* Laws made by parliament for the care and protection of people with mental illness. The Mental Health Act 1983 details the rights of patients with mental illness and the grounds for detaining mentally ill people against their will. It also outlines the provision of legal guardianship for such patients. In Scotland the Mental Welfare Commission is required to 'exercise protective functions in respect of persons who may by reason of mental disorder be incapable of adequately protecting their persons or interests'. This body also has the power of a court of law, having important functions with regard to detained patients, hospital care, treatment and discharge. It is also required to report annually to the Scottish Assembly. *Mental Health Act managers* NHS Trust non-executive directors who have power under the 1983 Mental Health Act to admit or discharge mentally ill patients. *M. Health Review Tribunal* a committee to whom persons detained under compulsory admission orders or taken into guardianship have the right of appeal at stated intervals for discharge from hospital. It consists of medical members, legal experts and lay members who include people with knowledge of social services. Also responsible to the Secretary of State for providing a Code of Practice for all mental health care practitioners. *M. health welfare* *officer* an approved social worker (ASW) who carries out the requirements of the Mental Health Acts. In Scotland the Mental Health Officer (MHO) is the equivalent professional to the ASW in England and Wales. *M. mechanism* an unconscious and indirect manner of gratifying a repressed desire.

**mentor** 1. a wise or trusted adviser or guide. 2. in nursing, a professional colleague who assists with the career development of a colleague, and facilitates and encourages that person's professional growth and awareness; mentorship.

**mercury** *symbol* Hg. Quicksilver; a heavy liquid metallic element. Previously, used in the manufacture of various types of thermometer and manometer. Poisoning from mercury (mercurialism) can occur in people in close contact with the metal over a period of time. This may present with a variety of symptoms ranging from gastrointestinal and dental problems, ataxia, visual and auditory disturbances.

**meridian** a conceptual channel along which qi energy flows in the body. *See* ACUPUNCTURE.

**mesentery** a fold of the peritoneum which connects the intestine to the posterior abdominal wall.

**mesmerism** *F.A. Mesmer, Austrian physician, 1734–1815.* Hypnotism.

**mesoderm** the middle of the three primary layers of cells in the embryo from which the connective tissues develop.

**mesometrium** the broad ligament connecting the uterus with the abdominal wall.

**mesomorph** a stocky individual of medium height with well-developed muscles.

**mesothelioma** a rapidly growing tumour of the pleura, peritoneum or pericardium which may be seen in patients with asbestosis. However,

this tumour may also occur in people who have no history of exposure to asbestos.

**messenger RNA** abbreviated mRNA. The ribonucleic acid which acts as a template for the linking of amino acids during the formation of protein in the cells.

**meta-analysis** an attempt to improve the findings of research by combining and analysing the results of all discoverable trials on the same subject.

**metabolic** referring to metabolism.

**metabolism** the sum of the physical and chemical processes by which living organized substance is built up and maintained (anabolism), and by which large molecules are broken down into smaller molecules to make energy available to the organism (catabolism). Essentially, these processes are concerned with the disposition of the nutrients absorbed into the blood after digestion. *Basal m.* the minimal energy expended for the maintenance of respiration, circulation, peristalsis, muscle tonus, body temperature, glandular activity and the other vegetative functions of the body. *Inborn error of m.* a genetically determined biochemical disorder in which a specific enzyme defect produces a metabolic block that may have pathological consequences at birth, as in phenylketonuria, or in later life.

**metabolite** any product or substance taking part in metabolism. *Essential m.* a substance that is necessary for normal metabolism, e.g. a vitamin.

**metacarpal** one of the five bones of the hand which join the fingers to the wrist.

**metacarpophalangeal** relating to the metacarpal bones and the phalanges.

**metacarpus** the five bones of the hand uniting the carpus with the phalanges of the fingers.

**metamorphosis**  a structural change or transformation.

**metaphase**  the second stage of mitosis or cell division.

**metaphysis**  the junction of the epiphysis with the diaphysis in a long bone.

**metaplasia**  abnormal change in the structure of a tissue. May be indicative of malignant change.

**metastasis**  the transfer of a disease from one part of the body to another, through the blood vessels, via the lymph channels or across the body cavities. Secondary deposits may occur from a primary malignant growth. Septic infection may arise in other organs from some original focus.

**metatarsal**  one of the five bones of the foot which join the tarsus to the toes.

**metatarsalgia**  pain in the metatarsal bones.

**metatarsus**  the five bones of the foot uniting the tarsus with the phalanges of the toes.

**Metazoa**  the division of the animal kingdom that includes the multicellular animals, i.e. all animals except the PROTOZOA.

**methadone**  a powerful analgesic with no sedative action. Similar in action to morphine, it is used to relieve pain in terminal illness and also in withdrawal programmes for heroin addicts. Methadone is addictive, but less socially disabling than heroin. Amidone.

**methaemalbumin**  a compound of haem with plasma albumin found in the blood in some types of anaemia.

**methaemoglobin**  an altered form of haemoglobin found in the blood and usually produced by the action of a drug on the red blood corpuscles, causing a reduction in their oxygen-carrying ability. May be associated with the use of phenacetin and other aniline derivatives.

**methaemoglobinaemia**  cyanosis and inability of the red blood cells to transport oxygen owing to the presence of methaemoglobin.

**methane**  marsh gas; an inflammable explosive gas produced by decomposition of organic matter.

**methicillin-resistant** *Staphylococcus aureus*  abbreviated MRSA. A strain of *S. aureus* that is resistant to methicillin and flucloxacillin but may be sensitive to other antimicrobial (antibiotic) drugs, such as vancomycin and teicoplanin. MRSA can affect people in different ways. People can carry the organism in the nose or on the skin without showing any symptoms of illness. This is called MRSA colonization. MRSA can also cause infections, especially in hospitalized patients and particularly in those who are elderly, seriously ill or who have an open wound (such as a pressure ulcer) or an indwelling urinary or intravenous catheter. Various types of infections occur, including skin, wound and surgical site infections, bone infections, pneumonia and severe life-threatening bloodstream infections. MRSA is almost always transmitted by direct physical contact, and not through the air. Transmission may also occur through indirect contact by touching objects (fomites) contaminated by the infected skin of a person with MRSA, e.g. towels, sheets, wound dressings, clothes or medical equipment. The most common means by which MRSA is transmitted between patients in hospital is by the contaminated hands of nurses, doctors and other health care workers. Standard infection prevention precautions (*see* Appendix 12), including meticulous attention to hand decontamination, can effectively reduce the risk of MRSA transmission during health care activities. Visitors should always wash their hands before and after visiting someone in hospital.

**methionine** 1. a sulphur-containing essential amino acid occurring in proteins that is a vital component of the diet. 2. a drug used orally in the treatment of paracetamol poisoning.

**methoxamine** a sympathomimetic amine used for its vasopressor effects in restoring blood pressure during anaesthesia.

**methyl salicylate** a compound used externally for rheumatic pains, lumbago, etc. Oil of wintergreen.

**methylated spirit** a mixture of 95% ethyl alcohol and 5% methyl alcohol. An industrial spirit which, taken as a drink, is poisonous.

**methylcellulose** a bulk-forming drug used as a laxative and to control diarrhoea.

**metra** the uterus.

**metre** *symbol* m. The fundamental SI unit of length.

**metritis** inflammation of the uterus.

**metrocolpocele** the protrusion of the uterus into the vagina, the wall of the latter also being pushed forwards.

**metrorrhagia** irregular uterine bleeding not associated with menstruation.

**mg** milligram(s).

**Mg** Symbol for *magnesium*.

**MHRA** Medicines and Healthcare products Regulatory Agency.

**microbe** a minute living organism, especially one causing disease. A microorganism.

**microbiology** the study of microorganisms and their effect on living cells.

**microcephalic** having an abnormally small head.

*Micrococcus* a genus of bacteria, each of which has a spherical shape. The bacteria occur in pairs or in groups and are Gram-positive. Found in soil and water.

**microcythaemia** the presence of abnormally small red cells in the blood; microcytosis.

**micrognathia** failure of development of the lower jaw, causing a receding chin.

**microgram** *symbol* μg. One millionth of a gram.

**micrometre** *symbol* μm. One millionth of a metre. Formerly called micron.

**micron** *see* MICROMETRE.

**micronutrient** a dietary element essential only in small quantities.

**microorganism** a minute animal or vegetable, particularly a virus, a bacterium, a fungus, a rickettsia or a protozoon.

**microphage** a minute phagocyte.

**microphthalmos** a condition in which one or both eyes are smaller than normal. Their function may or may not be impaired.

**microscope** an instrument which produces a greatly enlarged image of objects that are normally invisible to the human eye. *Electron m.* a microscope in which a beam of electrons is used instead of a light beam, allowing magnification of as much as 500 000 diameters.

**microscopic** visible only by means of the microscope. The opposite of macroscopic.

*Microsporum* a genus of fungi. The cause of some skin diseases, especially ringworm.

**microsurgery** the carrying out of surgical procedures using a binocular microscope with pedal-operated magnification and focusing. Microsurgery has been developed to enable operating, e.g. on the eye or in the ear, on delicate and previously inaccessible tissues, nerves and blood vessels.

**micturition** the act of passing urine.

**midbrain** that portion of the brain that connects the cerebrum with the pons and cerebellum.

**midlife crisis** experienced by many people during the fifth decade of life, resulting in doubt, anxiety and sometimes depression. During this time men and women may reflect on their lives, review the past and be aware of physiological deterioration associated with ageing. Any children are growing up, moving away from home and establishing their own adult relationships. Empty nest syndrome.

**midwife** the International Confederation of Midwives 1972 and International Federation of Gynaecologists and Obstetricians 1973 defined a midwife as 'a person who, having been regularly admitted to a midwifery education programme, duly recognised in the country in which it is located, has successfully completed the prescribed course of studies and acquired the requisite qualifications to be registered and/or legally licensed to practise midwifery, able to give the necessary supervision, care and advice to women during pregnancy, labour and the postpartum period, conduct deliveries on her [or his] own responsibility and care for the newborn and the infant; care includes preventative measures, detection of abnormal conditions in mother and child, procurement of medical assistance and execution of emergency measures in the absence of medical help. The midwifery practitioner has an important task in health counselling and health education, ... antenatal education and preparation for parenthood and ... certain areas of gynaecology, family planning and child care. The midwife may practise in hospitals, clinics, health units, domiciliary conditions or in any other service.'

**midwifery** the art and science of caring for women undergoing normal pregnancy, labour and the period following childbirth (usu-

ally 6–8 weeks). *M. process* the application of the nursing process to midwifery. It is the systematic, cyclical method of organizing midwifery care, and is carried out by the assessment of actual and potential problems, and the planning, implementation and evaluation of care.

**migraine** paroxysmal attacks of severe headache, often with nausea, vomiting and visual disturbance.

**milestone** one of the norms against which the motor, social and psychological development of a child is measured.

**milia** small white spots usually occuring in clusters around the nose and cheeks resulting from obstruction of a sebaceous gland. May occur in young adults. *M. neonatorum* milia occuring in the newborn, which are harmless and quickly disappear if left alone.

**miliaria** prickly heat, an acute itching eruption common among white people in tropical and subtropical areas.

**miliary** resembling millet seed. *M. tuberculosis see* TUBERCULOSIS.

**milieu** the environment or setting. *M. interieur* the internal physical and chemical environment experienced by individual cells. *M. therapy* a psychiatric intervention in which the physical surroundings and social setting are used as important elements in the therapeutic process.

**milk** 1. secretion of the mammary gland. 2. a liquid (emulsion or suspension) resembling the secretion of the mammary gland. *Human breast m.* contains lipids, 98% as triglycerides, which provide more than 50% of the calorific requirements; carbohydrates, mainly lactose, giving 40% of the calorific needs; whey-dominant protein; vitamins; minerals; trace elements; and anti-infective factors, such as leucocytes, immunoglobulins, lysozyme, lactoferrin, bifidus factor, hormones and growth factor. *Pasteurized m.* A process whereby milk is held at 72°C for 30 minutes and then rapidly cooled and bottled; this method kills non-spore bearing pathogenic organisms without affecting flavour or food properties of the milk. *Sterilized m.* milk heated to 100°C for 15 minutes to render it free from bacteria. *Tuberculin-tested m.* milk from cows certified free from tuberculosis and subject to strict bacteriological tests. *M. teeth* the first set of a child's teeth.

**Miller–Abbott tube** *T.G. Miller, American physician, 1886–1981; W.O. Abbott, American physician, 1902–1943.* A double-channel intestinal tube for treating obstruction, especially that due to paralytic ileus of the small intestine. It has an inflatable balloon at its distal end.

**milligram** *symbol* mg. One thousandth of a gram.

**millilitre** *symbol* ml. One thousandth of a litre (one cubic centimetre).

**millimetre** *symbol* mm. One thousandth of a metre.

**millimole** *symbol* mmol. The amount of a substance that balances or is equivalent in combining power to 1 mg of hydrogen. A method of assessing the body's acid–base balance or needs during electrolyte upset.

**Milwaukee brace** a brace consisting of a leather girdle and neck ring connected by metal struts; used to brace the spine in the treatment of SCOLIOSIS.

**mineralocorticoid** a hormone produced by the adrenal cortex. Its function is to maintain the salt and water balance in the body.

**miosis** contraction of the pupil of the eye, as in reaction to a bright light; meiosis.

**miscarriage** abortion; the expulsion of the fetus before the 24th week of pregnancy, i.e. before it is legally viable.

**Misuse of Drugs Act 1971** Regulations 1985. Controls the possession, prescription and sale of certain habit-forming drugs, including narcotic drugs such as papaveretum (Omnopon), cocaine, morphine, diamorphine, cannabis indica and amphetamines. These are called controlled drugs and are available for treatment only on medical prescription. Heavy penalties invariably follow the illegal sale or supply of these drugs.

**mite** a minute animal, frequently parasitic on humans and animals, and causing various forms of dermatitis.

**mitochondrion** a body which is found in the cytoplasm of cells and is concerned with energy production and the oxidation of food.

**mitosis** a method of multiplication of cells by a specific process of division.

**mitral** shaped like a mitre. *M. incompetence* the result of a defective mitral valve, when there is a back flow, or regurgitation, after closure of the valve. *M. stenosis* the formation of fibrous tissue, causing a narrowing of the valve; usually due to rheumatic heart disease and endocarditis. *M. valve* the bicuspid valve between the left atrium and left ventricle of the heart. *M. valvotomy* an operation for overcoming stenosis by dividing the fibrous tissue to free the cusps.

**mittelschmerz** pain occurring between the menses, accompanying ovulation.

**ml** symbol for *millilitre(s)*.

**MLNS** mucocutaneous lymph node syndrome.

**MLSO** medical laboratory scientific officer.

**mm** symbol for *millimetre(s)*.

**mmol** symbol for *millimole(s)*.

**MMR**   measles mumps rubella vaccine.

**Mn**   symbol for *manganese*.

**mobilization**   the bringing back into mobility of a limb, joint or person following illness or injury.

**model**   a conceptual paradigm, framework or theory which can be used as an example to illustrate a problem, process or situation.

**modelling**   providing an example that can be imitated, and used as a means of teaching others to learn new behaviour.

**modem**   a device for converting digital and analogue signals, especially to allow a computer to be connected to a telephone line to access the internet.

**MODS**   multiple organ dysfunction syndrome.

**molar**   a back tooth used for grinding. There are three on either side of each jaw, making 12 in all (only eight in children). *M. solution* the concentration of a solution expressed in terms of the weight of the dissolved substance in grams per litre divided by its molecular weight.

**mole**   1. the molecular weight of a substance expressed in grams. 2. a pigmented naevus or dark-coloured growth on the skin. Moles are of various sizes, and are sometimes covered with hair. 3. a uterine tumour. *Carneous m.* an organized blood clot surrounding a shrivelled fetus in the uterus. *Hydatidiform m.* (*vesicular m.*) a condition in pregnancy in which the chorionic villi of the placenta degenerate into clusters of cysts like hydatids. Malignant growth may follow if any remnants are left in the uterus. *See* CHORIOCARCINOMA.

**molecular**   pertaining to or composed of molecules. *M. weight* the weight of a molecule of a substance compared with that of an atom of carbon.

**molecule**   the chemical combination of two or more atoms which form a specific chemical substance, e.g. $H_2O$ (water). The smallest amount of a substance that can exist independently.

**molluscum**   a skin disease characterized by the development of soft, round tumours. *M. contagiosum* a benign tumour arising in the epidermis caused by a virus, transmitted by direct contact or fomites.

**monarticular**   referring to one joint only.

*Monilia*   former name for the genus of fungi now known as *Candida*.

**monitor**   1. to check constantly on a given condition, state or phenomenon, e.g. blood pressure, heart, respiration rate or standards of care. 2. an apparatus by which such conditions or phenomena can be constantly observed and recorded. *Patient m.* the use of electrodes or transducers attached to the patient so that information such as temperature, pulse, respiration and blood pressure can be seen on a screen or automatically recorded.

**monoamine oxidase**   an enzyme that breaks down noradrenaline and serotonin in the body. *M. o. inhibitor* abbreviated MAOI. A drug that prevents the breakdown of serotonin and leads to an increase in mental and physical activity.

**monochromatism**   colour-blindness. The patient sees all colours as black, grey or white.

**monoclonal**   derived from a single cell. *M. antibodies* antibodies derived from a single clone of cells. All the antibody molecules are identical and will react with the same antigenic site.

**monocular**   pertaining to, or affecting, one eye only.

**monocyte**   a white blood cell having one nucleus, derived from the reticular cells, and having a phagocytic action.

**mononucleosis** an excessive number of monocytes in the blood; monocytosis. *Infectious m.* an infectious disease due to the Epstein-Barr virus; glandular fever.

**monoplegia** paralysis of one limb or of a single muscle or a group of muscles.

**monosaccharide** a simple sugar. The end result of carbohydrate digestion. Examples are glucose, fructose and galactose.

**monosodium glutamate** a chemical food flavour enhancer commonly added to Chinese dishes. May result in nausea, faintness, facial flushing and headache (sometimes called the Chinese restaurant syndrome).

**monosomy** a congenital defect in the number of human chromosomes. There is one less than the normal 46.

**mons** a prominence or mound. *M. pubis* or *m. veneris* the eminence, consisting of a pad of fat, that lies over the pubic symphysis in the female.

**Montgomery's glands or tubercles** *W.F. Montgomery, Irish obstetrician, 1797–1859.* Sebaceous glands around the nipple, which grow larger during pregnancy.

**mood** emotional reaction. Variations in mood are natural, but in certain psychiatric conditions there is severe depression in some cases and wild excitement in others, or alternations between both.

**moon face** one of the features occurring in Cushing's syndrome and as a result of prolonged treatment with steroid drugs.

**morbid** diseased, or relating to an abnormal or disordered condition.

**morbidity** the state of being diseased. *M. rate* a figure that shows the susceptibility of a population to a certain disease. Usually shown statistically as the number of cases which occur annually per 1000 or other unit of population.

**morbilli** measles.

**morbilliform** resembling measles.

**moribund** in a dying condition.

**morning sickness** nausea and vomiting which sometimes occurs in early pregnancy.

**Moro reflex** *E. Moro, German paediatrician, 1874–1951.* The reaction to loud noise or sudden movement which should be present in the newborn. Startle reflex.

**morphine** the principal alkaloid obtained from opium and given mainly to relieve severe pain. It is a drug of addiction. Morphia.

**mortality** the state of being liable to die. *M. rate* the number of deaths, per 1000 or other unit of population, occurring annually from a certain disease or condition.

**mortification** gangrene or death of tissue; necrosis.

**morula** an early stage of development of the ovum when it is a solid mass of cells.

**mosaic** an individual who has cells of varying genetic composition.

**motile** capable of movement.

**motion** 1. the process of moving. 2. evacuation of the bowels; defecation. *M. sickness* sickness occurring as the result of travel by land, sea or air. Appears to be caused by excessive stimulation of the vestibular apparatus within the inner ear.

**motivation** the reason or reasons, conscious or unconscious, behind a particular attitude or behaviour.

**motive** the incentive that determines a course of action or its direction.

**motor** something that causes movement. *M. end-plate* the nuclei and cytoplasm of muscle fibres at the termination of motor nerves. *M. nerve* one of the nerves which convey an impulse from a nerve centre to a muscle or gland to promote activity. *M. neurone disease* a disease in which there is progressive degeneration of the anterior cells in the spinal cord, the motor nuclei of cranial nerves and the corticospinal tracts. The cause is unknown.

**mould** 1. a species of fungus. 2. the plastic shell used to immobilize a part of the body, usually the head, during radiotherapy.

**moulding** the alteration in shape of the infant's head as it is forced through the maternal passages during labour.

**mountain sickness** dyspnoea, headache, rapid pulse and vomiting, which occur on sudden change to the rarefied air of high altitudes.

**mourning** see BEREAVEMENT.

**mouth** an opening, particularly the external opening (in the face) of the alimentary canal. *M. ulcers* painful, greyish-white sores occurring inside the mouth. Most are of unknown cause and usually disappear after a few days. Aphthous ulcers. *M.-wash* a solution for rinsing the mouth.

**movement** 1. an act of moving; motion. 2. an act of defecation. *Active m.* movement produced by the person's own muscles. *Associated m.* movement of parts that act together, as the eyes. *Passive m.* a movement of the body or of the extremities of a patient performed by another person without voluntary motion on the part of the patient. *Vermicular m's* the worm-like movements of the intestines in peristalsis.

**MRI** magnetic resonance imaging.

**MRSA** methicillin-resistant *Staphylococcus aureus*.

**mucinase** an enzyme which acts upon mucin. Contained in some aerosols and useful in the treatment of cystic fibrosis.

**mucocele** a mucous tumour. *Lacrimal m.* a distension of the lacrimal sac caused by a blockage of the nasolacrimal duct. *M. of the gallbladder* occurs if a stone obstructs the cystic duct.

**mucocutaneous** pertaining to mucous membrane and skin. *M. lymph node syndrome* abbreviated MLNS. Usually reported in babies and children. See KAWASAKI DISEASE.

**mucoid** resembling mucus.

**mucopurulent** containing mucus and pus.

**mucosa** mucous membrane.

**mucous** pertaining to or secreting mucus. *M. membrane* a membrane that secretes mucus and lines many of the body cavities, particularly those of the respiratory and alimentary tracts.

**mucoviscidosis** fibrocystic disease of the pancreas. See FIBROCYSTIC.

**mucus** the viscous secretion of mucous membrane.

**multicellular** consisting of many cells.

**multidisciplinary** involving two or more professional disciplines.

**multigravida** a pregnant woman who has had two or more pregnancies.

**multilocular** having many locules. *M. cyst* a cyst, usually in the ovary, containing many compartments.

**multinuclear** possessing many nuclei.

**multipara** a woman who has had two or more children.

**multiple** manifold, occurring in many parts of the body at once. *M. myeloma* malignant disease of the plasma cells which invade the bone marrow and suppress its functioning. *M. sclerosis* see SCLEROSIS.

**multiple organ dysfunction syndrome** abbreviated MODS. a situation usually precipitated by shock or trauma in which the functioning of interdependant body systems is severely affected, e.g. respiration, gastrointestinal tract, kidneys, blood circulation and coagulation. This multiple organ failure causes physiological disturbance requiring vital system support to maintain life. Other systems too may be compromised.

**multivariate analysis** the analysis of data collected on several different variables but all having a relevance to the study; e.g. in a survey of the provision of community nursing services for a specific population, data may be collected on age, family size and previous use of the services. In analysing the data the effect of each of these variables and their interaction can be examined and considered.

**mumps** a communicable paramyxovirus disease, which is statutorily notifiable. Incubation period 2–3 weeks. It attacks one or both of the parotid glands, the largest of the three pairs of salivary glands; also called epidemic parotitis or epidemic parotiditis. Most common amongst children; characterized by inflammation and swelling of the parotid glands. The symptoms are fever, and a painful swelling in front of the ears, making mastication difficult.

**Münchhausen's syndrome** *Baron von Münchhausen, 16th-century German traveller noted for his lying tales.* Habitual seeking of hospital treatment for apparent acute illness, the patient giving a plausible and dramatic history, all of which is false. *M. s. by proxy* a situation in which a parent (usually the mother) or both parents fabricate symptoms or signs in a child, who is then presented for hospital treatment; overlaps with other forms of child abuse, and fatal outcomes have been reported.

**murmur** a sound, heard on auscultation, usually originating in the cardiovascular system. *Aortic m.* one indicating disease of the aortic valve. *Diastolic m.* one heard after the second heart sound. *Friction m.* one present when two inflamed surfaces of serous membrane rub on each other. *Mitral m.* a sign of incompetence of the mitral valve. *Systolic m.* one heard during systole.

**muscae volitantes** [L.] *flying flies.* Black spots floating before the eyes. They do not obscure the sight.

**muscle** strong tissue composed of fibres which have the power of contraction, and thus produce movements of the body. *Cardiac m.* muscle composed of partially striped interlocking cells. Not under the control of the will. *M. relaxant* one of a group of drugs used to reduce muscular spasm and also to relax the muscles during surgery. *Smooth* or *non-striated m.* involuntary muscle of spindle-shaped cells, e.g. that of the intestinal wall. Contracts independently of the will. *Striped* or *striated m.* voluntary muscle. Transverse bands across the fibres give the characteristic appearance. It is under the control of the will.

**muscular** 1. pertaining to muscle. 2. well provided with strong muscles. *M. dystrophy* one of a number of inherited diseases in which there is progressive muscle wasting. *See* DUCHENNE DYSTROPHY.

**musculocutaneous** referring to the muscles and the skin. *M. nerve* one of the nerves which supply the muscles and the skin of the arms and legs.

**musculoskeletal** referring to both the osseus and muscular systems.

**mutant** 1. in genetics, a variation owing to genetic changes. 2. produced by mutation.

**mutation** a chemical change in the genes of a cell causing it to show a new characteristic. Some produce evolutional changes, others disease.

**mute** without the power of speech. *Deaf m.* one who cannot hear and therefore cannot speak.

**mutilation** deliberate infliction of bodily injury.

**mutism** inability or refusal to speak. In almost all cases, mutes are unable to speak because deafness has prevented them from hearing the spoken word. Speech is learned by imitating the speech of others. May also result from disease, the most common being a stroke.

*Elective m.* psychological disorder of childhood.

**myalgia** pain in the muscles.

**myalgic encephalomyelitis** abbreviated ME. *See* CHRONIC FATIGUE SYNDROME.

**myasthenia** muscle weakness. *M. gravis* an extreme form of muscle weakness which is progressive. There is a rapid onset of fatigue, thought to be due to the too rapid destruction of acetylcholine at the neuromuscular junction. Commonly affected muscles are those of vision, speaking, chewing and swallowing.

**mycetoma** a chronic fungus infection of the tissues, both external and internal but most commonly affecting the hands and feet. There is swelling and the formation of sinuses. Madura foot.

*Mycobacterium* a genus of slender, rod-shaped, acid-fast, Gram-positive bacteria that cause a variety of diseases. *M. leprae* the causative organism of leprosy. *M. tuberculosis* the cause of tuberculosis.

**mycology** the study of fungi.

**mycosis** any disease that is caused by a fungus. *M. fungoides* a rare malignant lymphoreticular neoplasm of the skin which later progresses to the lymph nodes and viscera.

**mydriasis** abnormal dilatation of the pupil of the eye. Usually caused by injury to the pupil sphincter or by the use of mydriatic drugs.

**mydriatic** any drug that causes mydriasis. Used in examination of the eye and in the treatment of inflammatory conditions.

**myelin** the fatty covering of medullated nerve fibres.

**myelitis** 1. inflammation of the spinal cord, causing pain in the back and sometimes numbness and paralysis of the legs and the lower part of the trunk. 2. inflammation of the bone marrow; osteomyelitis.

**myeloblast** a primitive cell in the bone marrow, from which develop the granular leukocytes.

**myelocyte** a cell of the bone marrow, derived from a myeloblast.

**myelography** radio-graphic examination of the spinal cord after the introduction of a radio-opaque substance into the subarachnoid space by means of lumbar puncture.

**myeloid** 1. pertaining to, derived from or resembling bone marrow. 2. pertaining to the spinal cord. 3. having the appearance of myelocytes, but not necessarily derived from bone marrow. *M. leukaemia* a malignant disease in which there is excessive production of leukocytes in the bone marrow. *M. tissue* red bone marrow.

**myeloma** a tumour composed of plasma cells. *Multiple m.* a primary malignant tumour of plasma cells, usually arising in bone marrow, and usually associated with anaemia and with a paraprotein in the blood or Bence Jones protein in the urine.

**myelomatosis** a malignant disease of the bone marrow in which multiple myelomas are present.

**myelomeningocele** meningomyelocele.

**myiasis** infestation of wounds or body openings by fly larvae (maggots); more commonly seen in the tropics.

**myocardial** pertaining to the myocardium. *M. infarction* necrosis of a part of the myocardium, usually following a coronary thrombosis. Ventricular fibrillation may occur, followed by death.

**myocarditis** inflammation of the myocardium.

**myocardium** the muscle tissue of the heart.

**myoclonus** spasmodic contraction of the muscles.

**myofibrosis** a degenerative condition in which there is some replacement of muscle tissue by fibrous tissue.

**myohaemoglobin** a substance, resembling haemoglobin, which is present in muscle cells. It is a pigment and is responsible for the colour of muscle. It acts as an oxygen store. Myoglobin.

**myokymia** a benign condition in which there is persistent quivering of the muscles.

**myoma** a benign tumour of muscle tissue. *See* FIBROMYOMA.

**myomectomy** removal of a myoma; usually referring to a uterine fibroma.

**myometrium** the muscular tissue of the uterus.

**myoneural** relating to both muscle and nerve. *M. junction* the point at which nerve endings terminate in a muscle; neuromuscular junction.

**myopathy** any disease of the muscles. Muscular dystrophy is one of a group of inherited myopathies in which there is wasting and weakness of the muscles.

**myopia** shortsightedness. The light rays focus in front of the retina and a biconcave lens is needed to focus them correctly.

**myoplasty** any operation in which muscle is detached and utilized, as may be done to correct deformities.

**myosarcoma** a sarcomatous tumour of muscle.

**myosin** muscle protein.

**myositis** inflammation of a muscle. *M. ossificans* a condition in which bone cells deposited in

muscle continue to grow and cause hard lumps. It may occur after fractures.

**myotomy** the division or dissection of a muscle.

**myotonia** lack of muscle tone. *M. congenita* a hereditary disease in which the muscle action has a prolonged contraction phase and slow relaxation.

**myringa** the eardrum or tympanic membrane.

**myringitis** inflammation of the tympanic membrane.

**myringoplasty** a plastic operation to repair the tympanic membrane. *See* TYMPANOPLASTY.

**myringotome** an instrument for puncturing the tympanic membrane in myringotomy.

**myringotomy** incision of the tympanic membrane to drain fluid from an infected middle ear.

**myxoedema** a condition, caused by hypothyroidism, which is marked by mucoid infiltration of the skin. There is oedematous swelling of the face, limbs and hands, dry and rough skin, loss of hair, slow pulse, subnormal temperature, slowed metabolism and mental dullness. *Congenital m.* cretinism.

**myxoma** a benign mucous tumour of connective tissue.

**myxosarcoma** a sarcoma containing mucoid tissue.

**myxovirus** the group name of a number of related viruses, including the causal viruses of influenza, parainfluenza, mumps and Newcastle disease (of fowl).

**N** symbol for *nitrogen* and *newton*.

**Na** symbol for *sodium*.

**nadir** the lowest out of a series of measurements, e.g. the lowest level to which the viral load falls after starting antiretroviral treatment. The opposite is ZENITH.

**naevus** a birthmark; a circumscribed area of pigmentation of the skin due to dilated blood vessels. A haemangioma. *N. flammeus* a flat bluish-red area, usually on the neck or face; popularly known as 'port wine stain'. *N. pilosus* a hairy naevus. *Spider n.* a small red area surrounded by dilated capillaries. *Strawberry n.* a raised tumour-like structure of connective tissue containing spaces filled with blood.

**Nägele's rule** rule for calculating the estimated date of labour; subtract 3 months from the first day of the last menstrual period and add 7 days.

**NAI** non-accidental injury.

**nail** the keratinized portion of epidermis covering the dorsal extremity of the fingers and toes. *Hang n.* a strip of epidermis hanging at one side or at the root of a nail. *Ingrowing n.* a condition in which the flesh overhangs the edge of the nail, a sharp corner of which may pierce the skin, causing a wound which may become septic. *N. bed* the skin underlying a nail. *N. biting* a sign of nervousness or tension which occurs in childhood and may persist into adult life. It is a common problem and the most frequent habitual manipulation of the body but is rarely of psychopathological significance. *Spoon n.* a nail with a depression in the centre and raised edges. *See* KOILONYCHIA.

**named nurse** a qualified nurse, midwife or health visitor who is known to the patient or client by name and is accountable for planning and the delivery of care. The aim is to provide maximum continuity and coordination in care for the individual patient or client in a variety of health care settings.

**NANDA** North American Nursing Diagnosis Association.

**nanometre** *symbol* nm. A unit of measurement equal to one billionth ($10^{-9}$) of a metre, or more commonly used to describe a measure equal to one thousandth ($10^{-3}$) of a micrometre (µm). Nanometres are used to describe the smallest particles in nature, e.g. atoms, small molecules, viruses, electromagnetic radiation such as X-rays, and computer chips (CPUs). A nanometre is approximately the length of three to six atoms placed side by side, or the width of a single strand of DNA; the thickness of a human hair is between 50 000 and 100 000 nm and represents the smallest feature an unaided human eye can see.

**nape** the back of the neck.

**napkin rash** an erythematous rash which may occur in infants in the napkin area. The many causes include the passage of frequent loose stools, thrush, ammoniacal dermatitis and allergy to washing powders and detergents.

**narcissism** the stage of infant development when children are mainly interested in themselves and their own bodily needs. In adults it may be a symptom of mental disorder. The term is derived from the Greek myth of Narcissus.

**narcoanalysis** a form of psychotherapy in which an injection of a narcotic drug produces a drowsy, relaxed state during which a patient will talk more freely, and in this way much repressed material may be brought to consciousness.

**narcolepsy** a condition in which there is an uncontrollable desire for sleep.

**narcosis** a state of unconsciousness produced by a narcotic drug. *Basal n.* a state of unconsciousness produced prior to surgical anaesthesia.

**narcosynthesis** the inducement of a hypnotic state by means of drugs. An aid to psychotherapy.

**narcotic** a drug that produces narcosis or unnatural sleep.

**nares** the nostrils. *Posterior n.* the opening of the nares into the nasopharynx.

**nasal** pertaining to the nose.

**nascent** 1. at the time of birth. 2. incipient.

**nasoduodenal** related to the nose and duodenum. *N. tube* a fine-bore tube passed through the nose into the duodenum and used for enteral nutrition.

**nasogastric** referring to the nose and stomach. *N. tube* one passed into the stomach via the nose.

**nasojejunal feeding** a method in which a silicone-coated catheter is passed through the nose into the jejunum to provide sufficient nutrition to a sick baby on a ventilator

or receiving continuous inflating pressure (CIP) by mask or nasal tube. It is used to prevent the dangers of aspiration with a nasogastric tube feed.

**nasolacrimal** concerning both the nose and lacrimal apparatus. *N. duct* the duct draining the tears from the inner aspect of the eye to the inferior meatus of the nose.

**nasopharynx** the upper part of the pharynx; that above the soft palate.

**nasosinusitis** inflammation of the nose and adjacent sinuses.

**National Audit Office** (NAO) This is an independent Parliamentary body in the United Kingdom, responsible for auditing all central government departments, government agencies and non-departmental bodies. The NAO reports to the Comptroller and Auditor General in Parliament, these reports are reviewed by the Public Accounts Committee, a select committee of the House of Commons. The Audit Commission performs a similar function for local government in England and the English NHS Trusts. Audit Scotland performs both the roles of the Audit Commission and the NAO auditing the Scottish Executive and its public bodies. The Wales Audit Office is responsible for auditing the Welsh Assembly Government, its public bodies and local government in Wales. The Northern Ireland Audit Office performs similar functions in Northern Ireland.

**national confidential enquiries** system for examining clinical performance and serious avoidable events. Information is furnished on a confidential basis from around the NHS. The National Institute for Clinical Excellence supports the confidential enquiries. In 1998 the UK government announced that participation in the enquiries would be compulsory for all relevant clinicians. The four enquiries are: (a) national confidential enquiry into perioperative deaths (NCEPOD); (b) confidential enquiry into stillbirths and deaths in infancy (CESDI); (c) confidential enquiry into maternal deaths (CEMD); and (d) confidential enquiry into suicide and homicide by people with mental illness (CISH). *See* CONFIDENTIAL ENQUIRY.

**National Institute for Clinical Excellence** abbreviated NICE. A special health authority, providing formal advice for NHS clinicians and managers on the clinical and cost effectiveness of new and existing technologies such as medicines. It provides and disseminates clinical guidance and guidelines based on the relevant evidence, clinical audit methodologies and information on good practice.

**National Patient Safety Agency** organization that runs a mandatory reporting system for logging errors and near misses across the NHS, so as to improve safety by reducing the risk of harm. The aim is to create a more blame-free NHS, where lessons are shared and learnt.

**national service frameworks** abbreviated NSFs. Spells out what patients/clients can expect to receive from the NHS in a major care area or disease group. They are evidence-based and are drafted by expert reference groups. NSFs set national standards, define service models, include programmes to support implementation and set out performance measures against which to assess progress. There are several published NSFs which include paediatric intensive care, mental health, coronary heart disease, cancer, older people, maternity, and diabetes. *See* Appendix 14.

**National Vocational Qualifications** abbreviated NVQs. Nationally recognized work-related qualifications that are coordinated by the National Council for Vocational Qualifications. NVQs are based on a system of credits earned after a work-based assessment of skills and the level of competence attained.

**natural childbirth** a term used to describe an approach to LABOUR and delivery in which the parents are prepared for the event so that the mother is awake and co-operative and the father is able to assume an active and supportive role during the birth of their child. The underlying concept for all methods of natural childbirth is avoidance of medical interference and analgesia in labour, and education of the parents so that they can actively participate in and share the experience of childbirth.

**natural killer cells** abbreviated NK. A type of lymphocyte involved in natural killing (apoptosis) and forming part of the non-specific body defences. NK cells target viral infected cells and tumour cells.

**nature–nurture debate** the debate surrounding the issue of to what extent human behaviour is the result of hereditary or innate influences (nature) or is determined by the environment and learning (nurture).

**naturopathy** a drugless system of healing by a combination of diet, fasting, exercise, hydrotherapy and positive thinking.

**nausea** a sensation of sickness with an inclination to vomit.

**navel** the umbilicus.

**navicular** boat-shaped. *N. bone* one of the tarsal bones of the foot.

**nebula** a slight opacity or cloudiness of the cornea, caused by injury or by corneal ulceration.

**nebulizer** an apparatus for reducing a liquid to a fine spray. An atomizer.

**NEC** necrotizing enterocolitis.

**neck** 1. the narrow part of an organ or bone. 2. the part of the body which connects the head and the trunk. *Derbyshire n.* simple goitre. *Wry n.* torticollis.

**necrobiosis** localized death of a part as a result of degeneration.

**necropsy** autopsy; a postmortem examination of a body.

**necrosis** death of a portion of tissue.

**necrotizing enterocolitis** abbreviated NEC. A condition of neonates in which there is severe diarrhoea and blood in the stools. It occurs in preterm or low-birth-weight neonates. Exact cause is not known but is often associated with infection.

**necrotizing fasciitis** a bacterial infection of *Streptococcus* type A underneath the skin in the fascia layer; produces necrosis and toxins, resulting in shock and organ failure. Urgent treatment is required with antibiotics and surgical excision of the infected tissues.

**needlestick injury** an accidental injury with a needle that is contaminated with blood or body fluids. The term is also used sometimes to include other sharps injuries. The injuries have been reported as a means of infecting the nurse or health care professional with hepatitis or human immunodeficiency virus (HIV). A risk assessment procedure, training policies and clinical guidelines should be in place in all health care situations for staff to follow, should such an injury occur.

**need analysis** exercise often undertaken by NHS Trusts, service organizations and agencies of a target population to assess a service or situation with a view to change, e.g alteration in clinic times. Multiple research methods and techniques for data collection and analysis may be used in the process.

**needling** discission, the operation for cataract of lacerating and splitting up the lens so that it may be absorbed.

**needs** *see* MASLOW'S HIERARCHY OF NEEDS.

**negative** the opposite of positive. The absence of some quality or substance.

**negativism** a symptom of mental illness in which the patient does the opposite of what is required and so presents an uncooperative attitude. Common in schizophrenia.

**negligence** in law, the failure to do something that a reasonable person of ordinary prudence would do in a certain situation or the doing of something that such a person would not do. Negligence may provide the basis for a lawsuit when there is a legal duty, as in the duty of a doctor or nurse to provide reasonable care to patients, and when the negligence results in damage to the patient.

*Neisseria* *A.L.S. Neisser, German bacteriologist, 1855–1916.* A genus of paired, spherical, Gram-negative bacteria. *N. gonorrhoeae* the causative organism of gonorrhoea. *N. meningitidis* the cause of meningococcal meningitis.

**Nematoda** a phylum of worms, including the genus *Ascaris* or roundworm and the genus *Enterobius* or threadworm.

**neoadjuvant therapy** chemotherapy given prior to radiation treatment or surgery to reduce the size of a tumour.

**neoglycogenesis** the formation of liver glycogen from non-carbohydrate sources. Glyconeogenesis.

**neologism** the formation of new words, either completely new ones or ones formed by contraction of two separate words. This is done particularly by schizophrenic patients.

**neonatal** referring to the first month of life. *N. mortality rate* the number of deaths of infants up to 4 weeks old per 1000 live births in any one year. *N. period* the interval from the birth to 28 days of age and the period of greatest risk to the infant. *N. screening* see SCREENING. *N. intensive care unit* see INTENSIVE CARE UNIT.

**neonate** newborn; specifically pertaining to a baby under 1 month old.

**neonatologist** a medically qualified person specializing in the management, assessment, diseases and intensive care of newborn babies, especially those of low birthweight and those with congenital abnormalities.

**neonatology** the branch of medicine dealing with disorders of the newborn infant.

**neoplasm** a morbid new growth; a tumour. It may be benign or malignant.

**nephrectomy** excision of a kidney.

**nephritis** inflammation of the kidney; a focal or diffuse proliferative or destructive disease that may involve the glomerulus, tubule or interstitial renal tissue. Formerly called Bright's disease. The most usual form is glomerulonephritis.

**nephroblastoma** a rapidly developing malignant mixed tumour of the kidneys, made up of embryonic cells, and occurring chiefly in children before the fifth year; Wilms' tumour.

**nephrocalcinosis** a condition in which there is deposition of calcium in the renal tubules, resulting in calculi formation and renal insufficiency.

**nephrocapsulectomy** an operation for removal of the capsule of the kidney.

**nephrolith** stone in the kidney; renal calculus.

**nephrolithiasis** the presence of a calculus or of gravel in the kidney.

**nephrolithotomy** removal of a renal calculus by incising the kidney or by extracorporeal shock wave lithotripsy.

**nephroma** tumour of the kidney.

**nephron** the functional unit of the kidney, comprising Bowman's capsule, the proximal and distal tubules, the loop of Henle and the collecting duct, which conveys urine to the renal pelvis.

**nephropexy** the fixation of a floating (mobile) kidney, usually by sutures to neighbouring muscle.

**nephroptosis** downward displacement, or undue mobility, of a kidney.

**nephropyeloplasty** any plastic operation on the pelvis of the kidney.

**nephrosclerosis** constriction of the arterioles of the kidney. Seen in benign and malignant hypertension and in arteriosclerosis in old age.

**nephrosis** any disease of the kidney, especially that characterized by oedema, proteinuria and a low plasma albumin. Caused by noninflammatory degenerative lesions of the tubules.

**nephrostomy** creation of a permanent opening into the renal pelvis.

**nephrotic** referring to or caused by nephrosis. *N. syndrome* a clinical syndrome in which there is proteinuria, low plasma protein and gross oedema. The result of increased capillary permeability in the glomeruli. It may occur as a result of acute glomerulonephritis, in subacute nephritis, diabetes mellitus, amyloid disease, systemic lupus erythematosus and renal vein thrombosis.

**nephrotomy** incision of the kidney.

**nephrotoxic** poisonous or destructive to the cells of the kidney.

**nephroureterectomy** surgical removal of the kidney and the ureter.

**nerve** a bundle of conducting fibres enclosed in a sheath called the epineurium. Its function is to transmit impulses between any part of the body and a nerve centre. *Motor (efferent) n.* one that conveys impulses causing activity from a nerve centre to a muscle or gland. *N. block* a method of producing regional anaesthesia by injecting a local anaesthetic into the nerves supplying the area to be operated on. *N. fibre* the prolongation of the nerve cell, which conveys impulses. Each fibre has a sheath. Medullated nerve fibres have an insulating myelin sheath. *N. gas* a gas that interferes with the functioning of the nerves and muscles. Such gases may cause death from respiratory paralysis; some of them act through the skin and cannot be avoided by the use of gas masks. *Sensory (afferent) n.* one that conveys sensation from an area to a nerve centre.

**nervous** 1. pertaining to, or composed of, nerves. 2. apprehensive. *N. breakdown* a popular and misleading term for any type of mental illness that interferes with a person's normal activities. A so-called 'nervous breakdown' can include any of the mental disorders, including NEUROSIS, PSYCHOSIS or DEPRESSION, but is usually used to describe neurosis.

**nervousness** excitability of the nervous system, characterized by a state of mental and physical unrest.

**nesting** the provision of an enclosed space bounded by a small blanket roll encircling the sick or preterm infant in a cot or incubator. This helps to provide a supportive, calming environment for the infant.

**nettle rash** an allergic skin condition; urticaria.

**network** 1. an interconnected group or system of voluntary organizations or of colleagues with similar interests. 2. a system of interconnected computer terminals in which the user has access to others using the system for sharing data, etc. **Clinical n.** a group of health professionals and organizations from primary, secondary and tertiary care working together in a managed and coordinated way that is not constrained by existing organizational or professional boundaries. The aim is to deliver a patient-focused service that highlights quality of care and clinical effectiveness. These networks may be grouped by function (pathology, accident and emergency services), client group (children, the elderly), disease (cancer, coronary heart disease) or specialty (vascular surgery, cardiology).

**networking** 1. forming and maintaining professional connections and contacts through informal social meetings. 2. the interconnection of two or more computer networks in different places.

**neural** pertaining to the nerves. *N. arch* the bony arch on each vertebra which encloses the spinal cord. *N. tube defect* any of a group of congenital malformations involving the neural tube, including anencephaly, hypocephalus and spina bifida.

**neuralgia** a sharp stabbing pain, usually along the course of a nerve, owing to neuritis or functional disturbance.

**neurapraxia** an injury to a nerve resulting in temporary loss of function and paralysis. It is usually caused by compression of the nerve, and there is no lasting damage.

**neurasthenia** an outdated term in which there is much mental and physical fatigue, inability to concentrate, loss of appetite and initative with sometimes a failure of memory.

**neurectomy** excision of part of a nerve.

**neurilemma** the membranous sheath surrounding a nerve fibre.

**neurinoma** a benign tumour arising in the neurilemma of a nerve fibre.

**neuritis** inflammation of a nerve, with pain, tenderness and loss of function. *Multiple n.* that involving several nerves; polyneuritis.

*Nutritional (alcoholic) n.* that which may be caused by alcoholism or lack of vitamin B complex. *Optic n.* that affecting the optic disc or nerve. *Peripheral n.* that involving the terminations of nerves. *Sciatic n.* sciatica. *Traumatic n.* that which results from an injury to a nerve.

**neuroblast** an embryonic nerve cell.

**neuroblastoma** a malignant tumour of immature nerve cells, most often arising in the very young.

**neurodermatitis** a localized prurigo of somatic and psychogenic origin. It irritates, and rubbing causes thickening and pigmentation of the skin.

**neurodevelopmental therapy** an approach to the rehabilitation of patients with neurological problems based on current research findings into motor development and neurophysiology.

**neuroepithelioma** a malignant tumour of the retina of the eye, which may spread into the brain.

**neurofibroma** a benign tumour of nerve and fibrous tissue.

**neurofibromatosis** von Recklinghausen's disease. A generalized hereditary disease in which there are numerous fibromas of the skin and nervous system.

**neurogenic** derived from or caused by nerve stimulation. *N. bladder* a disorder of the urinary bladder caused by a lesion of the nervous system. *N. shock* shock originating in the nervous system.

**neuroglia** the special form of connective tissue supporting nerve tissues.

**neurological assessment** evaluation of the health status of a patient with a nervous system disorder or dysfunction. Purposes of the assessment include establishing nursing goals to guide the nurse in planning and implementing nursing measures to help the patient cope effectively with daily living activities. Nursing assessment of a patient's neurological status is concerned with identifying functional disabilities that interfere with the person's ability to provide self-care and lead an active life. A functionally oriented nursing assessment includes: (a) consciousness; (b) mental functions; (c) motor function; and (d) sensory function. Evaluation of these functions gives the nurse information about the patient's ability to perform everyday activities such as thinking, remembering, seeing, eating, speaking, moving, smelling, feeling and hearing. A patient with an acute and life-threatening alteration in neurological function is evaluated and monitored in four general areas: (a) level of consciousness; (b) sensory and motor function; (c) pupillary changes; and (d) vital signs and pattern of respiration.

**neurologist** a medical practitioner specializing in neurology.

**neurology** 1. the scientific study of the nervous system. 2. the branch of medicine concerned with diseases of the nervous system.

**neuroma** a tumour consisting of nervous tissue.

**neuromuscular** appertaining to nerves and muscles. *N. junction* the small gap between the end of the motor nerve and the motor end-plate of the muscle fibre supplied. This gap is bridged by the release of acetylcholine whenever a nerve impulse arrives.

**neuromyelitis** neuritis associated with myelitis. It is a condition akin to multiple sclerosis. *N. optica* a disease in which there is bilateral optic neuritis and paraplegia.

**neurone** a nerve cell. *Lower motor n.* the anterior horn cell and its neurone which convey impulses to the appropriate muscles. *Upper motor n.* that in which the cell is in the cerebral cortex and the fibres conduct impulses to associated cells in the spinal cord. Also called neuron.

**neuroparalysis** paralysis due to disease of a nerve or nerves.

**neuropathy** a disease process of nerve degeneration and loss of function. *Alcoholic n.* neuropathy due to thiamine deficiency in chronic alcoholism. *Diabetic n.* that associated with diabetes. *Entrapment n.* any of a group of neuropathies, e.g. carpal tunnel syndrome, due to mechanical pressure on a peripheral nerve. *Ischaemic n.* that caused by a lack of blood supply.

**neuroplasticity** the capacity for nerve cells to regenerate and recover function.

**neuroplasty** the surgical repair of a damaged nerve.

**neuropsychiatry** the medical specialism concerned with the effects on mind and behaviour of organic disorders of the nervous system, combining both neurology and psychiatry.

**neurorrhaphy** the operation of suturing a divided nerve.

**neurosis** now an outdated term for a mental health disorder, which does not affect the whole personality, characterized by exaggerated anxiety and tension. *Anxiety n.* persistent anxiety and the accompanying symptoms of fear, rapid pulse, sweating, trembling, loss of appetite and insomnia. *Obsessive-compulsive n.* one characterized by compulsions and obsessional rumination.

**neurosurgery** that branch of surgery dealing with the brain, spinal cord and nerves.

**neurosyphilis** a manifestation of third stage syphilis in which the nervous system is involved. Symptoms of the disease may not occur for 20 years or so after the primary infection. The three most common forms are: (a) meningovascular syphilis, affecting the blood vessels to the meninges; (b) tabes dorsalis (see ATAXIA); and (c) general paralysis of the insane.

**neurotoxic** poisonous or destructive to nervous tissue.

**neurotransmitter** a substance (e.g. noradrenaline, acetylcholine, dopamine) that is released from the axon terminal to produce activity in other nerves.

**neurotripsy** the surgical bruising or crushing of a nerve.

**neurotropic** having an affinity for nerve tissue. *N. viruses* (rabies, poliomyelitis, etc.) those that particularly attack the nervous system.

**neutropenia** a decrease in the number of neutrophils in the blood.

**neutrophil** a polymorphonuclear leukocyte that has a neutral reaction to acid and alkaline dyes.

**next of kin** technically a person's closest living relative, whose name is often required health care information. Patients should be asked whom they wish to nominate as their 'next-of-kin' or 'significant other' in accordance with their own personal situation.

**NHS Direct** a nurse-led telephone health advice service providing 24-hour access to health care assessment and health information. The service: (a) is a private, confidential, reliable and consistent source of professional advice; (b) is speedy with simple access to a comprehensive range of the latest health and health-related information; (c) improves quality, increases cost effectiveness and reduces demands on other NHS services; and (d) allows professionals to develop their role in enabling patients to be partners in self-care. **NHS Direct Online (www.nhsdirect.nhs.uk)** an interactive website that provides: a self-help guide to treating common problems in the home; a health encyclopaedia of over 400 topics; personal responses to specific requests for information; a searchable database of hospitals, community health services, GPs, dentists, opticians and pharmacies.

**niacin** nicotinic acid.

**nicotine** a poisonous alkaloid in tobacco. *N. replacement therapy* preparations containing nicotine that are used in place of cigarettes to assist people to stop smoking. Preparations are available in a variety of forms, e.g. as patches, sublingual tablets, chewing gum or nasal sprays, these therapies double the chances of smokers quitting successfully. Available on NHS prescription. Some side-effects may occur, e.g. nausea, headaches, palpitations and flu-like symptoms.

**nicotinic acid** niacin. A water-soluble vitamin in the B complex. A deficiency of this vitamin causes pellagra.

**nidation** implantation of the fertilized ovum in the uterus.

**nidus** 1. a nest. 2. a place in which an organism finds conditions suitable for its growth and development. 3. the focus of an infection.

**Niemann–Pick disease** *A. Niemann, German paediatrician, 1880–1921; F. Pick, German physician, 1868–1935.* A rare inherited disease occurring primarily in Jewish children and resulting in learning difficulties. There is lipoid storage abnormality and widespread deposition of lecithin in the tissues.

**night blindness** nyctalopia; difficulty in seeing in the dark. This may be a congenital defect or be caused by a vitamin A deficiency. Also occurs as a result of retinal degeneration.

**nightmare** a frightening or unpleasant dream that occurs during REM (rapid eye movement) sleep usually in the middle to later part of the night. The dreamer wakes completely, remembering the dream. Most common in young children; in adults may be a side-effect of certain drugs, e.g. beta-blockers, or associated with a traumatic experience.

**night sweat** profuse perspiration during sleep, associated with an acute feverish illness or the menopause.

**night terror** an unpleasant experience in which the subject, usually a young child, screams while asleep and seems terrified. On waking the individual is unable to remember the cause of the fear.

**nihilism** in psychiatry, a term used to describe feelings of not existing and hopelessness, that all is lost or destroyed.

**nipple** the small conical projection at the tip of the breast, through which, in the female, milk can be withdrawn. *Accessory n.* a rudimentary nipple anywhere in a line from the breast to the groin. *Depressed n.* one that does not protrude. *N. shield* a shield fitted with a rubber teat which covers the areola of a nursing mother when her nipple is sore or not sufficiently protractile for the baby to suck. *Retracted n.* one that is drawn inwards. It may be a sign of cancer of the breast.

**nit** the egg of the head louse, attached to the hair near the scalp.

**nitrate drugs** a group of coronary vasodilator drugs used to treat angina pectoris, e.g. glyceryl trinitrate and isosorbide. These drugs provide rapid relief of symptoms and improve exercise tolerance. They may be given as tablets to be chewed or dissolved sublingually, as skin patches, gel or sublingual sprays.

**nitrogen** *symbol* N. A gaseous element. Air is largely composed of nitrogen, and it is one of the essential constituents of all protein foods. *N. balance* the state of the body in regard to the rate of protein intake and protein utilization. A negative nitrogen balance occurs when more protein is utilized by the body than is taken in. A positive nitrogen balance implies a net gain of protein in the body. Negative nitrogen balance can be caused by such factors as malnutrition, debilitating disease, blood loss and glucocorticoids. A positive balance can be caused by exercise, growth hormone and testosterone.

**nitrous oxide** $N_2O$. An inhalation anaesthetic ensuring a brief spell of unconsciousness.

**NK** *see* NATURAL KILLER CELLS.

**NMC** Nursing and Midwifery Council.

**NNT** numbers needed to treat.

**nociassociation** the discharge of nervous energy which occurs unconsciously in trauma, as in surgical shock. *See* ANOCI-ASSOCIATION.

**noctambulation** sleep walking; somnambulism.

**nocturia** the production of large quantities of urine at night.

**nocturnal** referring to the night. *N. enuresis* bed-wetting; incontinence of urine during sleep.

**node** a swelling or protuberance. *Atrioventricular n.* the specialized tissue between the right atrium and the ventricle, at the point where the coronary vein enters the atrium, from which is initiated the impulse of contraction down the atrioventricular bundle. *N. of Ranvier* a constriction occurring at intervals in a nerve fibre to enable the neurilemma with its blood supply to reach and nourish the axon of the nerve. *Sinoatrial n.* known as the pacemaker of the heart. A group of specialized cells situated at the opening of the superior vena cava into the right atrium. These cells emit regular electric impulses which initiate and control the heart beat.

**nodule** a small swelling or protuberance.

**noma** a gangrenous condition of the mouth; cancrum oris.

**nominal** the level of measurement that simply assigns data into categories that are mutually exclusive.

**nomogram** a graph with several scales arranged so that a ruler laid on the graph intersects the scales at related values of the variables; the values of any two variables can be used to find the values of the others. Increasingly used in the determination of drug therapy dosage, e.g. in paediatrics.

**non compos mentis** [L.] *not of sound mind*. Applied to people whose mental state is such that they are unable to manage their own affairs.

**non-accidental injury** abbreviated NAI. Injuries inflicted upon children or infants by those looking after them, usually the parents. The injuries are usually physical (beating, burnings, biting) but the term includes the giving of poisons and dangerous drugs, sexual abuse, starvation and any other form of physical assault.

**non-compliance** describes the decision made by a patient not to comply with a drug regimen, even though fully understanding the rationale for such therapy.

**non-experimental research design** a research design in which an investigator observes a phenomenon without manipulating the independent variable(s).

**non-invasive** any medical procedure that does not penetrate the skin or organ of the body, e.g. CT scanning or blood pressure monitoring using a sphygmomanometer and stethoscope. The term may also be used to describe non-cancerous tumours that do not metastasize.

**non-maleficence** the concept in the health care services of the duty to avoid harm to the interests of others.

**non-shivering thermogenesis** the use of brown adipose tissue by the neonate to produce heat in times of stress. Brown fat is stored in the mediastinum, around the nape of the neck, between the scapulae and around the kidneys and suprarenal glands.

**non-specific** 1. not due to any single known cause. 2. not directed against a particular agent, but rather having a general effect. *N. urethritis* abbreviated NSU. A common, sexually transmitted disease which may be due to a variety of agents, e.g. *Chlamydia trachomatis* which causes 40% of cases. Also called non-gonococcal urethritis.

**non-steroidal anti-inflammatory drugs** abbreviated NSAIDs. A group of drugs with analgesic, antipyretic and anti-inflammatory activity due to their ability to inhibit the synthesis of prostaglandins. It includes aspirin, phenylbutazone, indomethacin, tolmetic, ibuprofen and related drugs.

**non-union** in a fracture, failure of the two pieces of bone to unite.

**noradrenaline** a hormone present in extracts of the suprarenal medulla and at synapses in the peripheral sympathetic nervous system. It causes vasoconstriction and raises both the systolic and the diastolic blood pressure.

**norm** a fixed standard or value against which values are measured.

**normal** conforming to a standard; regular or usual. *N. distribution* in statistics, a symmetrical 'bell-shaped' distribution or curve that forms in the plotting of the scores. The most probable scores are concentrated around the mean or average with progressively less probable scores occurring further from the mean. *N. flora* bacteria which normally live on body tissues and have a beneficial effect. *N. saline* isotonic solution of sodium chloride. Physiological solution.

**normoblast** a nucleated precursor red blood cell in bone marrow. *See* ERYTHROCYTE.

**normochromic** normal in colour. Applied to the blood when the haemoglobin level is within normal limits.

**normocyte** a red blood cell that is normal in size, shape and colour.

**normoglycaemia** normal blood sugar level.

**normotension** normal tone, tension or pressure. Usually used in relation to blood pressure.

**North American Nursing Diagnosis Association** abbreviated NANDA. Formed as a professional organization of registered nurses in 1982. The purpose of NANDA is 'to develop, refine and promote a taxonomy of nursing diagnostic terminology of general use to the professional'. Meets at regular intervals to review previously approved nursing diagnoses and to further develop the classification systems.

**Norton scale** *See* PRESSURE ULCER ASSESSMENT SCALES.

**nose** the organ of smell and the airway for respiration.

**nosocomial** pertaining to, or acquired in hospital. *N. disease* for the patient, a new disorder, not related to the original disease, that is caused or precipitated during hospitalization. *N. infection* an infection acquired in hospital at least 72 hours after admission. Also called hospital-acquired infection (HAI). *Contact transmitted infection* is the most important and frequent mode of transmission of nosocomial infections and may be either direct or indirect. *Direct contact transmitted infections* involve direct body surface-to-body surface contact, such as occurs in patient care activities, e.g. bathing a patient. Direct contact can also occur between two patients, with one serving as the source of infectious microorganisms, the other being a susceptible host. *Indirect contact transmitted infections* involve contact of a susceptible host with a contaminated intermediate object, usually inanimate (*see* FOMITES), e.g. contaminated instruments, needles, dressings or gloves that are not changed between patients. Unwashed, contaminated hands may also be a source of nosocomial infection.

**nosology** the classification of disease into groups by criteria, based on (expert) agreement of the boundaries of the groups, e.g. by the DELPHI TECHNIQUE.

**nostril** one of the anterior orifices of the nose.

**notifiable** applied to such diseases as must by law be reported to the health authorities. These include measles, scarlet fever, typhus and typhoid fever, cholera, diphtheria, tuberculosis, dysentery and food poisoning.

**NPF** Nurse Prescribers' Formulary.

**NSAIDs** non-steroidal anti-inflammatory drugs.

**NSU** non-specific urethritis.

**nuclear** pertaining to a nucleus. *N. medicine* that branch of medicine concerned with the use of radionuclides in the diagnosis and treatment of disease. *N. family see* FAMILY.

**nuclear magnetic resonance** abbreviated NMR. A phenomenon exhibited by atomic nuclei having a magnetic moment, i.e. those nuclei that behave as if they are tiny bar magnets. In the absence of a magnetic field these magnets are arranged randomly but when a strong magnetic field is applied they align with the field. These signals can be analysed and used for chemical analysis (NMR spectroscopy) or for imaging (magnetic resonance imaging).

**nuclease** an enzyme that breaks down nucleic acids.

**nucleic acids** deoxyribonucleic acid (abbreviated DNA) and ribonucleic acid (abbreviated RNA), both of which are found in cell nuclei; RNA is also found in the cytoplasm. They are composed of series of nucleotides.

**nucleolus** a small dense body in the cell nucleus which contains ribonucleic acid. It disappears during mitosis.

**nucleoprotein** a compound of nucleic acid and protein.

**nucleotide** a compound formed from pentose sugar, phosphoric acid and a nitrogen-containing base (a purine or a pyrimidine).

**nucleotoxic** applied to drugs, toxins, viruses and other agents that are toxic to cell nuclei.

**nucleus** 1. the essential part of a cell, governing nutrition and reproduction, its division being essential for the formation of new cells. 2. the positively charged centre portion of an atom. 3. a group of nerve cells in the central nervous system. *Caudate n.* and *lenticular n.* part of the basal ganglia. *N. pulposus* the jelly-like centre of an intervertebral disc.

**null hypothesis** a research concept indicating that there is no significant relationship between an independent variable and a dependent variable, and that the observed experimental results can therefore be attributed to chance alone.

**numbers needed to treat** abbreviated NNT. A measure of clinical significance in medicine and pharmacolgy. It is used to make decisions between treatment options being based upon the number of subjects receiving the medication before one subject has a positive outcome.

**nullipara** a woman who has never given birth to a child.

**nurse** 1. a person who is qualified in the art and science of nursing and meets certain prescribed standards of education and clinical competence. Is registered with the Nursing and Midwifery Council (NMC) if practising in the UK. The person so registered is entitled legally to use the title of nurse (*see also* NURSING (PRACTICE)). 2. to provide services that are essential to or helpful in the promotion, maintenance and restoration of health and wellbeing. 3. to nourish at the breast (*see also* BREAST (FEEDING)). *N. consultant* an experienced nurse practitioner educated to a Master's level, with advanced skills in a clinical area, e.g. mental health, neonatology or dermatology. The role is relatively new and developing, but involves considerable patient contact. The nurse consultant will be expected to promote research and evaluation in practice, demonstrate leadership skills, participate in the education and development of staff and the service delivery in the clinical area. *N. practitioner* a nurse with specific preparation and development to function at an advanced level who works in the primary care setry or in an acute care setting, e.g. accident and emergency services, orthopaedic clinics and minor injuries departments. The patients have a choice of seeing either the doctor or the nurse when they attend. *N. prescribing* registered nurses who have undertaken a specialist qualification and demonstrated prescribing competency may prescribe,

and therefore are accountable for prescribing for patients from the Nurse Prescribers' Formulary. *Practice n.* a qualified nurse who works with a general practitioner (GP), or with a group of GPs, in a health centre or surgery. *Primary n.* a named nurse who is responsible for the overall coordination of the patient's care. *Registered n.* in the UK, one whose name is on the register held by the NMC. *Wet n.* a woman who breast feeds the infant of another.

**Nurse Prescribers' Formulary** abbreviated NPF. A formulary from which nurses who are appropriately qualified may prescribe for patients.

**nursing** the profession of performing the functions of a nurse. *N. assessment* the systematic collection and analysis of patient data pertaining to the individual's health status, abilities and preferences for care and treatment. The first step of the nursing process leading to a clinical nursing judgement. *See* ASSESSMENT. *N. audit* a systematic procedure for assessing the quality of nursing care rendered to a specific patient population. *N. auxiliary* a health care assistant. *N. care plan* devised by a nurse and based upon a nursing assessment and nursing diagnosis for an individual patient. The plan has four essential components: (a) identification of the nursing care problems; (b) an outline of the means/methods of solving these; (c) a statement of the anticipated benefit to the patient; and (d) an account of the specific actions used to achieve the goals specified. *N. diagnosis* a statement of a health problem or of a potential health problem in the patient's/client's health status that a nurse is professionally competent to treat. *N. goal* the objective that the nurse hopes to achieve through nursing interventions and activities related to the patient's health status, needs and abilities, e.g. the development of self-care skills. *N. history* a written record providing data for assessing the nursing care needs of a patient. *N. models* a conceptual framework of nursing practice based on knowledge, ideas and beliefs. A model or theory of nursing clarifies the meaning of nursing, provides criteria for policy and gives direction to team nursing, thereby obviating conflicts in approach and giving the framework for continuity of care. It identifies the nurse's role, highlights areas of practice where research is needed. These models are traditionally named after the nurse theorist who first developed them, e.g. Roy's model or the Roper, Logan and Tierney model. *N. practice* the performance or compensation of any act in the observation, care and counsel of the ill, injured or infirm, or in the maintenance of health or prevention of illness of others, or in the supervision and teaching of other personnel, or in the administration of medications and treatments as prescribed by a doctor or dentist. This requires substantial specialized judgement and skill and is based on knowledge and application of the principles of biological, physical and social sciences. *N. process* a systematic approach to nursing care derived from many occupational groups. The system itself is not specific to nursing. It has been used as a framework for nursing care by American nurses and subsequently its principles have been adapted to the UK's culture and health care system by British nurses. It is an organized approach to the identification of a patient's nursing care problems and the utilization of nursing actions that effectively alleviate, minimize or prevent the problems being presented or from developing.

**Nursing and Midwifery Council (NMC)** The statutory regulatory body for nursing, midwifery and health visiting. Its prime purpose is to protect the public through establishing and monitoring professional standards. The council replaces the former UKCC and National Boards. It: (a) maintains a register of qualified staff; (b) sets standards for professional education, practice and conduct; (c) provides advice for nurses, midwives and health visitors on professional standards; (d) considers allegations of misconduct or unfitness to practice because of illness; and (e) publishes professional conduct rules and other documents to guide professional practice.

**nutation** uncontrollable nodding of the head.

**nutrient** food; any substance that nourishes. The six classes of nutrient are fats, carbohydrates, proteins, vitamins, minerals and water.

**nutrition** 1. the sum of the processes involved in taking in nutriments and assimilating and utilizing them. 2. nutriment. Nutrition is particularly concerned with those properties of food that build sound bodies and promote health. Good nutrition means a balanced diet containing adequate amounts of the essential nutritional elements that the body must have to function normally. The essential ingredients of a balanced diet are proteins, vitamins, minerals, fats and carbohydrates. The body can manufacture sugars from fats, and fats from sugars and proteins, depending on the need, but it cannot manufacture proteins from sugars and fats. *See* Appendix I *Enteral n.* the provision of nutrients in fluid form to the alimentary tract by mouth, nasogastric tube or via an opening into the tract such as through a gastrostomy. *N. disease* one that is due to the continued absence of a necessary food factor. *Parenteral n.* a technique for meeting a patient's nutritional needs by means of intravenous feedings; sometimes called hyperalimentation.

**nutritional status** the condition of the body as a result of its receiving and using nutrients. Nutritional status may also be affected by biochemical individuality as well as environmental factors.

**nyctalopia** night blindness. *See* HEMERALOPIA.

**nymphomania** excessive sexual desire in a woman.

**nystagmus** an involuntary, rapid movement of the eyeball. It may be hereditary or result from disease of the semicircular canals or of the central nervous system. It can occur from visual defect or be associated with other muscle spasms.

**O** symbol for *oxygen*.

**obese** very fat; corpulent.

**obesity** corpulence; excessive development of fat throughout the body. A body mass index (BMI) of over 30.

**objective** 1. in microscopy, the lens nearest the object being looked at. 2. a purpose; a desired end result. 3. concerning matters outside oneself. *O. signs* signs that the observer notes, as distinct from symptoms of which the patient complains (subjective).

**oblique** slanting. *O. muscles* 1. a pair of muscles, the inferior and the superior, which turn the eye upwards and downwards, and inwards and outwards. 2. muscles found in the wall of the abdomen.

**observation** the act or faculty of closely noticing and paying attention to someone or something. In nursing this is an active process whereby the nurse uses the senses for the purpose of collecting patient data for developing a nursing diagnosis or care plan.

**observational study** a research methodology in which the researcher is a non-participant observer and records behaviour without influencing it.

**obsession** an idea which persistently recurs to an individual, although resisted and regarded as being senseless. A compulsive thought. *See* COMPULSION.

**obsessive compulsive disorder (OCD)** a mental health condition characterized by obsessional thoughts and/or ideas associated often with compulsive acts which may interfere with daily living.

**obstetrician** one who is trained and specializes in obstetrics.

**obstetrics** the branch of medicine and surgery dealing with pregnancy, labour and the puerperium.

**obstipation** intractable constipation.

**obstruction** the act of blocking or clogging; the state of being clogged. *Intestinal o.* any hindrance to the passage of faeces.

**obturator** that which closes an opening. *O. foramen* the large hole in the hip bone, closed by fascia and muscle.

**obtusion** weakening or blunting of normal sensations, a condition produced by certain diseases.

**occipital** relating to the occiput. *O. bone* the bone forming the back and part of the base of the skull.

**occipitoanterior** referring to the position of the fetal occiput when it is to the front of the maternal pelvis as it comes through the birth canal. The opposite of occipitoposterior.

**occipitoposterior** referring to the position of the fetal occiput when it is to the back of the maternal pelvis as it comes through the birth canal. The opposite of occipitoanterior.

**occiput** the back of the head.

**occlusion** closure, applied particularly to alignment of the teeth in the jaws. *Coronary o.* obstruction of the lumen of a coronary artery. *O. of the* *eye* covering a good eye to improve the visual acuity of the other, lazy eye. *O. of the pupil* may be congenital or occur in iridocyclitis or after injury.

**occult** hidden, concealed. *O. blood* blood excreted in the stools in such a small quantity as to require chemical tests to detect it.

**occupational** relating to work and working conditions. *O. disease* one likely to occur among workers in certain trades. An industrial disease. *O. health nurse* provides immediate care to ill or injured workers in the workplace and follows up the return to work of the sick and injured. Develops accident prevention programmes and promotes good health amongst the work force. Also has an educational role and a health and safety obligation. *O. health nursing* the branch of nursing that is concerned with the health of people in the workplace. *O. medicine* the branch of medicine concerned with people at work and the effects of work on health. Essentially a branch of preventative or environmental medicine. It is concerned with ensuring that health and safety in the workplace is maintained and legislation complied with. *O. therapy* treatment by provision of interesting and congenial work within the limitations of the patient in cases of mental disability and in order to re-educate and coordinate muscles in physical defect.

**ocular** relating to the eye. *O. myopathy* a gradual bilateral loss of mobility of the eyes. *O. myositis* inflammation of the orbital muscles.

**oculogyric** causing movements of the eyeballs. *O. crisis* involuntary, violent movements of the eye, usually upwards.

**oculomotor** relating to movements of the eye. *O. nerves* the third pair of cranial nerves, which control the eye muscles.

**odontoid** resembling a tooth. *O. process* a tooth-like projection from the axis vertebra upon which the head rotates.

**odontoma** a tumour of tooth structures.

**oedema** an excessive amount of fluid in the body tissues. If the finger is pressed upon an affected part, the surface pits and slowly regains its original contour. *Angio o.* characterized by the sudden appearance of urticaria which may involve the skin of the face, hands, feet or genitalia, and with swelling of the mucosal membrane of mouth and throat, oedema of the glottis may be fatal. The swelling may be due to an allergic reaction to food (most common) moulds, pollens, or other allergens, infection or a reaction to an insect bite or sting. In many cases no identifiable cause can be found. *Cardiac o.* a manifestation of congestive heart failure, due to increased venous and capillary pressures and often associated with renal sodium retention. *Dependent o.* oedema affecting most severely the lowermost parts of the body. *Famine o.* that due to protein deficiency. *O. neonatorum* a disease of preterm and feeble infants resembling sclerema, marked by spreading oedema with cold, livid skin. *Pitting o.* oedema in which pressure leaves a persistent depression in the tissues. *Pulmonary o.* diffuse extravascular accumulation of fluid in the tissues and air spaces of the lung due to changes in hydrostatic forces in the capillaries or to increased capillary permeability.

**Oedipus complex** the suppressed sexual desire of a son for his mother, with hostility towards his father. It is a normal stage in the early development of the child, but may become fixed if the child cannot solve the conflict during his early years or during adolescence. Named after a mythical Greek hero.

**oesophageal** pertaining to the oesophagus. *O. atresia* a congenital abnormality in which the oesophagus is not continuous between the pharynx and the stomach. May be associated with a fistula into the trachea. *O. varices* varicose veins of the lower oesophagus secondary to portal hypertension.

**oesophagitis** inflammation of the oesophagus. *Reflux o.* caused by regurgitation of acid stomach contents through the cardiac sphincter.

**oesophagojejunostomy** an operation to create an anastomosis of the jejunum with the oesophagus after a total gastrectomy.

**oesophagus** the canal that extends from the pharynx to the stomach. It is about 23 cm long. The gullet.

**oestradiol** the chief naturally occurring female sex hormone produced by the ovary. Prepared synthetically, it is used to treat menopausal conditions and amenorrhoea.

**oestrogen** one of several steroid hormones, including oestradiol, all of which have similar functions. Although they are largely produced in the ovary, they can also be extracted from the placenta, the adrenal cortex and the testis. They control female sexual development.

**olecranon** the curved process of the ulna which forms the point of the elbow.

**oleum** [L.] *oil.*

**olfactory** relating to the sense of smell. *O. nerves* the first pair of cranial nerves; those of smell.

**oligohydramnios** a deficiency in the amount of amniotic fluid.

**oligomenorrhoea** 1. a diminished flow at the menstrual period. 2. infrequent occurrence of menstruation.

**oligospermia** a diminished output of spermatozoa.

**oliguria** a deficient secretion of urine.

**olivary** shaped like an olive. *O. body* a mass of grey matter situated behind the anterior pyramid of the medulla oblongata.

**ombudsman** a person appointed to receive complaints about unfair administration. The officer in the NHS, appointed as 'ombudsman' or Health Service Commissioner, investigates complaints about failures in the health services not resolved locally, and issuing a regular report. Is not able to pass judgement on clinical matters. *See* HEALTH SERVICE COMMISSIONER.

**omentum** a fold of peritoneum joining the stomach to other abdominal organs. *Greater o.* the fold reflected from the greater curvature of the stomach and lying in front of the intestines. *Lesser o.* the fold reflected from the lesser curvature and attaching the stomach to the undersurface of the liver.

**omnivorous** eating food of both plant and animal origin.

**omphalitis** inflammation of the umbilicus.

**omphalocele** an umbilical hernia.

*Onchocerca* a genus of filarial worms, found in tropical parts of Africa and America, which may give rise to skin and subcutaneous lesions and attack the eye.

**onchocerciasis** a tropical skin disease caused by infestation with *Onchocerca.*

**oncogenesis** the causation and formation of tumours.

**oncogenic** giving rise to tumour formation.

**oncology** the scientific and medical study of tumours.

**onychia** inflammation of the matrix of a nail, with suppuration, which may cause the nail to fall off.

**onychogryphosis** enlargement of the nails, with excessive ridging and curvature, most commonly affecting the elderly.

**onycholysis** loosening or separation of a nail from its bed.

**onychomycosis** infection of the nails by a fungus.

**oöcyte** the immature egg cell or ovum in the ovary.

**oögenesis** the development and production of the ovum.

**oöphorectomy** excision of an ovary; ovariectomy.

**oöphorocystosis** the development of one or more ovarian cysts.

**oöphoron** an ovary.

**opacity** cloudiness, lack of transparency. Opacities occur in the lens of an eye when a cataract is forming. They also occur in the vitreous humour and appear as floating objects.

**open ended items** questions that the respondent may answer in their own words.

**operant conditioning** a form of behaviour therapy in which a reward is given when the subject performs the action required. The reward serves to encourage repetition of the action.

**operation** a surgical procedure in which instruments or hands are used by the operator upon a part or organ of the body.

**operational definition** the measurements used to observe or measure a variable; delineates the procedures or operations required to measure a concept.

**ophthalmia** severe inflammation of the eye or of the conjunctiva or deeper structures of the eye. *O. neonatorum* any hyperacute purulent conjunctivitis which may be caused by the gonococcus, *Escherichia coli*, staphylococci or *Chlamydia trachomatis*, occurring within the first 21 days of life. This condition is notifiable except in Scotland. *Sympathetic o.* granulomatous inflammation of the uveal tract of the uninjured eye following a wound involving the uveal tract of the other eye, resulting in bilateral granulomatous inflammation of the entire uveal tract. Also called sympathetic uveitis.

**ophthalmologist** a specialist in diseases of the eye.

**ophthalmology** the study of the eye and its diseases.

**ophthalmoscope** an instrument fitted with a light and lenses by which the interior of the eye can be illuminated and examined.

**opiate** any medicine containing opium.

**opisthotonos** a muscle spasm causing the back to be arched and the head retracted, with great rigidity of the muscles of the neck and back. This condition may be present in acute cases of meningitis, tetanus and strychnine poisoning.

**opium** a drug derived from dried poppy juice and used as a narcotic. It produces deep sleep, slows the pulse and respiration, contracts the pupils and checks all secretions of the body except sweat. It is a highly addictive drug. Opium derivatives include apomorphine, codeine, morphine and papaverine.

**opponens** [L.] *opposing.* A term applied to certain muscles controlling the movements of the fingers. *O. pollicis* a muscle that adducts the thumb so that it and the little finger can be brought together.

**opportunistic** 1. taking advantage of immediate opportunities. 2. denoting a microorganism that does not ordinarily cause disease but becomes pathogenic under certain circumstances. 3. denoting a disease or infection caused by such an opportunistic pathogen.

**opsonic index** a measurement of the bactericidal power of the phagocytes in the blood of an individual.

**opsonin** an antibody, present in the blood, which renders bacteria more easily destroyed by the phagocytes. Each kind of bacterium has its specific opsonin.

**optic** relating to vision. *O. atrophy* degeneration of the optic nerve. *O. chiasma* the crossing of the fibres of the optic nerves at the base of the brain (*see* Figure). *O. disc* the point where the optic nerve enters the eyeball. *O. foramen* the opening in the posterior part of the orbit through which pass the optic nerve and the ophthalmic artery. *O. nerve* a bundle of nerve fibres running from the optic chiasma in the brain to the optic disc on the eyeball.

**optical** pertaining to sight. *O. density* the refractive power of the transparent tissues through which light rays pass, changing the direction of the ray.

**optician** a professional trained in the detection of refractive errors

and the dispensing of appropriate spectacles or contact lenses.

**optimum** the best and most favourable.

**optometry** assessing and measuring visual acuity for the fitting of glasses or contact lenses to correct visual defects.

**ora** [L.] *a margin. O. serrata* the jagged edge of the retina.

**oral** 1. pertaining to the mouth; taken through or applied in the mouth, as an oral medication or oral hygiene. 2. denoting that aspect of the teeth which faces the oral cavity or tongue. *O. contraceptive pill* a drug preparation taken orally containing one or more synthetic female hormones taken as part of the monthly cycle to prevent pregnancy. *O. hairy leukoplakia* an unusual form of leukoplakia that is seen only in human immunodeficiency virus (HIV) infected persons. It consists of fuzzy (hairy) patches on the tongue and, less frequently, elsewhere in the mouth. Hairy leukoplakia may be one of the first signs of HIV infection. *See* LEUKOPLAKIA. *O. rehydration therapy* abbreviated ORT. *See* REHYDRATION. *O. syringe* a calibrated device with a plunger that is used to administer small doses of oral liquid medications to young children. The dose is drawn up into the syringe via the plunger and then squirted onto the inside of the cheek.

**orbit** 1. the bony cavity containing the eyeball. 2. the path of an object moving around another object.

**orchidectomy** excision of a testicle. *Bilateral o.* the operation of castration.

**orchidopexy** an operation to free an undescended testicle and place it in the scrotum.

**orchiepididymitis** inflammation of a testicle and its epididymis.

**orchitis** inflammation of a testicle.

**ordinal scale** a measurement scale in which the data is arranged in order

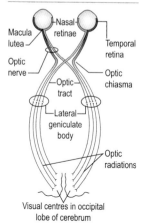

OPTIC CHIASMA

Macula lutea
Nasal retinae
Temporal retina
Optic nerve
Optic chiasma
Optic tract
Lateral geniculate body
Optic radiations
Visual centres in occipital lobe of cerebrum

of size or magnitude but where there is no standard measure of difference between the data given.

**orf** a virus infection transmitted from sheep to humans. It may give rise to a boil-like lesion on the hands of meat handlers.

**organ** a part of the body designed to perform a particular function. *O. of Corti* a spiral structure situated in the inner ear. It contains the basilar membrane that converts sound waves into nerve impulses that are then transmitted to the brain via the cochlear nerve.

**organelle** a structure within a cell that has specialized functions, e.g. nucleus, endoplasmic reticulum, mitochondrion, etc.

**organic** 1. pertaining to the organs. 2. pertaining to chemicals containing carbon. *O. disease* disease of an organ, accompanied by structural changes.

**organism** an individual living being, animal or vegetable.

**orgasm** the climax of sexual excitement.

**orientation** a sense of direction. 1. the ability of a person to estimate position in regard to time, place and persons. 2. the imparting of relevant information at the onset of a course or conference so that its content and objects may be understood. *Reality o.* the way in which older people who may be confused or mentally ill are assisted in keeping in touch with the world around them on a day-to-day basis. This may be achieved in a variety of ways, with large clocks, calendar boards, signs on doors and daily newspapers.

**orifice** any opening in the body.

**origin** 1. the point of attachment of a muscle. 2. the point at which a nerve or a blood vessel branches from the main stem.

**ornithosis** a virus disease of birds, usually pigeons, that may be transmitted to humans in a form resembling bronchopneumonia.

**orogenital** pertaining to the mouth and external genitalia.

**oropharynx** the lower portion of the pharynx behind the mouth and above the oesophagus and larynx.

**orphan** a child whose parents are dead. *O. drugs* those that have been found to be useful in the treatment of rare diseases but which are not commercially produced usually because of high costs involved in manufacture and minimal demand. *O. viruses* those that have been isolated in the laboratory but which do not appear to be associated with any particular disease.

**orthodontics** dentistry that deals with the prevention and correction of malocclusion and irregularities of the teeth.

**orthodox sleep** *see* SLEEP.

**Orthomyxovirus** RNA viruses belonging to the family of *Orthomyxoviridae* which cause influenza in humans and other mammals, e.g. birds and swine. *See* AVIAN FLU AND SWINE FLU. These viruses originated in aquatic birds and crossed the species barrier (*See Zoonosis*) about 10 000 years ago to infect humans.

**orthopaedics** the science dealing with deformities, injuries and diseases of the bones and joints.

**orthopnoea** difficulty in breathing unless in an upright position, e.g. sitting up in bed.

**orthoptics** the practice of treating by non-surgical methods (usually eye exercises) abnormalities of vision such as strabismus (squint).

**orthostatic** pertaining to or caused by standing erect. *O. albuminuria* see ALBUMINURIA. *O. hypotension* low blood pressure, occurring when the person stands up.

**orthotic** serving to protect or to restore or improve function.

**orthotics** the use or application of an orthosis (a supportive appliance that can be applied to or around the body in the care/treatment of physical impairment or disability).

**orthotist** a person skilled in orthotics and practising its application in individual cases.

**Ortolani's sign** *M. Ortolani, 20th-century Italian orthopaedic surgeon.* A test performed soon after birth to detect possible congenital dislocation of the hip. A 'click' is felt on reversing the movements of abduction and rotation of the hip while the child is lying with knees flexed.

**os** [L.] 1. (*pl.* ora) any body orifice. 2. (*pl.* ora) the mouth. 3. (*pl.* ossa) a bone.

**oscillation** 1. a backwards and forwards motion. 2. vibration.

**oscilloscope** an apparatus using a cathode-ray tube to depict visibly data fed into it electronically, e.g. the way in which the heart is performing.

**Osler's nodes** *Sir W. Osler, Canadian physician, 1849–1919.* Small painful swellings which occur in or beneath the skin, especially of the extremities in subacute bacterial endocarditis, caused by minute emboli. They usually disappear in 1–3 days.

**osmoreceptor** one of a group of specialized nerve cells which monitor the osmotic pressure of the blood and the extracellular fluid. Impulses from these receptors are relayed to the hypothalamus.

**osmosis** the passage of fluid from a low concentration solution to one of a higher concentration through a semipermeable membrane.

**osmotic** pertaining to osmosis. *O. pressure* the pressure exerted by large molecules in the blood, e.g. albumin and globulin proteins, which draws fluid into the bloodstream from the surrounding tissues. *O. diuretics* diuretics, e.g. mannitol, given intravenously to reduce elevated pressure in cerebral oedema or glaucoma, or to produce a diuresis in drug overdose.

**osseous** bony.

**ossicle** a small bone. *Auditory o.* one of the three bones in the middle ear: the malleus, incus and stapes.

**ossification** the process by which bone is developed; osteogenesis.

**osteitis** inflammation of bone. *O. deformans* Paget's disease. *O. fibrosa cystica* or *parathyroid o.* defects of ossification, with fibrous tissue production, leading to weakening and deformity. It affects children chiefly, and is associated with parathyroid tumour, removal of which checks it.

**osteoarthritis** often described as degenerative joint disease (DJD). *See* ARTHRITIS.

**osteoarthrotomy** surgical excision of the jointed end of a bone.

**osteoblast** a cell that develops into an osteocyte and turns into bone.

**osteochondritis** inflammation of bone and cartilage, particularly a degenerative disease of an epiphysis, causing pain and deformity. *O. of the hip* Perthes' disease. *O. of the tarsal scaphoid bone* Köhler's disease. *O. of the tibial tuberosity* Osgood–Schlatter disease.

**osteochondroma** a tumour consisting of both bone and cartilage.

**osteoclasis** 1. the surgical fracture of bones to correct a deformity such as bow-leg. 2. the restructuring of bone by osteoclasts during growth or the repair of damaged bone.

**osteoclast** 1. a large cell that breaks down and absorbs bone and callus. 2. an instrument designed for surgical fracture of bone.

**osteocyte** a bone cell.

**osteodystrophy** a metabolic disease of bone.

**osteogenesis** the formation of bone. *O. imperfecta* a congenital disorder of the bones, which are very brittle and fracture easily. Fragilitas osseum.

**osteoma** a benign tumour arising from bone.

**osteomalacia** a disease characterized by painful softening of bones. Due to vitamin D deficiency.

**osteomyelitis** inflammation of bone, localized or generalized, due to a pyogenic infection. It may result in bone destruction, stiffening of joints, and, in extreme cases occurring before the end of the growth period, in the shortening of a limb if the growth centre is destroyed. Acute osteomyelitis is caused by bacteria that enter the body through a wound, spread from an infection near the bone, or come from a skin or throat infection. The infection usually affects the long bones of the arms and legs and causes acute pain and fever. It most often occurs in children and adolescents.

**osteopath** one who practises osteopathy.

**osteopathy** a system of diagnosis and treatment of disease which involves massage, palpation and manipulation. Osteopathic treatment is aimed at freeing and loosening joints and re-establishing proper relationships of the spinal column, its component bones with the pelvis and limb bones on the basis that many diseases are associated with disorders of the musculoskeletal system.

**osteoperiostitis** inflammation of bone and periosteum.

**osteopetrosis** (Albers–Schönberg disease). A rare congenital disease in which the bones become abnormally dense.

**osteophyte** a small outgrowth of bone, usually in a joint damaged by osteoarthritis.

**osteoporosis** abnormal rarefaction of bone which may be idiopathic or secondary to other conditions. The disorder leads to thinning of the skeleton and decreased precipitation of lime salts. There may also be inadequate calcium absorption into the bone and excessive bone resorption. The principal causes are lack of physical activity, lack of oestrogens or androgens, and nutritional deficiency. There is almost always some degree of osteoporosis that occurs with ageing. Symptoms include pathological fractures and collapse of the vertebrae without compression of the spinal cord. Management involves minimizing bone loss with vitamin D, dietary calcium and regular sustained exercise to build and maintain bone strength. Long-term hormone replacement therapy can prevent osteoporosis in postmenopausal women.

**osteosarcoma** an osteogenic sarcoma; a malignant bone tumour.

**osteosclerosis** an increase in density and a hardening of bone. *O. congenita* achondroplasia. *O. fragilis* osteopetrosis.

**osteotomy** the cutting into or through a bone, sometimes performed to correct deformity. *O. of the hip* a method of treating osteoarthritis by cutting the bone and altering the line of weight-bearing (*see* Figure on p. 289).

**ostium** an opening or entrance. *Abdominal o.* the opening at the end of the uterine tube into the peritoneal cavity.

**otoacoustic emission (OAE)** a computer linked hearing test used for screening infants in the first few weeks of life to ascertain hearing levels.

**OTC drugs** *see* OVER-THE-COUNTER DRUGS.

**otic** relating to the ear.

**otitis** inflammation of the ear. *Aviation o.* a symptom complex resulting from fluctuations between atmospheric pressure and air pressure in the middle ear; also called

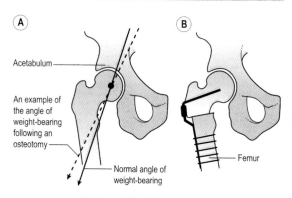

Acetabulum

An example of the angle of weight-bearing following an osteotomy

Normal angle of weight-bearing

Femur

Osteotomy of hip: A showing weight-bearing angle, and B showing an example of an osteotomy with fixator

OSTEOTOMY OF THE HIP

barotitis media. *Furuncular o.* the formation of furuncles in the external ear. *O. externa* inflammation of the external ear. *O. interna, o. labyrinthica* labyrinthitis. *O. media* inflammation of the middle ear, occurring most often in infants and young children, and classified as serous, secretory and suppurative.

**otolith** 1. a calculus in the middle ear. 2. one of a number of small calcareous concretions of the inner ear, at the base of the semicircular canals.

**otomycosis** a fungal infection of the auditory canal.

**otorrhoea** discharge from the ear, especially of pus.

**otosclerosis** the formation of spongy bone in the labyrinth of the ear, causing the auditory ossicles to become fixed and less able to pass on vibrations when sound enters the ear. The cause of otosclerosis is still unknown. It may be hereditary, or perhaps related to vitamin deficiency or otitis media. An early symptom is ringing in the ears, but the most noticeable symptom is progressive loss of hearing.

**otoscope** an auriscope; an instrument for examining the ear.

**ototoxic** anything that has a deleterious effect on the eighth cranial nerve or on the organs of hearing.

**outbreak** an epidemic of an infectious disease limited to a localized increase in the incidence of the disease, e.g. in a village, town or institution. *See* EPIDEMIC.

**outcome** a consequence or objective for a health care intervention, e.g. a patient goal. The implications are that the outcome is (a) measurable and (b) can be expected as a result of the planned intervention. *O. indicator* measurement of the success of a clinical treatment/intervention in terms of the impact on the health of the individual.

**outlet** a means or route of exit or egress. *Pelvic o.* the inferior opening of the pelvis; literally that bounded by the ischial spines, lower border of the symphysis pubis and the sacrococcygeal joint.

**out-of-the-body experience** a sensation of leaving one's body and travelling through tunnels and lights onto another plane of experience. The condition has been attributed to anoxia of the brain following anaesthesia or severe illness.

**outpatient** a patient who has a medical consultation or receives treatment at a hospital but who does not require to stay overnight in a hospital bed.

**output** the yield or total of something produced by a system. *Cardiac o.* the effective volume of blood expelled by either ventricle of the heart per unit of time (usually volume per minute); it is equal to the stroke output multiplied by the number of beats per the time unit used in the computation. *Fluid o.* the amount of urine passed, usually measured in comparison to oral fluid intake.

**outreach** health care services provided within a community setting, e.g. a specialized clinic held in a general practitioner's surgery, village hall or other public building enabling patients and/or clients to access care more conveniently and avoid long or difficult journeys.

**ovarian** relating to an ovary. *O. cyst* a tumour of the ovary containing fluid.

**ovariectomy** oöphorectomy; excision of an ovary.

**ovariotomy** 1. surgical removal of an ovary. 2. excision of an ovarian tumour.

**ovary** one of a pair of glandular organs in the female pelvis. They produce ova, which pass through the uterine tubes into the uterus,

and steroid hormones which control the menstrual cycle.

**over-the-counter drugs** abbreviated OTC drugs. Drugs that can be purchased from a pharmacy without a prescription from a doctor. The list of derestricted drugs available to the public is growing and includes corticosteroid ointments, antihistamines, aciclovir, ibuprofen and nicotine patches.

**overbite** an overlapping of the lower teeth by the upper teeth.

**overcompensation** a mental mechanism by which people try to assert themselves by aggressive behaviour or by talking or acting 'big' to compensate for a feeling of inadequacy.

**overuse injury** injury due to the repetitive movement of a joint or part of the body. See REPETITIVE STRAIN INJURY.

**oviduct** a uterine tube.

**ovulation** the process of rupture of the mature Graafian follicle when the ovum is shed from the ovary.

**ovum** [L.] *an egg.* The reproductive cell of the female.

**oxidization** oxidation. The process by which combustion occurs and breaking up of matter takes place, e.g. oxidization of carbohydrates gives carbon dioxide and water: $C_6H_{12}O_6 + 6 O_2 = 6 CO_2 + 6 H_2O$. The opposite of reduction.

**oximeter** a photoelectric cell used to determine the oxygen saturation of blood. *Ear o.* one attached to the ear by which the oxygen content of blood flowing through the ear can be measured.

**oxygen** *symbol* O. A colourless, odourless gas constituting one-fifth of the atmosphere. It is stored in cylinders at high pressure or as liquid oxygen. It is used medicinally to enrich the air when either respiration or circulation is impaired. *O. deficit* a physiological state that exists in cells during episodes of temporary oxygen shortage. *O. saturation* the amount of oxygen bound to haemoglobin in the blood. *O. tent* a large plastic canopy that encloses the patient in a controlled environment; used for oxygen therapy, humidity therapy or aerosol therapy. *O. therapy* supplementary oxygen administered for the purpose of relieving hypoxaemia and preventing damage to the tissue cells as a result of oxygen lack.

**oxygenation** saturation with oxygen; a process which occurs in the lungs to the haemoglobin of blood, which is saturated with oxygen to form oxy-haemoglobin.

**oxygenator** a machine through which the blood is passed to oxygenate it during open heart surgery. *Pump o.* a machine which pumps oxygenated blood through the body during heart surgery.

**oxyhaemoglobin** haemoglobin that has been oxygenated, as in arterial blood.

**oxyntic** acid-forming. *O. cell* a parietal cell of the gastric glands which secretes hydrochloric acid.

**oxytocic** any drug that stimulates uterine contractions and may be used to hasten delivery.

**oxytocin** a pituitary hormone which stimulates uterine contractions and the ejection of milk. Synthetically prepared, it is used to induce labour and to control postpartum haemorrhage.

**oxyuriasis** infestation by threadworms of the genus *Enterobius*.

**ozena** a severe form of rhinitis in which the mucus membrane of the nose atropies. This is associated with a thick offensive nasal discharge that crusts and often results in severe halitosis.

**ozone** an intensified form of oxygen containing three O atoms to the molecule (i.e. $O_3$), and often discharged by electrical machines, such as X-ray apparatus. In medicine it is employed as an antiseptic and oxidizing agent. *O. sickness* sometimes experienced by jet travellers due to the levels of ozone in the aircraft.

**Pa** symbol for *pascal*.

**pacemaker** an object or substance that controls the rate at which a certain phenomenon occurs. The natural pacemaker of the heart is the sinoatrial node. *Electronic cardiac p.* an electrically operated mechanical device which stimulates the myocardium to contract. It consists of an energy source, usually batteries, and electrical circuitry connected to an electrode which is in direct contact with the myocardium. Pacemakers may be temporary or permanent. Temporary ones usually have an external energy source, whereas permanent ones have a subcutaneously implanted one. The rate at which the pacemaker delivers pulses may be either fixed or on demand. *Fixed* pacing means that pulses are delivered to the heart at a predetermined rate irrespective of any cardiac activity. A *demand* pacemaker is programmed to deliver pulses only in the absence of spontaneous cardiac activity. The need for replacement batteries is usually indicated when the rate of the pulse slows by five beats or more.

**pachydermia** an abnormal thickening of the skin. *P. laryngis* chronic hypertrophy of the vocal cords.

**pachyonychia** abnormal thickening of the nails.

**pacing** a series of techniques used by occupational therapists to assist people to perform tasks within their health limitations and to reduce adverse effects such as pain, joint stress and fatigue. Using a contractual arrangement with the patient, the aim is to maximize performance and to meet personal objectives in achieving the desired task.

**PACT** prescribing analyses and cost.

**paediatric advanced life support (PALS)** *see* Appendix 2 and ADVANCED LIFE SUPPORT.

**paediatrician** a medically qualified person specializing in the diseases of children.

**paediatrics** the branch of medicine dealing with the care and development of children and with the treatment of diseases that affect them.

**paedophilia** a sexual attraction towards children.

**Paget's disease** *Sir J. Paget, British surgeon, 1814–1899.* 1. a chronic disease of bone in which overactivity of the osteoblasts and osteoclasts leads to dense bone formation with areas of rarefaction. Osteitis deformans. 2. an inflammation of the nipple caused by cancer of the milk ducts of the breast.

**pain** a feeling of distress, suffering or agony, caused by stimulation of specialized nerve endings. Its purpose is chiefly protective; it acts as a warning that tissues are being damaged and induces the sufferer to remove or withdraw from the source. Pain is a subjective experience and one person's pain cannot be compared to another's experience. *Bearing-down p.* pain accompany-

# 293 PAL

ing uterine contractions during the second stage of labour. *False p's* ineffective pains during pregnancy which resemble labour pains, but not accompanied by cervical dilatation; also called false labour. *See also* BRAXTON HICKS CONTRACTIONS. *Gas p's* pains caused by distension of the stomach or intestine from accumulations of air or other gases. *Hunger p.* pain coming on at the time of feeling hunger for a meal; a symptom of gastric disorder. *Intermenstrual p.* pain accompanying ovulation, occurring during the period between the menses, usually about midway. Also called mittelschmerz. *Labour p's* the rhythmic pains of increasing severity and frequency due to contraction of the uterus at childbirth. *See also* LABOUR. *Lancinating p.* sharp, darting pain. *P. assessment* the measurement of a patient's pain and its psychosocial and biological impact upon the individual's personal situation is especially difficult to assess where the patient is unable to articulate their distress, e.g. children, infants and some adults. A number of assessment tools are available for use with children and adults; they are primarily longitudinal scales which list 'no pain' at one end to 'intense pain' at the other. *Phantom p.* pain felt as if it were arising in an absent (amputated) limb. *See also* AMPUTATION. *Referred p.* pain in a part other than that in which the cause that produced it is situated. Referred pain usually originates in one of the visceral organs but is felt in the skin or sometimes in another area deep inside the body. Referred pain probably occurs because pain signals from the viscera travel along the same neural pathways used by pain signals from the skin. The person perceives the pain but interprets it as having originated in the skin rather than in a deep-seated visceral

organ. *Rest p.* a continuous burning pain due to ischaemia of the lower leg, which begins or is aggravated after reclining and is relieved by sitting or standing.

**painful arc syndrome** a condition in which pain occurs when the arm is raised from the side between 45 and 160 degrees. The most usual cause is an inflamed tendon or bursa around the shoulder joint that is being squeezed between the scapula and humerus on movement. *See* FROZEN SHOULDER.

**palate** the roof of the mouth. *Artificial p.* a plate made to close a cleft palate. *Cleft p.* a congenital deformity where there is lack of fusion of the two bones forming the palate. *Hard p.* the bony part at the front. *Soft p.* a fold of mucous membrane that continues from the hard palate to the uvula.

**palliative** treatment that relieves, but does not cure, disease. *P. care* the active total care of patients whose disease no longer responds to curative treatment; should neither hasten nor postpone death. It pays equal attention to the physical, psychological, social and spiritual aspects of care of patients and those close to them.

**pallor** abnormal paleness of the skin.

**palmar** relating to the palm of the hand. *Deep p. arches* the deep and superficial palmar arches are the chief arterial blood supply to the hand, formed by the junction of the ulnar and radial arteries. *P. fascia* the arrangement of tendons in the palm of the hand. *Superficial p. arches* see DEEP P. ARCHES above.

**palpation** the examination of the organs by touch or pressure of the hand over the part.

**palpebral** referring to the eyelids. *P. ligaments* a band of ligaments which stretches from the junction of the upper and lower lid to the orbital bones, both medially and laterally.

**palpitation**   rapid and forceful contraction of the heart of which the patient is conscious.

**PALS**   Patient Advocacy Liaison Service.

**palsy**   a historical term for paralysis. *Bell's p.* paralysis of the facial muscles on one side, supplied by the seventh cranial nerve. *Crutch p.* paralysis due to pressure of a crutch on the radial nerve, and a cause of 'dropped wrist'. *Shaking p.* Parkinsonism; paralysis agitans.

**panacea**   a remedy for all diseases.

**panarthritis**   inflammation of all the joints or of all the structures of a joint.

**pancreas**   an elongated, dual-purpose racemose gland about 15 cm long, lying behind the stomach, with its head in the curve of the duodenum and its tail in contact with the spleen (*see* Figure). It secretes a digestive fluid (pancreatic juice) containing ferments which act on all classes of food. The fluid enters the duodenum by the pancreatic duct, which joins the common bile duct. The pancreas also secretes the hormones insulin and glucagon.

**pancreatectomy**   surgical excision of the whole or a part of the pancreas.

**pancreatin**   an extract from the pancreas containing the digestive enzymes. Used to treat deficiency, as in cystic fibrosis, and after pancreatectomy.

**pancreatitis**   inflammation of the pancreas. *Acute p.* a severe condition usually associated with alchohol misuse or biliary disease in which the patient experiences sudden pain in the upper abdomen and back. The patient often becomes severely shocked. *Chronic p.* chronic inflammation occurring after acute attacks. Pancreatic failure may lead to diabetes mellitus.

**pancreozymin**   a hormone of the duodenal mucosa that stimulates the external secretory activity of the pancreas, especially its production of amylase.

**pancytopenia**   a reduction in number of all types of blood cell due to failure of bone marrow formation.

PANCREAS

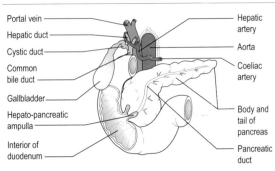

Portal vein

Hepatic duct

Cystic duct

Common bile duct

Gallbladder

Hepato-pancreatic ampulla

Interior of duodenum

Hepatic artery

Aorta

Coeliac artery

Body and tail of pancreas

Pancreatic duct

295 **PAR**

**pandemic** an epidemic spreading over a wide area, sometimes all over the world.

**panic** an unreasoning and overwhelming fear or terror. It may occur in anxiety states and acute schizophrenia. *P. attack* a brief period of acute anxiety, distress and fear of dying or of losing one's reason. It may be recognized by the person that this experience is associated with specific situations, e.g. being confined in a small space. Usually associated with other anxiety disorders or mental health problems. *P. disorder* a type of mental health disorder that is characterized by recurrent panic attacks of intense anxiety and distressing physical symptoms.

**pannus** increased vascularity of the cornea leading to granulation tissue formation and impaired vision. It occurs in trachoma after inflammation of the cornea.

**panophthalmia** panophthalmitis; inflammation of all the tissues of the eyeball.

**Papanicolaou test** *G.N. Papanicolaou, Greek physician, anatomist and cytologist, 1883–1962.* A smear test to detect diseases of the uterine cervix and endometrium. Also called Pap test.

**papilla** a small nipple-shaped protuberance. *Circumvallate p.* one surrounded by a ridge. A number are found at the back of the tongue arranged in a V-shape, and containing taste buds. *Filiform p.* one of the fine, slender filaments on the main part of the tongue which give it its velvety appearance. *Fungiform p.* a mushroom-shaped papilla of the tongue. *Optic p.* the optic disc, where the optic nerve leaves the eyeball. *Tactile p.* a projection on the true skin which contains nerve endings responsible for relaying sensations of pressure to the brain. A touch corpuscle.

**papillitis** 1. inflammation of the optic disc. 2. inflammation of a papilla.

**papilloedema** oedema and hyperaemia of the optic disc, usually associated with increased intracranial pressure; also called choked disc.

**papilloma** a benign growth of epithelial tissue, e.g. a wart.

**papillomatosis** the occurrence of multiple papillomas.

**papovavirus** a family of DNA-producing viruses which cause tumours, usually benign, such as warts.

**papule** a pimple, or small solid elevation of the skin.

**papulopustular** descriptive of skin eruptions of both papules and pustules.

**papulosquamous** descriptive of skin eruptions that are both papular and scaly. They include such conditions as lichen planus, pityriasis and psoriasis.

**paracentesis** puncture of the wall of a cavity with a hollow needle in order to draw off excess fluid or to obtain diagnostic material.

**paracusis** a perverted sense of hearing. *P. of Willis* an improvement in hearing when surrounded by noise.

**paradigm** an example or representative instance of a concept or theoretical approach.

**paradoxical sleep** rapid eye movement (REM) sleep. *See* SLEEP.

**paraesthesia** an abnormal tingling sensation. 'Pins and needles'.

*Paragonimus* a genus of trematode parasites. The flukes infest the lungs and are found mainly in tropical countries.

**paralysis** loss or impairment of motor function in a part owing to a lesion of the neural or muscular mechanism; also, by analogy, impairment of sensory function (sensory paralysis). Paralysis is a symptom of a wide variety of physical and emotional disorders rather than a disease in itself. *P. agitans* Parkinsonism. **Bulbar p. (labio-glossopharyngeal p.)** paralysis due to changes in the motor centre of the medulla oblongata. It affects the muscles of the mouth, tongue and pharynx. **Facial p. (Bell's palsy)** paralysis that affects the muscles of the face and is due to injury or to inflammation of the facial nerve. **Flaccid p.** loss of tone and absence of reflexes in the paralysed muscles. **General p. of the insane** abbreviated GPI. Paralytic dementia occurring in the late stages of syphilis. **Infantile p.** the major form of POLIOMYELITIS. **Spastic p.** paralysis characterized by rigidity of affected muscles.

**paralytic** affected by or relating to paralysis. *P. ileus* obstruction of the ileum due to absence of peristalsis in a portion of the intestine.

**paramedian** situated on the side of the median line.

**paramedic** a person employed in the paramedical services especially ambulance personnel qualified to provide pre-hospital procedures and care.

**paramedical** associated with the medical profession and the delivery of health care. The paramedical services include trained ambulance personnel, occupational and speech therapy, physiotherapy, radiography and social work.

**parametritis** inflammation of the parametrium; pelvic cellulitis.

**parametrium** the connective tissue surrounding the uterus.

**paramnesia** a defect of memory in which there is a false recollection. The patient may fill in the forgotten period with imaginary events, which are often described in great detail.

**paranoia** a mental disorder characterized by delusions of grandeur or persecution which may be fully systematized in logical form, with the personality remaining fairly well preserved.

**paranoid** resembling paranoia. Delusions of persecution are a marked feature. Associated with behaviour that denotes suspicion of others. *P. schizophrenia see* SCHIZOPHRENIA.

**paraparesis** an incomplete paralysis affecting the lower limbs.

**paraphimosis** retraction of the prepuce behind the glans penis, with inability to replace it, resulting in a painful constriction.

**paraphrenia** schizophrenia occurring for the first time in later life and not accompanied by deterioration of the personality.

**paraplegia** paralysis of the lower extremities and lower trunk. All parts below the point of lesion in the spinal cord are affected. It may be of sudden onset from injury to the cord or may develop slowly as the result of disease.

**parapraxia** describes minor aberrations of behaviour as forgetfulness, the misplacing of things, verbal errors known also as a 'Freudian slips' or 'senior moments' commonly associated with ageing.

**paraprofessional** 1. a person who is specially trained in a particular field or occupation to assist a professional. 2. an allied health professional. 3. pertaining to a paraprofessional.

**parapsychology** the branch of psychology dealing with psychical effects and experiences that appear to fall outside the scope of physical laws, e.g. telepathy and clairvoyance.

**paraquat** a poisonous compound used as a contact herbicide. Contact with concentrated solutions causes irritation of the skin, cracking and shedding of the nails, and delayed healing of cuts and wounds. After ingestion renal and hepatic failure may develop, followed by pulmonary insufficiency and death.

**parasite** any animal or vegetable organism living upon or within another, from which it derives its nourishment.

**parasiticide** a drug that kills parasites.

**parasuicide** a suicidal action such as self-mutilation or the taking of a drug overdose which is motivated by a need to attract attention and seek help rather than commit suicide. Also known as deliberate self-harm (DSH).

**parasympathetic nervous system** the craniosacral part of the autonomic nervous system.

**parasympatholytic** anticholinergic; an agent that opposes the effects of the parasympathetic nervous system.

**parathormone** the endocrine secretion of the parathyroid glands.

**parathyroid gland** one of four small endocrine glands, two of which are associated with each lobe of the thyroid gland, and sometimes embedded in it. The secretion from these has some control over calcium metabolism, and lack of it is a cause of tetany.

**paratyphoid** a notifiable infection caused by *Salmonella* of all groups except *S. typhi*. The disease is usually milder and has a shorter incubation period, more abrupt onset and lower mortality rate than typhoid. Clinically and pathologically, the two diseases cannot be distinguished. Also called paratyphoid fever.

**paravertebral** near or alongside the vertebral or spinal column. *P. block anaesthesia* induced by the infiltration of a local anaesthetic around the spinal nerve roots emerging from the intervertebral foramina. *P. injection* an injection of local anaesthetic into the sympathetic chain. May be used as a test in ischaemic limbs to ascertain if a sympathectomy would be a useful treatment.

**parenchyma** the essential active cells of an organ, as distinguished from its vascular and connective tissue.

**parent–infant relationship** the unique relationship that develops between parents and their infant(s), sometimes referred to as 'bonding', which endures throughout life. Promoted by early touching, fondling, speech with eye-to-eye contact and breast feeding.

**parenteral** apart from the alimentary canal. Applied to the introduction into the body of drugs or fluids by routes other than the mouth or rectum, e.g. intravenously or subcutaneously. *P. feeding see* NUTRITION.

**paresis** partial paralysis.

**parietal** relating to the walls of any cavity. *P. bones* the two bones forming part of the roof and sides of the skull. *P. cells* the oxyntic cells in the gastric mucosa that secrete hydrochloric acid. *P. pleura* the pleura attached to the chest wall.

**parity** the classification of a woman with regard to the number of children that have been born live to her.

**Parkinson's disease** *J. Parkinson, British physician, 1755–1824.* Parkinsonism; paralysis agitans. A slowly progressive disease usually occurring in later life, characterized pathologically by degeneration within the nuclear masses of the extrapyramidal system, and clinically by mask-like facies (*see* FACIES (PARKINSON)), a characteristic tremor of resting muscles, a slowing of voluntary movements, a festinating gait, peculiar posture and muscular weakness. When this symptom complex occurs secondarily to another disorder, the condition is called Parkinsonism.

**paronychia** an abscess near the fingernail; a whitlow or felon. *P. tendinosa* a pyogenic infection that involves the tendon sheath.

**parotid** situated near the ear. *P. glands* two salivary glands, one in front of each ear.

**parotitis** inflammation of a parotid gland. Caused usually by ascending infection via its duct, when hygiene of the mouth is neglected or when the natural secretions are lessened, especially in severe illness or after operation. *Epidemic p.* mumps.

**parous** having borne one or more children.

**paroxysm** a sudden attack, worsening or recurrence of symptoms of a disease. A spasm or seizure.

**paroxysmal** occurring in paroxysms. *P. cardiac dyspnoea* cardiac asthma. Recurrent attacks of dyspnoea associated with pulmonary oedema and left-sided heart failure. *P. tachycardia* recurrent attacks of rapid heart beats that may occur without heart disease.

**parrot disease** *see* PSITTACOSIS.

**particle** a minute piece of substance.

**partnership working** the relationship between central government, NHS Trusts, Primary Care Trusts, local authorities and patient representatives that has been developed to provide coordinated health care and social services to those in need. This approach aims to achieve improved health for all in the community with the coordinated and collaborative working between all involved agencies.

**parturient** giving birth; relating to childbirth.

**parturition** the act of giving birth.

**pascal** *symbol* Pa. The SI unit of pressure.

**passive** not active. *P. immunity see* IMMUNITY. *P. movements* in massage, manipulation by a physiotherapist without the help of the patient. *P. smoking* inhaling tobacco smoke exhaled by others; associated with a significant risk of increase in lung cancer.

**passivity** in psychiatry, a delusional feeling that a person is under some outside control and must therefore be inactive.

*Pasteurella* L. Pasteur, French chemist and bacteriologist, 1833–1895. A genus of short Gram-negative bacilli. *P. pestis* the causative organism of plague transmitted by rat fleas to humans.

**pasteurization** the process of heating foods to destroy disease causing micro-organisms, and to reduce the numbers of micro-organisms responsible for fermentation and putrefaction. The Pasteurization process using moist heat is also used to disinfect medical instruments and other equipment.

**patch test** a test of skin sensitivity in which a number of possible allergens are applied to the skin under a plaster. The causal agent of the allergy will produce an inflammation.

**patella** the small, circular, sesamoid bone forming the kneecap.

**patellar** belonging to the patella. *P. reflex* a knee jerk obtained by tapping the tendon below the patella.

**patellectomy** excision of the patella.

**patent** open or unobstructed. *P. ductus arteriosus* failure of the ductus arteriosus to close, causing a shunt of blood from the aorta to the pulmonary artery and producing a continuous heart murmur.

**paternity testing** the use of blood samples to assist in establishing the paternity of a child. Blood taken from the suspected father, the child and sometimes the mother are tested to ascertain blood grouping, histocompatibility antigens and similarities in DNA.

**pathogen** a microorganism that can cause disease, e.g. *Clostridium tetani* causing tetanus.

**pathogenicity** the ability of a microorganism to cause disease.

**pathognomonic** specifically characteristic of a disease. A sign or symptom by which a pathological condition can positively be identified.

**pathological** 1. pertaining to pathology. 2. causing or arising from disease. *P. fracture* a fracture occurring in diseased bone where there has been little or no external trauma.

**pathology** the branch of medicine that deals with the essential nature of disease, especially of the structural and functional changes in tissues and organs of the body which cause or are caused by disease.

**patient** a person who is ill or is undergoing treatment for a health care problem and/or is registered with a general practitioner. *P. advocate*, *P. representative*, a person who acts on behalf of an incapacitated patient. *P. allocation*: see ALLOCATION. *P. pathway* the route followed by the patient into, through and out of NHS and social care services. It can involve referral from primary care to hospital, visits to hospital departments and specialties, a pathway through a clinical network, or the experience of joint NHS and social care in the community.

**Patient Advocacy Liaison Services** abbreviated PALS. A service for patients in NHS Trusts and Primary Care Trusts providing on-the-spot help and information about the health services to patients, their families and carers. PALS also monitors trends, highlighting gaps within the service and provides reports for action to the trust managers. It also represents patients' complaints and concerns to the trust management and board.

**patients' forum** a body set up in each NHS Trust and Primary Care Trust to represent the views of patients and users of the services provided. They have extensive powers to inspect all aspects of health service work.

**patients' rights** the three basic rights of patients: namely, the right to know, the right to privacy and the right to treatment. The first two are moral rights while the third is, in the UK, both a moral and legal right.

**Paul–Bunnell test** *J.R. Paul, American physician, 1893–1971; W.W. Bunnell, American physician, 1902–1966.* An agglutination test which, if positive, confirms the diagnosis of glandular fever.

**Pavlov's method** *I.P. Pavlov, Russian physiologist, 1849–1936.* A method for the study of the conditioned reflexes. Pavlov noticed that his experimental dogs salivated in anticipation of food when they heard a bell ring.

**PCT** Primary Care Trust.

**peau d'orange** [Fr.] a dimpled appearance of the overlying skin. Blockage of the skin lymphatics causes dimpling of the hair follicle openings which resembles orange skin. Particularly associated with breast cancer.

**pecten** 1. the middle third of the anal canal. 2. a ridge on the pubic crest to which the inguinal ligament is attached.

**pectoral** relating to the chest. *P. muscles* two pairs of muscles, pectoralis major and pectoralis minor, which control the movements of the shoulder and upper arm.

**pectus** the chest.

**pedicle** the stem or neck of a tumour. *P. graft* a tissue graft that is partially detached and inserted in its new position while temporarily still obtaining its blood supply from the original source.

**pediculosis** the condition of being infested with lice.

*Pediculus* a genus of lice. *P. humanus* a species that feeds on human blood and is an important vector of relapsing fever, typhus and trench fever. Two subspecies are recognized: *P. humanus* var. *capitis* (head louse), found on the scalp hair, and *P. humanus* var. *corporis* (body or clothes louse), found elsewhere on the body.

**peduncle** a narrow part of a structure acting as a support. *Cerebellar p.* one of the collections of nerve fibres connecting the cerebellum with the medulla oblongata.

**PEEP** positive end-expiratory pressure.

**peer.** *P. review* a basic component of a quality assurance (see QUALITY) programme in which the results of health and/or nursing care given to a specific patient population are evaluated according to defined criteria established by the peers of the professionals delivering the care. Peer review is focused on the patient and on the results of care given by a group of professionals rather than on individual professional practitioners. *P. support* the social support provided by one's peer group.

**Pel–Ebstein syndrome** *P.K. Pel, Dutch physician, 1852–1919; W. Ebstein, German physician, 1836–1912.* A recurrent pyrexia, having a cycle of 15–21 days, which occurs in cases of lymphadenoma.

**pellagra** a syndrome caused by a diet seriously deficient in niacin (or by failure to convert tryptophan to niacin). Most patients with pellagra also suffer from deficiencies of vitamin $B_2$ (riboflavin) and other essential vitamins and minerals. The disease also occurs in persons suffering from alcoholism and drug addiction. Characterized by debility, digestive disorders, peripheral neuritis, ataxia, mental disturbance and erythema with exfoliation of the skin.

**pelvic** pertaining to the pelvis. *P. exenteration* removal of all the pelvic organs. *P. floor exercises* a programme of exercises to strengthen the muscles and tighten the ligaments at the base of the abdomen which form the pelvic floor. *P. girdle* the ring of bone to which the lower limbs are jointed. It consists of the two hip bones and the sacrum and coccyx. *P. inflammatory disease* persistent infection of the internal reproductive organs of the female, often resulting in infertility.

**pelvimetry** measurement of the pelvis.

**pelvis** a basin-shaped cavity. *Bony p.* the pelvic girdle, formed of the hip bones and the sacrum and coccyx. *Contracted p.* narrowing of the diameter of the pelvis. It may be of the true conjugate or the diagonal. Effective antenatal care will recognize this condition, and caesarean section may be necessary. *False p.* the part formed by the concavity of the iliac bones above the ileopectineal line. *Renal p.* the dilatation of the ureter which, by enclosing the hilum, surrounds the pyramids of the kidney substance. *True p.* the basin-like cavity below the false pelvis, its upper limit being the pelvic brim.

**pemphigoid** 1. resembling pemphigus. 2. a bullous disease of the elderly with the blisters arising beneath the epidermis. The skin and the mucosa are affected, and sometimes the conjunctiva.

**pemphigus** a distinctive group of rare but serious diseases characterized by successive crops of large bullae ('water blisters'); the name is derived from the Greek word for blister, *pemphix*. Clusters of blisters usually appear first near the nose and mouth (sometimes inside them) and then gradually spread over the skin of the rest of the body. When the blisters burst, they leave round patches of raw and tender skin. Pemphigus is considered to be an autoimmune disorder.

**pendulous** hanging down. *P. abdomen* the hanging down of the abdomen over the pelvis, due to weakness and laxity of the abdominal muscles.

**penicillin** an antibiotic cultured from certain moulds of the genus *Penicillium*. The drug is used in various forms to treat a wide variety of bacterial infections, it was first used therapeutically in 1941. Varieties of the drug include: benethamine penicillin, benzylpenicillin, benzathine penicillin, procaine penicillin, cloxa-cillin, ampicillin and amoxycillin.

**penicillinase** an enzyme that inactivates penicillin. Many bacteria, particularly staphylococci, produce this enzyme.

*Penicillium* a genus of mould-like fungi, from some of which the penicillins are derived. Some species are pathogenic to humans.

**penis** the male organ of copulation and urination.

**pentose** a monosaccharide containing five carbon atoms in a molecule.

**pepsin** an enzyme found in gastric juice. It partially digests proteins in an acid solution.

**pepsinogen** the precursor of pepsin, activated by hydrochloric acid.

**PEP** post-exposure prophylaxis.

**peptic** relating to pepsin or the action of the gastric juices in promoting digestion. *P. ulcer* an ulcer, usually in the stomach or the duodenum, caused by an erosion of the surface to expose the muscle wall by the stomach acid and digestive enzymes. It is often precipitated by *Helicobacter pylori* organisms.

**peptide** any of a class of compounds of low molecular weight that yield two or more amino acids on hydrolysis. Peptides form the constituent parts of proteins.

**peptone** a substance produced by the action of pepsin on protein.

**per os** [L.] *by the mouth.*

**percentile** a term used in statistics to show how common some characteristic is. The line represents the percentage of the population who have this characteristic. The 90th percentile (or centile) for height means that 90% of the population will be no taller than the figure. The 50th percentile is the median or average.

**percept, perception** an awareness and understanding of an impression that has been presented to the senses. The mental process by which we perceive.

**percussion** a method of diagnosis by tapping with the fingers or with a light hammer upon any part of the body. Information can thus be gained as to the condition of underlying organs.

**percutaneous** through the skin. *P. endoscopic gastrostomy (PEG)* a gastrostomy tube inserted endoscopically through the abdominal wall to allow feeding and the passage of drugs. *See* ARTIFICIAL (FEEDING) and Appendix 1.

**perforation** a hole or break in the containing walls or membranes of an organ or structure of the body. Perforation occurs when erosion, infection or other factors create a weak spot in the organ and internal pressure causes a rupture. It may also result from a deep penetrating wound.

**performance assessment** The current performance framework for NHS and social care organizations came into effect in 2005, and replaced star ratings. The 'annual health check' sets out the level of quality that all organizations providing NHS care – including Foundations Trusts and those in the private and voluntary sectors – are expected to meet or aspire to. It is administered by the Healthcare Commission.

**performance indicators** abbreviated PIs. A 'package' of routine statistics derived nationally by the Department of Health and visually presented in ways that highlight the relative efficiency of health services. Performance indicators are intended to compare services and identify aspects that merit further scrutiny locally with a view to changes in organization or practice.

**perfusion** the passage of liquid through a tissue or an organ, particularly the passage of blood through the lung tissue.

**perianal** surrounding or located around the anus. *P. abscess* a small subcutaneous pocket of pus near the anal margin.

**periarteritis** inflammation of the outer coat and surrounding tissues of an artery.

**periarthritis** inflammation of the tissues surrounding a joint.

**pericarditis** inflammation of the pericardium. *Adhesive p.* the presence of adhesions between the two layers of pericardium owing to a thick fibrinous exudate. *Bacterial p.* inflammation of the pericardium due to bacterial infection. *Chronic constrictive p.* thickening and sometimes calcification of the pericardium, which inhibits the action of the heart. *Rheumatic p.* pericarditis due to rheumatic fever.

**pericardium** the smooth membranous sac enveloping the heart, consisting of an outer fibrous and an inner serous coat. The sac contains a small amount of serous fluid.

**perichondrium** the membrane covering cartilaginous surfaces.

**pericranium** the periosteum of the cranial bones.

**perilymph** the fluid that separates the bony and the membranous labyrinths of the ear.

**perimeter** 1. the line marking the boundary of any area or geometrical figure; the circumference. 2. an instrument for measuring the field of vision.

**perimetrium** the peritoneal covering of the uterus.

**perinatal** relating to the period shortly before and 7 days after birth. *P. mortality rate* the number of stillbirths plus deaths of babies under 7 days old per 1000 total births in any one year.

**perinatologist** a medically qualified person specializing in perinatology.

**perinatology** the branch of medicine (obstetrics and paediatrics) dealing with the fetus and infant during the perinatal period.

**perineal** relating to the perineum.

**perineum** the tissues between the anus and external genitals. *Lacerated p.* a torn perineum, which may result from childbirth but is often forestalled by performing an episiotomy. Treatment is by suturing of the laceration.

**periodic** recurring at regular or irregular intervals. *P. apnoea of the newborn* occurring in the normal full-term infant, periodic episodes of rapid breathing followed by a brief period of apnoea which is associated with rapid eye movements. *P. syndrome* recurrent head, limb or abdominal pains in children for which no organic cause can be found. It often leads to migraine in adult life.

**periodontitis** inflammation of the periodontium.

**periodontium** the connective tissue between the teeth and their bony sockets.

**perioperative** pertaining or relating to the period immediately before or after an operation, as in perioperative care.

**periosteal** pertaining to or composed of periosteum. *P. elevator* an instrument for separating the periosteum from the bone.

**periosteum** the fibrous membrane covering the surface of bone. It consists of two layers: the inner or osteogenetic layer, which is closely adherent and forms new cells (by which the bone grows in girth); and, in close contact with it, the fibrous layer richly supplied with blood vessels.

**periostitis** inflammation of the periosteum, usually as a result of injury.

**peripheral** relating to the periphery. *P. iridectomy* excision of a small piece of iris from its peripheral edge. *P. nervous system* those parts of the nervous system lying outside the central nervous system. *P. neuritis* inflammation of terminal nerves. *P. resistance* the resistance in the walls of the arterioles, which is a major factor in the control of blood pressure.

**periphery** the outer surface or circumference.

**peristalsis** a wave-like contraction, preceded by a wave of dilatation, that travels along the walls of a tubular organ, tending to press its contents onwards. It occurs in the muscle coat of the alimentary canal. *Reversed p.* a wave of contraction in the alimentary canal which passes *towards* the mouth. *Visible p.* a wave of contraction in the alimentary canal that is visible on the surface of the abdomen.

**peritoneal** referring to the peritoneum. *P. cavity* the cavity between the parietal and the visceral peritoneum. *P. dialysis* a method of removing waste products from the blood by passing a cannula into the peritoneal cavity, running in a dialysing fluid, and after an interval, draining it off.

**peritoneoscopy** visual examination of the peritoneum by means of a peritoneoscope.

**peritoneum** the serous membrane lining the abdominal cavity and forming a covering for the abdominal organs. *Parietal p.* that which lines the abdominal cavity. *Visceral p.* the inner layer which closely covers the abdominal organs and includes the mesenteries.

**peritonitis** inflammation of the peritoneum. This may be produced by inflammation of abdominal organs, by irritating substances from a perforated gallbladder or gastric ulcer, by rupture of a cyst, or by irritation from blood, as in cases of internal bleeding. Less frequently, it may result from long-standing irritation caused by the presence in the abdomen of a foreign body, such as gunshot, or by chronic peritoneal dialysis.

**peritonsillar** around the tonsil. *P. abscess* quinsy.

**perlèche** [Fr.] inflammation with fissuring at the angles of the mouth; often due to vitamin B deficiency, poorly fitting dentures or thrush infection.

**permeability** the degree to which a fluid can pass from one structure through a wall or membrane to another.

**pernicious** highly destructive; fatal. *P. anaemia* an anaemia due to lack of absorption of vitamin $B_{12}$ for the formation of red blood cells.

**perniosis** a condition, resulting from persistent exposure to cold, which produces vascular spasm in the superficial arterioles of the hands and feet, causing thrombosis and necrosis. Perniosis includes chilblains and Raynaud's disease.

**peroral** by the mouth.

**perseveration** the constant recurrence of an idea or the tendency to keep repeating the same words or actions.

**persistent vegetative state** a long-term dependent state that may last for weeks, months or years. Caused by damage to the cerebral cortex of the brain that controls higher mental functions, while the brainstem controlling respiration and circulation remains undamaged. The individual appears awake but is totally dependent on others for all care and remains unresponsive.

**persona** what one presents of one's self, to be perceived by others.

**personal development plan** a planned process whereby an individual develops skills and knowledge that is beneficial to themselves and their career. This is part of a life long learning commitment for nurses and other health professionals.

**personality** the sum total of heredity and inborn tendencies, with influences from environment and education, which forms the mental make-up of a person and influences attitude to life. *Antisocial p.* a personality disorder in which repetitive antisocial behaviour is associated with ego eccentricity, lack of guilt or anxiety, and imperviousness to punishment. Also called sociopathic (psychopathic) personality. *Double p., dual p.* multiple personality. *Multiple p.* a dissociative reaction in which an individual adopts two or more personalities alternatively, in none of which is there awareness of the experiences of the other(s). *Psychopathic p.* antisocial personality, sociopathic personality. *Schizoid p.* a personality disorder marked by timidity, self-consciousness, introversion, feelings of isolation and loneliness, and failure to form close interpersonal relationships; the individual is frequently ambitious, meticulous and a perfectionist.

**perspiration** sweat or the act of sweating. *Insensible p.* water evaporation from the moist surfaces of the body, such as the respiratory tract and skin, that is not due to the activity of the sweat glands. It occurs at a constant rate of about 500 ml/day. When treating dehydration this loss must be taken into account. *Sensible p.* sweat that is visible as droplets on the skin. Part of the mechanism for regulation of body temperature.

**Perthes' disease** *G.C. Perthes, German surgeon, 1869–1927.* Osteochondritis of the head of the femur. Pseudocoxalgia (Legg–Calvé–Perthes disease).

**pertussis** *See* WHOOPING COUGH.

**perversion** morbid diversion from a normal course. *Sexual p.* abnormal sexual desires and behaviour. A deviation.

**pes** the foot, or any foot-like structure. *P. cavus* a foot with an abnormally high arch. Claw foot. *P. malleus valgus* hammer toe. *P. planus* flat foot.

**pessary** 1. a plastic or metal ring-shaped device which is inserted in the vagina to support a prolapsed uterus. 2. a medicated suppository inserted into the vagina for antiseptic or contraceptive purposes.

**PET** positron emission tomography.

**petechia** a small spot due to an effusion of blood under the skin, as in purpura.

**petit mal** a mild form of epilepsy common in children and characterized by a sudden and brief loss of consciousness.

**pétrissage** [Fr.] a kneading action used in massage.

**petrositis** inflammation of the petrous portion of the temporal bone, usually spread from a middle-ear infection.

**Peyer's glands or patches** *J. C. Peyer, Swiss anatomist, 1653–1712.* Small lymph nodules situated in the mucous membrane of the lower part of the small intestine.

**Peyronie's disease** induration of the corpora cavernosa of the penis, producing a fibrous chordee leading to painful erection.

**pH** a measure of the hydrogen ion concentration, and so the acidity or alkalinity of a solution. Expressed numerically 1 to 14; 7 is neutral, and below this is acid and above alkaline. *See* HYDROGEN (ION CONCENTRATION).

**phaeochromocytoma** a rare tumour of the adrenal medulla which gives rise to paroxysmal hypertension.

**phage** bacteriophage. A virus that lives on bacteria but is confined to a particular strain. *P.-typing* the identification of certain bacterial strains by determining the presence of strain-specific phages. Used in detecting the causative organisms of epidemics, especially food poisoning.

**phagocyte** a blood cell that has the power of ingesting bacteria, protozoa and foreign bodies in the blood.

**phagocytosis** the engulfing and destruction of microorganisms and foreign bodies by phagocytes in the blood.

**phalanges** the bones of the fingers or toes.

**phallus** the penis.

**phantasy** *see* FANTASY.

**phantom** 1. an image or impression not evoked by actual stimuli. 2. a model of the body or of a specific part thereof. 3. a device for simulating the in vivo interaction of radiation with tissues. *P. pain* pain felt as if it were arising in an absent (amputated) limb also known as p. limb pain/experience. *P. pregnancy see* PSEUDOCYESIS. *P. tumour* a tumour-like swelling of the abdomen caused by contraction of the muscles or by localized gas.

**pharmacist** a person professionally qualified to carry out pharmacy. The traditional role of giving advice, dispensing prescriptions and selling over-the-counter medicines from the 10 000 community pharmacies in England has been supplemented by the appointment of pharmacy advisers to strategic health authorities and Primary Care Trusts and new services such as medicines management for the patient.

**pharmacogenetics** the study of genetically determined variations in drug metabolism and the response of the individual.

**pharmacokinetics** the study of how drugs are processed within the body, including their absorption, distribution, metabolism and excretion.

**pharmacology** the science of the nature and preparation of drugs and particularly of their effects on the body.

**pharmacopoeia** an authoritative publication that gives the standard formulae and preparations of drugs used in a given country. *British P.* that authorized for use in the UK.

**pharmacy** 1. the activity or study of medicine preparations. 2. the art of preparing, compounding and dispensing medicines. 3. the place where drugs are stored and dispensed.

**pharyngeal** relating to the pharynx. *P. pouch* dilatation of the lower part of the pharynx.

**pharyngitis** inflammation of the pharynx.

**pharyngolaryngeal** referring to both the pharynx and larynx.

**pharyngotympanic tube** the tube that joins the middle ear to the pharynx; the eustachian tube.

**pharynx** the muscular tube, lined with mucous membrane, situated at the back of the mouth. It leads into the oesophagus, and also communicates with the nose through the posterior nares, with the ears through the pharyngotympanic (eustachian) tubes, and with the larynx. *See*

LARYNGOPHARYNX, NASOPHARYNX and OROPHARYNX.

**phenol** carbolic acid. A disinfectant derived from coal tar.

**phenomenon** 1. an objective sign or symptom. 2. A noteworthy occurrence.

**phenomenology** an approach in research, as the study of the lived experience of people or a way of thinking about what life experiences are like for people.

**phenotype** the characteristics of an individual that are due both to the environment and to genetic make-up.

**phenylalanine** an essential amino acid which cannot be properly metabolized in persons suffering from phenylketonuria.

**phenylketonuria** abbreviated PKU. A disease due to a defect in the metabolism of the amino acid phenylalanine. The condition is hereditary. It results from lack of an enzyme, phenylalanine hydroxylase, necessary for the conversion of phenylalanine into tyrosine. Thus there is accumulation of phenylalanine in the blood, with eventual excretion of phenylpyruvic acid in the urine. If untreated, the condition results in learning difficulties and other abnormalities. The condition can be detected soon after birth, and screening of newborns for PKU entails a simple blood test. A sample of blood is taken from the infant at approximately 2 weeks. Phenylalanine levels are assessed (Guthrie test) and treatment is with a diet low in phenylalanine if necessary. A special diet is usually recommended throughout life and especially during pregnancy as high phenylalanine levels in the mother's blood can damage the fetus.

**phenylpyruvic acid** an abnormal constituent of the urine present in phenylketonuria.

**pheromone** a chemical substance with specific odour secreted externally by an organism and affecting the behaviour or physiology of members of the same species. These substances may be involved in the physiological communication within a species and provide an influence upon sexual behaviour.

**phimosis** constriction of the prepuce so that it cannot be drawn back over the glans penis. The usual treatment is circumcision.

**phlebectomy** excision of a vein or a portion of a vein.

**phlebitis** inflammation of a vein, usually in the leg, which tends to lead to the formation of a thrombus. The symptoms are pain and swelling, and redness along the course of the vein, which is felt later as a hard, tender cord.

**phlebography** 1. radiographic examination of a vein containing a contrast medium. 2. the graphic representation of the venous pulse.

**phlebothrombosis** obstruction of a vein by a blood clot, without local inflammation. It is usually in the deep veins of the calf of the leg, causing tenderness and swelling. The clot may break away and cause an embolism.

*Phlebotomus* a genus of sandflies, the various species of which transmit leishmaniasis in its many forms, and also sandfly fever.

**phlebotomy** the puncture of a vein for the withdrawal of blood. Venesection.

**phlegm** mucus secreted by the lining of the air passages.

**phlegmatic** calm and unemotional.

**phlycten** 1. a small blister caused by a burn. 2. a small vesicle occurring in the conjunctiva or cornea of the eye. Often associated with tuberculosis.

**phobia** an irrational fear produced by a specific situation or object that the patient attempts to avoid.

**phocomelia** a rare congenital deformity in which the long bones of the limbs are minimal or absent and the individual has stump-like limbs of various lengths. The drug thalidomide, used in the 1960s in early pregnancy, was associated with this deformity.

**phonation** the art of uttering meaningful vocal sounds.

**phonocardiogram** a record of the heart sounds made by a phonocardiograph.

**phonocardiograph** an instrument that graphically records heart sounds and murmurs.

**phonology** the study of speech sounds, their production and the relationship between sounds as elements of language.

**phosphatase** one of a group of enzymes involved in the metabolism of phosphate. *Alkaline p.* an enzyme formed by osteoblasts in the bones and by liver cells and excreted in the bile.

**phosphate** a salt or ester of phosphoric acid.

**phospholipid** a lipid of glycerol fats found in cells, especially those of the nervous system.

**phosphorus** *symbol* P. An essential element in the diet. It is a major component of bone, is involved in almost all metabolic processes and also plays an important role in cell metabolism. It is obtained by the body from milk products, cereals, meat and fish. Its use by the body is controlled by vitamin D and calcium. *See* Appendix 1.

**phosphorylase** an enzyme, found in the liver and kidneys, that catalyses the breakdown of glycogen into glucose 1-phosphate.

**photocoagulation** the use of a powerful light source to induce inflammation of the retina and choroid to treat retinal detachment.

**photophobia** intolerance of light. It can occur in many eye conditions, including conjunctivitis, corneal ulceration, iritis and keratitis.

**photophthalmia** inflammation of the eye due to overexposure to bright light, especially to ultraviolet light.

**photopic** pertaining to bright light. *P. vision* vision in bright light when the cones of the retina provide the visual appreciation of colour and shape.

**photopsia** a sensation of flashes of light sometimes occurring in the early stages of retinal detachment.

**photosensitivity** an abnormal degree of sensitivity of the skin to sunlight.

**phototherapy** treatment using fluorescent light, containing a high output of blue light, to reduce the amount of unconjugated bilirubin in the skin of a jaundiced neonate.

**phrenic** 1. relating to the mind. 2. pertaining to the diaphragm. *P. avulsion* the surgical excision of a part of the phrenic nerve. *P. nerve* one of a pair of nerves controlling the muscles of the diaphragm.

*Phthirus pubis* the crab louse.

**phthisis** pulmonary tuberculosis. *P. bulbi* a shrinking of the eyeball following inflammation or injury.

**physical** in medicine, relating to the body as opposed to the mental processes. *P. abuse. See* ABUSE. *P. examination* examination of the bodily state of a patient by ordinary physical means, such as inspection, palpation, percussion and auscultation. *P. handicap* a term used when a physical disadvantage is due to impairment of physiological or anatomical structure of function. *P. medicine* the treatment and rehabilitation of patients with physical disabilities. It includes physiotherapy and manipulation. *P. signs* those observed by inspection, percussion, etc.

**physician** a medically qualified person who practises medicine as opposed to surgery. *Community p.* a doctor who practises community medicine (*see* MEDICINE). *Consultant p.* senior doctor in overall charge of patients within a specialist medical field, and responsible for directing junior medical staff working for the same firm. *House p.* a junior doctor, resident in hospital while on duty, acting under the orders of a consultant physician.

**physiological** relating to physiology. Normal, as opposed to pathological. *P. jaundice see* JAUNDICE. *P. solutions* those of the same salt composition and same osmotic pressure as blood plasma.

**physiology** the science of the functioning of living organisms.

**physiotherapy** a health care profession concerned with function and movement as well as maximizing mobility potential. It provides treatment for physical problems due to accident, illness or disability, promotes normal function and mobility, using skills of manipulation, electrotherapy with appropriate exercise programmes as necessary. Physiotherapists are also involved in preventative health care and rehabilitation and committed to reviewing evidence that informs its practice and delivery.

**physique** the structure of the body.

**pia mater** [L.] the innermost membrane enveloping the brain and spinal cord, consisting of a network of small blood vessels connected by areolar tissue. This dips down into all the folds of the nerve substance.

**pica** an unnatural craving for strange foods and for things not fit to be eaten. It may occur in pregnancy, and sometimes in children with learning disabilities.

**Pickwickian syndrome** (named after the fat boy 'Joe' in *Pickwick Papers*). A condition in which extreme obesity is associated with severe congestive cardiac failure.

**picornavirus** a family of small RNA-containing viruses including echoviruses and rhinoviruses.

**PICU** paediatric intensive care unit.

**PID** prolapse of an intervertebral disc.

**pie chart** a circular graph divided into sectors proportional to the magnitudes of the quantities represented.

**pigeon breast** a deformity in which the sternum is unduly prominent. *P. toed* walking with the toes of one foot or of both feet turned inwards.

**pigment** colouring matter. *Bile p's* bilirubin and biliverdin. *Blood p.* haemoglobin. *Melanotic p.* melanin.

**pigmentation** the deposition of pigment in the tissues. In some conditions, e.g. jaundice or albinism, there is either an excess or a lack of pigmentation.

**pile** a haemorrhoid.

**pill** a rounded mass of one or more drugs, sometimes coated with sugar. Taken orally.

**pilomotor** capable of moving the hair. *P. nerves* sympathetic nerves which control muscles in the skin connected with hair follicles. Stimulation causes the hair to be erected, and also the condition of 'goose-flesh' of the skin.

**pilonidal** having a growth of hair. *P. cyst* a congenital infolding of hair-bearing skin over the coccyx. It may become infected and lead to sinus formation.

**pilot study** a small-scale version of a planned experiment or observation used initially to test the design of the larger study. A pilot study is helpful to see if any difficulties or problems arise in order that they can be clarified before embarking on the larger study, thus saving time and resources. A pilot study may also indicate possible extensions to the study or suggest restrictions of those aspects likely to be unhelpful.

**pimple** a small papule or pustule.

**pineal** shaped like a pine cone. *P. body* a small cone-shaped structure attached by a stalk to the posterior wall of the third ventricle of the brain and composed of glandular substance.

**pinguecula** [L.] a small, benign, yellowish spot on the bulbar conjunctiva, seen usually in the elderly. Caused by degeneration of the elastic tissue of the conjunctiva.

**pinkeye** acute contagious conjunctivitis.

**pinna** the projecting part of the external ear; the auricle.

**pinta** a non-venereal skin infection caused by *Treponema carateum* which is similar to the causative agent of syphilis. It is prevalent in the West Indies and Central America.

**pinworm** a threadworm; *Enterobius vermicularis*.

**pituitary** an endocrine gland suspended from the base of the brain and protected by the sella turcica in the sphenoid bone. It consists of two lobes: (a) the anterior, which secretes a number of different hormones, including adrenocorticotrophic hormone (ACTH), gonadotrophin, thyroid-stimulating hormone (TSH) and prolactin; (b) the posterior, which secretes oxytocin and vasopressin.

**pityriasis** a skin disease characterized by fine scaly desquamation. *P. alba* a condition, common in children, in which white scaly patches appear on the face. *P. capitis* dandruff. *P. rosea* an inflammatory form, in which the affected areas are macular and ring-shaped.

**PKU** phenylketonuria.

**place of safety order** a court order whereby a child is arbitrarily removed from the care of its parents in the interests of the child's safety.

**placebo** [L.] a substance given to a patient as medicine or a procedure performed on a patient that has no intrinsic therapeutic value and relieves symptoms or helps the patient in some way only because the patient believes or expects that it will. A placebo may be prescribed to satisfy a patient's psychological need for drug therapy and may also be given during controlled experiments. *P. effect* after the administration of a drug or treatment, a change (usually temporary) in a patient's physical or emotional condition following publicity or media interest in the drug or treatment. The placebo response is due more to the patient's expectations or to the expectations of the person giving the drug or treatment than to the result of any direct physiological or pharmacological substance response.

**placenta** the afterbirth. A vascular structure inside the pregnant uterus, supplying the fetus with nourishment through the connecting umbilical cord. The placenta develops in about the third month of pregnancy and is expelled after the birth of the child. *Battledore p.* one in which the cord is attached to the margin and not the centre. *P. praevia* one attached to the lower part of the uterine wall. It may cause severe antepartum haemorrhage. *See also* ABRUPTIO PLACENTAE.

**plagiocephaly** asymmetry of the head resulting from the irregular closing of the sutures.

**plague** an acute, febrile, infectious, highly fatal disease caused by the bacillus *Yersinia pestis*. It is a notifiable disease. Transmitted to humans by the bites of fleas that have derived the infection from diseased rats. **Bubonic p.** a type in which the lymph glands are infected and buboes form in the groins and arm-pits. Known in medieval times as 'The Black Death'. **Pneumonic p.** a type in which the infection attacks chiefly the lung tissues. A fatal form. **Septicaemic p.** a very severe and fatal form when the infection enters the bloodstream.

PLANES

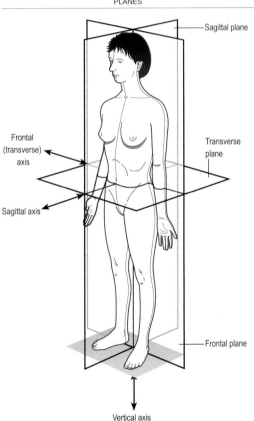

**plan** a detailed proposal for doing or achieving something.

**planes** used in the description of location and movement of parts of the body. Three planes are perpendicular to each other passing through the middle of the body. These are defined: *sagittal* – vertical, front-to-back; *frontal* – vertical, side-to-side; *transverse* – horizontal (*see* Figure on p. 310). *See* AXIS.

**planned parenthood** the practice of measures including contraception that limit the number and the spacing of pregnancies.

**planning** the second stage of the nursing process in which the nurse and the patient together consider the goals to achieve in meeting the patient's identified or potential problems in daily life and produce an individual care plan. A forward date is also set for evaluation of whether or not the goals have been achieved.

**plantar** relating to the sole of the foot. *P. arch* the arch made by anastomosis of the plantar arteries. *P. flexion* bending of the toes downwards and so arching the foot. *P. reflex* contraction of the toes on stroking the sole of the foot. *P. wart* a common wart located on the sole of the foot. Plantar warts are epidermal tumours caused by a virus that may be picked up by going barefoot. Also called verruca plantaris.

**plaque** 1. a flat patch on the skin. 2. a deposit of food and bacteria on the enamel of teeth which may produce tartar and caries.

**plasma** the fluid portion of the blood in which corpuscles are suspended. Plasma is to be distinguished from serum, which is plasma from which the fibrinogen has been separated in the process of clotting. *P. proteins* those present in the blood plasma: albumin, globulin and fibrinogen. *P. volume*

*expander* a solution transfused instead of blood to increase the volume of fluid circulating in the blood vessels. Also called artificial plasma extender. *Reconstituted p.* dried plasma when again made liquid by addition of distilled water.

**plasmapheresis** a method of removing a portion of the plasma from circulation. Venesection is performed, the blood is allowed to settle, the plasma is removed, and the red blood cells are returned to the circulation. Used in the treatment of those diseases caused by antibodies circulating in the patient's plasma.

**plasmid** deoxyribonucleic acid (DNA) present in the cytoplasm of some bacteria. This genetic material can be transferred during bacterial reproduction thus permitting the genes of antibiotic resistance to be passed on.

**plasmin** a fibrinolytic, found in blood plasma, which can dissolve fibrin clots.

**plasminogen** the inactive precursor of plasmin.

*Plasmodium* a genus of protozoan parasites in the red blood cells of animals and humans. Four species, *P. falciparrum, P. malariae, P. ovale* and *P. vivax*, cause the four specific types of human malaria.

**plaster** 1. a mixture of materials that hardens; used for immobilizing or making impressions of body parts. 2. an adhesive substance spread on fabric or other suitable backing material for application to the skin. *Bohler's p.* plaster for Pott's fracture. A leg splint of plaster of Paris, in which is embedded an iron stirrup extending below the foot, which enables the patient to walk without putting weight on the joint. *Corn p.* an adhesive strip or patch impregnated with salicylic acid and applied to corns on the feet. *Frog p.* a plaster of Paris splint used to maintain the position after correction of the deformity due to congenital dislocation of the hip. *P. of Paris* calcium sulphate or gypsum which sets hard when water is added to it; it is used to form a plaster cast to immobilize a part, and in dentistry for making dental impressions.

**plastic** 1. constructive; tissue-forming. 2. capable of being moulded; pliable. *P. lymph* the exudate which, in wounds and inflamed serous tissues, is organized into fibrous tissue and promotes healing. *P. surgery* the branch of surgery that deals with the repair and reconstruction of deformed or injured parts of the body, including their replacement, by tissue grafting or other means.

**platelet** a disc-shaped structure present in the blood and concerned in the process of clotting. A thrombocyte.

**play** an occupation, for either children or adults, which is voluntary and may be a spontaneous or an organized activity providing enjoyment, entertainment, amusement or a diversion. Play is important in childhood as a necessary part of psychological and physical development. *Normative p.* is by children that is spontaneous and child led, being pleasurable with no intrinsic goals. *P. group* a session of care and activities for preschool children. It can be organized by any interested person at home or in other premises, but it must be registered by the social services department. *P. specialist* a person who is qualified to use play constructively to help children come to terms with illness and hospitalization. *P. therapist* one trained in the skills of play therapy. *P. therapy* a technique used in child psychotherapy in which play is used to reveal unconscious material. Play is the natural way in which children express and work through unconscious conflicts; thus play therapy is analogous to the technique of free association used in adult psychotherapy.

**pleoptics** an orthoptic method of improving the sight in cases of strabismus by stimulating the use of the macular part of the retina.

**plethora** a general term denoting a red, florid complexion or, specifically, an excessive amount of blood.

**plethysmography** the measurement of changes in the volume of organs or limbs due to alterations in blood pressure.

**pleura** the serous membrane lining the thorax and enveloping each lung. *Parietal p.* the layer that lines the chest wall. *Visceral p.* the inner layer which is in close contact with the lung.

**pleurisy, pleuritis** inflammation of the pleura; it may be caused by infection, injury or tumour. It may be a complication of lung diseases, particularly of pneumonia, or sometimes of tuberculosis, lung abscess or influenza. The symptoms are cough, fever, chills, sharp, sticking pain that is worse on inspiration, and rapid shallow breathing. *Dry p., fibrinous p.* pleurisy in which the membrane is inflamed and roughened, but no fluid is formed. *P. with effusion* wet pleurisy. A type that is characterized by inflammation and exudation of serous fluid into the pleural cavity. *Purulent p.* empyema. The formation of pus in the pleural cavity. An operation for drainage is usually necessary. *Wet p.* pleurisy with effusion.

**pleurodynia** pain in the intercostal muscles, probably rheumatic in origin.

**plexus** a network of veins or nerves. *Auerbach's p.* the nerve ganglion situated between the longitudinal and circular muscle fibres of the intestine. The nerves are motor nerves. **Brachial p.** the network of nerves of the neck and axilla. **Choroid p.** a capillary network situated in the ventricles of the brain which forms the cerebrospinal fluid. **Coeliac p.** solar plexus. **Meissner's p.** the sensory nerve ganglion situated in the submucous layer of the intestinal wall. **Rectal p.** the network of veins that surrounds the rectum and forms a direct communication between the systemic and portal circulations. **Solar p.** coeliac plexus. The network of nerves and ganglia at the back of the stomach, which supply the abdominal viscera.

**plication** the taking of tucks in a structure to shorten it; a folding to decrease the size of a structure or organ during a surgical procedure.

**pluripotent stem cells** bone marrow cells that have the potential to develop into many other types of mature cells, e.g. erythrocytes, lymphoctyes, granulocytes and thrombocytes.

**pneumaturia** the passing of flatus with the urine owing to a vesicointestinal fistula and air from the bowel entering the bladder.

**pneumococcus** the causative agent of a range of illnesses described as pneumococcal disease, e.g. pneumonia, septicaemia and meningitis. A Gram-positive, ovoid diplococcus, *Streptococcus pneumoniae*. Immunization with pneumococcal vaccine helps prevent pneumococcal disease, and is recommended for people over the age of 80 years and those with certain medical conditions, e.g. diabetes, heart and lung conditions.

**pneumoconiosis** an industrial disease of the lung due to inhalation of dust particles over a period of time. *See* ANTHRACOSIS, ASBESTOSIS and SILICOSIS.

*Pneumocystis carinii* is an atypical fungus acquired by the airborne route which frequently causes pneumonia (abbreviated PCP) in people with human immunodeficiency virus (HIV) infection and in other immunosuppressed persons.

**pneumodynamics** the mechanics of respiration.

**pneumoencephalography** *See* ENCEPHALOGRAPHY.

**pneumogastric** pertaining to lungs and stomach. *P. nerve* the tenth cranial nerve to the lungs, stomach, etc. The vagus nerve.

**pneumomycosis** infection of the lung by microfungi, e.g. candidiasis or aspergillosis.

**pneumonectomy** partial or total removal of a lung.

**pneumonia** inflammation of the lung with consolidation and exudation. *Aspiration p.* an acute condition caused by the aspiration of infected material into the lungs. *Hypostatic p.* a form that occurs in weak, bedridden patients. *Lobar p.* an acute infectious disease caused by a pneumococcus and affecting whole lobes of either or both lungs. *Virus p.* inflammation of the lung occurring during some virus disease and secondary to it.

**pneumonitis** an imprecise term denoting any inflammatory condition of the lung.

**pneumoperitoneum** the presence of air or gas in the peritoneal cavity, occurring pathologically or introduced intentionally for diagnostic or therapeutic purposes.

**pneumoradiography** radiographic examination of a cavity or part after air or a gas has been injected into it.

**pneumotaxic** regulating the rate of respiration. *P. centre* the centre in the pons that influences inspiratory effort during respiration.

**pneumothorax** accumulation of air or gas in the pleural cavity, resulting in collapse of the lung on the affected side. The condition may occur spontaneously, as in the course of a pulmonary disease, or it may follow trauma to, and perforation of, the chest wall. *Artificial p.* a surgical procedure sometimes used in the treatment of tuberculosis or after pneumonectomy. *Spontaneous p.* sometimes occurs when there is an opening on the surface of the lung allowing leakage of air from the bronchi into the pleural cavity. *Tension p.* a particularly dangerous form of pneumothorax that occurs when air escapes into the pleural cavity from a bronchus but cannot regain entry into the bronchus. As a result, continuously increasing air pressure in the pleural cavity causes progressive collapse of the lung tissue.

**podagra** gout, particularly of the big toe.

**podalic** relating to the feet. *P. version* a method of changing the lie of a fetus so that its feet will present.

**podarthritis** inflammation of any of the joints of the foot.

**podiatry** chiropody. The examination, diagnosis, treatment and prevention of diseases and malfunction of the foot, lower limb and related structures. Now a health care profession under regulation by the Health Professions Council, the main role of the podiatrist or chiropodist, is to assess and treat abnormalities and diseases of the foot, and to give advice on proper care of the foot and the prevention of foot problems.

**pointillage** [Fr.] a method of massage using the tips of the fingers.

**poison** any substance that, applied to the body externally or taken internally, can cause injury to any part or cause death.

**poisoning** the morbid condition produced by a poison. The poison may be swallowed, inhaled (see CARBON (MONOXIDE)), injected by a stinging insect as in a BEE STING, or spilled or otherwise brought into contact with the skin.

**polioencephalitis** acute inflammation of the cortex of the brain.

**poliomyelitis** an acute, notifiable, infectious viral disease that attacks the central nervous system, injuring or destroying the nerve cells that control the muscles and sometimes causing paralysis; also called polio or infantile paralysis. Paralysis most often affects the limbs but can involve any muscles, including those that control breathing and swallowing. Since the development and the use of vaccines against poliomyelitis, the disease has been virtually eliminated in wealthier countries, where vaccination rates are high, but is still common in many other parts of the world. See IMMUNIZATION SCHEDULE.

**poliovirus** a small RNA-containing virus which causes poliomyelitis.

**pollinosis** hay fever; an allergy caused by various kinds of pollen. Pollinosis.

**pollution** 1. the act of destroying the purity of or contaminating something. 2. contamination of the environment by poisons, radioactive substances, accidental chemical spillage, microorganisms or other wastes from industrial activity, vehicle exhausts or untreated sewage. Pollution into the environment has been linked at many levels as being injurious to good health. Air pollution causes respiratory problems while noise pollution has been linked to hearing loss, insomnia and poor concentration.

**polyarteritis** inflammatory changes in the walls of the small arteries.

**polyarthralgia** pain in several joints.

**polyarthritis** inflammation of several joints at the same time, as seen in rheumatoid arthritis.

**polycoria** a congenital abnormality in which there are one or more holes in the iris in addition to the pupil.

**polycystic** containing many cysts. *P. ovary disease* Stein–Leventhal syndrome. *P. renal disease* a hereditary disease in which there is massive enlargement of the kidney with the formation of many cysts. Severe bleeding into cysts can occur. End-stage renal disease can affect many members of one family.

**polycythaemia** an abnormal increase in the number of red cells in the blood. Erythrocythaemia. *P. vera* a rare disease in which there is a greatly increased production of red blood cells and also of leukocytes and platelets. The skin becomes flushed, with cyanosis, thrombosis and splenomegaly.

**polydactylism** the condition of having more than the normal number of fingers or toes.

**polydipsia** abnormal thirst. It may be a symptom of diabetes.

**polyhydramnios** *see* HYDRAMNIOS.

**polymorphonuclear** 1. having nuclei of many different shapes. 2. a polymorphonuclear leukocyte.

**polymorphous** occurring in several or many different forms.

**polymyalgia rheumatica** persistent aching pain in the muscles, often involving the shoulder or the pelvic girdle and spine. Associated with morning stiffness. More common in older people.

**polymyositis** a generalized inflammation of the muscles with weakness and joint stiffness, particularly around the hips and shoulders.

**polyneuritis** inflammation of many nerves at the same time.

**polyneuropathy** a number of disease conditions of the nervous system.

**polyopia** the perception of two or more images of the same object. Multiple vision.

**polyp** a pedunculated tumour of mucous membrane. A polypus.

**polypharmacy** 1. the administration of many drugs together. This increases the likelihood of side-effects from drug interactions and of non-compliance by the patient. The taking of 'over-the-counter' medications and the use of complimentary therapies may enhance the problem. 2. the administration of excessive medication.

**polyposis** the presence of many polyps in an organ. *Familial p.* a hereditary condition in which large numbers of polyps develop in the colon, which may become malignant.

**polyuria** an abnormally large output of urine due either to an excessive intake of liquid or to disease, often diabetes.

**pompholyx** an intensely pruritic skin condition in which vesicles appear on the hands and feet, particularly on the palms and soles. Typically occurring in repeated, self-limiting attacks.

**pons** a bridge of tissue connecting two parts of an organ. *P. varolii* the part of the brain that connects the cerebrum, cerebellum and medulla oblongata.

**Pontiac fever** an influenza-like illness with little or no pulmonary involvement, caused by *Legionella pneumophila*. It is not life-threatening, as is the pulmonary form known as legionnaires' disease.

**popliteal** relating to the posterior part of the knee joint.

**poppers** a street name for nitrite inhalants generally or amyl nitrite in particular taken in substance misuse to achieve 'an elevated mood' or 'high'.

**population** 1. the total number of persons inhabiting a given geographical area or location. 2. in statistics the aggregate of individuals or items from which a sample for a study is drawn. 3. any group that is distinguished by a particular trait or situation.

**pore** a minute circular opening on a surface. *Sweat p.* an opening of a sweat gland on the skin surface.

**porphyria** an inborn error in the metabolism of porphyrins, resulting in porphyrinuria. Two general types of porphyria are known: erythropoietic porphyrias, which are concerned with the formation of erythrocytes in the bone marrow; and hepatic porphyrias, which are responsible for liver dysfunction. The manifestations of porphyria include gastrointestinal, neurological and psychological symptoms, cutaneous photosensitivity, pigmentation of the face (and later of the bones) and anaemia, with enlargement of the spleen.

**porphyrin** one of a number of pigments used in the production of the haem portion of haemoglobin.

**porphyrinuria** the presence of an excess of porphyrin in the urine.

**porta** an opening in an organ through which pass the main vessels.

**portacaval** pertaining to the portal vein and the inferior vena cava. *P. anastomosis* the joining of the portal vein to the inferior vena cava so that much of the blood bypasses the liver. It is used in the treatment of portal hypertension.

**portage system** a method of behaviour modification taught to family members to enable them to assist a handicapped child in development and acquiring skills for everyday living.

**portfolio** a collection of competency evidence assembled by the practitioner/student which demonstrates the owner's professional development. The portfolio may include such material as journals, marked assessments, evidence of reflective practice or other examples that document the acquisition of new skills,

knowledge, understanding and achievements relevant to professional practice. *See* PROFILE.

**position** attitude or posture. *Dorsal p.* lying flat on the back. *Genupectoral* or *knee–chest p.* resting on the knees and chest with arms crossed above the head. *Lithotomy p.* lying on the back with thighs raised and knees supported and held widely apart. *Prone p.* face down. *Sims' p.* or *semi-prone p.* lying on the left side with the right knee well flexed and the left arm drawn back over the edge of the bed. *Trendelenburg p.* lying down on a tilted plane (usually an operating table at an angle of 30°–45° to the floor), with the head lowermost, the shoulders supported and the legs hanging over the raised end of the table.

**positive** having a value greater than zero; indicating existence or presence, as chromatin positive or Wassermann positive; characterized by affirmation or cooperation. The opposite of negative.

**positive end-expiratory pressure** abbreviated PEEP. In mechanical ventilation, a positive airway pressure maintained until the end of expiration. A PEEP higher than the critical closing pressure holds alveoli open until the end of expiration and can markedly improve the arterial $Po_2$ in patients with a lowered functional residual capacity (FRC), as in acute respiratory failure.

**positron emission tomography** abbreviated PET. A diagnostic technique based upon the detection of positively charged particles with a short half-life known as positrons that are emitted by radioactive labelled substances introduced into the body. PET scanning produces three-dimensional images of the metabolic and chemical activity of tissues in the body, e.g. the brain.

**posseting** regurgitation of a small amount of milk by an infant immediately after a feed.

**Possum** patient-operated selector mechanism; a machine that can be operated with a very slight degree of pressure, or suction, using the mouth, if no other muscle movement is possible. It may transmit messages from a light panel or be adapted for telephoning, computing or working certain machinery.

**post-exposure prophylaxis** abbreviated PEP. The administration of antibiotics, antiviral agents, or active and/or passive vaccination following exposure to an infectious agent, e.g. antiretroviral drugs after exposure (usually occupationally, but may include sexual exposure) to human immunodeficiency virus (HIV).

**post-traumatic stress disorder** following the experience of a major incident – personal, such as injury, rape or drowning, or other serious event, such as a natural disaster – the person may experience insomnia, acute anxiety, nightmares and 'flashbacks' resulting in depression, loss of concentration, apathy and guilt. This reaction may be immediate or delayed, and may last for a variable time. Support and counselling are needed.

**postconcussional syndrome** constant headaches with mental fatigue, difficulty in concentration and insomnia that may persist after head injury.

**posterior** behind a part. Dorsal. The opposite of anterior. *P. chamber* that part of the aqueous chamber that lies behind the iris, but in front of the lens.

**postgastrectomy syndrome** *see* DUMPING.

**posthumous** occurring after death. *P. birth* one occurring after the death of the father, or by caesarean section after the death of the mother.

**postmature** a state in which the pregnancy is prolonged after the expected date of delivery. Owing to the many variables it is difficult to estimate, but may exist when a pregnancy has lasted 41–42 weeks from the last menstrual period. There is a danger of hypoxia to the fetus.

**postmenopausal** relating to or occurring in the period following the menopause. *See* MENOPAUSE.

**postmortem** after death. *P. examination* autopsy.

**postnatal** after childbirth. *P. care* includes the care of the mother for at least 6 weeks after delivery. *P. clinic* an examination centre where the patient can be examined (postnatally), preferably 6 weeks after childbirth: (a) regarding her general health; (b) specifically, to find out the state of the uterus, pelvic floor and vagina. *P. depression* the condition ranges from being a common, mild and short lived episode, (sometimes called the 'baby blues') to a rare and severe depressive psychosis. *P. exercises* taught to the mother by the midwife or physiotherapist during the puerperium to strengthen the pelvic floor and abdominal muscles but also includes deep breathing and leg exercises as preventive measures against respiratory tract infection and deep vein thrombosis. *P. period* a period of not less than 10 days and not more than 28 days after the end of labour, during which the continued attendance of a midwife on the mother and baby is mandatory. This is a rule of the Nursing and Midwifery Council.

**postpartum** occurring after labour.

**postprandial** occurring after a meal.

**postregistration education and practice (PREP)** The Nursing and Midwifery Council (NMC) Code of professional conduct (2008) requires that all nurses maintain their professional knowledge and competence in order that they can retain their registration. The Council expects that where possible, all care provided should be evidenced based, and that nurses have a duty to develop their professional competence throughout their working lives. In order to maintain their registered status with the NMC, at three yearly intervals from the time of registration a notification of practice form (NOP) must be completed by all nurses and midwives. To meet the practice standard the requirements for working is that a minimum of 100 days or 750 hours in the previous five years have been served in a capacity that requires the use of the nursing and midwifery qualifications held. Registered practitioners are also required to undertake and record all continuing professional development. This standard requires that the practitioner has undertaken a minimum of 35 hours learning activity during the three years prior to the renewal of registration. The NMC audits compliance with the standards monthly, 10% of registrants due for renewal are selected for audit. This audit form must be completed before registration can be renewed.

**postural** relating to a position or posture. *P. drainage* drainage of secretions from specific lobes or segments of the lung, aided by careful positioning of the patient.

**potassium** *symbol* K. A metallic alkaline element which is a constituent of all plants and animals. Its salts are widely used in medicine.

**Pott's disease** *P. Pott, British surgeon, 1714–1788.* Tuberculosis of the spine.

**Pott's fracture** a fracture-dislocation of the ankle, involving fracture of the lower end of the tibia, displacement of the talus and sometimes fracture of the medial malleolus.

**pouch** a pocket-like space or cavity. *Morison's p.* a fold of peritoneum below the liver. *P. of Douglas* the lowest fold of the peritoneum between the uterus and rectum.

**poultice** a soft, moist mass of about the consistency of cooked cereal, spread between layers of muslin, linen, gauze or towels and applied hot to a given area in order to create moist local heat or to counter irritation.

**Poupart's ligament** *F. Poupart, French anatomist, 1616–1708.* The inguinal ligament. The tendinous lower border of the external oblique muscle of the abdominal wall, which passes from the anterior spine of the ilium to the os pubis.

**poverty** the lack of sufficient material, economic and cultural resources to sustain an existence compatible with wellbeing. *Absolute p.* the situation of not having sufficient resources to maintain nutrition for good health or to provide shelter and living accommodation. *P. of speech* marked deficit in spontaneous speech; replies to questions are perfunctory, monosyllabic or unforthcoming. *P. trap* a situation whereby an increase in a person's income results in a loss of state benefits leaving them no better off. *Relative p.* where a person's living standards are below those of the community in which the person lives.

**power calculation** a measure of statistical power used in research. The likelihood of a study to produce statistically significant results.

**powerlessness** without power, or ability leading to a feeling of being without influence upon their personal situation. People may feel powerless in their dealings with health services and health care professionals.

**practice** the exercise of a profession. *P. nurse* a member of the primary health care team who is a registered nurse employed by general practitioners to work within the practice setting providing health care services to the population served by the practice. *Family p.* the medical specialty concerned with the planning and provision of comprehensive primary health care, regardless of age or sex, on a continuing basis.

**practitioner** a person who practices a profession. *See* NURSE (PRACTITIONER).

**pre-eclampsia** a condition occurring in late pregnancy. The symptoms include proteinuria, hypertension and oedema.

**preceptor** 1. a teacher, an instructor. 2. a first-level nurse, midwife or health visitor, with at least 12 months (or equivalent) experience in the relevant clinical field, who provides newly registered practitioners with support and guidance in making the transition from student to registered practitioner. Preceptors should be provided with specific preparation for their role.

**preceptorship** a period of support, given by a preceptor, of at least the first 4 months of registered practice for the newly registered nurse, midwife or health visitor practitioner or for those returning to nursing after a break of more than 5 years.

**precipitate labour** unusually rapid labour with extremely quick delivery. There is danger to the mother of severe perineal lacerations, and to the child of intracranial trauma as a result of the rapid passage through the birth canal.

**precocious** developed in advance of the norm, either mentally or physically or both.

**precognition** a direct perception of a future event which is beyond the reach of inference.

**precursor** something that precedes. In biological processes, a substance from which another, usually more active or mature, substance is formed. In clinical medicine, a sign or symptom that heralds another.

**prediabetes** a state which precedes diabetes mellitus, in which the disease is not yet clinically manifest. In pregnancy the diabetes may become evident, or the patient may remain well but give birth to an usually large child. Screening by urine testing can detect the condition.

**predisposition** susceptibility to a specific disease.

**pregnancy** being with child; the condition from conception to the expulsion of the fetus. The normal period is 280 days or 40 weeks counted from the first day of the last normal menstrual period. *Ectopic* or *extrauterine p.* pregnancy occurring outside the uterus, in the uterine tube (*tubal p.*) or very rarely in the abdominal cavity. *P. tests* tests used to demonstrate whether conception has occurred. These detect the human chorionic gonadotrophin (HCG) produced by the embryo 8 days after the first missed period. Immunologicallaboratory tests are more accurate and less likely to give a false positive result than an over-the-counter kit.

**prejudice** *see* BIAS.

**premature** occurring before the anticipated time. *P. contraction* a form of cardiac irregularity in which the ventricle contracts before its anticipated time. *See* SYSTOLE. *P. ejaculation* emission of semen before or at the beginning of sexual intercourse. *P. infant* preterm infant. A child born before the 37th completed week of gestation.

**premedication** drugs given preoperatively in order to reduce fear and anxiety and to facilitate the induction and maintenance of, and recovery from, anaesthesia.

**premenstrual** preceding menstruation. *P. endometrium* the hypertrophied and vascular mucous lining of the uterus immediately before the menstrual flow starts. *P. tension* feelings of nervousness, depression and irritability experienced by some women in the days before their menstrual periods. Emotional and physical symptoms usually disappear with the onset of menstruation.

**premolar teeth** a bicuspid tooth in front of the molars on each side of the upper and lower jaws. *See* DENTITION

**prenatal** preceding birth; antenatal. *P. care* of the pregnant woman before delivery of the infant.

**prepuce** foreskin; the loose fold of skin covering the glans penis.

**presbyopia** diminution of accommodation of the lens of the eye, due to a loss of elasticity, occurring normally with ageing and usually resulting in hyperopia, or farsightedness.

**prescribed diseases** a group of occupational diseases on an annually reviewed official listing, e.g. pneumoconiosis or occupational deafness, that give the sufferers legal entitlement to financial benefits.

**prescribing analyses and cost** abbreviated PACT. Data on the prescribing of drugs in primary care.

**prescription** a formula written by a medically qualified doctor, and in some instances a specially qualified nurse (*see* prescribing by nurses, midwives and specialist community public health nurses in Appendix 3), directing the pharmacist to supply the medication. Also contains instructions to the patient indicating how the medication is to be taken.

**prescription-only medicines** abbreviated POMs. Drugs and medicines that are not available 'over the counter' and can only be obtained by prescription from the pharmacist.

**presenile** prematurely aged in mind and body. *See* DEMENTIA.

**presentation** in obstetrics, that portion of the fetus that appears in the centre of the neck of the uterus (*see* Figure on p. 321).

**pressure** stress or strain. The force exerted by one object upon another. *P. areas* areas of the body where the tissues may be compressed between the bed and the underlying bone, especially the sacrum, greater trochanters and heels; the tissues become ischaemic (*see* Figure on p. 322). *P. garment* often used in the treatment of burns and scalds to reduce scarring. Made of Lycra (a strong, synthetic, slightly elastic fibre), the garment is worn by the patient to exert firm pressure on the affected area. *P. group* an organization or charitable association that seeks to pressurize local and central government to advance the interests of that group. *P. point* the point at which an artery can be compressed against a bone in order to stop bleeding (*see* Figure on p. 323). *P. ulcer* a decubitus ulcer; a bedsore. Ulceration of the skin due to pressure, which causes interference with the blood supply to the area. Causes localized damage to the skin and underlying tissue due to pressure, shear, friction or a combination of these. *P. ulcer assessment scales* regular assessment of the patient's nutrition, general condition especially of the skin and pressure areas, is focal in the prevention of pressure ulcers. Pressure ulcer risk assessment scales are used to monitor and record data for the nursing care plan. *Braden scale* a pressure ulcer assessment scale mainly used in North America, similar to the Norton scale. *Norton scale* pressure ulcer risk assessment scale devised by Norton, McLaren and Exton Smith in the UK. Used primarily in the care of elderly patients and reviewed on a weekly basis. It comprises five health state components, each with a four-point descending scale. Maximum points are 20 and the minimum five; a 'score' of 14 and below indicates

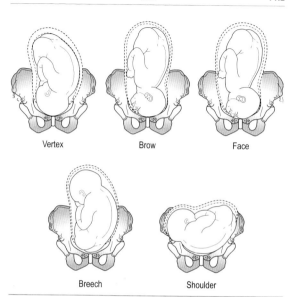

Vertex          Brow          Face

Breech          Shoulder

FETAL PRESENTATIONS

that the patient is at risk of developing pressure sores and needs 1–2-hourly changes of posture and the use of pressure-relieving aids. *Waterlow scale* a comprehensive scale which recognizes that there are many factors influencing the development of pressure ulcers. Waterlow's scale includes such factors as physique (weight/height), mobility, sex, age and other influencing factors such as medication, surgery and neurological deficits.

**presystole** the period in the cardiac cycle just before systole.

**preterm** before term, i.e. before the 37th completed week of pregnancy. *P. infant* baby born before 37 weeks' gestation. The baby will be of low birth weight, but may also be small for gestational age. Gestational age is assessed using the Dubowitz score. Preterm infants are prone to respiratory distress syndrome, feeding problems due to immature sucking, swallowing and coughing reflexes, hypothermia, jaundice and infection. There is also the risk of a poor maternal–infant relationship due to the baby's prolonged admission to the neonatal intensive care unit. *P. labour* labour that occurs before 37 weeks' gestation. It may occur spontaneously as a result of changing hormone levels, an overstretched uterus or weak cervix or due to infection; the obstetrician may attempt to

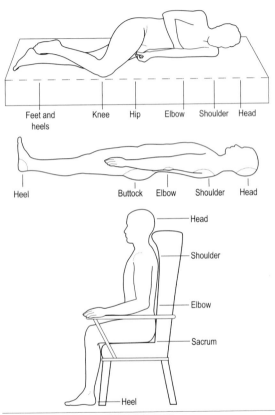

PRESSURE AREAS

arrest labour by the administration of tocolytic drugs until conditions are more favourable for the baby to be born. Labour may be induced before term because of poor maternal or fetal health, and thus the extrauterine environment will be less hazardous for the infant.

**prevalence** the number of persons who have a specific disease

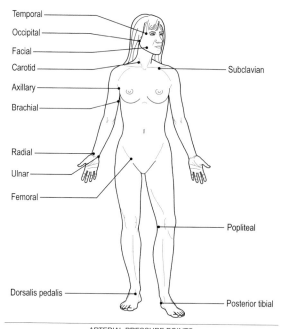

Temporal
Occipital
Facial
Carotid
Axillary
Brachial
Radial
Ulnar
Femoral
Dorsalis pedalis

Subclavian
Popliteal
Posterior tibial

ARTERIAL PRESSURE POINTS

or condition that are present in a defined population at one specific point in time. *See* INCIDENCE.

**preventative** serving to avert the occurrence of; prophylactic.

**priapism** persistent erection of the penis, usually without sexual desire. It may be caused by local or spinal cord injury.

**prickly heat** miliaria; heat rash. A skin eruption characterized by minute red spots with central vesicles.

**primary** first in order of time or importance.

**primary care** the level of care in the HEALTH CARE SYSTEM that consists of initial care outside institutions. *P. C. Trusts* abbreviated PCTs. A grouping of general practitioners and their services within a defined area. PCTs provide a direct means by which general practitioners (and their primary care teams) and community nurses working in cooperation with other health and social care professionals will lead the process of securing appropriate, high-quality care for local people. Responsible also for the commissioning of health services as well as the promotion of good health, combating inequalities in health in partnership with other agencies, developing and planning primary care services and integrating primary, community and social services.

**primary health care** the care given to individuals in the community at the first point of contact with the primary health care team. First contact may be the general practitioner, a health visitor, paramedic or a district nurse. *P. h. c. team* usually made up of a general practitioner, district nurse, health visitors and paramedical staff, such as a physiotherapist. They may serve a geographical area and be based in a health centre or a general practice area.

**primary nurse** a nurse who is responsible for the planning, implementation and evaluation of nursing care for assigned patients and their families for the duration of the patients' stay in hospital. The primary nurse delegates to an associate nurse when off duty but the primary nurse remains responsible and accountable for the patient's nursing care.

**primary nursing** a system for delivering nursing care that consists of four design elements: (a) allocation and acceptance of individual responsibility for decision-making to/by one individual; (b) individual assignment of daily care; (c) direct communication channels; and (d) one person responsible for the quality of care administered to patients on a unit 24 hours a day, 7 days a week.

**primary source** in a research study, the original source of data, e.g. manuscripts, documents or firsthand accounts. Primary sources are preferred over secondary sources because of the reduced potential for bias and distortion beyond the control of the researcher.

**primigravida** a woman who is pregnant for the first time.

**primipara** a woman who has given birth to her first child.

**prion** tiny protein-based infectious agent similar to a virus. Prions transmit diseases, including Creutzfeldt–Jakob disease in humans and bovine spongiform encephalopathy (BSE) in cattle. Prions do not contain nucleic acids and are difficult to destroy.

**Private Finance Initiative** abbreviated PFI. An agreement between the private and public sector whereby a health care facility, e.g. a hospital, is built using private funding. The facility is then leased to the NHS Trust. The lease agreement may also contain provision for the delivery of on-site services.

**probability** a statistical term meaning the likelihood of an association between variables being due to chance.

**probity** honesty and decency: one of the three foundations of public service. There should be an absolute standard of honesty in dealing with the assets of the NHS.

**problem-oriented record** a multiprofessional approach to patient care record-keeping that focuses on the patient's specific health problems requiring immediate attention, and the structuring of a health care plan designed to cope with the identified problems.

**process** in anatomy, a prominence or outgrowth of any part. *P. of nursing see* NURSING (PROCESS).

**procidentia** complete prolapse of an organ, particularly the uterus so that the cervix extrudes through the vagina.

**proctalgia** pain in the rectum and anus; proctodynia.

**proctitis** inflammation of the rectum.

**proctosigmoiditis** inflammation of the rectum and sigmoid colon.

**prodrome** a symptom that appears before the true diagnostic signs of a disease.

**prodrug** a compound that, on administration, must undergo chemical conversion by metabolic processes before becoming an active pharmacological agent, thus avoiding gastrointestinal side-effects.

**profession** 1. an avowed, public declaration or statement of intention or purpose. 2. a calling or vocation requiring specialized knowledge, methods and skills, as well as preparation, in an institution of higher learning, in the scholarly, scientific and historical principles underlying such methods and skills. Members of a profession are committed to continuing study, to enlarging their body of knowledge, to placing service above personal gain and to providing practical services vital to human and social welfare. A profession functions autonomously and is committed to higher standards of achievement and conduct.

**professional** 1. pertaining to one's profession or occupation. 2. one who is a specialist in a particular field or occupation. *Allied health p.* a person with special training, and licensed when necessary, who works closely with other health professionals with responsibilities bearing on patient care. *P. disciplinary process* complaints against nurses from members of the public or an employer are reported to the statutory regulatory body (*see* P. SELF-REGULATION below). The professional conduct of the nurse is then investigated and judged by peers. The ultimate sanction is that the nurse is removed from the professional register. *P. organization* an organization formed to deal with issues of mutual concern for its members who share common goals and professional status (*see* PRESSURE GROUP). *P. self-regulation* the means whereby a profession monitors its own standards for quality and continuing professional and educational development. Professional regulatory bodies include the General Medical Council for medically qualified practitioners, the Nursing and Midwifery Council for nurses and midwives and the Health Professions Council for dieticians, physiotherapists, etc.

**profile** 1. a simple outline, as of the side view of the head or face; by extension, a graph representing quantitatively a set of characteristics determined by tests. 2. a record of achievements developed during a course of study, or subsequently. *See* PORTFOLIO.

**progeny** issue. Descendants.

**progeria** premature ageing the signs of which appear in childhood.

**progesterone** a hormone of the corpus luteum which plays an important part in the regulation of the menstrual cycle and in pregnancy.

**progestogen** one of a group of steroid hormones having an action similar to that of progesterone.

**prognathism** enlargement and protrusion of one or both jaws.

**prognosis** a forecast of the probable course and outcome of an attack of disease and the prospects of recovery, as indicated by the nature of the disease and the symptoms of the case. *Nursing p.* the application of information obtained during a nursing assessment in order to determine the prospect for altering, through nursing intervention, a client's/patient's response to illness or injury. The prognosis provides a rationale for setting priorities for meeting a particular client's/patient's nursing care needs and enhances continuity of nursing care by clearly indicating agreed priorities.

**projectile vomiting** *see* VOMITING.

**projection** in psychology, an unconscious process by which painful thoughts or impulses are made acceptable by transferring them on to another person or object in the environment.

**prolactin** a milk-producing hormone of the anterior lobe of the pituitary body which stimulates the mammary gland.

**prolapse** the downward displacement of an organ or part of one. *P. of the cord* expulsion of the umbilical cord before the fetus presents. *P. of an intervertebral disc* abbreviated PID. Displacement of part of an intervertebral disc; 'slipped disc'. *P. of the iris* protrusion of a part of the iris through a wound in the cornea. *P. of the rectum* protrusion of the mucous membrane through the anal canal to the exterior. *P. of the uterus* descent of the cervix or of the whole uterus into the vagina owing to a weakening of its supporting ligaments.

**proliferation** rapid multiplication of cells, as may occur in a malignant growth and in wound healing.

**prominence** in anatomy, a projection, usually on a bone.

**pronation** turning the palm of the hand downwards.

**prone** lying face downwards *See* SUPINE.

**prophylactic** 1. relating to prophylaxis. 2. a drug used to prevent a disease developing. *See* PREVENTATIVE.

**prophylaxis** measures taken to prevent a disease.

**proprietary name** the name assigned to a drug or device by the manufacturer that first made it.

**proprioceptor** one of the sensory end-organs that provide information about movements and position of the body. They occur chiefly in the muscles, tendons, joint capsules and labyrinth.

**proptosis** forward displacement of the eyeball; exophthalmus.

**prostaglandin** one of several hormone substances produced in many body tissues, including the brain, lungs, uterus and semen. They are active in many ways, having cardiac, gastric and respiratory effects and causing uterine contractions. They are sometimes used for the induction of abortion. Chemically they are fatty acids.

**prostate** the gland surrounding the male urethra at its junction with the bladder; during ejaculation it produces a fluid which forms part of the semen. It often becomes enlarged after middle age and may require removal if it causes obstruction to the outflow of urine. *P. cancer* of unknown cause and one of the most common cancers in men, usually occuring in older men. Treatments include surgery, radiotherapy, chemotherapy and hormone therapy. *P. screening* routine examination and blood testing for prostate-specific antigen (PSA) in older men, as a means to detect cancer of the prostate at an early stage.

**prostatectomy** surgical removal of the whole or a part of the prostate gland. *Retropubic p.* removal of the gland by incising the capsule of the prost after making a suprapubic abdominal incision. *Transurethral p.* resection of the gland through the urethra using a resectoscope. *Transvesical p.* removal of the gland by incising the bladder after making a low abdominal incision.

**prostatitis** inflammation of the prostate gland.

**prosthesis** 1. the replacement of an absent part by an artificial substitute. 2. an artificial substitute for a missing part.

**prostration** a condition of extreme exhaustion.

**protease** a proteolytic enzyme in the digestive juices that causes the breakdown of protein.

**protective isolation** a type of ISOLATION designed to prevent contact between potentially pathogenic microorganisms and uninfected persons who have seriously impaired resistance. Also called reverse isolation.

**protein** one of a group of complex organic nitrogenous compounds formed from amino acids and occurring in every living cell of animal and vegetable tissue. *Bence Jones p.* an abnormal protein found in the urine of patients suffering from multiple myeloma. *First-class p.* one that provides the essential amino acids. Sources are meat, poultry, fish, cheese, eggs and milk. *P.-bound iodine* the iodine in the plasma that is combined with protein. Measurement of this is made when assessing thyroid function. *P.-losing enteropathy* a condition in which protein is lost from the lumen of the intestine. This causes hypoproteinaemia and oedema. *Second-class p.* one that comes from a vegetable source (e.g. peas, beans and whole cereal) that cannot supply all the body's needs.

**proteinuria** an excess of serum proteins in the urine.

**proteolysis** the processes by which proteins are reduced to an absorbable form by digestive enzymes in the stomach and intestines.

**proteolytic** 1. pertaining to, characterized by, or promoting proteolysis. 2. a proteolytic enzyme.

*Proteus* a genus of Gram-negative bacteria common in the intestines of humans and animals and in decaying matter. They are frequently to be found in secondary infections of wounds and in the urinary tract.

**prothrombin** a constituent of blood plasma, the precursor of thrombin, which is formed in the presence of calcium salts and thrombokinase when blood is shed. *P. time* a test to measure the activity of clotting factors. Deficiency of any of these factors leads to a prolongation of clotting time. This test is widely used for the establishment and maintenance of anticoagulant therapy.

**protocol** a term used by researchers to indicate the method or overall plan for procedures to be carried out in a particular study. Commonly used to indicate a specific programme to be followed or with exclusion criteria for the study.

**protoplasm** the essential chemical compound of which living cells are made.

**prototype** the original form from which all other forms are derived.

**Protozoa** a phylum comprising the unicellular eukaryotic organisms; most are free-living but some lead commensalistic, mutualistic or parasitic existences. Pathogenic protozoa include *Entamoeba histolytica* (cause of amoebic dysentery) and *Plasmodium vivax* (cause of malaria). *See* METAZOA.

**protuberance** in anatomy, a rounded projecting part.

**proud flesh** excessive granulation tissue in a wound or ulcer.

**provider** in the health services, a person, group of people or organization supplying a service.

**provitamin** a precursor of a vitamin. *P. 'A'* carotene. *P. 'D'* ergosterol.

**proxemics** the study of how the use of personal space and other spatial aspects affects human behaviour and interactions.

**proximal** in anatomy, nearest that point which is considered the centre of a system; the opposite to distal.

**prurigo** a chronic skin disease with an irritating papular eruption.

**pruritus** great irritation of the skin. It may affect the whole surface of the body, as in certain skin diseases and nervous disorders, or it may be limited in area, especially involving the anus and vulva.

**pseudoangina** false angina. Precordial pain occurring in anxious individuals without evidence of organic heart disease.

**pseudoarthrosis** a false joint formed when the two parts of a fractured bone have failed to unite together.

**pseudocoxalgia** osteochondritis of the head of the femur. Perthes' disease.

**pseudocyesis** false pregnancy; development of all the signs of pregnancy without the presence of an embryo.

**pseudogynaecomastia** the deposition of adipose tissue in the male breast which may give the appearance of enlarged mammary glands.

**pseudohermaphroditism** a congenital abnormality in which the external genitalia are characteristic of the opposite sex and confusion may arise as to the true sex of the individual.

*Pseudomonas* a genus of Gramnegative motile bacilli commonly found in decaying organic matter. *P. aeruginosa* found in pus from wounds ('blue pus') and also in urinary tract infections. Also called *P. pyocyanea.*

**pseudomyopia** spasm of the ciliary muscle causing the same focusing defect as in myopia.

**psittacosis** a disease of parrots and budgerigars due to *Chlamydia psittaci,* communicable to humans. The symptoms resemble paratyphoid fever with bronchopneumonia.

**psoas** a long muscle originating from the lumbar spine and inserting into the lesser trochanter of the femur. It flexes the hip joint. *P. abscess* one that arises in the lumbar region and is due to spinal caries as a result of tuberculous infection.

**psoriasis** a chronic, recurrent skin disease characterized by reddish marginated patches with profuse silvery scaling on extensor surfaces, such as the knees and elbow, but which may be more widespread and may be associated with arthritis of the joints. It is non-infectious and the cause is unknown. It tends to occur in families; about one-third of cases are believed to be related to a hereditary factor. Psoriasis may present in different forms. The most common is discoid or plague psoriasis in adults. Guttate psoriasis occurs most commonly in children, consisting of small patches that may develop over a wide area of the body. Pustular psoriasis is characterized by small pustules.

**psyche** the mind, both conscious and unconscious.

**psychedelic** mind-altering; a term applied to hallucinatory or psychotomimetic drugs capable of profound effects upon the nature of the perception and conscious experience. *See also* HALLUCINOGEN.

**psychiatrist** a medically qualified doctor who specializes in psychiatry.

**psychiatry** the branch of medicine that deals with the treatment and prevention of mental illness.

**psychoanalysis** 1. a method of investigating mental processes, developed by Sigmund Freud, which uses the techniques of free association, interpretation and dream analysis. 2. a system of theoretical psychology, formulated by Freud, based on the recognition of unconscious mental processes, such as resistance, repression and transference, and of the importance of infantile experience as a determinant of adult behaviour. 3.

a method of psychotherapy based on the psychoanalytic method and psychoanalytical psychology.

**psychoanalyst** one who specializes in psychoanalysis.

**psychodrama** group PSYCHOTHERAPY in which patients dramatize their individual conflicting situations of daily life.

**psychodynamics** the understanding and interpretation of psychiatric symptoms or abnormal behaviour in terms of unconscious mental mechanisms.

**psychogenic** originating in the mind. *P. illness* a disorder that has a psychological as opposed to an organic origin.

**psychologist** one who studies normal and abnormal mental processes, development and behaviour.

**psychology** the study of the mind and mental processes.

**psychometrics** the measurement of mental characteristics by means of a series of tests.

**psychomotor** related to the motor effects of mental activity. The term is applied to those mental disorders that affect muscular activity.

**psychoneurosis** a mental disorder characterized by an abnormal mental response to a normal stimulus. The psychoneuroses include anxiety states, depression, hysteria and obsessive-compulsive neurosis.

**psychopath** see PERSONALITY (ANTI-SOCIAL).

**psychopathic disorder** a persistent disorder or disability of the mind (whether or not including significant impairment of intelligence) which results in abnormally aggressive or seriously irresponsible conduct on the part of the patient (Mental Health Act 1983).

**psychopathology** the study of the causes and processes of mental disorders.

**psychopharmacology** the study of drugs that have an action on the

mind, and how such action is produced.

**psychoprophylaxis** 1. a psychological technique used to prevent emotional disturbances and mental health problems. 2. a technique involving breathing control and exercises used to relieve pain during childbirth.

**psychosexual** relating to the mental aspects of sex. *P. development* the stages through which an individual passes from birth to full maturity, especially in regard to sexual urges, in the total development of the person. *P. counselling* a service provided primarily outside the NHS for otherwise 'healthy' people who seek help because of failure to achieve emotional and sexual satisfaction within a relationship.

**psychosis** any major mental disorder of organic or emotional origin, marked by derangement of the personality and loss of contact with reality, often with delusions, hallucinations or illusions. Psychoses are usually classified as functional psychoses, those for which no physical cause has been discovered, and organic psychoses, which are the result of organic damage to the brain.

**psychosomatic** relating to the mind and the body. *P. disorders* those illnesses in some individuals in which emotional factors (either causative or aggravating) have a profound influence, including anorexia nervosa and asthma respectively.

**psychotherapy** any of a number of related techniques for treating mental illness by psychological methods. These techniques are similar in that they all rely mainly on establishing communication between the therapist and the patient as a means of understanding and modifying the patient's behaviour. On occasion, drugs may be used, but only in order to make this communication easier.

**psychotrophic** pertaining to drugs that have an effect on the psyche. These include antidepressants, stimulants, sedatives and tranquillizers.

**ptosis** 1. drooping of the upper eyelid due to paralysis of the third cranial nerve. It may be congenital or acquired. 2. prolapse of an organ.

**ptyalin** an enzyme (amylase) in saliva which metabolizes starches.

**puberty** the period during which secondary sexual characteristics develop and the reproductive organs become functional. Generally between the 12th and 17th years.

**pubes** pubic hair or the area on which it grows.

**pubic** pertaining to the pubis.

**pubis** the anterior part of a hip bone. The left and right pubic bones meet at the front of the pelvis at the pubic symphysis.

**public domain** intellectual property, e.g. published documents, programs or files, usually from government sources and other organizations, that have been released for unconditional access and use by the public.

**public health** the field of medicine that is concerned with safeguarding and improving the physical, mental and social wellbeing of the community as a whole. Environmental aspects are the responsibility of the district local authority, whereas communicable disease control is supervised by the Medical Officer for Environmental Health, from the District Health Authority. Central government formulates national policy and is responsible for international aspects. *P. h. laboratory service* a central service which aims to protect the public from infection and prevent the spread of infectious disease through a network of over 50 laboratories in the UK that provide the necessary resources for investigation, diagnosis and testing in suspected cases or in outbreaks of infectious disease. *See* HEALTH PROTECTION AGENCY. *P. h. nurse* one who works within a community service in a variety of settings promoting good health and the prevention of ill health, e.g. a health visitor, school nurse or practice nurse.

**pudendal block** a form of local analgesia induced by injecting a solution of 0.5% or 1% lignocaine around the pudendal nerve. Used mainly for episiotomy and forceps delivery.

**pudendum** the external genitalia, especially those of a woman.

**puerperal** pertaining to childbirth. *P. fever* or *sepsis* infection of the genital tract following childbirth.

**puerperium** a period of about 6 weeks following childbirth when the reproductive organs are returning to their normal state.

*Pulex* a genus of fleas. *P. irritans* those parasitic on humans. The type that infests rats may transmit plague to humans.

**pulmonary** pertaining to or affecting the lungs. *P. embolism* obstruction of the pulmonary artery or one of its branches by an embolus. *P. hypertension* an increase of blood pressure in the lungs, usually as a result of disease of the lung. *P. oedema* an excess of fluid in the lungs. *P. stenosis* a narrowing of the passage between the right ventricle of the heart and the pulmonary artery. The condition is frequently congenital. *P. tuberculosis see* TUBERCULOSIS. *P. valve* the valve at the point where the pulmonary artery leaves the heart.

**pulp** any soft, juicy animal or vegetable tissue. *Digital p.* the soft pads at the ends of the fingers and toes. *P. cavity* the centre of a tooth containing blood tissue and nerves.

*Splenic p.* the reddish-brown tissue of the spleen.

**pulsation**    a beating or throbbing.

**pulse**    the local rhythmic expansion of an artery, which can be felt with the finger, corresponding to each contraction of the left ventricle of the heart. It may be felt in any artery sufficiently near the surface of the body, which passes over a bone, and the normal adult rate is about 72 beats/min. In childhood it is more rapid, varying from 130 in infants to 80 in older children. *Alternating p.* alternate strong and weak beats; pulsus alternans. *High-tension p.* cordy pulse. The duration of the impulse in the artery is long, and the artery feels firm and like a cord between the beats. *Paradoxical p.* pulsus paradoxus; the pulse rate slows on inspiration and quickens on expiration. It may occur in constrictive pericarditis. *P. deficit* a sign of atrial fibrillation; the pulse rate is slower than the apex beat. *P. oximetry* a non-invasive method for measuring haemoglobin oxygen saturation in the body using a sensor from an oximeter that is attached, usually to a finger but may be elsewhere, e.g. nose, finger or ear lobe. *Running p.* there is little distinction between the beats. It occurs in haemorrhage. *Thready p.* thin and almost imperceptible pressure. *Venous p.* that felt in a vein; it is usually taken in the right jugular vein.

**pulseless disease**    progressive obliteration of the vessels arising from the aortic arch, leading to loss of the pulse in both arms and carotids and to symptoms associated with ischaemia of the brain, eyes, face and arms.

**punctate**    dotted. *P. erythema* a rash of very fine spots.

**punctum**    a point or small spot. *P. lacrimalis* one of the two openings of the lacrimal ducts at the inner canthus of the eye.

**puncture**    1. the act of piercing with a sharp object. 2. the wound so produced. *Cisternal p.* the withdrawal of fluid from the cisterna magna. *Lumbar p.* the removal of cerebrospinal fluid by puncture between the third and fourth lumbar vertebrae. *Sternal p.* the withdrawal of bone marrow from the manubrium of the sternum. *Ventricular p.* the withdrawal of cerebrospinal fluid from a cerebral ventricle.

**pupil**    the circular aperture in the centre of the iris, through which light passes into the eye. *Argyll Robertson p.* absence of response to light but not to accommodation; characteristic of syphilis of the central nervous system. *Artificial p.* one made by cutting a piece out of the iris when the centre part of the cornea or the lens is opaque. *Fixed p.* one that fails to respond to light or convergence. *Multiple p.* two or more openings of the iris. *Tonic p.* one that reacts slowly to light or to convergence or both.

**pupillary**    referring to the pupil.

**purchaser**    in the health services, a budget-holder (e.g. a Primary Care Trust) who agrees to buy a service from a PROVIDER. *See* COMMISSIONING

**purgative**    a laxative; an aperient drug. Purgatives may be: (a) irritants, like cascara, senna, rhubarb and castor oil; (b) lubricants, like liquid paraffin; (c) mechanical agents that increase bulk, like bran and agar preparations.

**purine**    a heterocyclic compound that is the nucleus of the purine bases such as adenine and guanine, which occur in DNA and RNA. *See* PYRIMIDINE.

**purpura**    a condition characterized by extravasation of blood in the skin and mucous membranes, causing purple spots and patches.

There are two general types of purpura: primary or idiopathic (usually autoimmune) thrombocytopenic purpura, in which the cause is unknown; and secondary or symptomatic thrombocytopenic purpura, which may be associated with exposure to drugs or other chemical agents, systemic diseases such as systemic lupus erythematosus, diseases affecting the bone marrow, such as leukaemia, and infections such as septicaemia and viral infections. *Allergic p.*, anaphylactic *p.* Schönlein–Henoch purpura; also called Henoch–Schönlein. *Idiopathic thrombocytopenic p.* abbreviated ITP. An acquired thrombocytopenia which may be acute or chronic in its course. Acute ITP is common in young children. The disorder is usually self-limiting and rarely fatal. Chronic ITP is more insidious in onset, and is more common in young adult women. *P. senilis* dark purplish-red ecchymoses occurring on the forearms and backs of the hands in the elderly; the platelet count is normal. *Schönlein–Henoch p.* non-thrombocytopenic purpura of unknown cause, most often seen in children; associated with various clinical symptoms, such as urticaria and erythema, arthropathy and arthritis, gastrointestinal symptoms and renal involvement. *Steroid p.* purpura secondary to prolonged use of steroids. The platelet count is normal, the basic defect being the loss of supporting connective tissue. *Thrombocytopenic p.* purpura associated with a decrease in the number of platelets in the blood.

**purulent** containing or resembling pus.

**pus** a thick, yellow semiliquid substance consisting of dead leukocytes and bacteria, debris of cells, and tissue fluids. It results from inflammation caused by invading bacteria, mainly *Staphylococcus aureus* and *Streptococcus haemolyticus*, which have destroyed the phagocytes and set up local suppuration. *Blue p.* that produced by infection with *Pseudomonas pyocyanea.*

**pustule** a small pimple or elevation of the skin containing pus. *Malignant p. see* ANTHRAX.

**putative** supposed, reputed. *P. father* the man believed to be the father of an illegitimate child.

**putrefaction** decomposition of animal or vegetable matter under the influence of microorganisms, usually accompanied by an offensive odour due to gas formation.

*P* **value** the symbol used to denote the probability of test results occurring by chance.

**pyaemia** a condition resulting from the circulation of pyogenic microorganisms from some focus of infection. Multiple abscesses occur, the development of which causes rigor and high fever. *Portal p.* pylephlebitis.

**pyarthrosis** suppuration in a joint.

**pyelography** *see* UROGRAPHY.

**pyelolithotomy** the surgical removal of a stone from the renal pelvis.

**pyelonephritis** inflammation of the renal pelvis and renal substance, characterized by fever, acute loin pain and increased frequency of micturition, with the presence of pus and albumin in the urine.

**pyeloplasty** plastic repair of the renal pelvis.

**pylephlebitis** inflammation of the portal vein which gives rise to severe symptoms of septicaemia or pyaemia.

**pyloric** relating to the pylorus. *P. stenosis* stricture of the pyloric orifice. It may be: (a) hypertrophic, when there is thickening of normal tissue; this is congenital and occurs in infants from 4–7 weeks old, usually males and first babies; (b) cicatricial, when there is ulceration or a malignant growth near the pylorus.

**pyloromyotomy** Ramstedt's operation; an incision of the pylorus performed to relieve congenital pyloric stenosis.

**pyloroplasty** plastic operation on the pylorus to enlarge the outlet. A longitudinal incision is made and it is resutured transversely (*see* Figure).

**pylorospasm** forceful muscle contraction of the pylorus which delays emptying of the stomach and causes vomiting.

**pylorus** the opening into the duodenum at the lower end of the stomach. It is surrounded by a circular muscle, the *pyloric sphincter*, which contracts to close the opening.

**pyoderma** any purulent skin disease, e.g. impetigo.

**pyogenic** producing pus.

**pyorrhoea** a discharge of pus. *P. alveolaris* pus in the sockets of the teeth; suppurative periodontitis.

**pyramidal** of pyramid shape. *P. cells* cortical cells shaped like a pyramid from which originate nerve impulses to voluntary muscle. *P. tract* the nerve fibres that transmit impulses from pyramidal cells through the cerebral cortex to the spinal cord.

**pyrexia** fever; a rise of body temperature to any point between 37 and 40°C; above this is hyperpyrexia.

**pyrimidine** a nitrogen-containing organic compound. Thymine and cytosine are essential constituents of DNA, and uracil and cytosine of RNA. *See* PURINE.

**pyrixodine** vitamin $B_6$. This vitamin is concerned with protein metabolism and blood formation. It is found in many types of food and deficiency is rare.

**pyrogen** a substance that can produce fever.

PYLOROPLASTY

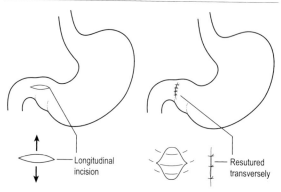

Longitudinal incision

Resutured transversely

**pyromania** an irresistible desire to set things on fire.

**pyrosis** heartburn; a symptom of indigestion marked by a burning sensation in the stomach and oesophagus with eructation of acid fluid.

**pyuria** the presence of pus in the urine; more than three leukocytes per high-power field on microscopic examination.

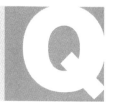

**QALY** quality adjusted life year.

**Q fever** an acute infectious disease of cattle which is transmitted to humans, usually by infected milk. It is caused by a rickettsia, *Coxiella burnetii*, and has symptoms resembling pneumonia.

**qi energy** in Chinese medicine, the energy believed to be present in all living things. Qi energy is considered to flow through 12 meridian channels in the body mainly connected to the internal organs, and considered essential to good health and wellbeing. This concept is used in a variety of complementary therapies, e.g. reflexology and acupuncture. Complementary therapy practitioners consider that any disturbance or blockage to the flow of qi energy results in illness or bodily and mental disturbance but that with manipulation, e.g. through acupuncture, the qi flow can be increased. Also called chi, prana and aura.

**QRS complex** a group of waves depicted on an electrocardiogram; also called the QRS wave. It actually consists of three distinct waves created by the passage of the cardiac electrical impulse through the ventricles and occurs at the beginning of each contraction of the ventricles (*see* Figure on p. 336). In a normal ELECTROCARDIOGRAM the R wave is the most prominent of the three; the Q and S waves may be extremely weak and are sometimes absent.

**quadriceps** four-headed. *Q. femoris muscle* the principal extensor muscle of the thigh.

**quadriplegia** paralysis in which all four limbs are affected; tetraplegia.

**quadruplets** four children born at the same labour. Once very rare, but now more common with the use of fertility drugs.

**qualitative research** a research method widely used in sociology, psychology and anthropology. It is a method that uses a systematic subjective approach to describe life experiences and to give them meaning. In nursing and health care it is used to promote understanding of human experiences of pain, caring and comfort. *See also* QUANTITATIVE RESEARCH.

**quality** 1. a distinguishing characteristic, property or attribute. 2. a degree or standard of excellence. *Q. adjusted life year* abbreviated QALY. A measure which assesses variations in the quality of life for the patient resulting from an intervention, in relation to cost and length of life. Used for measuring the clinical and cost effectiveness of interventions. *Q. assurance* in the health care field, a pledge to the public by those within the various health disciplines that they will work towards the goal of an optimal achievable degree of excellence that is measured and evaluated in the services rendered to every patient. *See* COST EFFECTIVENESS

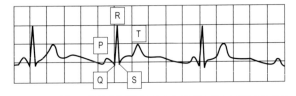

A NORMAL ELECTROCARDIOGRAM SHOWING THE QRS COMPLEX

and PERFORMANCE INDICATORS. **Q. Assurance Agency** organization which approves higher education institutions offering courses and awards. Monitors delivery of subjects in universities. Has established codes of practice and guidance for programme development, and a contract with the Department of Health to carry out subject review in England. **Q. circle** a group of health care workers from differing levels within an organization who meet regularly to discuss ways in which they can improve their service and raise standards. **Q. indicator** a defined, measurable variable used to monitor the quality or appropriateness of an important aspect of care. Indicators may be activities, events, occurrences or outcomes. **Q. systems audit** International and British Standards in Quality Systems. An audit programme used to monitor quality in organizations providing health care.

**quality and outcomes framework** a system of standards, incentives and assessment for GP practices.

**quango** a form of government agency used to provide services or to carry out other duties determined by government. Originally an acronym for 'quasi-autonomous non-governmental organization', which initially comprised voluntary and non-profit organizations but became increasingly dependent upon government grants.

**quantitative research** a formal objective systematic approach to research in which numerical data are utilized to obtain information. It is used to describe variables, examine relationships among variables and to determine cause and effect interactions between variables. Some researchers believe this form of research provides a sounder knowledge base to nursing and midwifery practice than QUALITATIVE RESEARCH.

**quarantine** the period of isolation of an infectious or suspected case, to prevent the spread of disease. For contacts, this is the longest incubation period known for the specific disease.

**quartan** 1. recurring in 4-day cycles (every third day). 2. a variety of intermittent fever of which the paroxysms recur on every third day (see MALARIA).

**Queckenstedt's test** *H.H.G. Queckenstedt, German physician, 1876–1918.* A test, carried out during lumbar puncture, by compression of the jugular veins. When normal there is a sharp rise in pressure, followed by a fall as the compression is released. Blockage of the spinal canal or thrombosis of the jugular vein will result in an absence of rise, or only a sluggish rise and fall.

**quickening** the first perceptible fetal movement, felt by the mother usually between the fourth and fifth months of pregnancy.

**quiescent** inactive or at rest. Descriptive of a time when the symptoms of a disease are not evident.

**quinsy** a peritonsillar abscess; acute inflammation of the tonsil and surrounding cellular tissue with suppuration.

**quintuplets** five children born at the same labour.

**quotidian** recurring every day. *Q. fever* a variety of malaria in which the fever recurs daily.

**quotient** a number obtained by dividing one number by another.

*Intelligence q.* abbreviated IQ. The degree of intelligence estimated by dividing the mental age, reckoned from standard tests, by the age in years. *Respiratory q.* the ratio between the carbon dioxide expired and the oxygen inspired during a specified time.

**qwerty** the standard typewriter keyboard layout that is also used for computers with some additions.

# R

**R** symbol for the *roentgen* unit.

**Ra** symbol for *radium*.

**rabid** infected with rabies.

**rabies** hydrophobia; an acute notifiable infectious disease of the central nervous system of animals, especially dogs, foxes, wolves and bats. The virus is found in the saliva of infected animals and is usually transmitted by a bite. Symptoms include fever, muscle spasms and intense excitement, followed by convulsions and paralysis, and death usually occurs. Vaccines are available.

**race** a term formerly used to describe a group of people sharing the same culture, language, values and beliefs. The preferred terms are now ethnic group or ethnicity.

**racemose** grape-like *R. gland* a compound gland composed of a number of small sacs, e.g. the salivary gland.

**racism** the belief that races are inherently different from one another. A belief that is usually associated with the view that one race has an intrinsic superiority over others, leading to stereotyping, prejudice and discrimination. Also called racialism.

**radiant** emitting rays.

**radiation** the emanation of energy in the form of electromagnetic waves, including gamma rays, X-rays, infrared and ultraviolet rays, and visible light rays. Radiation may cause damage to living tissues, e.g. in sunburn. *R. dosimetry* the method used to calculate the amount of radiation received by an individual. Also called radiation monitoring. *Ionizing r.* a form of radiation that destabilizes an atom to produce highly reactive ions, e.g. X-rays, gamma rays and particle radiation. When used therapeutically ionizing radiation needs careful control and monitoring as it can cause tissue damage. *R. pneumonitis* inflammatory changes in the alveoli and interstitial tissue caused by radiation and which may lead to fibrosis later. *R. sickness* a toxic reaction of the body to radiation. Any or all of the following may be present: anorexia, nausea, vomiting and diarrhoea.

**radical** dealing with the root or cause of a disease. *R. cure* one which cures by complete removal of the cause.

**radioactivity** disintegration of certain elements to ones of lower atomic weight, with the emission of alpha and beta particles and gamma rays. *Induced r.* that brought about by bombarding the nuclei of certain elements with neutrons.

**radiobiology** the branch of medical science that studies the effect of radiation on live animal and human tissues.

**radiocolloid** a radioactive isotope, in the form of a large molecule solution, which can be instilled into the body cavities to treat malignant ascites.

**radiodermatitis** a late skin complication of radiotherapy in which there is atrophy, scarring, pigmentation and telangiectases of the skin.

**radiograph** skiagram; the picture obtained, on specially sensitized film, by passing X-rays through the body.

**radiographer** a professional health care worker in a diagnostic X-ray department (diagnostic radiographer) or in a radiotherapy department (therapy radiographer).

**radiography** the making of film records (radiographs) of internal structures of the body by exposure of film specially sensitized to X-rays or gamma rays. *Body-section r.* a special technique to show in detail images and structures lying in a predetermined plane of tissue, while blurring or eliminating detail in images in other planes; various mechanisms and methods for such radiography have been given various names, e.g. laminagraphy, tomography, etc. *Double-contrast r.* a technique for revealing an abnormality of the intestinal mucosa; it involves injection and evacuation of a barium enema, followed by inflation of the intestine with air under light pressure. *Neutron r.* that in which a narrow beam of neutrons from a nuclear reactor is passed through tissues; especially useful in visualizing bony tissue. *Serial r.* the making of several exposures of a particular area at arbitrary intervals.

**radioisotope** an isotope of an element that emits radioactivity. These isotopes may occur naturally or be produced artificially by bombardment with neutrons.

**radiologist** a medically qualified doctor who specializes in the science of radiology.

**radiology** the science of radiation. Using X-rays and other allied imaging techniques in the diagnosis and treatment of disease.

**radiomimetic** producing effects similar to those of ionizing radiations.

**radionuclide** a radioactive substance which is inherently unstable. It is used in both radiodiagnosis and in radiotherapy. *R. scanning* a diagnostic technique based on the detection of radiation emitted by radioactive substances introduced into the body. These substances are taken up by different tissues thus allowing specific organs to be studied, e.g. the thyroid gland following the administration of a radionuclide-tagged dose of iodine.

**radioscopy** the examination of X-ray images on a fluorescent screen.

**radiosensitive** pertaining to those structures that respond readily to radiotherapy.

**radiotherapist** a medically qualified doctor specializing in radiotherapy.

**radiotherapy** a method of treating disease and eradicating tumour cells by aiming to deliver a therapeutic dose of radiation while preserving normal tissue function and structure.

**radium** *symbol* Ra. A radioactive element, obtained from uranium ores, which gives off emanations of great radioactive power. Used in the treatment of some malignant diseases.

**RAI** relatives assessment interview.

**raised intracranial pressure** abbreviated RIP. May be associated with a variety of conditions, e.g. haemorrhage, oedema, brain tumour, head injury or disturbance to the flow of cerebrospinal fluid.

**râle** an abnormal rattling sound, heard on ausculation of the chest during respiration when there is fluid in the bronchi.

**Ramstedt's operation** *W.C. Ramstedt, German surgeon, 1867–1963.* A pyloroplasty for congenital stricture of the pylorus in which the fibres of the sphincter muscle are divided, leaving the mucous lining intact (*see* Figure on p. 333).

**random sample** a sample from a population, obtained by ensuring that each member of that population has an equal chance of being selected. The sample selected should then demonstrate the same profile as the parent population.

**randomized clinical trial** a study in which experimental and control groups are randomly selected for research. There are also a number of other synonyms for this term such as randomized trial, controlled clinical trial and true experiment.

**ranula** a retention cyst, usually under the tongue when blockage occurs in a submaxillary or sublingual duct, or in a mucous gland.

**rape** sexual assault or abuse; criminal forcible sexual intercourse (i.e. penetration) without the consent of the adult or child. Many cases are not reported because of feelings of shame, guilt, embarrassment or fear. Although rape can occur between men, it is usually associated with victims who are female.

**raphe** a seam or ridge of tissue indicating the junction of two parts.

**rapport** in psychiatry, a satisfactory relationship based upon respect, understanding and mutuality between two persons, either the doctor and patient or nurse and patient, or the patient with any significant other.

**rarefaction** the process of becoming less dense, e.g. in bone disease.

**rash** a superficial eruption on the skin, frequently characteristic of some specific fever.

**rate** the speed or frequency with which an event or circumstance occurs per unit of time, population, or other standard of comparison. *Basal metabolic r.* abbreviated BMR. An expression of the rate at which oxygen is utilized in a fasting subject at complete rest as a percentage of a value established as normal for such a subject. *Birth r.* the number of live births in a population in a specified period of time (crude birth rate), for the female population (refined birth rate), or for the female population of childbearing age (true birth rate), usually expressed per year per 1000 of the estimated mid-year population. *Death r.* the number of deaths per stated number of persons (1000, 10 000 or 100 000) in a certain region in a certain time (crude death rate). The death rate calculated with allowances made for age and sex distribution in the population is termed the standardized death rate. Also called *mortality rate. Glomerular filtration r.* an expression of the quantity of glomerular filtrate formed each minute in the nephrons of both kidneys, calculated by measuring the clearance of specific substances, e.g. insulin or creatinine.

**ratio** an expression of the quantity of one substance or entity in relation to that of another; the relationship between two quantities expressed as the quotient of one divided by the other. *Lecithin–sphingomyelin r.* the ratio of lecithin to sphingomyelin in amniotic fluid.

**rationalization** in psychiatry, the mental process by which individuals explain their behaviour, giving reasons that are advantageous to themselves or are socially acceptable. It may be a conscious or an unconscious act.

**Raynaud's phenomenon or disease** *M. Raynaud, French physician, 1834–1881.* Raynaud's phenomenon is characterized by episodic digital ischaemia provoked by stimuli such as emotion, cold, trauma, hormones and drugs. It includes both Raynaud's disease, where no underlying cause can be found, and Raynaud's syndrome, where there is an associated underlying disorder. These disorders include scleroderma, mixed connective tissue disease, systemic lupus erythematosus, polymyositis, rheumatoid arthritis, neurovascular entrapment syndromes and occlusive arterial disease.

**reaction** counteraction; a response to the application of a stimulus. *R. time* the interval between the stimulus and the response.

**reactive** in psychiatry, used to describe a mental condition brought about by adverse external circumstances. *R. depression* one that arises in this way and is not endogenous.

**reagent** a substance employed to produce a chemical reaction.

**reality** agreed as an absolute by members of the same culture as the total of all things related to perception, meaning and behaviour. Not imaginary, fictitious or pretended. *R. orientation see* ORIENTATION.

**real-time scanner** an ultrasound scanner that gives a moving visual display.

**recall** to bring back to consciousness.

**receptor** 1. a sensory nerve ending that receives stimuli for transmission through the sensory nervous system. 2. a molecule on the surface or within a cell that recognizes and binds with specific molecules, producing some effect in the cell.

**recessive** tending to recede. The opposite to dominant. *R. gene* a gene that will produce its characteristics only when present in a homozygous state; both parents need to possess the particular gene, and there is a 1 in 4 chance of a child inheriting it homozygously.

**recipient** one who receives, as a blood transfusion, or a tissue or organ graft. *Universal r.* a person thought to be able to receive blood of any 'type' without agglutination of the donor cells.

**recombinant** 1. a new cell or individual that results from genetic recombination. 2. pertaining or relating to such cells or individuals. *R. DNA technology* the process of taking a gene from one organism and inserting it into the DNA of another. Also called gene splicing.

**recommended daily allowance (RDA)** a standard for the daily intake of individual nutrients and calories for groups of people. See Appendix 1.

**recommended international non-proprietary name** a system whereby all drugs have a recommended non-proprietary name that is used internationally.

**reconstituted family** *see* FAMILY (BLENDED).

**recrudescence** renewed aggravation of symptoms after an interval of abatement.

**rectal** relating to the rectum. *R. examination* inspection by insertion of a glove-covered finger or with the aid of a proctoscope. *R. varices* haemorrhoids.

**rectopexy** the operation for fixation of a prolapsed rectum.

**rectovaginal** concerning the rectum and vagina.

**rectovesical** concerning the rectum and bladder.

**rectum** the lower end of the large intestine from the sigmoid flexure to the anus.

**recumbent** lying down in the dorsal position.

**recuperation** convalescence; recovery of health and strength.

**recurrent** liable to recur. *R. fever* relapsing fever.

**reduction** 1. the correction of a fracture, dislocation or hernia.

2. removal of oxygen or the addition of hydrogen to a substance or, more generally, the gain of electrons; the opposite of oxidization. *Closed r.* the manipulative reduction of a fracture without incision. *Open r.* reduction of a fracture after incision into the fracture site.

**referred pain** that which occurs at a distance from the place of origin due to the sensory nerves entering the cord at the same level, e.g. the phrenic nerve supplying the diaphragm enters the cord in the cervical region, as do the nerves from the shoulder, and so an abscess on the diaphragm may cause pain in the shoulder. *See* SYNALGIA.

**reflection** 1. a turning or bending back, as in the folds produced when a membrane passes over the surface of an organ and then passes back to the body wall that it lines. 2. in nursing and health care practice, conscious and systematic thinking about one's actions; the review, analysis and evaluation of those situations that have occurred, usually after but maybe during an event. An active process by which the practitioner learns from situations with a view to improving future practice.

**reflective practice** an active process by which the health care professional is able to review, analyse and evaluate events or situations. This conscious monitoring process can be based on any conceptual model, and may utilize supervision of peers in the process. The aim is to facilitate and enhance professional practice.

**reflex** reflected or thrown back. *Accommodation r.* the alteration in the shape of the lens according to the distance of the image viewed. *Conditioned r.* that which is not natural, but is developed by association and frequent repetition until it appears natural. *Corneal r.* the automatic reaction of closing the eyelids after exertion of light pressure on the cornea. This is a test for unconsciousness which is absolute when there is no response. *Deep r.* a muscle reflex elicited by tapping the tendon or bone of attachment. *Light r.* alteration of the size of the pupil in response to exposure to light. *R. action* an involuntary action following immediately upon some stimulus, e.g. the knee jerk, or the withdrawal of a limb from a pin-prick. *R. arc* the sensory and motor neurones, together with the

REFLEX ARC

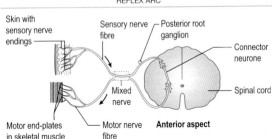

Skin with sensory nerve endings

Sensory nerve fibre

Posterior root ganglion

Connector neurone

Mixed nerve

Spinal cord

Motor end-plates in skeletal muscle

Motor nerve fibre

**Anterior aspect**

connector neurone, which carry out a reflex action (*see* Figure on p. 342). *R. zone therapy* a system of complementary therapy, similar to reflexology, in which it is believed the body is divided into ten longitudinal and three transverse zones, with corresponding divisions in the feet. Reflex zone therapy can be used to identify areas of disorder or disease in the body and a sophisticated grip technique is used to massage the feet and so treat the problem. The therapy can also be performed on the hands, which correspond closely to the feet, the tongue, the face and the back.

**reflexology** a technique of deep massage to the soles of the feet, and occasionally the palms of the hands, to relieve somatic symptoms, and promote health and wellbeing. A complementary therapy.

**reflux** a backward flow; regurgitation.

**refraction** 1. the bending or deviation of rays of light as they pass obliquely through one transparent medium and penetrate another of different density. 2. in ophthalmology, the testing of the eyes to ascertain the amount and variety of refractive error that may be present in each of them.

**refractory** not yielding to, or resistant to, treatment. *R. period* the period immediately after some activity during which a nerve or muscle is unable to react to a fresh impulse.

**regeneration** renewal, as in new growth of tissue in its specific form after injury.

**regimen** a regulated system, programme or schedule such as diet, therapy or exercise intended to promote health or achieve another beneficial effect for a person's wellbeing. Regimen is used in preference to the word regime, which usually refers to a political system or structure.

**register** an epidemiological term meaning an index or file of all cases with a particular disease or condition in a defined population.

**Registered Nurse** a qualified practitioner whose name appears on the central register of the Nursing and Midwifery Council. The title is protected by law in the UK and other countries too. *See* NURSE.

**registrar** 1. an official keeper of records. 2. in British hospitals, a doctor training to be a specialist. *R. of births, marriages and deaths* the official recorder of births, marriages and deaths. In England and Wales, the office comes under the Office for National Statistics. Local registry offices are available in most towns. Births should be registered within 6 weeks in England and Wales (21 days in Scotland). Without a death certificate, which indicates that the death has been registered, it is illegal to dispose of a body.

**registration** the act of recording; in dentistry, the making of a record of the jaw relations, present or desired, in order to transfer them to an articulator to facilitate proper construction of a dental prosthesis.

**regression** 1. a return to a previous state of health. 2. in psychiatry, a tendency to return to primitive or child-like modes of behaviour. Some degree of regression frequently accompanies physical illness and hospitalization. Patients who are mentally ill may exhibit regression to an extreme degree, reverting all the way back to infantile behaviour (atavistic regression).

**regulatory bodies** organizations responsible for defining and monitoring preparation and practice of a specific professional group, e.g. Nursing and Midwifery Council, General Medical Council and the Health Professions Council. *See* PROFESSIONAL SELF-REGULATION.

**regurgitation** backward flow, e.g. of food from the stomach into the mouth. Fluids regurgitate through the nose in paralysis affecting the soft palate. *Aortic r.* backward flow of blood into the left ventricle when the aortic valve is incompetent. *Mitral r.* mitral incompetence. *See* MITRAL.

**REHAB** rehabilitation evaluation of Hall and Baker.

**rehabilitation** reeducation, particularly where an individual has been ill or injured, to enable them to become capable of useful activity. *R. centre* one which provides for organized employment within the capacity of the patient, and with especial regard to the physical influence of the work. *R. evaluation of Hall and Baker* abbreviated REHAB. An assessment system for identifying the patient's level of normal, everyday living and work skills, and of any disturbed behaviour.

**rehydration therapy** the treatment of dehydration by administering fluid and salts by mouth (oral rehydration) or by intravenous infusion. *See* FLUID BALANCE.

**reinforcement** the increasing of force or strength. In behavioural science, the process of presenting a reinforcing stimulus to strengthen a response. *See* CONDITIONING. A positive reinforcer is a stimulus that is added to the environment immediately after the desired response. It serves to strengthen the response: that is, to increase the likelihood of its occurring again. Examples of a positive reinforcer are food, money, a special privilege, or some other reward that is satisfying to the subject.

**Reiter's syndrome** *H. Reiter, German bacteriologist, 1881–1969.* A nonspecific urethritis, affecting males, in which there is also arthritis and conjunctivitis.

**rejection** 1. in immunology, the formation of antibodies by the host against transplanted tissue, with eventual destruction of the transplanted tissue. 2. in psychosocial terms, the denial of acceptance or affection, or the exclusion of another person.

**relapse** the return of a disease after an interval of convalescence.

**relapsing fever** one of a group of similar notifiable infectious diseases transmitted to humans by the bites of ticks. Marked by alternating periods of normal temperature and periods of fever relapse. The diseases in the group are caused by several different species of spirochaetes belonging to the genus *Borrelia.* Also called recurrent fever.

**relatives assessment interview** abbreviated RAI. An assessment tool used by mental health nurses and other staff to identify the perceptions and coping skills of relatives of patients with mental health problems. The data obtained forms an important component in the planning and delivery of care to the patient and the family. *R. A. I. for schizophrenia in a secure environment* abbreviated RAISSE. Adapted from the RAI for use in a secure environment, and used to examine the effects of a secure environment on the course of schizophrenia.

**relaxant** a drug or other agent that brings about muscle relaxation or relieves tension.

**relaxation** a lessening of tension, which may be observed when muscles slacken after they have contracted; it is characterized by feelings of peace and calmness. *R. therapy* classes in which patients are taught breathing and other exercises to use for the relief of pain, stress and tension. Used as part of the preparation for childbirth.

**relaxin** a hormone that is produced by the corpus luteum of the ovary; it softens the cervix and loosens the pelvic ligaments to aid the birth of the baby.

**releasing factor** a substance, produced in the hypothalamus, which causes the anterior pituitary gland to release hormones.

**reliability** the quality of being trustworthy or dependable. In research the consistency of a measure in a study and the likelihood of reproducing the same results, if used again in similar circumstances.

**REM** rapid eye movement, a phase of SLEEP associated with dreaming and characterized by rapid movements of the eyes. Paradoxical sleep.

**reminiscence therapy** measures to stimulate long-term elderly patients with memorabilia, films and songs meaningful to their generation. Used in conjunction with or as a prelude to reality orientation therapy. *See* ORIENTATION.

**remission** subsidence of the symptoms of a disease for a long time.

**remittent** decreasing at intervals. *R. fever* one in which a partial fall in the temperature occurs daily.

**remotivation** in psychiatry, a group therapy technique administered by the nursing staff in a psychiatric unit, which is used to stimulate the communication skills and an interest in the environment of long-term, withdrawn patients.

**renal** relating to the kidney. *R. calculus* stone in the kidney. *R. clearance tests* laboratory tests that determine the ability of the kidney to remove certain substances from the blood. *R. dialysis* the application of the principles of dialysis for treatment of renal failure (*see* below). *See also* HAEMODIALYSIS and PERITONEAL (DIALYSIS). *R. failure* inability of the kidney to maintain normal function. It may be *acute* or *chronic*. Acute renal failure is a sudden, severe interruption of kidney function. It is normally the complication of another disorder and is reversible. Chronic renal failure is a progressive loss of kidney function. In its early stage, renal function can remain adequate but the glomerular filtration rate (GFR) is depressed and plasma chemistry begins to show abnormalities as waste products accumulate. In the later stage, known as end-stage renal disease (ESRD), the GFR deteriorates and when uraemia becomes evident and the patient becomes symptomatic, dialysis is started or the patient receives a transplant. *R. threshold* the level of the blood sugar beyond which it is excreted in the urine; normally 10 mmol/litre (180 mg/100 ml). *R. tubule* the thin tubular part of a nephron. A uriniferous tubule.

**renin** a proteolytic enzyme released into the bloodstream when the kidneys are ischaemic. It causes vasoconstriction and increases the blood pressure.

**reorganization** healing by formation of new tissue identical to that which was injured or destroyed.

**reovirus** any of a group of RNA viruses isolated from healthy children, children with febrile and afebrile upper respiratory disease, or children with diarrhoea.

**repetitive strain injury** abbreviated (RSI) a soft-tissue disorder produced by repetitive use of muscle, especially if the muscle activity involves an awkward or uncomfortable position of the body. Particularly affects keyboard operators, musicians, packers and machine operators.

**replication** 1. the turning back of a tissue on itself. 2. the process by which DNA duplicates itself when the cell divides.

**replogle tube** a double-lumen aspiration catheter attached to low pressure suction apparatus.

**repression** 1. the act of restraining, inhibiting or suppressing. 2. in psychiatry, a defence mechanism whereby a person unconsciously banishes unacceptable ideas, feelings or impulses from consciousness. A person using repression to obtain relief from mental conflict is unaware that 'forgetting' unpleasant situations is a way of avoiding them (motivated forgetting).

**reproductive system** all those parts of the male and female body associated with the production of children.

**Rescue Remedy** one of the Bach Flower remedies, based on homoeopathic principles, and available in liquid form, which is particularly effective in reducing stress, panic, anxiety and hysteria. Useful for those who have a fear of needles for venepuncture and injections, for the transition stage of labour and at any other time when patients are especially anxious or nervous, e.g. before surgical intervention. Four drops of the remedy are given neat on the tongue or can be added to a small glass of water or applied to the temples or wrists. *See* BACH FLOWER REMEDIES.

**research** the purposeful, systematic study of sources, data and materials to establish and reach new conclusions. May also be used to find solutions to previously identified problems or to test theories. Nurses and other health care professionals use both qualitative and quantative research methods, with the ultimate aim being improved practice and better patient care.

**resection** surgical removal of a part. *Submucous r.* removal of part of a deflected nasal septum, from beneath a flap of mucous membrane, which is then replaced. *Transurethral r.* a method of removing portions of an enlarged prostate gland via the urethra.

**reservoir** 1. a storage place or cavity. 2. the host or environment in which an organism lives and from which it is able to infect susceptible individuals, e.g. hands, skin, nose and bowel.

**residential care** the provision of care for frail, elderly people in a variety of settings, e.g. local authority residential homes for the elderly or private residential homes.

**residual** remaining. *R. air* residual volume. The amount of air remaining in the lungs after breathing out fully. *R. urine* urine remaining in the bladder after voiding; seen with bladder outlet obstruction and disorders affecting nerves controlling bladder function. *R. volume* residual air.

**resistance** the degree of opposition to a force. 1. in electricity, the opposition made by a non-conducting substance to the passage of a current. 2. in psychology, the opposition, stemming from the unconscious, to repressed ideas being brought to consciousness. *Drug r.* the ability of a microorganism to withstand the effects of a drug that are lethal to most members of its species. *Peripheral r.* that offered to the passage of blood through small vessels and capillaries. *R. to infection* the natural power of the body to withstand the toxins of disease.

**resolution** 1. in medicine, the process of returning to normal. 2. the disappearance of inflammation without the formation of pus.

**resonance** the reverberating sound obtained on percussion over a cavity or hollow organ, such as the lung.

**respiration** the gaseous interchange between the tissue cells and the atmosphere. *Artificial r.* the production of respiratory movements by external effort. *External r.* breathing, which comprises inspiration, when the external intercostal muscles and the diaphragm contract and air is drawn into the lungs, and expiration, when the air is breathed out. *Intermittent positive pressure r.*

abbreviated IPPR. Respiration produced by a ventilator. *Internal r.* tissue respiration. The interchange of gases that occurs between tissues and blood through the walls of capillaries. *Laboured r.* that which is difficult and distressed. *Stertorous r.* snorting; a noisy breathing. *Tissue r.* internal respiration. *See* CHEYNE–STOKES RESPIRATION.

**respirator** an apparatus to qualify the air breathed through it, or a device for giving artificial respiration or to assist pulmonary ventilation (*see also* VENTILATOR).

**respiratory** pertaining to respiration. *Acute r. distress syndrome* abbreviated ARDS. A group of signs and symptoms resulting in acute respiratory failure; characterized clinically by tachypnoea, dyspnoea, tachycardia, cyanosis, and low Pao$_2$ that persists even with oxygen therapy. *R. distress syndrome of newborn* a condition occurring in preterm infants, full-term infants of diabetic mothers, and infants delivered by caesarean section, and associated with pulmonary immaturity and inability to produce sufficient lung surfactant. Also called hyaline membrane disease, idiopathic respiratory distress syndrome, infant respiratory distress syndrome (abbreviated IRDS). *R. failure* a life-threatening condition in which respiratory function is inadequate to maintain the body's need for oxygen supply and carbon dioxide removal while at rest; also called acute ventilatory failure. *R. insufficiency* a condition in which respiratory function is inadequate to meet the body's needs when increased physical activity places extra demands on it. *R. quotient* the ratio of the volume of expired carbon dioxide to the volume of oxygen absorbed by the lungs per unit of time. *R. shock* circulatory SHOCK due to interference with the flow of blood through the great vessels and chambers of the heart, causing pooling of blood in the veins and the abdominal organs and a resultant vascular collapse. The condition sometimes occurs as a result of increased intrathoracic pressure in patients who are being maintained on a mechanical ventilator. *R. syncytial virus* a virus isolated from children with bronchopneumonia and bronchitis, characteristically causing severe respiratory infection in very young children but less severe infections as the children grow older. *R. therapy* the technical specialty concerned with the treatment, management and care of patients with respiratory problems, including administration of medical gases.

**respite care** temporary care provided for those with disabilities or serious and terminal conditions to allow relief for the family and other carers. Provision may be on a daily or longer-term basis and in a variety of settings, e.g. in a hospice, nursing home, hostel or in the family home. *See* HOSPICE.

**restless legs syndrome** characterized by weakness and coldness in the lower limbs with an unpleasant feeling of a creeping tingling sensation, firstly in the lower legs but possibly extending to the thighs, arms and hands. Symptoms most commonly occur in patients in bed at night, or sometimes in those sitting in chairs for prolonged periods during the day. Occurs primarily in the elderly. The cause is unknown but maybe due to a vascular disorder.

**resuscitation** restoration to life or consciousness of one apparently dead, or whose respirations have ceased. *See also* ARTIFICIAL (RESPIRATION). *Cardiopulmonary r.* an emergency technique used in cardiac arrest to re-establish heart and lung function until more advanced life support is available. *See* Appendix 2.

**retardation** delay; hindrance; delayed development. *Mental r.* low general intellectual development, associated with impairment either of learning and social adjustment or of maturation, or of both. A term no longer used.

**retching** strong, involuntary effort to vomit.

**retention** holding back. *R. cyst see* CYST. *R. defect* a defect of memory. Inability to retain material in the mind so that it can be recalled when required. *R. of urine* inability to pass urine from the bladder, which may be due to obstruction or be of nervous origin.

**reticular** resembling a network. *R. formation* areas in the brain stem from which nerve fibres extend to the cerebral cortex.

**reticulocyte** a red blood cell that is not fully mature; it retains strands of nuclear material.

**reticulocytosis** the presence of an increased number of immature red cells in the blood, indicating overactivity of the bone marrow.

**reticuloendothelial system** a collection of endothelial cells in the liver, spleen, bone marrow and lymph glands that produce large mononuclear cells or macrophages. They are phagocytic, destroy red blood cells and have the power of making some antibodies.

**retina** the innermost coat of the eyeball, formed of nerve cells and fibres, from which the optic nerve leaves the eyeball and passes to the visual area of the cerebrum. The impression of the image is focused upon it.

**retinal** relating to the retina. *R. detachment* partial detachment of the retina from the underlying choroid layer, resulting in loss of vision. It may result from the presence of a tumour, from trauma or from high myopia.

**retinitis** inflammation of the retina.

**retinoblastoma** a malignant tumour arising from retinal cells. Occurs in infancy and may be hereditary. Treatment includes cryosurgery, irradiation and photocoagulation, but enucleation may be required.

**retinol** a light-absorbing molecule obtained from vitamin A. *See* RHODOPSIN.

**retinopathy** any non-inflammatory disease of the retina. *R. pigmentosa* a group of diseases, frequently hereditary, marked by progressive loss of retinal function, especially associated with contraction of the visual field and impairment of vision. The disorder often follows a slow course over a period of many years, but there is considerable variation in the progression of the disease. *Diabetic r.* a complication of diabetes. Retinal haemorrhages occur, resulting in permanent visual damage, and retinal detachment may follow. *Hypertensive r.* retinal change occurring as a result of high blood pressure.

**retrobulbar** pertaining to the back of the eyeball. *R. neuritis* dimness of vision due to inflammation of the optic nerve.

**retroflexion** a bending back, particularly of the uterus when it is bent backwards at an acute angle, the cervix being in its normal position. *See* RETROVERSION.

**retrograde** going backwards. *R. amnesia* forgetfulness of events occurring immediately before an illness or injury. *R. urography* radiographic examination of the kidney after the introduction of a radio-opaque substance into the renal pelvis through the urethra.

**retrolental fibroplasia** a fibrous condition of the anterior vitreous body which develops when a premature infant is exposed to high concentrations of oxygen. Both eyes are affected, seriously interfering with vision and leading to retinal detachment. Early treatment with a freezing probe (cryopexy) can prevent retinal detachment.

**retroperitoneal** behind the peritoneum.

**retropharyngeal** behind the pharynx.

**retrospection** a morbid dwelling on memories.

**retrospective** looking back on or dealing with past events. *R. study* one that examines data from the past, e.g. discharged patients' records, to discover causal factors relevant to outcomes.

**retrosternal** behind the sternum.

**retroversion** a lifting backwards, particularly of the uterus when the whole organ is tilted backwards. *See* RETROFLEXION.

**retrovirus** a group of viruses belonging to the family Retroviridae, principally infecting and frequently causing diseases in animals, but also including viruses that infect and cause disease in humans, e.g. HUMAN IMMUNODEFICIENCY VIRUS (HIV) and human T cell leukaemia/lymphoma/lympho-tropic virus type I (HTLV-I).

**Reverdin's graft** *J.L. Reverdin, Swiss surgeon, 1842–1929.* A form of skin graft in which pieces of skin are placed as islands over the area. *See* THIERSCH SKIN GRAFT.

**reverse isolation** *see* PROTECTIVE ISOLATION; also Appendix 12.

**Reye's syndrome** *R.D.K. Reye, 20th-century Australian pathologist.* An acute, potentially fatal illness that may follow a virus infection occurring in children; there is fatty degeneration of the liver and the brain and raised intracranial pressure, accompanied by vomiting, convulsions and coma. The cause of Reye's syndrome is unknown but administration of salicylates in children under the age of 16 years is not recommended. This follows evidence that aspirin may be a contributory factor in the development of Reye's syndrome.

**Rh factor** rhesus factor.

**rhabdomyosarcoma** a rare malignant growth of striated muscle. It grows rapidly and metastasizes early.

**rhagades** cracks or fissures in the skin, especially those round the mouth.

**rhesus factor** abbreviated Rh factor. The red blood cells of most humans carry a group of genetically determined antigens and are said to be rhesus positive (Rh+). Those that do not are said to be rhesus negative (Rh-). This is of importance as a cause of anaemia and jaundice in the newly born when the infant is Rh+ and the mother Rh-. The result of this incompatibility (isoimmunization) is the formation of an antibody which causes excessive haemolysis in the child's blood. *See* ANTI-RHESUS SERUM.

**rheumatism** any of a variety of disorders marked by inflammation, degeneration or metabolic derangement of the connective tissue structures, especially the joints and related structures, and attended by pain, stiffness or limitation of motion. *Acute r.* rheumatic fever. An acute fever associated with previous streptococcal infection and occurring most commonly in children. The onset is usually sudden, with pain, swelling and stiffness in one or more joints. There is fever, sweating and tachycardia, and carditis is present in most cases. Sometimes the symptoms are minor and ignored. This disease is the most common cause of mitral stenosis because scar tissue results from the inflammation.

**rheumatoid** resembling rheumatism. *R. arthritis see* ARTHRITIS.

**rheumatology** the branch of medicine dealing with disorders of the joints, muscles, tendons and ligaments.

**rhinitis** inflammation of the mucous membrane of the nose.

**rhinoplasty** a plastic operation on the nose; repairing a part of or forming an entirely new nose.

**rhinorrhoea** an abnormal discharge of mucus from the nose.

**rhinoscopy** examination of the interior of the nose. *Anterior r.* examination through the nostrils with the aid of a speculum. *Posterior r.* examination through the nasopharynx by means of a rhinoscope.

**rhinovirus** one of a genus of small RNA-containing viruses that cause respiratory diseases, including the common cold.

*Rhipicephalus* a genus of ticks that can transmit the rickettsiae which cause typhus and relapsing fever.

**rhodopsin** the visual purple of the retina, the formation of which is dependent upon vitamin A (retinol) in the diet. *See* RETINOL.

**rhonchus** a wheezing sound, produced in the bronchial tubes, which is caused by partial obstruction and can be heard on auscultation.

**rhythm** a regular recurring action. *Cardiac r.* the smooth action of the heart when systole is followed by diastole. *R. method* a contraceptive technique in which intercourse is limited to the 'safe period' (avoiding the 2–3 days immediately before and after ovulation).

**rib** any one of the 12 pairs of long, flat curved bones of the thorax, each united by cartilage to the spinal vertebrae at the back. *Cervical r.* a short extra rib, often bilateral. Pressure on this may cause impairment of nerve or vascular function. *See* SCALENUS (SYNDROME). *False r's* the last five pairs, the upper three of which are attached by cartilage to each other. *Floating r's* the last two pairs, connected only to the vertebrae. *True r's* the seven pairs attached directly to the sternum.

**riboflavin** a chemical factor in the vitamin B complex.

**ribonuclease** an enzyme from the pancreas which is responsible for the breakdown of nucleic acid.

**ribonucleic acid** abbreviated RNA. A complex chemical found in the cytoplasm of animal cells and concerned with protein synthesis. Certain viruses contain RNA.

**ribosome** an RNA- and protein-containing particle which is the site of protein synthesis in the cell.

**rickets** a condition of infancy and childhood caused by deficiency of vitamin D, which leads to altered calcium and phosphorus metabolism and consequent disturbance of ossification of bone, resulting in deformity, such as bowing of the legs. Since the action of sunlight on the skin produces vitamin D in the human body, rickets often occurs in parts of the world where the winter is especially long, and where smoke and fog constantly intercept the sun. *Adult r.* OSTEOMALACIA; a rickets-like disease affecting adults. *Fetal r.* achondroplasia. *Late r.* osteomalacia, that occurring in older children. *Vitamin D-resistant r.* a condition almost indistinguishable from ordinary rickets clinically but resistant to unusually large doses of vitamin D; it is often familial.

*Rickettsia* a genus of microorganisms which are parasitic in lice and similar insects. The bite of the host is thus the means of transmitting the organisms, some of which are responsible for the typhus group of fevers.

**rigidity** sustained muscle tension causing the affected part to be stiff and inflexible; may be due to stress, injury or neurological disease.

**rigor** an attack of intense shivering occurring when the heat regulation is disturbed. The temperature rises rapidly and may either stay elevated or fall rapidly as profuse sweating occurs. *R. mortis* stiffening of the body which occurs soon after death.

**Ringer's solution** *S. Ringer, British physiologist, 1835–1910.* A physiological solution of saline to which small amounts of calcium and potassium salts have been added. Used to replace fluids and electrolytes intravenously.

**ringworm** tinea. A contagious skin disease, characterized by circular patches, pinkish in colour with a desquamating surface, and due to a parasitic fungus.

**risk** hazard, or chance of developing a disease or of complications during or after treatment. This may arise because of inherent problems with the treatment itself (e.g. drug side-effects) or because of the frailty of the patient. *Relative r.* the likelihood of developing a disease after a given exposure; in epidemiological terms, calculated as incidence rate of disease in an exposed group divided by incidence rate in the non-exposed group. *R. assessment* 1. a study of a patient by a health care practitioner in which the details of the person's health record are considered together with other relevant factors to assess the likelihood of the development of a particular disease, or, if the disease is already present, the probability of exacerbation or remission. 2. an assessment of a situation or activity for risks with a view to prevention of any damaging effects upon health, e.g. procedures and environment related to manual lifting and handling. *R. factor* a factor which, when added to others, increases the likelihood of a disease or complication (e.g. smoking and obesity are risk factors for the development of coronary artery disease). *R. management* use of a structured approach to reduce identifiable risks in the health services before problems occur in order to protect the interests of the patients by improving the quality of care, reducing costs and potential litigation.

**rite of passage** the cultural ceremonies and rituals that may accompany the changes in status that occur in the course of a person's life, e.g. 18th birthday parties, bar mitzvah. These ceremonies serve to draw attention to changes in status and social identity and also to the management of the social tensions that such changes may involve.

**RNA** ribonucleic acid. *RNA viruses* viruses which contain ribonucleic acid as their genetic material.

**Road Traffic Act (NHS Charges)** responsibility for the collecting of NHS charges for the cost of treating road traffic victims has been transferred from hospitals to the Secretary of State for Health. There is a centralized system to support the collection of charges.

**Rocky Mountain spotted fever** a tick-borne infection caused by a *Rickettsia*, common in the USA, with rash, fever, muscle pain and often an enlarged liver. The disease lasts about 3 weeks.

**rod** a straight thin structure. *Retinal r.* one of the two types of light-sensitive end-organ of the retina, which contain rhodopsin and are responsible for night vision.

**role** a pattern of behaviour developed in response to the demands or expectations of others; the pattern of responses to the persons with whom an individual interacts in a particular situation. *R. play* an educational technique used in teaching interpersonal, communication and practice skills. Students are given roles (or parts) and asked to act these roles out. Some members of the group may be given observational tasks related to the exercise. At the end of the session there is an opportunity for the group to evaluate the exercise. This technique may also be used therapeutically, usually in the psychiatric setting. *Sick r.* the role played by people who have defined themselves as ill. Adoption of the sick role changes the behavioural expectations of others towards the sick person, who is exempted from normal social responsibilities and is not held responsible for the condition. The patient is obliged to 'want to get well' and to seek competent medical help.

**Romberg's sign** *M.H. Romberg, German physician, 1795–1853.* Inability to stand erect without swaying if the eyes are closed. A sign of tabes dorsalis.

**Rorschach test** *H. Rorschach, Swiss psychiatrist, 1884–1922.* A personality trait test that consists of ten inkblot designs, some in colours and some in black and white.

**rosacea** *see* ACNE (ROSACEA).

**roseola** 1. a rose-coloured rash. 2. roseola infantum. *R. infantum* a common acute viral disease that usually occurs in children under 24 months old; it attacks suddenly but disappears in a few days, leaving no permanent marks. *Syphilitic r.* an eruption of rose-coloured spots in early secondary syphilis.

**roughage** coarse vegetable fibres and cellulose that give bulk to the diet and stimulate peristalsis.

**rouleau** a rounded formation found in blood, caused by red cells piling on each other.

**roundworm** any of various types of parasitic nematode worm, somewhat resembling the common earthworm, which sometimes invade the human intestinal tract and multiply there. Very common among them is the pinworm, or threadworm.

**Rovsing's sign** *N.T. Rovsing, Danish surgeon, 1868–1927.* A test for acute appendicitis in which pressure in the left iliac fossa causes pain in the right iliac fossa.

**RSI** repetitive strain injury.

**rubefacient** an agent causing redness of the skin.

**rubella** German measles. An acute, notifiable virus infection of short duration, characterized by pyrexia, enlarged cervical lymph glands and a transient rash. The greatest risk from this disease is to the offspring of mothers who contract it during the early weeks of pregnancy. The child may be born with cataract or deformities, be a deaf mute or have other congenital defects. When a woman is exposed to rubella during the first 4 months of pregnancy, serum should be taken to test for immunity to rubella. If this shows immunity and no infection, reassurance can be given to continue the pregnancy. The second serum should be taken 4 weeks later, if the first showed no immunity. Only if this shows evidence of infection should termination of the pregnancy be considered. Rubella vaccination is given, in conjunction with immunization against mumps and measles (MMR) when an infant is approximately 1 year old. Rubella vaccination alone is repeated for all schoolgirls between the ages of 11 and 14 years. *See* Appendix 9.

**rumination** 1. recurring thoughts. 2. voluntary regurgitation of food, which is then chewed and swallowed again. *Obsessional r.* thoughts which persistently recur against the patient's will.

**rupture** 1. tearing or bursting of a part, as in rupture of an aneurysm; of the membranes during labour; or of a tubal pregnancy. 2. a term commonly applied to hernia.

**Ryle's tube** *G.A. Ryle, British physician, 1889–1950.* A thin tube with a weighted end, introduced into the stomach. It may be used for the withdrawal of gastric contents or for the administration of fluids.

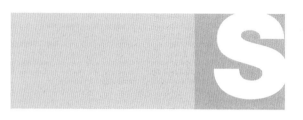

**Sabin vaccine** *A.B. Sabin, American biologist, 1906–1993.* A live oral attenuated poliovirus vaccine active against poliomyelitis. *See* Appendix.

**saccharide** one of a series of carbohydrates, including the sugars.

**saccule** a small sac, particularly the smaller of the two sacs within the membranous labyrinth of the ear.

**sacral** relating to the sacrum.

**sacroiliac** relating to the sacrum and the ilium.

**sacrum** a triangular bone composed of five united vertebrae, situated between the lowest lumbar vertebra and the coccyx. It forms the back of the pelvis.

**sadism** a form of sexual perversion in which the individual takes pleasure in inflicting mental and physical pain on others.

**SADS** seasonal affective disorder syndrome.

**safe motherhood initiative** The World Health Organization (WHO) campaign to reduce worldwide maternal mortality and morbidity with the implementation of simple, appropriate and cost effective strategies to enable mothers to have access to high quality, affordable care during pregnancy and childbirth. The campaign also seeks to improve the health, nutrition and the general well-being of girls and women of reproductive age and to the reduction of any long-term sequelae of childbirth which often result in lifelong disabilities.

**safer sex** preventative measures to reduce the risk of sexually transmitted infections; e.g. maintaining a monogamous sexual relationship and using a condom.

**sagittal** arrow-shaped. *S. suture* the junction of the parietal bones.

**salicylate** a salt of salicylic acid. *Methyl s.* the active ingredient in ointments and lotions for joint pains and sprains. *Sodium s.* the specific drug used for rheumatic fever. It reduces the pyrexia and relieves the pain but does not prevent cardiac complications.

**saline** a solution of sodium chloride and water. *Hypertonic s.* a greater than normal strength. *Hypotonic s.* a lower than normal strength. *Normal* or *physiological s.* a 0.9% solution which is isotonic with blood.

**saliva** the secretion of the salivary glands. When food is taken, saliva moistens and partially digests carbohydrates by the action of its enzyme, ptyalin (amylase).

**salivary** relating to saliva. *S. calculus* a duct. *S. fistula* an abnormal opening on the skin of the face, leading into a salivary duct or gland. *S. glands* the parotid, submaxillary and sublingual glands.

**salivation** 1. the process of salivating. 2. excessive salivation which may lead to soreness of mouth and gums.

**Salk vaccine** *J.E. Salk, American virologist, 1914–1995.* The first poliomyelitis vaccine of live viruses, given by injection. *See* VACCINE.

**Salmonella** any of the genus of Gram-negative, non-sporing, rodlike bacteria that are parasites of the intestinal tract of humans and animals. *S. typhi* and *S. paratyphi* are exclusively human parasites which cause typhoid and paratyphoid fevers.

**salmonellosis** infection with the genus *Salmonella*, usually caused by the ingestion of food containing salmonellae or their products. The organisms can be found in raw meats, raw poultry, eggs and dairy products; they multiply rapidly at temperatures between 7 and 46°C. Symptoms of salmonellosis include violent diarrhoea attended by abdominal cramps, nausea and vomiting, and fever. It is rarely fatal and can be prevented by adequate cooking.

**salpingectomy** excision of one or both of the uterine tubes.

**salpingitis** 1. inflammation of the uterine tubes. 2. inflammation of the pharyngotympanic (eustachian) tubes. *Acute s.* most often a bilateral ascending infection due to a streptococcus or a gonococcus. *Chronic s.* a less acute form that may be blood-borne.

**salpingography** radiographic examination of the uterine tubes after injection of a radio-opaque substance to determine their patency.

**salpingostomy** the making of a surgical opening in a uterine tube near the uterus to restore patency.

**salpinx** a tube. Applied to the uterine or pharyngotympanic (eustachian) tubes.

**salt** 1. sodium chloride, common salt, used in solution as a cleansing lotion, a stimulating bath, or for infusion into the blood, etc. 2. any compound of an acid with an alkali or base. 3. a saline purgative such as Epsom salts. *S. depletion* a loss of salt from the body due to sweating or persistent diarrhoea or vomiting. Common in hot climates when it may be prevented by the taking of salt tablets. *Smelling s's* aromatic ammonium carbonate. A restorative in fainting.

**sample** 1. a selection of individuals made for research purposes from a larger population and intended to reflect that population in all significant aspects. 2. a small part of anything intended as representative of the whole, e.g. blood specimen.

**sandfly** a very small fly of the genus *Phlebotomus*, common in tropical climates and the vector of most types of leishmaniasis. *S. fever* a fever transmitted by the bites of sandflies, and common in Mediterranean countries. Similar to dengue and sometimes known as three-day fever.

**sanguineous** pertaining to or containing blood.

**saphenous** relating to the saphena veins that carry blood from the foot upwards.

**sapphism** female homosexuality; lesbianism.

**sarcoid** 1. tuberculoid; characterized by non-caseating epithelioid cell tubercles. 2. pertaining to or resembling sarcoidosis. 3. sarcoidosis.

**sarcoidosis** a chronic, progressive, generalized disease resembling tuberculosis which may affect any part of the body but most frequently involves the lymph nodes, liver, spleen, lungs, skin, eyes and small bones of the hands and feet.

**sarcoma** a malignant tumour developed from connective tissue cells and their stroma. *Kaposi's s.* one principally involving the skin, although visceral lesions may be present; it usually begins on the distal parts of the extremities, most often on the toes or feet, as reddish-blue or brownish soft nodules and tumours. It is viral in origin and is frequently seen in AIDS. **Melanotic s.** a highly malignant type, pigmented with melanin. **Round-celled s.** a highly malignant growth, composed of a primitive type of cell.

**sarcomatosis** multiple sarcomatous growths in various parts of the body.

*Sarcoptes* a genus of mites. *S. scabiei* the cause of scabies.

**SARS** severe acute respiratory syndrome.

*sartorius* a long muscle of the thigh, which flexes both the thigh and the lower leg.

**satyriasis** abnormally excessive sexual appetite in men.

**scab** the crust on a superficial wound consisting of dried blood, pus, etc.

**scabies** 'the itch'; a contagious skin disease caused by the itch mite (*Sarcoptes scabiei*), the female of which burrows beneath the skin and deposits eggs at intervals. It is intensely irritating, and the rash is aggravated by scratching. The sites affected are chiefly between the fingers and toes, the axillae and groins. Acquired by close direct contact and highly contagious. All members of the family should be treated.

**scald** a burn caused by hot liquid or vapour.

**scale** 1. a scheme or instrument by which something can be measured. A pair of scales is a balance for measuring weight. 2. compact layers of dead epithelial tissue shed from the skin. 3. to scrape deposits of tartar from the teeth.

**scalenus** one of four muscles which move the neck to either side and raise the first and second ribs during inspiration. *S. syndrome* symptoms of pain and tenderness in the shoulder, with sensory loss and wasting of the medial aspect of the arm. It may be caused by pressure on the brachial plexus, by spasm of

the scalenus anterior muscle or by a cervical rib.

**scalp** the hairy skin that covers the cranium.

**scan** an image produced using a moving detector or a sweeping beam of radiation, as in scintiscanning, B-mode ultrasonography, scanography or computed tomography.

**scanning** 1. visual examination of an area. 2. a speech disorder that may be present in cerebellar disease. The syllables are inappropriately separated from each other and are evenly stressed with rhythmically occurring pauses between them.

**scaphoid** boatshaped. *S. bone* a boat-shaped bone of the wrist which articulates with the radius and with the trapezium and the trapezoid bones.

**scapula** the large flat triangular bone forming the shoulder-blade.

**scar** the mark left after a wound has healed with the formation of connective tissue.

**scarlet fever** scarlatina; an acute, notifiable, rare, infectious disease of childhood with an incubation period of 2–4 days. It is caused by a group A beta-haemolytic streptococcus. There is sore throat, high fever and a punctate rash. It is readily treated by antibiotics and the complications of nephritis and middle ear infection are less common.

**scattergram** used in research and statistics, where two variables are represented by a single plot against an x and y axis.

**Schilling test** *R.F. Schilling, American haematologist, b. 1919.* A test used to confirm the diagnosis of pernicious anaemia by estimating the absorption of ingested radioactive vitamin $B_{12}$.

*Schistosoma* a genus of minute blood flukes, some of which are parasitic in humans. *S. haematobium* a species that infests the urinary bladder; widely found in Africa and the Middle East, especially in Egypt. *S. japonicum* and *S. mansoni* species that infest the large intestine. They are found respectively in China, Japan and the Philippines, and in Africa, the West Indies and tropical America.

**schistosomiasis** a parasitic infection of the intestinal or urinary tract by *Schistosoma*. The parasite enters the skin from contaminated water, and causes diarrhoea, haematuria and anaemia. The secondary hosts are freshwater snails. Bilharziasis.

**schizoid** resembling schizophrenia. *S. personality* one that is marked by introspection, self-consciousness, solitariness and a failure in affection towards others. Some schizophrenics have this personality, but only a few who are schizoid become schizophrenic.

**schizophrenia** a general term encompassing a large group of mental disorders (the schizophrenic disorders) characterized by mental deterioration from a previous level of functioning and characteristic disturbances of multiple psychological processes, including delusions, loosening of associations, poverty of the content of speech, auditory hallucinations, inappropriate affect, disturbed sense of self and withdrawal from the external world. *Paranoid s.* predominance of delusions of a persecutory nature. *S. nursing assessment* used by mental health nurses to assess all family members including the patient as a means of identifying the main issues for care and treatment. *Simple s.* a progressive deterioration of the patient's efficiency with increasing social withdrawal.

**Schlemm's canal** *F. Schlemm, German anatomist, 1795–1858.* A venous channel at the junction of the cornea and sclera for the draining of aqueous humour.

**Schönlein–Henoch purpura** or **syndrome** *J.L. Schönlein, German physician, 1793–1864; E.H. Henoch, German paediatrician, 1820–1910.* See PURPURA.

**school health service** the provision of medical and dental inspection and treatment, immunization and health programmes in schools.

**school nurse** a registered nurse who has undertaken further education to specialize in the health care of school-age children. Responsibilities include health promotion and education, monitoring growth and development, screening and caring for those with special educational needs.

**sciatica** pain down the back of the leg in the area supplied by the sciatic nerve. It is usually caused by pressure on the nerve roots by a protrusion on an intervertebral disc.

**scintillography** the visual recording of the distribution of radioactivity in an organ after injection of a small dose of a radioactive substance specifically taken up by that organ.

**sclera** the fibrous coat of the eyeball, the white of the eye, which covers the posterior part and in front becomes the cornea.

**scleroderma** a disease marked by progressive hardening of the skin in patches or diffusely, with rigidity of the underlying tissues. It is often a chronic condition. *See* RAYNAUD'S PHENOMENON.

**sclerosis** the hardening of any part from an overgrowth of fibrous and connective tissue, often due to chronic inflammation.

**sclerotherapy** treatment of oesophageal varices, varicose veins and haemorrhoids by the injection of sclerosing solutions to produce fibrosis.

**sclerotic** 1. hard; indurated; affected by sclerosis. 2. pertaining to the sclera of the eye. *S. coat* the tough membrane forming the outer covering of the eyeball, except in front of the iris, where it becomes the clear horny cornea.

**sclerotomy** incision of the sclerotic coat, usually for the removal of a foreign body or for the relief of glaucoma.

**scoliosis** lateral curvature of the spine (*see* Figure). See LORDOSIS and KYPHOSIS.

**scotoma** a blind area in the field of vision, due to some lesion of the retina. It is also found in glaucoma and in detachment of the retina.

**screening** 1. fluoroscopy. 2. the carrying out of a test on a large

SCOLIOSIS

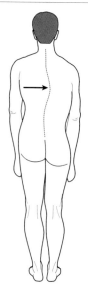

number of people to identify those that have a particular disease for which treatment may be available. Screening tests include: breast screening with mammography, testing for faecal occult blood, cervical cytology, blood pressure measurement, blood tests and ultrasound examination in pregnancy, testing for prostate specific antigen in men.

**scrotum** the pouch of skin and soft tissues containing the testicles.

**scurf** dandruff.

**scurvy** avitaminosis C. A deficiency disease caused by lack of vitamin C, which is found in raw fruits and vegetables. Clinical features include fatigue, oozing of blood from the gums and bruising. The condition rapidly improves with adequate diet.

**seasonal affective disorder syndrome** abbreviated SADS. A condition in which the person notices a change in mood or feelings according to the season of the year and hence the amount of exposure to (sun)light.

**sebaceous** fatty, or pertaining to the sebum. *S. cyst see* CYST. *S. glands* found in the skin, communicating with the hair follicles and secreting sebum.

**seborrhoea** a disease of the sebaceous glands, marked by an excessive secretion of sebum which collects on the skin in oily scales.

**sebum** the fatty secretion of the sebaceous glands.

**secondary** second in order of time or importance. *S. deposits see* METASTASIS. *S. intention* wound healing as the edges of a wound unite after the formation of granular tissue. *See* HEALING.

**secretin** the hormone originating in the duodenum which, in the presence of bile salts, is absorbed into the bloodstream and stimulates the secretion of pancreatic juice.

**secretion** a substance formed or concentrated in a gland and passed into the alimentary tract, the blood or to the exterior. The secretions of the endocrine glands include various hormones and are important in the overall regulation of body processes.

**sedation** the allaying of irritability, the relief of pain or mental distress, and the promotion of sleep, particularly by drugs.

**sedative** a drug or agent that lessens excitement and relieves tension. Sedative drugs are used to induce sleep.

**sedentary** pertaining to sitting; physically inactive.

**sedimentation** the deposit of solid particles at the bottom of a liquid. *Erythrocyte s. rate* abbreviated ESR. *See* ERYTHROCYTE.

**segregation** the separation during meiosis of allelic genes as the chromosomes migrate towards opposite poles of the cell.

**self** 1. a term used to denote an animal's own antigenic constituents, in contrast to 'not-self', denoting foreign antigenic constituents. 2. the complete being of an individual, comprising both physical and psychological characteristics, and including both conscious and unconscious components.

**self-actualization** a level of psychological development in which innate potential is realized to the full, allowing transcendence of the environment. *See* MASLOW'S HIERARCHY OF NEEDS.

**self-care** the personal care carried out by the patient, e.g. bathing, personal grooming, eating and toilet hygiene. May be with assistance or instruction from a health care worker. The aim of rehabilitative care is to maximize self-care and personal independence.

**self-catheterization** men, women and older children can be taught to pass a fine catheter into the urinary bladder to evacuate urine as required.

**self-esteem** a person's evaluation of their own worth as an individual.

**self-examination of breast** *see* BREAST.

**self-examination of testes** *see* TESTICULAR SELF-EXAMINATION.

**self-governing trusts** hospitals or other establishments or facilities which assume responsibility for their own ownership and management by 'opting out' of direct NHS control. Foundation Trust status is approved by the Secretary of State and each trust has a board of executive and non-executive directors and a chairperson who is approved by the Secretary of State.

**self-harm** deliberate damage to one's own body. People who self-harm are not usually attempting suicide, but are seeking to relieve intense emotional pressure, and may sometimes be associated with mental illness, bipolar disorders or anorexia. Most often occurs in young adults and is three times more common in women. Also referred to as self-injury or self-mutilation.

**self-image** an individual's concept of their own personality and abilities based on their own ideas and perceptions.

**self-limited** descriptive of a condition affecting health and wellbeing that runs a definite course regardless of external factors or influences, e.g. the common cold.

**self-retaining catheter** *See* CATHETER.

**sella turcica** a depression in the sphenoid body which protects the pituitary gland.

**semen** the secretion of the testicles containing spermatozoa, which is ejaculated from the penis during sexual intercourse. Seminal fluid.

**semicircular** formed in a half-circle. *S. canals* part of the labyrinth of the internal ear, consisting of three canals in the form of arches which contain fluid and are connected with the cerebellum by their nerve supply. Impressions of change of position of the body are registered in these canals by oscillation of the fluid, and are conveyed by the nerves to the cerebellum.

**semicomatose** in a condition of unconsciousness from which the patient can be roused.

**semilunar** shaped like a half-moon. *S. cartilages* two crescent-shaped cartilages in the knee joint. *S. valve* see VALVE.

**seminoma** a malignant tumour of the testis that is highly radiosensitive.

**semipermeable** of a membrane, permitting the passage of some molecules and hindering that of others.

**semiprone** partly prone. Applied to a position in which the patient is lying face down but the knees are turned to one side.

**senescence** the process of growing old.

**senile** related to the involutional changes associated with old age. *S. dementia* deterioration of mental activity in the elderly, associated with an impaired blood supply to the brain.

**sensation** a feeling resulting from impulses sent to the brain by the sensory nerves.

**sense** the faculty by which conditions and properties of things are perceived, e.g. hunger or pain. *S. organ* one that receives a sensory stimulus: for instance, the eyes and ears. *Special s.* any one of the faculties of sight, hearing, touch, smell, taste and muscle sense, through which the consciousness receives impressions from the environment.

**sensible** 1. capable of being perceived. 2. sensitive. *S. perspiration* that obvious on the skin as moisture.

**sensitization** 1. the process of rendering susceptible. 2. an increase in the body's response to a certain stimulus, as in the development of an allergy. *Protein s.* the condition occurring in an individual when a foreign protein is absorbed into the body, e.g. shellfish causing urticaria when eaten. *See* DESENSITIZATION.

**sensory** relating to sensation. *S. cortex* that part of the cerebral cortex to which information is relayed by the sensory nerves. *S. deprivation* the effecting of a major reduction of sensory information received by the body. This is damaging to the person's ability to function normally, which is dependent upon constant stimulation. *S. nerve* an afferent nerve conveying impressions from the peripheral nerve endings to the brain or spinal cord. *S. overload* exposure to bright lights, constant loud music and noise that may result in distress, confusion and headaches. May occur in intensive care units.

**sentiment** an emotion directed towards some object or person. Sentiments are acquired and profoundly influence a person's actions.

**separation anxiety disorder** developmentally, young children experience feelings of distress at separation from home, parents or carers to whom they have formed an attachment. If hospitalized at this time without a 'live-in' parent or carer the child may regress to a former stage of development with food refusal and incontinence. Separation anxiety usually diminishes by the age of 3 or 4 years but occasionally may occur in older children resulting in nightmares, complaints of somatic symptoms (e.g. headaches, nausea or vomiting) and refusal to attend school. May be associated with depression.

**sepsis** an infection of the body by pus-forming bacteria. *Focal s.* a local focus of infection which produces general symptoms. *Oral s.* infection of the mouth which causes general ill-health by absorption of toxins. *Puerperal s.* infection of the uterus occurring after labour.

**septic** referring to or produced by sepsis. *S. shock* a life-threatening condition in which there is tissue damage and a severe fall in blood pressure as a result of septicaemia. Toxic shock syndrome is one type of septic shock. *See* TOXIC SHOCK.

**septicaemia** the presence in the blood of large numbers of bacteria and their toxins. The symptoms are: a rapid rise of temperature, which is later intermittent, rigors, sweating, and all the signs of acute fever.

**septum** a division or partition. *Atrial s., atrioventricular s.* along with ventricular septum, the partitions dividing the various cavities of the heart. *Nasal s.* the structure made of bone and cartilage which separates the nasal cavities. *Ventricular s. see* ATRIAL SEPTUM above.

**sequela** a morbid condition occurring after a disease and resulting from it.

**sequestrum** a piece of dead bone. Inflammation in bone leads to thrombosis of blood vessels, resulting in necrosis of the affected part, which separates from the living structure.

**serious untoward incident** abbreviated SUI. Any incident on an NHS site or elsewhere, whilst in NHS-funded or NHS-regulated care, that involves: (a) patients, relatives or visitors; (b) staff; or (c) contractors, equipment, building or property. An SUI either or potentially could have: (a) caused death (including sucide) or serious injury or was life-threatening; (b) contributed to a pattern of reduced standard of care; (c) involved a hazard to public health; (d) involved the absconding of a patient detained under the Mental Health Act or a patient who poses a significant risk to themselves or others; (e) caused serious disruption to services; (f) caused significant damage to NHS assets or to the reputation of an NHS organization or its staff; (g) involved fraud or suspected fraud; (h) given rise to a significant claim for damages; (i) involved suspension of a member of staff or a student on care/clinical issues; or (j) raised concerns following an inquest.

**serological** relating to serum. *S. tests* those that are dependent on the formation of antibodies in the blood as a response to specific organisms or proteins.

**serology** the scientific study of serum.

**serosa** a serous membrane. It consists of two layers: the visceral, in close contact with the organ, and the parietal, lining the cavity.

**serotonin** an amine present in blood platelets, the intestine and the central nervous system, which acts as a vasoconstrictor. It is derived from the amino acid tryptophan and is inactivated by monoamine oxidase.

**serotype** the type of organism identified by the kinds of antigens present in the cell. Used to classify microorganisms.

**serous** related to serum. *S. effusion* an effusion of serous exudate.

**serum** the clear, fluid residue of blood, from which the corpuscles and fibrin have been removed. *S. hepatitis* jaundice caused by hepatitis B virus, usually after a blood transfusion or an inoculation with contaminated material. *S. sickness* an allergic reaction usually 8–10 days after a serum injection. It may be manifest by an irritating urticaria, pyrexia and painful joints. It readily responds to adrenaline and antihistaminic drugs. *See* ANAPHYLAXIS.

**severe acute respiratory syndrome** abbreviated SARS. An acute respiratory illness caused by a new variant of a previously unknown coronavirus (SARS Co-V) identified in March 2003. Infected persons develop high fever (>38°C) and cough and/or dyspnoea followed by rapidly progressive respiratory compromise. Infected persons may also experience chills, muscle aches, headache and loss of appetite. The SARS virus is highly contagious and is predominantly transmitted by droplets or by direct and indirect contact. Shedding of the virus in faeces and urine also occurs. Mortality rates vary depending on age and underlying medical conditions but may be as high as 50% in those aged 60 years or older. Treatment is symptomatic and intensive respiratory support may be required.

**sex** 1. either of the two divisions of organic organisms described respectively as male and female. 2. to discover the sex of an organism. *S. chromosome* a chromosome that determines sex. Women have two X chromosomes and men have one X chromosome and one Y chromosome. *S. hormone* a steroid hormone produced by the ovaries or the testes and controlling sexual development. *S.-limited* pertaining to a characteristic found in only one sex. *S.-linked* pertaining to a characteristic that is transmitted by genes that are located on the sex chromosomes, e.g. haemophilia.

**sexism** a belief in the intrinsic superiority of one sex over the other often accompanied by prejudice, stereotyping and discrimination on the basis of sex.

**sexual** pertaining to sex. *S. abuse see* ABUSE. *S. development* the biologi-

cal and psychosocial changes that lead to sexual maturity. *S. deviation* aberrant sexual activity; expression of the sexual instinct in practices which are socially prohibited or unacceptable, or biologically undesirable. *S. intercourse* coitus.

**sexuality** 1. the characteristic quality of the male and female reproductive elements. 2. the constitution of an individual in relation to sexual attitudes and behaviour.

**sexually transmitted infection** abbreviated STI. An infection transmitted either by means of sexual intercourse between heterosexual or homosexual individuals, or by intimate contact with the genitals, mouth and rectum. STIs include syphilis, gonorrhoea, human immunodeficiency virus (HIV) infection, acquired immunodeficiency syndrome (AIDS), chlamydial infection, genital herpes, non-specific urethritis, trichomoniasis, genital lice, scabies, genital warts, hepatitis B infection and yaws. 'Sexually transmitted infection' is now the preferred term for what was formerly known as sexually transmitted disease (STD).

**SGA** small for gestational age.

**SGOT** serum glutamic–oxalacetic transaminase, an enzyme excreted by damaged heart muscle. A raised serum level occurs in myocardial infarction.

**SGPT** serum glutamic–pyruvic transaminase, an enzyme excreted by the parenchymal cells of the liver. There is a raised blood level in infectious hepatitis.

**SHA** strategic health authority.

**shaken baby syndrome** the presence of unexplained fractures in the long bones, together with evidence of a subdural haematoma (bleeding under the membrane surrounding the brain) in a baby. These injuries are caused by the violent shaking of the baby which produces a whiplash effect and a rotational movement of the head resulting in vomiting, convulsions, irritability, coma and death. *See* ABUSE.

**shared care** the coordinated care of patients across the primary and secondary health care interface. In obstetrics, a term used to describe antenatal care carried out by an obstetrician and a general practitioner. *S. c. protocols* consenus protocols for the clinical management of patients across the interface of primary and secondary health care, e.g. for the prescribing of expensive drugs or the use cytotoxic therapy.

**shearing force** a strain produced by pressure in the structure of a substance so that each layer slides over the next. In the body this may occur when any part is on a gradient; the deeper tissues slide towards the lower gradient and the skin remains with the supporting contact, e.g. sheets on a bed or on a chair. In the presence of moisture this friction is exacerbated and the deeper tissues become ischaemic. *See* PRESSURE ULCER.

**sheath** 1. an enveloping tubular structure or part. 2. a condom, worn on the erect penis during sexual intercourse to trap seminal fluid, preventing the transmission of human immunodeficiency virus (HIV) and other viruses and also reducing the risk of pregnancy.

**shiatsu** a form of manipulation in which the practitioner uses the thumbs, fingers and palms of the hands, knees, forearms, elbows and feet to apply pressure to the client's body in order to promote and maintain health.

***Shigella*** a genus of Gram-negative rod-like bacteria. Some species cause bacillary dysentery. *S. flexneri* and *S. shigae* are common in Asia, *S. dysenteriae* in the USA and *S. sonnei* in Western Europe.

**shin** the bony front of the leg below the knee. The tibia.

**shingles** herpes zoster.

**Shirodkar's operation** *Shirodkar, Indian obstetrician.* A cervical cerclage operation to prevent abortion resulting from cervical incompetence. The internal os is closed by means of a nylon suture which is removed shortly before term, or earlier if labour should begin.

**shock** a condition produced by severe illness or trauma in which there is a sudden fall in blood pressure. This leads to lack of oxygen in the tissues and greater permeability of the capillary walls, so increasing the degree of shock by greater loss of fluid. The patient has a cold, moist skin, a feeble pulse and a low blood pressure, and is distressed, thirsty and restless. *Allergic* or *anaphylactic s.* shock produced by the injection of a protein to which the patient is sensitive. *Cardiogenic s.* shock as a result of an acute heart condition such as myocardial infarction. *Hypovolaemic s.* shock resulting from a reduction in the volume of blood in the circulation after haemorrhage or severe burns. *Neurogenic s.* shock due to nervous or emotional factors. *Septic s. see* SEPTIC. *Shell s.* a mental health condition caused by the stresses of warfare. *Toxic s. see* TOXIC.

**short-sightedness** myopia.

**shoulder** the junction of the clavicle and the scapula where the arm joins the body.

**show** the blood-stained discharge that occurs at the onset of labour.

**shunt** a diversion, particularly of blood, due to a congenital defect, disease or surgery.

**sialolith** a salivary calculus.

**sibling** one of a family of children having the same parents. Applied in psychology to one of two or more children of the same parent or substitute parent figure. *S. rivalry* jealousy, compounded of love and hate of one child for its sibling.

**sickle-cell anaemia** an inherited blood disease. See ANAEMIA.

**side effect** a result other than the one for which the drug or agent used is being given. Some side effects are predictable, e.g. hair loss with cytotoxic therapy but others are unpredictable, e.g skin eruptions or anaphylactic shock.

**siderosis** 1. chronic inflammation of the lung due to inhalation of particles of iron. 2. excess iron in the blood. 3. the deposit of iron in the tissues.

**SIDS** sudden infant death syndrome.

**sigmoid** shaped like the Greek letter sigma, Σ. *S. colon* or *flexure* that part of the colon in the left iliac fossa just above the rectum.

**sigmoidoscope** an instrument by which the interior of the rectum and sigmoid colon can be seen.

**sign** 1. any objective evidence of disease or dysfunction. 2. an observable physical phenomenon so frequently associated with a given condition as to be considered indicative of its presence. *S. language* hand and body language used by deaf people to communicate with others. *Vital s's* the signs of life, namely pulse, respiration and temperature.

**significant other** a person designated by the patient as the person who should be consulted in the event of an emergency or to contact when making arrangements for discharge.

**silicosis** fibrosis of the lung due to the inhalation of silica dust particles. It occurs in miners, stone masons and quarry workers.

**Sims' position** *J.M. Sims, American gynaecologist, 1813–1883.* A semiprone position. See POSITION.

**sinoatrial** situated between the sinus venosus and the atrium of the heart. *S. node* the pacemaker of the heart. See NODE.

**sinus** 1. a cavity in a bone. 2. a venous channel, especially within the cranium. 3. an unhealed passage leading from an abscess or internal lesion to the surface. *Air s.* a cavity in a bone containing air. *Cavernous s.* a venous sinus of the dura mater which lies along the body of the sphenoid bone. *Coronary s.* the vein that returns the blood from the heart muscle into the right atrium. *Ethmoidal s.* air spaces in the ethmoid bone. *Frontal s.* air spaces in the frontal bone. *S. arrhythmia see* ARRHYTHMIA. *S. thrombosis* clotting of blood in a cranial venous channel. In the lateral sinus it is a complication of mastoiditis. *Sphenoidal s.* air spaces in the sphenoid bone.

**sinusitis** inflammation of the lining of a sinus, especially applied to the bony cavities of the face.

**skeleton** the bony framework of the body, supporting and protecting the organs and soft tissues.

**skewed distribution** in statistics, the degree to which the distribution is asymmetric around the mean. The normal distribution is symmetric, thus having a zero skewness.

**skill mix** the ratio of staff employed in an area of health-care activity, whether qualified, trained or untrained, representing the availability of skills possessed by these staff.

**skin** the outer protective covering of the body. It consists of an outer layer, the epidermis or cuticle, and an inner layer, the dermis or corium, which is known as 'true skin'. *S. grafting* transplantation of pieces of healthy skin to an area where loss of surface tissue has occurred. *S. patch* a drug-impregnated adhesive patch which is applied to the skin. The drug is slowly absorbed, allowing its level in the blood to be maintained over a given period of time. *S. test* application of a substance to the skin, or intradermal injection of a substance, to permit observation of the body's reaction to it.

**skull** the bony framework of the head, consisting of the cranium and facial bones.

**sleep** a period of rest for the body and mind, during which volition and consciousness are in partial or complete abeyance and the bodily functions partially suspended. It occurs in a 24-hour biological rhythm. Sleep occurs in cycles which have two distinct phases. Each phase lasts approximately 60–90 minutes: orthodox or non-rapid eye movement sleep (NREM), and paradoxical or rapid eye movement sleep (REM). Sleeping requirements vary, with each individual averaging between 4–10 hours in a 24-hour period. The purpose of sleep is unknown but sleep deprivation is harmful.

**sleeping sickness** trypanosomiasis. A tropical fever occurring in parts of Africa, caused by a protozoal parasite (*Trypanosoma*) which is conveyed by the tsetse fly.

**slim disease** a term primarily used in Africa and other tropical countries for a progressive wasting disease associated with human immunodeficiency virus infection resulting in a loss of 10% or more of the baseline body weight. *See* AIDS and HUMAN IMMUNODEFICIENCY VIRUS.

**slipped disc** a prolapsed intervertebral disc which causes pressure on the spinal nerves. It may be very painful.

**slough** dead tissue caused by injury or inflammation. It separates from the healthy tissue and is ultimately washed away by exuded serum, leaving a granulating surface.

**slow** taking a long time before acting or showing signs of activity. *S.-acting drugs* those that are absorbed in the small intestine and have a sustained release over a period of time. Many of these drugs are now incorporated into skin patches. *S. viruses* those infective agents that produce infection after a latent period in the body which may last weeks to months. *See* PRION.

**small for gestational age** abbreviated SGA. Term for a baby who is smaller or lighter in weight than expected for its gestational age. There is some variance in definition, from inclusion of babies below the 10th percentile to only those below the 5th percentile.

**smallpox** once a highly infectious viral disease, associated with high mortality. Eradicated from the world in 1980. Smallpox vaccination is no longer required for travellers to any part of the world.

**smear** A specimen for microscopic examination that has been prepared by spreading a thin film of the material across a glass slide.

**smegma** the secretion of sebaceous glands of the clitoris and prepuce.

**smell** one of the five senses. Airborne particles are deposited and dissolved in the mucous membrane lining the nose, stimulating the endings of the olfactory nerve. The nose is able to distinguish a wide range of odours.

**smoking** the act of drawing into the mouth and puffing out the smoke of tobacco contained in a cigarette, cigar or pipe. A close relationship between smoking and lung cancer, heart disease and bronchitis and emphysema has been established. Smoking is also harmful in pregnancy because the inhaled carbon monoxide reduces oxygen transportation in the body and the nicotine causes vasoconstriction of the arterioles. *Anti-s. initiatives* a range of programmes stemming from the government white paper

*Smoking Kills*. They include the development of the smoking cessation programme, nicotine replacement therapy available on the NHS and the smoker's charter. **Passive s.** the involuntary inhalation of tobacco smoke by people who do not smoke. Passive smoking has been shown to increase the risks of chest infections, coronary disease and tobacco-induced cancers in adults. The infants of mothers who smoke are likely to suffer from fetal growth retardation and development may be delayed. Children exposed to passive smoking are prone to develop ear and chest infections and asthma. Smoking in the workplace and other public environments, e.g. restaurants, shops, also planes and buses, is regarded as an environmental health hazard and is banned throughout the UK.

**snake** a limbless reptile; a serpent. The bites of many snakes are poisonous to humans. **S. venom antitoxin** antivenin. A serum made from animals, usually horses, which have been immunized against the venom of a specific type of snake.

**Snellen's test types** *H. Snellen, Dutch ophthalmologist, 1834–1908.* Square-shaped letters on a chart, used for sight testing (*see* Figure).

**snow** frozen water vapour. **Carbon dioxide s.** solid $CO_2$, which is used as a refrigerant; 'dry ice'. **S. blindness** photophobia due to the glare of snow.

**snuffles** a chronic discharge from the nose, occurring in children, as a result of infection of the nasal mucous membrane.

**social** in health care, the prefix 'social' denotes a role, function or description to do with society, its peoples and its organization. **S. class** a category arising from the division of society into economic or occupa-

SNELLEN'S TEST TYPES

tional groupings. The most widely used grouping of social class or occupational scale in the UK is the Registrar General's Classification designed originally for use in the 1911 Census but extensively modified for use in later censuses (*see* Table on p. 366). Occupations are now coded to be comparable with the International Standard Classification of Occupations. **S. drift** the movement of people from one social class to another usually as

| NATIONAL STATISTICS SOCIO-ECONOMIC CLASSIFICATIONS | |
|---|---|
| Class | Occupation |
| 1.1 | Company directors, senior officials in government, senior executives in large organizations (e.g. NHS Trust Managers) |
| 1.2 | Doctors, lawyers, academics, accountants, pharmacists |
| 2 | Teachers, social workers, lower and middle managers (e.g. health care practice managers), physio and occupational therapists, radiographers, nurses and midwives, actors, musicians, sports players |
| 3 | Photographers, clerical officers, secretaries, nursing auxiliaries, medical technicians, paramedics and ambulance staff |
| 4 | All non-professional self-employed occupations, e.g. hoteliers, publicans, hairdressers, plumbers, carpenters, electricians |
| 5 | Plumbers, carpenters, electricians, motor mechanics, printers, train drivers, TV and telephone engineers |
| 6 | Dental nurses, care assistants, cooks, machinists, assemblers, sales assistants, hospital porters |
| 7 | Cleaners, hotel porters, drivers, labourers, waiters/waitresses, bar staff, hairdressers |

Reproduced with thanks to Professor David Rose, ISER, University of Essex.

a result of socioeconomic circumstances or as a result of morbid processes. Sometimes referred to as social mobility. *S. exclusion* people from groups which for a variety of reasons are not able to participate in community and mainstream activities, e.g. refugees and homeless people. *S.e. unit* a government unit set up to study and report on social exclusion and to identify means to reduce some of the issues, e.g. provision of improved hostel accomodation for young people. *S. norms* socially accepted patterns of behaviour within a community or population. *S. worker* a professional qualified in the treatment of individual and social problems of patients and their families. *See also* MEDICAL (SOCIAL WORKER).

**socialization** the process by which society integrates the individual,

and the individual learns to behave in socially acceptable ways.

**sociology** the scientific study of the development of human social relationships and organization, i.e. interpersonal and intergroup behaviour as distinct from the behaviour of an individual.

**sociopath** a person with an antisocial personality; a psychopath.

**sodium** *symbol* Na. A metallic alkaline element widely distributed in nature, and forming an important constituent of animal tissue. *S. aminosalicylate* an antituberculous drug used in conjunction with streptomycin and isoniazid. *S. bicarbonate* an antacid widely used to treat digestive disorders, especially flatulence. Repeated use can cause alkalosis. *S. chloride* common salt. Its presence in the diet is necessary to health. *S. citrate* compound used to prevent clotting of blood during blood transfusions. *S. cromoglycate* a drug used as an inhalant in the treatment of asthma. *S. fluoride* a salt used in the fluoridation of water and also in toothpastes to prevent the formation of caries. *S. hydroxide* caustic soda. A powerful corrosive drug used to destroy warts. It can cause severe chemical burns. *S. hypochlorite* a compound with germicidal properties used in solution to disinfect utensils, and diluted as a topical antibacterial agent in many environmental situations. *Salicylate* an antipyretic drug used in the treatment of rheumatic fever.

**soft tissue mobilization** *see* MASSAGE.

**software** computer data and programs containing instructions that detail how to use a specific computer facility.

**solar plexus** coeliac plexus. A network of sympathetic nerve ganglia in the abdomen; the nerve supply to abdominal organs below the diaphragm.

**solution** a liquid in which one or more substances have been dissolved.

**solvent** a liquid that dissolves or has power to dissolve. *S. abuse see* ABUSE.

**soma** 1. the body as distinct from the mind. 2. the body tissue as distinct from the germ cells.

**somatic** 1. relating to the body as opposed to the mind. 2. relating to the body wall as distinct from the viscera.

**somnambulism** walking and carrying out other complex activities during a state of sleep.

**Somogyi effect** *M. Somogyi, American biochemist, 1883–1971.* A rebound phenomenon occurring in diabetes mellitus; overtreatment with insulin induces hypoglycaemia, resulting in rebound hyperglycaemia and ketosis.

**Sonne dysentery** *C.O. Sonne, Danish bacteriologist, 1882–1948.*

Bacillary dysentery which is common in the UK. The symptoms are diarrhoea, vomiting and abdominal pain. The causative agent is *Shigella sonnei.*

**sonogram** a record or display obtained by ultrasonic scanning. *See* ULTRASONOGRAPHY.

**sonography** *see* ULTRASONOGRAPHY.

**sorbitol** a sweetening agent which is converted into sugar in the body although it is slowly absorbed from the intestine. It is used in some diabetic foods and in intravenous feeding.

**sordes** brown crusts which form on the teeth and lips of unconscious patients, or those suffering from acute or prolonged fevers.

**sore** a general term for any ulcer or open skin lesion. *Cold s.* herpes simplex. *Hard s.* a syphilitic chancre. *Pressure s.* a sore caused by pressure from the bed, chair (decubitus ulcer) or a splint. *Soft s.* a chancroid ulcer. *S. throat* inflammation of the larynx or pharynx, including tonsillitis.

**souffle** a blowing sound heard on auscultation. *Uterine s.* a sound due to the blood passing through the uterine arteries of the mother, particularly over the placental site. It is synchronous with the maternal pulse.

**soya bean** a legume that contains high-quality protein and little starch. *S. milk* used as a milk substitute for babies who cannot tolerate constituents of breast or cow's milk, e.g. lactose. Soya-based milk substitutes, containing only vegetable fats, are now available as infant formulae.

**spam** unsolicited advertising or 'junk' mail sent to an individual address via e-mail.

**Spansule** trade name for a delayed-release form of capsule.

**spasm** a sudden involuntary muscle contraction. *Carpopedal s.* spasm of the hands and feet. A sign of tetany. *Clonic s.* alternate muscle rigidity and relaxation. *Habit s.* a tic. *Nictitating s.* spasmodic twitching of the eyelid. *Tetanic s.* violent muscle spasms, including opisthotonos. *Tonic s.* a sustained muscle rigidity.

**spastic** 1. caused by spasm; convulsive. 2. one affected by spasticity; often applied to persons suffering from congenital paralysis due to some cerebral lesion or impairment. *S. colon* irritable bowel syndrome. *S. paralysis* paralysis associated with lesions of the upper motor neurone, as in cerebral vascular accidents, and characterized by increased muscle tone and rigidity.

**spasticity** marked rigidity of muscles.

**spatial** pertaining to space.

**SPC** statistical process control.

**special needs** a term generally used to describe the educational or learning needs of a child or adult with a learning disability. The expression may also be used in a wider context to describe the special educational needs of any child, e.g. one who is musically gifted.

**special health authorities** provide a service to the whole of England. They are independent but can be subject to ministerial direction. Examples include the National Institute for Health and Clinical Excellence and the Mental Health Act Commission. Some such authorities have UK-wide responsibilities.

**specific** 1. relating to a species. 2. a remedy that has a distinct curative influence on a particular disease, e.g. quinine in malaria. 3. related to a unit mass of a substance. *S. gravity* the density of fluid compared with that of an equal volume of water.

**specimen** a sample or part taken to show the nature of the whole, e.g. for chemical testing or microscopic survey.

**specular reflection** reflecting as from a surface. A term used in ultrasound to describe an interface which gives a strong reflection or echo, e.g. the fetal skull or bony prominence.

**speech** the act of communicating by sounds by means of a linguistic code. *Clipped s.* speech in which the words are cut short. *Deaf s.* the characteristic utterance of people with severe hearing loss. *Explosive s.* loud, sudden utterances; a sign of mental disorder. *Incoherent s.* disconnected utterances made when the sequence of thought is disturbed, as in delirium. *Oesophageal s.* speech produced after laryngectomy by swallowing air and using it to vibrate within the oesophagus against the closed cricopharyngeal sphincter. *Scanning s.* speech in which the syllables are inappropriately separated from each other and are evenly stressed. Characteristic of cerebellar damage. *S. therapist* a professional qualified to identify, assess and rehabilitate persons with speech or language disorders and feeding difficulties. *Staccato s.* speech in which each syllable is separately pronounced. Characteristic of multiple sclerosis.

**sperm** 1. a spermatozoon. 2. the semen. *S. count* a method of determining the concentration of spermatozoa in a semen sample. *S. donation* seminal fluid provided by donors for the fertilization of women whose partners are sterile.

**spermatocele** a cystic swelling in the epididymis, containing semen.

**spermatozoon** a mature male germ cell consisting of a flat-shaped head, a short middle part and a long tail. There are 300–500 billion spermatozoa in a normal ejaculate.

**spermicide** any agent that will destroy spermatozoa.

**sphenoid** wedge-shaped. *S. bone* the central part of the base of the skull.

**spherocytosis** the presence in the blood of erythrocytes that are more nearly spherical than biconcave. Characteristic of acholuric jaundice, it may also be hereditary.

**sphincter** a ring-shaped muscle, contraction of which closes a natural orifice.

**sphygmomanometer** an instrument for measuring the arterial blood pressure.

**spica** a bandage or plaster cast applied to a joint, e.g. shoulder spica, to hold it in the required position.

**spigot** a small peg or bung to close the opening of a tube.

**spina** spine; a slender, thorn-like projection that occurs on many bones. *S. bifida* a congenital defect of non-union of one or more vertebral arches, allowing protrusion of the meninges and possibly their contents. The condition can be detected during pregnancy by ultrasonography, or by testing the blood of the mother or the amniotic fluid for the presence of increased levels of alpha-fetoprotein. Associated with this condition is a folate deficiency in the diet of women of child bearing age who should be encouraged to take sufficient amounts in their diet. See APPENDIX 1, MENINGOCELE and MENINGOMYELOCELE.

**spinal** relating to the spine. *S. anaesthesia see* ANAESTHESIA. *S. canal* the hollow in the spine formed by the neural arches of the vertebrae. It contains the spinal cord, meninges and cerebrospinal fluid. *S. caries* disease of the vertebrae, usually tuberculous. *See* POTT'S DISEASE. *S. column* the backbone; the vertebral column. *S. cord see* CORD. *S. cord compression see* CORD. *S. curvature* abnormal curving of the spine. If associated with caries, it is known as Pott's disease. See

KYPHOSIS, LORDOSIS and SCOLIOSIS. *S. jacket* a support for the spine, made of plaster of Paris or other material, used to give rest after injury to or operation on the spine. *S. nerves* the 31 pairs of nerves which leave the spinal cord at regular intervals throughout its length. They pass out in pairs, one on either side between each of the vertebrae, and are distributed to the periphery. *S. puncture* lumbar or cisternal puncture.

**spine** 1. the backbone or vertebral column, consisting of 33 vertebrae, separated by fibrocartilaginous discs, and enclosing the spinal cord. 2. a sharp process of bone.

**Spinhaler** a nebulizing device which delivers a preset dose of the contained drug.

**spinnbarkeit** [Ger.] a thread of mucus secreted by the cervix uteri. Used to determine ovulation as this usually coincides with the time at which the mucus can be drawn out on a glass slide to its maximum length.

**spirochaete** one of a group of microorganisms in the form of a spiral, some of which are found in impure fresh or salt water. The group includes the species *Treponema*, *Borrelia* and *Leptospira*.

**spirograph** an instrument for registering respiratory movements.

**spirometer** an instrument for measuring the air capacity of the lungs.

**Spitz–Holter valve** *Spitz, American engineer; J.W. Holter, American engineer.* A device used in the treatment of hydrocephalus to drain the cerebrospinal fluid from the ventricles into the superior vena cava or the right atrium.

**splanchnic** pertaining to the viscera. *S. nerves* sympathetic nerves to the viscera.

**spleen** a large, vascular, glandlike but ductless organ, coloured a reddish purple and situated in the left hypochondrium under the border of the stomach. It manufactures lymphocytes and breaks down red blood corpuscles.

**splenectomy** excision of the spleen.

**splenomegaly** enlargement of the spleen.

**splint** an appliance used to support or immobilize a part while healing takes place or to correct or prevent deformity.

**spondylitis** inflammation of the vertebrae. *Ankylosing s.* a rheumatic disease, chiefly of young males, in which there is abnormal ossification with pain and rigidity of the intervertebral, hip and sacroiliac joints.

**spondylolisthesis** a sliding forwards or displacement of one vertebra over another, usually the fifth lumbar over the sacrum, causing symptoms such as low back pain, as a result of pressure on the nerve roots.

**spondylosis** ankylosis of the vertebral joints, usually caused by a degenerative disease of the intervertebral discs, such as osteoarthritis.

**spontaneous** occurring without apparent cause. Applied to certain types of fracture and to recovery from a disease without any specific treatment.

**sporadic** pertaining to isolated cases of a disease that occurs in various and scattered places (compare ENDEMIC and EPIDEMIC).

**spore** 1. a reproductive stage of some of the lowest forms of vegetable life, e.g. moulds. 2. a protective state which some bacteria are able to assume in adverse conditions, such as lack of moisture, food or heat. In this form the organism may remain alive, but inert, for years.

**sporulation** the formation of spores by bacteria, e.g. clostridia or bacilli.

**spotted fever** a febrile disease characterized by a skin eruption, such as Rocky Mountain spotted fever, and other infections due to tickborne rickettsiae.

**sprain** wrenching of a joint, producing laceration of the capsule or stretching of the ligaments, with consequent swelling, which is due to effusion of fluid into the affected part.

**spreadsheet** a computer program that aligns data in tables, rows and columns.

**sprue** a disease of malabsorption in the intestine, which may be tropical or non-tropical in form. There is steatorrhoea, diarrhoea, glossitis and anaemia.

**sputum** material expelled from the air passages through the mouth. It consists chiefly of mucus and saliva; in diseased conditions of the air passages it may be purulent, blood-stained and frothy and may contain many bacteria. It must always be regarded as highly infectious. *Rusty s.* that in which altered blood permeates the mucus. Characteristic of acute lobar pneumonia.

**squamous** scaly. *S. bone* the thin part of the temporal bone which articulates with the parietal and frontal bones. *S. cell carcinoma* a malignancy of the squamous cells of the bronchus. *S. epithelium* epithelium composed of flat and scale-like cells.

**squint** *see* STRABISMUS.

**staging** 1. the determination of distinct phases or periods in the course of a disease. 2. the classification of neoplasms according to the extent of the tumour. *TNM s.* staging of tumours according to three basic components: primary tumour (T), regional nodes (N) and metastasis (M). Subscripts are used to denote size and degree of involvement; for example, 0 indicates undetectable, and 1, 2, 3 and 4 a progressive increase in size or involvement.

**stammering** stuttering; a speech disorder in which the utterance is broken by hesitation and repetition or prolongation of words and syllables.

**standard deviation** in statistics, a measure of the dispersion of a random variable: the square root of the average squared deviation from the mean. For data that have a normal distribution, about 68% of the data points fall within one standard deviation from the mean and about 95% fall within two standard deviations.

**standard precautions** the current model of best practice in infection control, a synthesis of UNIVERSAL PRECAUTIONS and BODY SUBSTANCE ISOLATION (published 1999). Standard precautions are designed to reduce the risk of transmission of blood-borne and other pathogens in hospital, from both recognized and unrecognized sources of infection, and apply to all patients all the time. Their implementation requires that nurses and other health care professionals take appropriate measures, e.g. wear gloves, to avoid contact with (a) blood; (b) all body fluids, secretions and excretions except sweat, regardless of whether or not they contain visible blood; (c) non-intact skin; and (4) mucous membranes. Standard precautions are used in association with new concepts of TRANSMISSION-BASED PRECAUTIONS. *See also* INFECTION CONTROL and Appendix 12.

**standards** statements of the levels of service or care related to specific topics which staff agree to provide. Often accompanied by a description of the structure (staff, equipment, etc.) and process needed to attain specified observable outcomes. *S. of care* a measure by which a professional's conduct is compared, comprises a list of those acts that a prudent professional practitioner would have carried out (or not performed) in similar circumstances within health care.

**stapedectomy** removal of the stapes and insertion of a vein graft or other device to re-establish conduction of sound waves in otosclerosis.

**stapediolysis** an operation in which the footpiece of the stapes is mobilized to aid conduction in deafness from otosclerosis.

**stapes** the stirrup-shaped bone of the middle ear.

*Staphylococcus* a genus of Gram-positive non-mobile bacteria which, under the microscope, appear grouped together in small masses like bunches of grapes. They are normally present on the skin and mucous membranes. *S. pyogenes* (or *S. aureus*) is a common cause of boils, carbuncles and abscesses.

**staphyloma** a protrusion of the cornea or the sclerotic coat of the eyeball as the result of inflammation or a wound.

**starch** carbohydrates are stored as starch in many plants. Starch consists of linked glucose units in two forms, amylose and amylopectin, providing a valuable source of energy and fibre in the diet.

**startle reflex** *see* MORO REFLEX.

**stasis** the stagnation or stoppage of the flow of a fluid. *Intestinal s.* sluggish movement of faeces through the bowel, owing to partial obstruction or to impairment of the action of the intestinal muscles. *Venous s.* congestion of blood in the veins.

**statementing** the provision by a local authority of a statement following formal assessment of the special educational needs of a child with mental or physical disabilities to attend either a mainstream school with extra help, or a special school.

**statistical process control** abbreviated SPC. The use of statistical concepts which place the emphasis on the continuous monitoring of a process rather than the reliance on a single outcome as the sole measure for quality assurance in the delivery of a service.

**statistical significance** in research, a conclusion that the results achieved have little probability of occurring by chance alone. If the result is statistically significant, e.g. below 1 in 20 or the 0.05 level, then something other than chance produced the result.

**statistics** 1. numerical facts pertaining to a particular subject or body of objects. 2. the science dealing with the collection, tabulation and analysis of numerical facts.

**status** condition. *S. asthmaticus* a severe and prolonged attack of asthma. *S. epilepticus* a serious condition in which there is rapid succession of epileptic fits. *S. lymphaticus* a condition in which all lymphatic tissues are hypertrophied, especially the thymus gland.

**STD** sexually transmitted disease.

**steapsin** the fat-splitting enzyme (lipase) of the pancreatic juice.

**steatoma** 1. a sebaceous cyst. 2. a lipoma; a fatty tumour.

**steatorrhoea** the presence of an excess of fat in the stools owing to malabsorption of fat by the intestines.

**Stein–Leventhal syndrome** *I.F. Stein, American gynaecologist, 1887–1976; M.L. Leventhal, American gynaecologist, 1901–1971.* Condition affecting females in which obesity, hirsutism and sterility are associated with polycystic ovaries and menstrual irregularities.

**Steinmann pin** *F. Steinmann, Swiss surgeon, 1872–1932.* A fine metal rod, passed through a bone, by which extension is applied to overcome muscle contraction in certain fractures. *See* KIRSCHNER WIRE.

**stellate** star-shaped. *S. fracture* a radiating fracture of the patella. *S. ganglion* the inferior cervical ganglion. A star-shaped collection of nerve cells at the base of the neck.

**stenosis** abnormal narrowing or contraction of a channel or opening. *Aortic s.* narrowing of the opening of the aortic valve due to scar tissue formation as the result of inflammation. *Mitral s.* narrowing of the orifice of the mitral valve, usually following rheumatic fever. *Pulmonary s.* a congenital narrowing of the opening from the right ventricle of the heart into the pulmonary artery. *Pyloric s.* narrowing of the pyloric orifice of the stomach due to scar tissue, new growth or congenital hypertrophy.

**stent** a device or splint of rubber, stainless steel or plastic mesh or a coil of wire placed inside a canal, duct or artery to keep the passageway open.

**stercobilin** a brown-orange pigment derived from bile and present in faeces.

**stereognosis** the ability to visualize the shape of an object by touch alone.

**stereotype** an oversimplified generalization about a group or class of people which is often then applied to an individual. May form a basis for discrimination and prejudice.

**stereotypy** repetitive actions carried out or maintained for long periods in a monotonous fashion.

**sterile** 1. aseptic; free from microorganisms. 2. barren; incapable of producing young.

**sterility** 1. the state of being free from microorganisms. 2. the inability of a woman to become pregnant, or of a man to produce potent spermatozoa.

**sterilization** 1. rendering dressings, instruments, etc. aseptic by destroying or removing all microbial life. 2. rendering incapable of reproduction by any means.

**sterilizer** an apparatus in which objects can be sterilized. *See* AUTOCLAVE.

**sternotomy** the operation in which the sternum is cut through to enable the heart to be reached.

**sternum** the breastbone; the flat narrow bone in the centre of the anterior wall of the thorax.

**steroid** one of a group of hormones chemically related to cholesterol. They include oestrogen and androgen, progesterone and the corticosteroids. They may be naturally occurring or they may be synthesized.

**sterol** one of a group of steroid alcohols which includes cholesterol and ergosterol.

**stertorous** snore-like; applied to a snoring sound produced in breathing during sleep or in coma.

**stethoscope** the instrument used for listening to internal body sounds, especially from the heart and lung. It consists of a hollow tube, one end of which is placed over the part to be examined and the other at the ear of the examiner.

**Stevens–Johnson syndrome** *A.M. Stevens, American paediatrician, 1884–1945; F.C. Johnson, American paediatrician, 1894–1934.* A severe form of erythema multiforme in which the lesions may involve the oral and anogenital mucosa, eyes and viscera, associated with such constitutional symptoms as malaise, headache, fever, arthralgia and conjunctivitis.

**STI** sexually transmitted infection.

**stigma** any mark characteristic of a condition or defect, or of a disease.

May also be applied to any physical or social quality of a person that is perceived by others as a negative attribute.

**stillbirth** a baby which has issued forth from its mother after the 24th week of pregnancy and has not, at any time after being completely expelled from its mother, breathed or shown any sign of life. *S. certificate* a certificate issued to the parents by a registered medical practitioner who was present at the birth or examined the body.

**Still's disease** *Sir G.F. Still, British paediatrician, 1868–1941.* A form of rheumatoid arthritis in children, sometimes associated with enlargement of the lymph glands.

**stimulant** an agent that causes increased energy or functional activity of any organ.

**stimulus** *pl.* stimuli. Any agent, act or influence that produces functional or trophic reaction in a receptor or an irritable tissue. *Conditioned s.* a neutral object or event that is psychologically related to a naturally stimulating object or event and which causes a CONDITIONED RESPONSE (*see also* CONDITIONING). *Discriminative s.* a stimulus, associated with reinforcement, which exerts control over a particular form of behaviour; the subject discriminates between closely related stimuli and responds positively only in the presence of that stimulus. *Eliciting s.* any stimulus, conditioned or unconditioned, that elicits a response. *Structured s.* a well-organized and unambiguous stimulus, the perception of which is influenced to a greater extent by the characteristics of the stimulus than by those of the perceiver. *Threshold s.* a stimulus that is just strong enough to elicit a response.

*Unconditioned s.* any stimulus that is capable of eliciting an unconditioned response (*see also* CONDITIONING). *Unstructured s.* an unclear or ambiguous stimulus, the perception of which is influenced to a greater extent by the characteristics of the perceiver than by those of the stimulus.

**stitch** 1. a popular term used to describe a sudden sharp pain usually due to spasm of the diaphragm. 2. a suture. *S. abscess* pus from a formation where a stitch has been inserted.

**Stokes–Adams syndrome** *Sir W. Stokes, Irish surgeon, 1804–1878; R. Adams, Irish physician, 1791–1875.* Attacks of syncope or fainting due to cerebral anaemia in some cases of complete heart block. The heart stops temporarily but breathing continues. The syndrome is treated by using an artificial pacemaker.

**stoma** *pl.* stomata 1. a mouth or mouth-like opening. 2. an artificial opening in the skin surface leading into one of the tubes forming the alimentary canal. *See* COLOSTOMY and ILEOSTOMY.

**stomach** the dilated portion of the alimentary canal between the oesophagus and the duodenum, just below the diaphragm. *Bilocular* or *hourglass s.* one divided into two parts by a constriction. *S. pH electrode* apparatus used to measure gastric contents in situ. *S. pump* a pump that removes the contents of the stomach by suction. *S. tube* a flexible tube used for washing out the stomach or for the administration of liquid food.

**stomatitis** inflammation of the mouth, either simple or with ulceration, caused by a vitamin deficiency or by a bacterial or fungal infection. *Angular s.* cracking at the corners of the mouth, usually due to riboflavin deficiency. *Aphthous s.* that characterized by small, white, painful ulcers on the mucous membrane. *Ulcerative s.* painful shallow ulcers on the tongue, cheeks and lips. A severe type that may produce serious constitutional effects.

**stone** a calculus.

**stool** a motion or discharge from the bowels. *Fatty s.* that which contains undigested fat. *Hunger s.* stool passed by underfed infants: frequent, small and green. *Ricewater s.* the water stool, containing small white flakes, seen in cholera. *Tarry s.* a black tarry stool due to the presence of blood from a peptic ulcer.

**strabismus** squint; heterotropia. A deviation of the eye from its normal direction. It is called convergent when the eye turns in towards the nose, and divergent when it turns outwards. *Concomitant s.* a squint in which the angle of deviation stays constant.

**strabotomy** the division of ocular muscles in the treatment of strabismus.

**strain** 1. overuse or stretching of a part, e.g. a muscle or tendon. 2. a group of microorganisms within a species. 3. to pass a liquid through a filter.

**strangulated** compressed or constricted so that the circulation of the blood is arrested. *S. hernia see* HERNIA.

**strangulation** 1. choking caused by compression of the air passages. 2. arrested circulation to a part, which will result in gangrene.

**strangury** a painful, frequent desire to micturate, but in which only a few drops of urine are passed with difficulty.

**strategic health authority** abbreviated SHA. Ten SHAs in England act as the local headquarters of the NHS. They do not deliver services, but provide leadership, co-ordination and support across a defined geographical area in managing the performance of PCTs and NHS Trusts. Arrangements in Scotland, Wales and Northern Ireland are subject to local variation. SHAs are responsible for the recruitment, retention and development of NHS staff. They also work with partner organizations in local government, education and with the voluntary sector.

**stratified** arranged in layers. *S. tissue* a covering tissue in which the cells are arranged in layers. The germinating cells are the lowest, and as surface cells are shed there is continual replacement.

**stratum** a layer; applied to structures such as the skin and mucous membranes. *S. corneum* the outer, horny layer of the epidermis.

*Streptococcus* a genus of Grampositive spherical bacteria occurring in chains or pairs. Divided into various groups. The first group includes the beta-haemolytic human and animal pathogens; the second and third include alpha-haemolytic parasitic forms occurring as normal flora in the body; and the fourth is made up of saprophytic forms. *S. mutans* implicated in dental caries. *S. pneumoniae* pneumococcus, the most common cause of lobar pneumonia; also causes serious forms of meningitis, septicaemia, empyema and peritonitis. *S. pyogenes* beta-haemolytic, toxigenic, pyogenic streptococci causing septic sore throat, scarlet fever, rheumatic fever, puerperal fever and acute glomerulonephritis.

**streptokinase** an enzyme derived from a streptococcal culture and used to liquefy clotted blood and pus.

*Streptomyces* a genus of soil bacteria from which a large number of antibiotics are derived.

**stress** any factor, mental or physical, the pressure of which can adversely affect the functioning of the body. *S. disorders* those resulting from an individual's inability to withstand stress. *S. fracture* one that occurs as a result of repetitive jarring of a bone, e.g. metatarsal bones in the foot associated with long-distance running and walking, known as a 'march fracture'. *S. incontinence* incontinence, usually of urine, when the intra-abdominal pressure is raised, such as in coughing, sneezing or laughing. *S. ulcer* an acute peptic ulcer, which may be multiple and develop after severe burns, major injuries and occur sometimes during serious illness. The cause is unknown.

**stressor** any life event or change that causes a person stress and which in some circumstances may precipitate distress or deterioration in mental health. These factors may be physical, physiological or psychosocial, e.g. pain and hunger, loss of job, bereavement, divorce, etc.

**stria** *pl.* striae. A line or stripe. *Striae gravidarum* the lines that appear on the abdomen of pregnant women. They are red in first pregnancy, but white subsequently, and are due to stretching and rupture of the elastic fibres.

**striated** striped. *S. muscle* voluntary muscle. *See* MUSCLE.

**stricture** a narrowing or local contraction of a canal. It may be caused by muscle spasm, new growth, or scar tissue formation after inflammation.

**stridor** a harsh, vibrating, shrill sound, produced during respiration when there is partial obstruction of the larynx or trachea.

**stroke** a popular term to describe the sudden onset of symptoms, especially those of cerebral origin affecting movement, sensation, speech and vision. There may be paralysis and loss of sensation down one side of the body or one side of the face. *See* CERE-

BROVASCULAR ACCIDENT. **Heat s.** a hyperpyrexia accompanied by cerebral symptoms. It may occur in someone newly arrived in a very hot climate.

**stroma** the connective tissue forming the ground substance, framework or matrix of an organ, as opposed to the functioning part or parenchyma.

*Strongyloides* a genus of nematode worms, one of which, *S. stercoralis*, is common in tropical countries and causes diarrhoea and intestinal ulcers.

**strontium** *symbol* Sr. A metallic element. Isotopes of strontium are used in bone scanning to detect abnormalities. **S.-90** a radioactive isotope used in radiotherapy in the treatment of skin and eye malignancies.

**structuralism** in psychology, the view that the important influences on people's lives are the basic content of consciousness including intellect, feelings, memory and behaviour. Structuralist approaches in anthropology and sociology are concerned with the social structures within which people function.

**Stryker frame** an apparatus specially designed for care of patients with injuries of the spinal cord or paralysis. It is constructed of pipe and canvas and is designed so that one nurse can turn the patient without difficulty.

**study skills** a set of techniques, strategies and behaviour patterns which form a structured approach to learning.

**stupor** a state of semi-unconsciousness, occurring in the course of many varieties of mental illness, in which the patient does not move or speak, and usually only responds to noxious stimuli.

**Sturge–Weber syndrome** *W.A. Sturge, British physician, 1850–1919; Sir H.D. Weber, British physician, 1824–1918.* A congenital abnormality in which there is a port wine stain on the face with an angioma of the meninges on the same side. Common symptoms are epilepsy, hemiplegia and associated learning difficulties.

**stuttering** *see* STAMMERING.

**stye** *see* HORDEOLUM.

**stylet** a wire or rod for keeping clear the lumen of catheters, cannulae and hollow needles.

**styloid** like a pen. **S. process** a long pointed spine, particularly one projecting from the temporal bone. Also processes on the ulna and radius.

**styptic** an astringent which, applied locally, arrests haemorrhage, e.g. alum and tannic acid.

**subacute** moderately acute. Applied to a disease that progresses moderately rapidly, but does not become acute.

**subarachnoid** below the arachnoid. **S. haemorrage** bleeding into the subarachnoid space from a vessel in the brain. Commonly, due to a rupture of a cerebral aneurysm or to trauma. Blood is present in the cerebrospinal fluid. **S. space** between the arachnoid and pia mater of the brain and spinal cord, and containing cerebrospinal fluid.

**subclavian** beneath the clavicle. **S. artery** the main vessel of supply to the neck and arms.

**subclinical** without clinical manifestations; said of the early stages or a very mild form of a disease.

**subconscious** 1. not conscious yet able to be recalled to consciousness. 2. in psychoanalysis, the part of the mind that retains memories which cannot without much effort be recalled to mind.

**subculture** a subgroup that diverges from the dominant culture in a society but may retain some of its customs and values, while rejecting others.

**subcutaneous** beneath the skin. *S. injection* one given hypodermically.

**subdural** below the dura mater. *S. haematoma* a blood clot between the arachnoid and dura mater. It may be acute or arise slowly from a minor injury.

**subinvolution** incomplete or delayed return of the uterus to its pregravid size during the puerperium, usually as the result of retained products of conception and infection.

**subjective** related to the individual. *S. symptoms* those of which the patient is aware by sensory stimulation, but which cannot easily be seen by others. *See also* OBJECTIVE.

**sublimate** a substance obtained by sublimation.

**sublimation** 1. the vaporization of a solid and its condensation into a solid deposit. 2. in psychoanalysis, a redirecting of energy at an unconscious level. The transference into socially acceptable channels of tendencies that cannot be expressed. An important aspect of maturity.

**subliminal** below the threshold of perception.

**sublingual** beneath the tongue. *S. glands* two small salivary glands in the floor of the mouth.

**subluxation** partial dislocation of a joint.

**submaxillary** beneath the lower jaw. *S. glands* two salivary glands situated under the lower jaw.

**submucous** beneath mucous membrane. *S. resection* an operation to correct a deflected nasal septum.

**subnormal** below normal.

**subphrenic** beneath the diaphragm. *S. abscess* one that develops below the diaphragm, usually after peritonitis or from postoperative infection.

**substitution** the act of putting one thing in place of another. In psychology, this may be the nurse or foster mother in the place of the child's own mother. In psychotherapy, the nurse or therapist may be substituted for someone in the patient's background.

**substrate** a substance on which an enzyme acts.

**succus** a juice. *S. entericus* a digestive fluid secreted by intestinal glands. *S. gastricus* gastric juice.

**succussion** a method of determining when free fluid is present in a cavity in the body. A sound of splashing is heard when the patient moves or is deliberately moved.

**sucrose** a disaccharide obtained from cane or beet sugar.

**suction** 1. the process of sucking. 2. the removal of gas or fluid from a cavity or other container by means of reduced pressure. *Post-tussive s.* a sucking noise heard in the lungs just after a cough.

**sudamen** a small white vesicle formed in the sweat glands after prolonged sweating.

**sudden infant death syndrome** abbreviated SIDS. The sudden and unexpected death of an apparently healthy infant, typically occurring between the ages of 4 weeks and twelve months, and not explained by postmortem studies. Called crib or cot death because the infant often is found dead in the cot. The prone position, respiratory illness and infection, tobacco smoke and overheating have been found to be risk factors. Parents and carers are advised to put their babies to sleep on their backs at the foot of the cot to prevent them wriggling under the bed clothes, not to overheat the room, not to smoke in the same room and to seek advice from a health professional if the baby seems unwell.

**sudor** sweat; perspiration.

**sudorific** diaphoretic; an agent causing sweating.

**suffocation** asphyxiation; a cessation of breathing caused by occlusion of the air passages, leading to unconsciouness and ultimately to death.

**suffusion** a process of diffusion or overspreading, as in flushing of the skin; blushing.

**sugar** a group of sweet carbohydrates classified chemically as monosaccharides or disaccharides. The following are included: *beet s.* obtained from sugar beet; *cane s.* obtained from sugar cane; *fructose* fruit sugar; *grape s.* dextrose, glucose; *milk s.* lactose. *Muscle s.* inositol; a sugar-like compound found in animal tissue, particularly in muscle, and also in many plant tissues.

**suggestibility** inclination to act on suggestions of others.

**suggestion** a tool of psychotherapy in which an idea is presented to and accepted by a patient. *Posthypnotic s.* one implanted in a patient under hypnosis, which lasts after return to a normal condition.

**SUI** serious untoward incident.

**suicide** the intentional taking of one's own life. Legally, a death suspected of being due to violence that is self-inflicted is not termed a suicide unless the victim leaves positive evidence of the intention to commit suicide, or the method of death is such that a verdict of suicide is inevitable. Attitudes to suicide are culturally determined and vary from one group to another. Depression is the commonest cause of suicide and severely depressed people are always at risk.

**sulcus** a furrow or fissure; applied especially to those of the brain.

**sunburn** a dermatitis due to exposure to the sun's rays, causing burning and redness.

**sunstroke** a profound disturbance of the body's heat-regulating mechanism caused by prolonged exposure to excessive heat from the sun. Persons over 40 and those in poor health are most susceptible to it. *See* STROKE.

**superego** that part of the personality that is concerned with moral standards and ideals that are derived unconsciously from parents, teachers and environment, and influence the person's whole mental make-up, acting as a control on impulses of the ego.

**superfecundation** the fertilization of two or more ova, produced during the same menstrual cycle, by spermatozoa from separate coital acts.

**superfetation** the fertilization of a second ovum when pregnancy has already started, producing two fetuses of different maturity.

**supernumerary** 1. present in excess of the normal or required number; extra, as in supernumerary digit. 2. students and new staff placed in clinical areas for orientation and/or for supervised practice who are not included in the staffing numbers.

**superior** above; the upper of two parts.

**supine** 1. lying on the back, with the face upwards. 2. with the palm of the hand upwards. *See* PRONE.

**support** in the health care setting, the assistance and aid that is provided to patients and their families. This support may be physical, e.g. in assisting a patient to walk, or psychological, as when listening to the concerns of relatives. *S. worker* a nursing assistant or auxiliary, physiotherapy helper, foot care assistant or ward receptionist, etc. In clinical areas all these work under the supervision of a registered practitioner who is responsible for the support worker's practice and activities.

**suppository** a medicated solid substance, prepared for insertion into the rectum or vagina, which will dissolve at body temperature.

**suppression** 1. complete cessation of a secretion. 2. in psychology, conscious inhibition as distinct from repression, which is unconscious. *S. of urine* no secretion of urine by the kidneys.

**suppuration** the formation of pus.

**supracondylar** above the condyles. *S. fracture* one above the lower end of the humerus or femur.

**supraorbital** above the orbit of the eye.

**suprapubic** above the pubic bones. *S. cystotomy* surgical incision of the urinary bladder just above the pubic bones.

**suprarenal** above the kidney. *S. gland* adrenal gland. One of a pair of triangular endocrine glands situated on the upper surface of the kidneys. *See* ADRENAL.

**Sure Start** part of the government's drive to eradicate child poverty. The programme aims to improve the health and wellbeing of families and children before and from birth, so that children are ready to flourish when they go to school. Involves interagency collaboration and multidisciplinary partnership in working with disadvantaged families to achieve change.

**surfactant** a surface-active agent. A mixture of phospholipids that is secreted into the pulmonary alveoli and reduces the surface tension of pulmonary fluids, thus contributing to the elastic properties of pulmonary tissue. Surfactant can be instilled via a tracheal catheter as treatment for respiratory distress syndrome. *See also* RESPIRATORY (DISTRESS SYNDROME OF NEWBORN).

**surgeon** a medical practitioner who specializes in surgery. By custom the surgeon's title is Mr, Mrs, Miss or Ms, as opposed to physicians who are called Doctor.

**surgery** the branch of medicine that treats disease by operative measures.

**surrogate** a real or imaginary substitute for a person or object in someone's life. *S. mother* a woman who carries a child for another (the commissioning parent) with the intention that the child be handed over after birth.

**surveillance** the monitoring, recording, analysing and reporting of the occurrence of infectious outbreaks of disease, e.g. hospital-acquired infections, bacterial bloodstream infections and wound infection following orthopaedic surgery. The process can be applied to other incidences, e.g. the cases of notifiable disease in a population.

**survey** the systematic collection of information, not forming part of a scientific epidemiological study.

**susceptibility** lack of resistance to infection. The opposite to immunity.

**suspensory** supporting a part. *S. bandage* one applied to support a part of the body, particularly the scrotum or the lower jaw. *S. ligament* a ligament that supports or suspends an organ, e.g. that of the lens of the eye.

**suture** 1. a stitch or series of stitches used to close a wound (*see* Figure on p. 380). 2. the jagged line of junction of the bones of the cranium. *Atraumatic s.* a suture fused to the needle to obtain a single thickness through each puncture of the needle. *Continuous s.* a form of oversewing with one length of suture. *Coronal s.* the junction between the frontal and parietal bones. *Everting s.* a type of mattress stitch that turns the edges outwards to give a closer approximation. *Fascial s.* a strip of fascia taken from the patient and used to form a suture. *Interrupted s.* a series of separate sutures. *Lambdoid s.* the

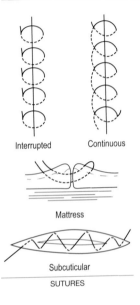

Interrupted     Continuous

Mattress

Subcuticular

SUTURES

junction between the parietal and occipital bones. *Mattress s.* one in which each suture is taken twice through the wound, giving a loop one side and a knot the other. *Purse-string s.* a circular continuous suture round a small wound or appendix stump. *Sagittal s.* the junction between the two occipital bones. *Subcuticular s.* a continuous suture placed just below the skin. *Tension s.* or *relaxation s.* one taking a large bite and relieving the tension on the true stitch line.

**swab** 1. a small piece of cotton wool or gauze. 2. in pathology, a dressed sterile stick used in taking bacteriological specimens.

**swallowing** the taking in of a substance through the mouth and into the oesophagus. It is a combination of a voluntary act and a series of reflex actions. Once begun, the process operates automatically. Also called deglutition.

**sweat** perspiration; a clear watery fluid secreted by the sweat glands. *S. glands* coiled tubular glands situated in the dermis with long ducts to the skin surface.

**Swine influenza** a highly contagious respiratory disease of pigs caused by infection with the swine fever influenza viruses (SIV). A (H1N1) virus. Infected swine can infect and cause symptomatic disease in humans with fever of sudden onset, cough or shortness of breath associated with headache, tiredness, aching muscles, sneezing and runny nose. Currently there is no vaccine developed for this strain of virus. Treatment is with antiviral drugs to minimise complications. *See* INFLUENZA, AVIAN INFLUENZA and ORTHOMYXOVIRUS.

**sycosis** a pustular inflammation of the hair follicles, usually of the beard and moustache.

**Sydenham's chorea** *T. Sydenham, English physician, 1624–1689.* A disorder of the central nervous system closely linked with rheumatic fever; called also St Vitus's dance. The condition, usually self-limited, is characterized by purposeless, irregular movements of the voluntary muscles that cannot be controlled by the patient.

**symbiosis** in parasitology, an intimate association between two different organisms for the mutual benefit of both.

**symblepharon** adhesion of an eyelid to the eyeball.

**symbolism** in psychology, an abnormal mental condition in which events or objects are interpreted as symbols of the patient's own thoughts. In psychiatry, the re-entry into consciousness of repressed material in an acceptable form.

**sympathectomy** division of autonomic nerve fibres which control specific involuntary muscles. An operation performed for many conditions, among them Raynaud's disease.

**sympathetic** 1. exhibiting sympathy. 2. relating to the autonomic nervous system. *S. nervous system* one of the two divisions of the autonomic nervous system. It supplies involuntary muscle and glands; it stimulates the ductless glands and the circulatory and respiratory systems, but inhibits the digestive system. *S. ophthalmia* inflammation leading to loss of sight in the opposite eye after a perforating injury in the ciliary region.

**sympathomimetic** pertaining to drugs that produce effects similar to those caused by a stimulation of the sympathetic nervous system.

**symphysis** a cartilaginous joint along the line of union of two bones. *S. pubis* the cartilaginous junction of the two pubic bones.

**symptom** any indication of disease perceived by the patient. *Cardinal s's* 1. symptoms of greatest significance to the doctor, establishing the identity of the illness. 2. the symptoms shown in the temperature, pulse and respiration. *Dissociation s.* anaesthesia to pain and to heat and cold, without impairment of tactile sensibility. *Objective s.* one perceptible to others than the patient, such as pallor, rapid pulse or respiration, restlessness, etc. *Presenting s.* the symptom or group of symptoms about which the patient complains or from which relief is sought. *Signal s.* a sensation, aura or other subjective experience indicative of an impending epileptic or other seizure. *Subjective s.* one perceptible only to the patient, as pain, pruritus, vertigo, etc. *Withdrawal s's* symptoms that follow sudden abstinence from a drug on which a person is dependent.

**symptomatology** 1. the study of the symptoms of a disease. 2. the symptoms of a particular disease, taken together.

**synalgia** pain felt in one part of the body but caused by inflammation of or injury to another part. *See* REFERRED PAIN.

**synapse** the junction between the termination of an axon and the dendrites of another nerve cell. Chemical transmitters pass the impulse across the space.

**syncope** a simple faint or temporary loss of consciousness due to cerebral ischaemia, often caused by dilatation of the peripheral blood vessels and a sudden fall in blood pressure.

**syndactylism** possessing webbed fingers or toes. A condition in which two or more fingers or toes are joined together.

**syndrome** a group of signs or symptoms typical of a distinctive disease, which frequently occur together and form a distinctive clinical picture.

**synergist** 1. a muscle that works in conjunction with another muscle. 2. a drug that works in combination with another drug, the two drugs having a greater effect when taken together than when taken separately.

**synovectomy** excision of a diseased synovial membrane to restore joint movement.

**synovial fluid** the fluid that surrounds a joint and is secreted by the synovial membrane. It is a thick, colourless, lubricating substance.

**synovial membrane** a serous membrane lining the articular capsule of a movable joint and terminating at the edge of the articular cartilage.

**synovitis** inflammation of a synovial membrane, usually with an effusion of fluid within the joint.

**synthesis** the building up of a more complex structure from simple components. This may apply to drugs or to plant or animal tissues.

**syphilis** a sexually transmitted infection caused by the spirochaete *Treponema pallidum;* the incidence is currently on the increase in the UK. Primary syphilis is with the first appearance of a painless sore, appearing either on the genitals, anus, rectum, lips, throat or fingers, which heals within a few weeks. A rash then ensues, which may be transient, recurrent or last for months. Other symptoms include lymphadenopathy, malaise, headaches, fever and fatigue. Following the symptomatic phase, the disease becomes latent for a few years or sometimes indefinitely. For untreated cases the disease progresses to the development of gummatous lesions involving the cardiovascular and neurological systems. Syphilis can be vertically transmitted from mother to fetus from 9 weeks of gestation, causing miscarriage, stillbirth, neonatal death and long-term morbidity. All pregnant women are offered serological screening, initially with the Venereal Disease Research Laboratory if the results are positive, treatment with penicillin is effective. Practising safer sex can help to prevent syphilis infection. People with syphilis are infectious in the early stages but not in the latent and final stages.

**syringe** an instrument for injecting fluids or for aspirating or irrigating body cavities. It consists of a hollow tube with a tight-fitting piston. A hollow needle or a thin tube can be fitted to the end.

**syringomyelia** the formation of cavities filled with fluid inside the spinal cord. Impairment of muscle function and sensation result at the level of and below the lesion. Painless injury may be the first symptom. It is a progressive disease.

**syringomyelitis** inflammation of the spinal cord, as the result of which cavities are formed in it.

**syringomyelocele** a type of spina bifida in which the protruded sac of fluid communicates with the central canal of the spinal cord.

**systematic** describing a process that is carried out according to a method or a system. *S. review* a methodical approach to literature reviews that reduces random error and bias. This requires a review of clinical literature in a particular field that has set explicit tests for whether research is valuable enough to be included in an overview of the area. This is often combined with a statistical meta-analysis of clinical trial results. *S. sampling* a type of sampling in which a convenient number is chosen, e.g. every tenth or fourth member of the population is selected into the sample.

**Système International d'Unités** [Fr.] *SI units.* The international system for measurement in science, industry and general use. It was agreed in 1960, and it is now illegal in the UK to prescribe or dispense drugs in any other units.

**systemic** pertaining to or affecting the body as a whole. *S. circulation* circulation of the blood throughout the whole body, other than the pulmonary circulation. *See* SCLEROSIS.

**systole** the period of contraction of the heart. *See* DIASTOLE. *Atrial s.* the contraction of the heart by which the blood is pumped from the atria into the ventricles. *Extra-s.* a premature contraction of the atrium or ventricle, without alteration of the fundamental rhythm of the pacemaker. *Ventricular s.* the contraction of the heart by which the blood is pumped into the aorta and pulmonary artery.

**systolic** relating to a systole. *S. murmur* an abnormal sound produced during systole in heart infections. *S. pressure* the highest pressure of the blood reached during systole.

**T**   symbol for *thymine*.

**T cell**   a lymphocyte which is derived from the thymus and is responsible for cell-mediated immunity. *T. helper cells*   T cells that activate B lymphocytes to release antibodies and T killer cells to destroy cells having a specific antigenic profile. *T. killer cells*   T cells that are activated by circulating T helper cells in the blood and lymphatic systems, and which recognize body cells displaying antigens to which they have become sensitized, targeting those which are viral or bacterially infected, triggering cell-mediated immunity. *T. suppressor cells*   T cells that keep the immune response at an appropriate level and also stop or slow down the activity of B lymphocytes and other T cells once the immune response has dealt with the antigen.

**tabes**   a wasting away. *T. dorsalis* locomotor ataxia. A slowly progressive disease of the nervous system affecting the posterior nerve roots and spinal cord. It is a late manifestation of syphilis.

**taboo**   any ritual prohibition of certain activities, e.g. incest in many societies, or the open discussion of death and dying.

**tachycardia**   abnormally rapid action of the heart and consequent increase in pulse rate. See BRADYCARDIA. *Paroxysmal t.* spasmodic increase in cardiac contractions of sudden onset lasting a variable time, from a few seconds to hours.

**tachyphasia, tachyphrasia**   extreme volubility of speech. It may be a sign of mental disorder.

**tachyphrenia**   hyperactivity of the mental processes.

**tachypnoea**   rapid, shallow respirations; a reflex response to stimulation of the vagus nerve endings in the pulmonary vessels.

**tactile**   relating to the sense of touch.

*Taenia*   a genus of tapeworms. *T. saginata* the beef tapeworm. The most common type of tapeworm found in the human intestine. *T. solium* the pork tapeworm. Can also be parasitic in humans, causing cysticercosis. See TAPEWORM.

**taeniasis**   an infestation with tapeworms.

**t'ai chi**   a system of movement, breathing and concentration, Chinese in origin, promoting general health and wellbeing.

**talipes**   clubfoot. A deformity caused by a congenital or acquired contraction of the muscles or tendons of the foot (see Figure on p. 384). *T. calcaneus* the heel alone touches the ground on standing. *T. equinus* the toes touch the ground but not the heel. *T. valgus* the inner edge of the foot only is in contact with the ground. *T. varus* the person walks on the outer edge of the foot.

**talus**   the astragalus or ankle bone.

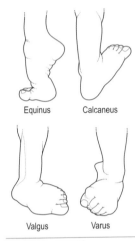

Equinus   Calcaneus

Valgus   Varus

TALIPES

**tampon** a plug of absorbent material inserted in the vagina, the nose or other orifice to restrain haemorrhage or absorb secretion.

**tamponade** the surgical use of tampons. *Cardiac t.* impairment of heart action by haemorrhage or effusion into the pericardium; may be due to a stab wound or follow surgery.

**tantrum** an outburst of ill temper. *Temper t.* a behaviour disorder of childhood. A display of bad temper in which the child performs uncontrolled actions in a state of emotional stress.

**tapeworm** any of a group of cestode flatworms, including the *Taenia* genus, which are parasitic in the intestines of humans and many animals. The adult consists of a round head with suckers or hooklets for attachment (scolex). From this,

numerous segments (proglottids) arise, each of which produces ova capable of independent existence for a considerable length of time. Treatment is by anthelmintic drugs.

**tapotement** [Fr.] a tapping movement used in massage.

**tapping** *see* PARACENTESIS.

**target cells** abnormal flat red blood cells seen in liver and spleen disease and in the haemoglobinopathies. The haemoglobin is distributed as a small inner mass with a pale outer ring.

**tarsal** relating to a tarsus. *T. bones* the seven small bones of the ankle and instep. *T. cyst* Meibomian cyst; chalazion. *T. glands* Meibomian glands of the eyelids. *T. plates* small cartilages in the upper and lower eyelids.

**tarsalgia** pain in the foot.

**tarsorrhaphy** stitching of the eyelids together to protect the cornea or to allow healing of an abrasion.

**tartar** a hard incrustation deposited on the teeth and on dentures.

**task allocation** a method of organizing care whereby each specific type of care is carried out by a separate nurse or health care assistant for the same patient.

**taste** the sense by which it is possible to identify what is eaten and drunk. Taste receptors (buds) lie on the tongue and give the sensations of sweet, sour, salt and bitter.

**tattoo** a permanent discoloration of the skin due to a foreign pigment.

**tattooing** the deliberate (usually for decorative purposes) or accidental, perhaps as a result of an explosion, insertion of coloured material into the deeper layers of the skin.

**taxis** manipulation by hand to restore any part to its normal position. It can be used to reduce a hernia or a dislocation.

**taxonomy** the theory and practice of the classification of animals and plants.

**team nursing** method of organizing care based on the allocation of each nurse to a team that cares for a group of patients, usually for a number of shifts.

**tears** the watery, slightly alkaline and saline secretion of the lacrimal glands that moistens the conjunctiva. Tears contain lyozyme, a bactericidal enzyme. *Artifical t.* preparations used to supplement tear production in patients with dry eye associated with autoimmune disorder, e.g. rheumatoid arthritis, or to relieve irritation.

**teat** 1. a nipple of the breast. 2. a manufactured nipple used on infants' feeding bottles.

**technetium** *symbol* Tc. A metallic element. *Radioactive t.* an isotope ($^{99m}$Tc) used in a number of diagnostic tracer tests. As it has a short half-life (6 hours), a high dose may be given for scanning organs, but the patient receives only a low radiation dose.

**teeth** *see* DENTITION.

**tegument** the skin.

**telangiectasis** a group of dilated capillary blood vessels, web-like or radiating in form.

**telangioma** a tumour of the blood capillaries.

**telemedicine** the use of communications systems (such as electronic networks and VDUs) to provide remote diagnosis, advice, treatment and monitoring. Being used widely in both primary and acute care settings.

**telepathy** the transmission of thought without any normal means of communication between two persons.

**telereceptor** a sensory nerve ending which can respond to distant stimuli. Those of the eyes, ears and nose are examples. Teleceptor.

**telophase** the last stage in the division of cells when the chromosomes have been reconstituted in the nuclei at either end of the cell and the cell cytoplasm divides to form two new cells.

**temperament** a person's nature; the habitual and emotional attitude, as distinct from mood which is temporary.

**temperature** the degree of heat of a substance or body as measured by a thermometer. *Normal t.* the normal temperature of the human body is 37°C, with a slight decrease in the early morning and a slight increase at night. It indicates the balance between heat production and heat loss.

**template** a mould or pattern. In radiotherapy, a map of the area of the patient requiring treatment and of those areas to be protected from radiation.

**temple** the region on either side of the head above the zygomatic arch.

**temporal** pertaining to the side of the head. *T. arteritis* giant cell arteritis. A chronic inflammatory condition of the carotid arterial system, occurring usually in elderly people. There is persistent headache and partial or total blindness may result. *T. bone* one of a pair of bones on either side of the skull containing the organ of hearing. *T. lobe* the part of the cerebrum below the lateral sulcus.

**temporomandibular** relating to the temporal bone and the mandible. *T. joint* the hinge of the lower jaw. *T. joint syndrome* painful dysfunction of the temporomandibular joint, marked by a clicking or grinding sensation in the joint; commonly caused by malocclusion of the teeth.

**tenacious** thick and viscid, as applied to sputum or other body fluids.

**tendinitis** inflammation of a tendon and its attachments.

**tendon** a band of fibrous tissue forming the termination of a muscle and attaching it to a bone. *Achilles t.* that inserted into the calcaneum.

*T. grafting* an operation which repairs a defect in one tendon by a graft from another. *T. insertion* the point of attachment of a muscle to a bone which it moves. *T. reflex* the muscular contraction produced on percussing a tendon.

**tenesmus** a painful, ineffectual straining to empty the bowel or bladder.

**tennis elbow** a painful disorder which affects the extensor muscles of the forearm at their attachment to the external epicondyle.

**tenorrhaphy** the suturing together of the ends of a divided tendon.

**tenosynovitis** inflammation of a tendon sheath.

**TENS** abbreviation for transcutaneous electrical nerve stimulation. A method of treating persistent pain by passing small electrical currents into the spinal cord or sensory nerves by means of electrodes applied to the skin. TENS is noninvasive and non-addictive, with no known side-effects. The NMC has approved the use of TENS by midwives and first-level nurses on their own responsibility, provided they have been instructed in its use.

**tension** the act of stretching or the state of being stretched. *Arterial t.* the pressure of blood on the vessel wall during cardiac contraction. *Intraocular t.* the pressure of the contents of the eye on its walls, measured by a tonometer. *Intravenous t.* the pressure of blood within the veins. *Premenstrual t.* symptoms of abdominal distension, headache, emotional lability and depression, occurring a few days before the onset of menstruation. *See* PREMENSTRUAL. *Surface t.* tension or resistance which acts to preserve the integrity of a surface, particularly the surface of a liquid.

**teratogen** an agent or influence that causes physical defects in the developing embryo.

**teratoma** a solid tumour containing tissues similar to those of a dermoid cyst. Found most often in the ovaries and testes, many of these tumours are malignant.

**term** the end of pregnancy, normally calculated as 280 days or 40 weeks from the date of the last normal menstrual period but considered to be any time after the 37th week of pregnancy.

**termination of pregnancy (TOP)** abortion that is induced, legally or illegally.

**tertiary** third. *T. care* care and treatment that is given in a large regional hospital providing specialist care, e.g cardiac surgery, intensive, neonatal, oncological services. *T. prevention* prevention of ill health, mitigating the effects of illness and disease that have already occurred.

**test** 1. an examination or trial. 2. analysis of the composition of a substance by the use of chemical reagents, and/or to determine the presence or absence of a substance.

**testicle** a testis; one of the two glands in the scrotum which produce spermatozoa. *Undescended t.* a condition in which the organ remains in the pelvis or inguinal canal.

**testicular self-examination** should be performed regularly once a month for the detection of early tumours of the testis, which are highly curable if detected at an early stage. Self-examination should take place after a warm bath or shower, which relaxes the scrotal skin. It is performed as follows: standing in front of a mirror, look for any swelling. One testicle may appear larger than the other or hang lower; this is usually perfectly normal. Examine each testicle with both hands and gently roll each testicle between the fingers and thumb. A small lump is felt for and, if found, almost always occurs in only one testis and is usually

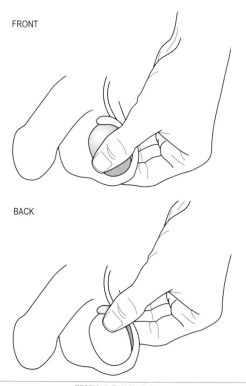

FRONT

BACK

TESTICLE EXAMINATION

painless (*see* Figure). A cord-like structure found on the top and back of each testicle should be found and examined for any swelling.

**testis** a testicle.

**testosterone** the hormone produced by the testes which stimulates the development of sex characteristics. It can now be made synthetically, and is used medicinally in cases of failure of sex function and as a palliative treatment in some cases of advanced metastatic breast cancer in females.

**tetanus** an acute disease of the nervous system caused by the contamination of wounds by the spores of a soil bacterium, *Clostridium tetani*. Muscle stiffness around the site of the wound occurs, followed by rigidity of face and neck muscles; hence 'lockjaw'. All muscles are then affected and opisthotonos may occur. *T. antitoxin* a serum that gives a short-term passive immunity and may be used with penicillin for immediate treatment of a case of tetanus. *T. vaccine* or *toxoid* will give an active immunity.

**tetany** an increased excitability of the nerves due to a lack of available calcium, accompanied by painful muscle spasm of the hands and feet (carpopedal spasm). The cause may be hypoparathyroidism or alkalosis owing to excessive vomiting or hyperventilation.

**tetralogy** a series of four. *T. of Fallot* see FALLOT'S TETRALOGY.

**tetraplegia** quadriplegia. Paralysis of all four limbs.

**thalamus** a mass of nerve cells at the base of the cerebrum. Most sensory impulses from the body pass to this area and are transmitted to the cortex.

**thalassaemia** a group of haemolytic anaemias where there is interference with the synthesis of haemoglobin resulting in anaemia. Several types are recognized, according to the symptoms. Thalassaemia is prevalent in the Mediterranean, Middle East and Southeast Asian regions, and occurs in families from these regions as the disease is genetically inherited. There is no known cure and genetic counselling is advised for the parents or other close relatives of a child with thalassaemia and also for any person with thalassaemia trait.

**thalassotherapy** treatment involving sea bathing or a sea voyage.

**thanatology** 1. the study of death and dying. 2. the forensic study of the causes of death.

**theca** a sheath, such as the covering of a tendon. *T. folliculi* the covering of a Graafian follicle. *T. vertebralis*

the membranes enclosing the spinal cord; the dura mater.

**thenar** 1. the palm of the hand. 2. the fleshy part at the base of the thumb.

**therapeutic** pertaining to therapeutics or treatment of disease; curative. *T. abortion* see ABORTION. *T. community* any treatment setting (usually psychiatric) which provides a living–learning situation through group processes emphasizing social, environmental and personal interactions and which encourages the individual to learn socially from these processes. *T. drug monitoring* abbreviated TDM. Some drugs require that blood levels are maintained within a certain range (often called a therapeutic window) to avoid inefficacy as a result of low blood levels and producing side-effects for the patient as a result of levels in the blood being too high. To do this blood levels of the drug concerned need to be measured at appropriate intervals and medication regimes altered as necessary. *T. index* the margin of difference between the desired and safe effect that a drug dose achieves, and the dose that is known to produce toxic effects. This measure varies between people, who all process drugs differently, but it does alert the prescriber to the margins of safety in the use of a particular drug. *T. touch* techniques that are used to facilitate healing and wellbeing of a person based on the concept that the body is an energy field and that this field can be influenced from outside itself. Body energies can be transferred to and through the hands of a therapist who has been trained to assume the role of healer. *See* MASSAGE. *T. use of self* the ability of the psychiatric nurse to use therapy and experimental knowledge along with self-awareness and the ability to explore, and use, one's personal impact on others. *T. window* range of blood level in the use of certain drugs. *See* TDM above.

**therapeutics** the science and art of healing and the treatment of disease.

**therapy** the treatment of disease.

**thermal** relating to heat.

**thermocautery** the deliberate destruction of tissue by means of heat. *See* CAUTERY.

**thermography** a method of measuring the amount of heat produced by different areas of the body, using infrared photography. Used as a diagnostic aid in the detection of breast tumours and the assessment of rheumatic joints; also used in the study of pain.

**thermolysis** the loss of body heat by radiation, by excretion and by the evaporation of sweat.

**thermometer** an instrument for measuring temperature. *Clinical t.* one used to measure the body temperature.

**thermoreceptor** a nerve ending that responds to heat and cold.

**thermoregulation** the normal regulation of body temperature by the maintenance of the balance between heat production and heat loss.

**thermotherapy** the treatment of disease by application of heat.

**thiamine** vitamin B₁, or aneurine. An essential vitamin involved in carbohydrate metabolism. A deficiency causes beriberi. The source is liver and unrefined cereals.

**Thiersch skin graft** *I. Thiersch, German surgeon, 1822–1895.* The transplantation of areas of partial thickness skin. *See* GRAFT.

**thirst** an uncomfortable sensation of dryness of the mouth and throat with a desire for oral fluids. *Abnormal t.* polydipsia.

**Thomas splint** *H.O. Thomas, British orthopaedic surgeon, 1834–1891.* A splint consisting of an oval iron ring that fits over the lower limb.

Attached to the ring are two round iron rods which are bent into a **W** shape at the lower end. It is used to support the limb and move the weight from the knee joint to the pelvis.

**thoracic** relating to the thorax. *T. duct* the large lymphatic vessel situated in the thorax along the spine. It opens into the left subclavian vein.

**thoracocentesis** puncture of the wall of the thorax to allow aspiration of pleural fluid.

**thoracoscopy** examination of the pleural cavity by means of an endoscopic instrument.

**thoracotomy** a surgical incision into the thorax.

**thorax** the chest; a cavity containing the heart, lungs, bronchi and oesophagus. It is bounded by the diaphragm, the sternum, the thoracic vertebrae and the ribs. *Barrel-shaped t.* a development in emphysema, when the chest is malformed like a barrel.

**threadworm** a species of roundworm, *Enterobius vermicularis*, parasitic in the large intestine, particularly of children.

**threonine** one of the essential amino acids.

**thrill** a tremor discerned by palpation.

**throat** 1. the anterior surface of the neck. 2. the pharynx. *Clergyman's sore t.* laryngitis. *Sore t.* pharyngitis.

**thrombin** an enzyme that converts fibrinogen to fibrin during the later stages of blood clotting.

**thromboangiitis** inflammation of blood vessels with clot formation. *T. obliterans* inflammation of the arteries, usually of the legs of young males, causing intermittent claudication and gangrene. Buerger's disease.

**thrombocyte** a disc-shaped blood platelet; essential for the clotting of shed blood.

**thrombocytopenia** a reduction in the number of platelets in the blood; bleeding may occur. Destruction of platelets can be caused by infections, certain drugs, transfusion-related purpuras, idiopathic thrombocytopenic purpura and disseminated intravascular coagulation.

**thrombocytosis** an increase in the number of platelets in the blood.

**thromboembolism** a clot or embolism, which has become detached from a thrombus formed in another site that is carried in the blood flow to obstruct a blood vessel elsewhere in the body.

**thrombokinase** thromboplastin. A lipid-containing protein, activated by blood platelets and injured tissues, which is capable of activating prothrombin to form thrombin, which, combined with fibrinogen, forms a clot.

**thrombolysis** the disintegration or dissolving of a clot by the infusion of an enzyme such as streptokinase into the blood.

**thrombophlebitis** the formation of a clot, associated with inflammation of the lining of a vein.

**thromboplastin** *see* THROMBOKINASE.

**thrombosis** the formation of a thrombus. *Cavernous sinus t.* thrombosis of the cavernous sinus, usually the result of infection of the face, when the veins in the sinus are affected via ophthalmic vessels. *Cerebral t.* the occlusion of a cerebral artery, the most common cause of cerebral infarction (a 'stroke'). *Coronary t.* the occlusion of a coronary vessel, by which the heart muscle is deprived of blood, causing myocardial ischaemia and often leading to myocardial infarction (a 'heart attack'). *See* DEEP VEIN T. *Lateral sinus t.* a complication of mastoiditis when infection of the lateral sinus of the dura mater occurs and there is clot formation.

**thrombus** a stationary blood clot caused by coagulation of the blood in the heart or in an artery or a vein.

**thrush** an infection of the mucous membranes, most commonly of the mouth and vagina, by a fungus, *Candida albicans. See* CANDIDIASIS.

**thymectomy** surgical removal of the thymus.

**thymine** symbol T. One of the pyrimidine bases found in DNA.

**thymus** a gland-like structure situated in the upper thorax and neck. Present in early life, it reaches its maximum development during puberty and continues to play an immunological role throughout life, even though its function declines with age.

**thyroglossal** relating to the thyroid and the tongue. *T. cyst see* CYST.

**thyroid** 1. shaped like a shield. 2. pertaining to the thyroid gland. *Intrathoracic* or *retrosternal t.* position of the gland low in the neck and wholly or in part behind the sternum. *T. cartilage* the largest cartilage of the larynx. It forms the 'Adam's apple' in the front of the throat. *T. gland* a ductless gland, consisting of two lobes, situated in front and on either side of the trachea. It secretes the hormones thyroxine and triiodothyronine which are concerned in regulating the metabolic rate. *T.-stimulating hormone* abbreviated TSH. Thyrotrophin; a hormone, produced by the anterior pituitary gland, which controls the activity of the thyroid gland.

**thyroidectomy** partial or complete removal of the thyroid gland.

**thyroiditis** inflammation of the thyroid. Acute thyroiditis, usually due to a virus infection, is characterized by sore throat, fever and painful enlargement of the gland. *Hashimoto's t.* a progressive autoimmune disease of the thyroid gland with degeneration of its epithelial elements and replacement by lymphoid and fibrous tissue.

**thyrotoxicosis** hyperthyroidism. The symptoms arise when there is overactivity of the thyroid gland. The metabolism is speeded up and there is enlargement of the gland and exophthalmos.

**thyrotrophin** *see* THYROID-(STIMULA-TING HORMONE).

**thyroxine** one of the two hormones secreted by the thyroid gland. It is used in the treatment of hypothyroidism.

**TIA** transient ischaemic attack.

**tibia** the shin bone; the larger of the two bones of the leg, extending from knee to ankle.

**tic** a spasmodic twitching of certain muscles, usually of the face, neck or shoulder. *T. douloureux* paroxysmal trigeminal neuralgia.

**tick** a blood-sucking parasite which may transmit the organisms of disease.

**tidal volume** the amount of gas passing into and out of the lungs in each respiratory cycle.

**tincture** a medical substance dissolved in alcohol.

**tinea** a group of skin infections caused by a variety of fungi and named after the area of the body affected, thus: *T. barbae*, the beard; *T. capitis*, the head; *T. circinata* or *T. corporis*, the body; *T. cruris*, the groin; and *T. pedis*, the feet. *See* RINGWORM.

**tinnitus** a ringing, buzzing or roaring sound in the ears.

**tissue** a group or layer of similarly specialized cells that together perform certain special functions.

**titration** determination of a given component in solution by addition of a liquid reagent of known strength until a given endpoint, e.g. change in colour, is reached, indicating that the component has been consumed by reaction with the reagent.

**tobacco** the dried leaves of the plant *Nicotiana tabacum*, containing the drug nicotine, which may be smoked, chewed or inhaled. All these activities are potentially dangerous to health. Cigarette smoking in particular is responsible for an increase in cancer of the lungs and mouth and bronchitis. Smoking increases the likelihood of emphysema and coronary artery disease. It is also harmful during pregnancy, leading to smaller and less healthy babies. *T. withdrawal syndrome* a change in mood or behaviour associated with the stopping of or reduction in cigarette smoking. *See* PASSIVE SMOKING.

**tocography** the measurement of alterations in the intrauterine pressure during labour.

**tocopherol** vitamin E, present in wheatgerm, green leaves and milk.

**token economy programme** a behavioural approach to modifying troublesome behaviours and restoring lost self-help behaviours by the systematic rewarding of desired behaviour by giving tokens which may be exchanged for goods or privileges.

**tolerance** the ability to endure without effect or injury. *Exercise t. test* to determine how much oxygen a patient's myocardium requires during exercise. The results indicate the patient's capacity for exercise and in the estimation of the extent of coronary disease. *Drug t.* decrease of susceptibility to the effects of a drug due to its continued administration. *Immunological t.* specific non-reactivity of lymphoid tissues to a particular antigen caused, under other conditions, of inducing immunity.

**tomography** body section radiography in which X-rays or ultrasound waves are used to produce an image of a layer of tissue at any depth.

**tone** 1. the normal degree of tension, e.g. in a muscle. 2. a particular quality of sound.

**tongue** a muscular organ attached to the floor of the mouth and concerned in taste, mastication, swallowing and speech. It is covered by a mucous membrane from which project numerous papillae.

**tonic** 1. a term popularly applied to any drug supposed to brace or tone up the body or any particular part or organ. 2. possessing tone in a state of contraction, e.g. muscles. *T. spasm* a prolonged contraction of one or several muscles, as seen in epilepsy, for example. *See* CLONIC.

**tonography** the measurement made by an electric tonometer recording the intraocular pressure and so, indirectly, the drainage of aqueous humour from the eye.

**tonsil** a mass of lymphoid tissue, particularly one of two small, almond-shaped bodies, situated one on each side between the pillars of the fauces. It is covered by mucous membrane, and its surface is pitted with follicles. *Pharyngeal t.* the lymphadenoid tissue of the pharynx between the pharyngotympanic tubes. Adenoids. *T. test* a small sample of tonsil obtained in suspected cases of CREUTZFELDT–JAKOB DISEASE (CJD) for the identification of the prion found in new variant CJD, a spongiform encephalopathy.

**tonsillectomy** excision of one or both tonsils.

**tonus** the normal state of partial contraction of the muscles.

**tooth** a structure in the mouth designed for the mastication of food. Each is composed of a crown, neck and root with one or more fangs. The main bulk is of dentine enclosing a central pulp; the crown is covered with a hard white substance called enamel. *See* DENTITION.

**tophus** a small, hard, chalky deposit of sodium urate in the skin and cartilage, occurring in gout and sometimes appearing in the auricle of the ear.

**topical** relating to a particular spot; local. *T. lotion* one for local or external application.

**topography** the study of the surface of the body in relation to the underlying structures.

**torpor** a sluggish condition in which response to stimuli is absent or very slow.

**torsion** twisting: (a) of an artery to arrest haemorrhage; (b) of the pedicle of a cyst, which produces venous congestion in the cyst and consequent gangrene (a possible complication of ovarian cyst).

**torso** the body, excluding the head and the limbs; the trunk.

**torticollis** wryneck, a contracted state of the cervical muscles, producing torsion of the neck. The deformity may be congenital or secondary to pressure on the accessory nerve, to inflammation of glands in the neck, or to muscle spasm.

**total** complete, the whole number or amount. *T. body irradiation* abbreviated TBI. The complete exposure of the patient's body to radiotherapy, used in the treatment of some cancers and prior to bone marrow transplantation. *T. lung capacity* abbreviated TLC. The volume of air held in the lungs following deep inspiration. *T. parenteral nutrition* abbreviated TPN. The supplying of all essential nutrients to a patient via the intravenous route. *See* Appendix 1. *T. patient care* 1. the inclusion of all aspects of care for a patient, i.e. physical, psychological, spiritual and social aspects of care. 2. a planned care programme for a patient to which members of several different professional groups have contributed. *T. quality management* an approach to management based upon the idea that quality of service depends upon the active involvement of all members of staff in achieving and maintaining high standards of care throughout the organization.

**tourniquet** a constrictive band applied to a limb to arrest arterial haemorrhage. No longer used in first aid because its use may cause permanent damage to muscles or nerve supply.

**toxaemia** poisoning of the blood by the absorption of bacterial toxins. *T. of pregnancy* a condition affecting pregnant women and characterized by albuminuria, hypertension and oedema, with the possibility of pre-eclampsia and eclampsia developing.

**toxic** 1. poisonous, relating to a poison. 2. caused by a toxin. *T. shock syndrome* a severe illness characterized by high fever of sudden onset, vomiting, diarrhoea and, in severe cases, death. A sunburn-like rash with peeling of the skin occurs.

**toxicity** the degree of virulence of a poison.

**toxicology** the science dealing with poisons.

**toxin** any poisonous compound, usually referring to that produced by bacteria.

*Toxocara* a genus of nematode worms, parasitic in the intestines of dogs and cats, which may also infest humans, especially children. The spleen, liver and lungs are most often affected but the parasite may also infest the retina, causing inflammation and granulation.

**toxoid** a toxin which has been deprived of some of its harmful properties but is still capable of

producing immunity and may be used in a vaccine.

*Toxoplasma* a genus of protozoa which infests birds and animals and may be transmitted from them to humans.

**toxoplasmosis** a disease due to *Toxoplasma gondii* carried by cats, birds and other animals and in contaminated soil. The congenital form is marked by central nervous system lesions, which may lead to blindness, brain defects and death. The acquired infection is often asymptomatic but may result in pneumonia, skin rashes and nephritis. Can cause severe multisystem disease in immunocompromised people.

**TPN** total parenteral nutrition.

**trabecula** a dividing band or septum, extending from the capsule of an organ into its interior and holding the functioning cells in position.

**trabeculectomy** an operation to lower the intraocular pressure in glaucoma that cannot be controlled by medication.

**trace element** an element that is essential in the diet, for the normal functioning of the body, but is required only in minute amounts, e.g. zinc, manganese, fluorine, etc.

**tracer** a means by which something may be followed, as (a) a mechanical device by which the outline or movements of an object can be graphically recorded, or (b) a material by which the progress of a compound through the body may be observed, e.g. a radioactive isotope tracer.

**trachea** the windpipe; a cartilaginous tube lined with ciliated mucous membrane, extending from the lower part of the larynx to the commencement of the bronchi.

**tracheitis** inflammation of the trachea causing pain in the chest, with coughing.

**tracheobronchitis** acute infection of the trachea and bronchi due to viruses or bacteria.

**tracheostomy** a surgical opening into the third and fourth cartilage rings of the trachea. *T. tubes* those used to maintain an airway after tracheotomy, either permanently or until the normal use of the air passages is regained.

**tracheotomy** surgical incision of the trachea. *High t.* superior tracheotomy. *Inferior* or *low t.* that in which the opening is made below the thyroid isthmus. *Superior t.* high tracheotomy. That in which the opening is made above the thyroid isthmus.

**trachoma** a chronic infectious disease of the conjunctiva and cornea, producing photophobia, pain and lacrimation, caused by an organism once thought to be a virus but now classified as a strain of the bacterium *Chlamydia trachomatis*. Trachoma is more prevalent in Africa and Asia than in other parts of the world.

**traction** 1. the exertion of a pulling force, such as that applied to a fractured bone or dislocated joint or to relieve muscle spasm, to maintain proper position and facilitate healing. 2. in obstetrics, that along the axis of the pelvis to assist in delivery of a fetal part, or the placenta and membranes. *Hamilton–Russell t.* a form of traction of the leg. *Head t.* traction exerted on the head in the treatment of cervical injury. *Skeletal t.* a method of keeping the fractured ends of bone in position by traction on the bone. A metal pin or wire is passed through the distal fragment or adjacent bone to overcome muscle contraction.

**trait** an inherited or developed physical or mental characteristic.

**trance** a condition of semiconsciousness of hysterical, cataleptic or hypnotic origin. It is not due to organic disease.

**tranquilizer** a drug which allays anxiety, relieves tension and has a calming effect on the patient.

**transactional analysis** a theory of personality structure and a psychotherapeutic method. The human personality is viewed as consisting of three ego states: the parent, the adult and the child. The aim is to allow the adult ego to take control over the child and parent egos.

**transaminase** one of a group of enzymes which catalyse the transfer of an amine group from one amino acid into another. Transaminases include *glutamic-oxalacetic t.* (GOT) and *glutamic-pyruvic t.* (GPT).

**transcendental meditation** a technique for attaining a state of physical relaxation and psychological calm by the regular practice of a relaxation procedure which entails the repetition of a mantra. Has been successfully used by some patients to reduce hypertension.

**transcultural nursing** being aware of the patient's cultural health beliefs and values and incorporating these into the agreed care plan with the patient.

**transcutaneous blood gas monitors** the application to the skin of a probe which is heated to a temperature of 44°C and enables measurements of $Po_2$ and $Pco_2$ to be made. Accuracy depends on the quality of the peripheral circulation, thus transcutaneous blood gas monitoring is usually used in conjunction with intermittent arterial sampling.

**transcutaneous electrical nerve stimulation** *see* TENS.

**transdermal** through the skin. *T. patch* a sticky adhesive patch which has been coated with a dose of a drug. This patch can be applied to the skin and over a period of time the drug is absorbed into the body.

**transference** in psychiatry, the unconscious transfer by the patient on to the psychiatrist of feelings that are appropriate to other people significant to the patient.

**transferrin** a glycoprotein that acts as a carrier for iron in the bloodstream.

**transfusion** the introduction of whole blood or a blood component into a vein, performed in cases of severe loss of blood, shock, septicaemia, etc. It is used to supply actual volume of blood, or to introduce constituents, such as clotting factors or antibodies, that are deficient in the patient. *Direct t.* the transfer of blood directly from a donor to a recipient. *Exchange t.* replacement transfusion. The removal of most or all of the recipient's blood and its replacement with fresh blood. Used with infants suffering from erythroblastosis. See RHESUS FACTOR. *Feto-maternal t.* from fetus to mother via the placenta; transplacental transfusion (TPT). *Intra-arterial t.* the passing of blood into an artery under positive pressure in cases where large quantities are required rapidly, as in cardiovascular surgery. *Replacement t.* exchange transfusion.

**transient ischaemic attack** abbreviated TIA. A sudden episode of temporary or passing symptoms, caused by diminished blood flow through the carotid or vertebrobasilar blood vessels.

**transillumination** the illumination of a translucent body structure by a strong light as an aid to diagnosis, particularly of tumours of the retina and of abnormalities in the ethmoidal and frontal sinuses.

**translocation** in morphology, the transfer of a segment of a chromosome to a different site on the same chromosome or to a different chromosome. It can be a cause of congenital abnormality.

**translucent** allowing light rays to pass through indistinctly.

**transmigration** a movement from one place to another, as in the passage of blood cells through the walls of the capillaries. Diapedesis. *External t.* the passage of an ovum from its ovary to the uterine tube on the opposite side. *Internal t.* the movement of an ovum from one uterine tube to the other through the uterus.

**transmission-based precautions** precautions, designed to be applied to patients known or suspected to be infected with pathogens that are highly transmissible or epidemiologically important, and for which additional measures beyond STANDARD PRECAUTIONS are needed to interrupt transmission in hospital. There are three types of transmission-based precaution: airborne, droplet and contact precautions. They may be combined for diseases that have multiple routes of transmission. When employed either singly or in combination, they are used in addition to standard precautions.

**transplacental** across the placenta. Movement may be from mother to fetus or vice versa. *T. infection* may affect the unborn child.

**transplant** 1. an organ or tissue taken from the body and grafted into another area of the same individual or another individual. 2. to transfer tissue from one part to another or from one individual to another.

**transplantation** the transfer of living organs from one part of the body to another (autotransplant) or from one individual to another (allograft). Transplantation is often called grafting, though the latter is more commonly used to refer to the transfer of skin.

**transposition** 1. displacement of any of the viscera to the opposite side of the body. 2. the operation which partially removes a piece of tissue from one part of the body to another, complete severance being delayed until it has become established in its new position. *T. of the great vessels* a congenital abnormality of the heart in which the positions of the pulmonary artery and aorta are reversed.

**transsexualism** a disturbance of gender identity; there is a persistent conviction that the person's true gender is opposite to the actual anatomical sex.

**transudate** any fluid that passes through a membrane.

**transverse** cross-wise. *T. presentation* position of the fetus whereby it lies across the pelvis; this position must be corrected before normal birth can take place.

**transvestite** a person who experiences a habitual and strongly persistent desire to dress as a member of the opposite sex ('cross-dressing'), often for reasons of sexual gratification. The majority are male and have no desire to physically change sex.

**trauma** injury. *Birth t.* an injury to the infant sustained during the process of being born. In some psychiatric theories, the psychological shock produced in an infant by the experience of being born. *Psychological t.* an emotional shock that makes a lasting impression.

**treatment** the mode of dealing with a patient or disease. *Active t.* that in which specific medical or surgical treatment is undertaken. *Conservative t.* that which aims at preserving and restoring injured parts by natural means, e.g. rest, fluid replacement, etc., as opposed to radical or surgical methods. *Empirical t.* treatment based on observation of symptoms and not on science. *Palliative t.* that which relieves distressing symptoms but does not cure the disease.

*Prophylactic t.* that which aims at the prevention of disease.

**Trematoda** a class of fluke worms, some of which are parasitic in humans. Many of them have freshwater snails as secondary hosts.

**tremor** an involuntary, muscular quivering which may be due to fatigue, emotion or disease. Tremor, first of one hand, and later affecting the other limbs, is the first symptom of Parkinsonism. *Intention t.* one that occurs on attempting a movement, as in disseminated sclerosis.

**Trendelenburg's position** *F. Trendelenburg, German surgeon, 1844–1924. See* POSITION.

**Trendelenburg's sign** a test of the stability of the hip. The patient stands on the affected leg and flexes the other knee and hip. If there is dislocation the pelvis is lower on the side of the flexed leg, which is the reverse of normal.

*Treponema* a genus of spirochaetes. Anaerobic bacteria, they are motile, spiral and parasitic in humans and animals. *T. carateum* the causative agent of pinta. *T. pallidum* the causative agent of syphilis. *T. immobilization test* a serological test for syphilis. *T. pertenue* the causative agent of yaws (framboesia).

**tri-iodothyronine** a hormone produced by the thyroid gland together with thyroxine.

**triage** [Fr.] 1. choosing, classifying or sorting. 2. a process by which a patient is assessed upon arrival to determine the urgency of the problem, and to designate appropriate health care resources to care for the identified problem. *T. nurse* a registered nurse with specialist skills and knowledge who carries out the assessment and classification of casualties according to the type and severity of their injuries in order to assign them for treatment in the accident and emergency department.

**triceps** having three heads. *T. muscle* that situated on the back of the upper arm, which extends the forearm.

**trichiasis** 1. a condition of ingrowing hairs about an orifice, or ingrowing eyelashes. 2. the appearance of hair-like filaments in the urine.

**trichinosis** a disease caused by eating underdone pork containing a parasite, *Trichinella spiralis*. This becomes deposited in muscle and causes stiffness and painful swelling. There may also be nausea, diarrhoea and fever. Trichiniasis.

**trichology** the study of hair.

*Trichomonas* a genus of flagellate protozoa that are parasitic to humans. *T. hominis* infests the bowel and may cause dysentery. *T. tenax* infests the mouth and may be present in cases of pyorrhoea. *T. vaginalis* is commonly present in the vagina and may cause leukorrhoea and vaginitis.

**trichomoniasis** infestation with a parasite of the genus *Trichomonas*.

*Trichophyton* a genus of fungi that affect the skin, nails and hair.

**trichophytosis** infection of the skin, nails or hair with one of the genus *Trichophyton*. See TINEA.

**trichosis** any abnormal growth of hair.

**trichuriasis** infestation by the whipworm.

*Trichuris* a genus of nematode worms that may infest the colon and cause diarrhoea. A whipworm.

**tricuspid** having three flaps or cusps. *T. valve* that at the opening between the right atrium and the right ventricle of the heart.

**trifocal** pertaining to a spectacle lens that has three foci, one for distant, one for intermediate and one for near vision.

**trigeminal** divided into three. *T. nerves* the fifth pair of cranial nerves, each of which is divided into three main branches and supplies one side of the face. *T. neuralgia* pain in the face which is confined to branches of the trigeminal nerve. Tic douloureux.

**trigger finger** a stenosing of the tendon sheath at the metacarpophalangeal joint, allowing flexion of the finger but not extension without assistance, when it 'clicks' into position.

**triglyceride** 'human fat', an ester of glycerol and three fatty acids.

**trigone** a triangular area. *T. of the bladder* the triangular space on the floor of the bladder, between the ureteric openings and the urethral orifice.

**trimester** a period of 3 months. *First t. of pregnancy* the first 3 months, during which rapid development is taking place.

**triple vaccine** a combined dose of diphtheria, tetanus and pertussis immunization.

**triplets** three children carried in the uterus at once and born at one labour. Incidence formerly about 1 in 6400 births; now, as a result of treatment of infertility, more common.

**triplopia** a condition in which three images of an object are seen at the same time.

**trismus** lockjaw; a tonic spasm of the muscles of the jaw.

**trisomy** the presence of an extra chromosome in each cell in addition to the normal paired set of 46. The cause of several chromosome disorders including Down's syndrome and Klinefelter's syndrome.

**trochanter** either of two bony prominences below the neck of the femur. *Greater t.* that on the outer side forming the bony prominence of the hip. *Lesser t.* that on the inner side at the neck of the femur.

**trochlea** any pulley-shaped structure, but particularly the fibrocartilage near the inner angular process of the frontal bone through which passes the tendon of the superior oblique muscle of the eye.

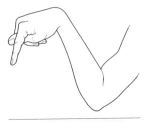

TROUSSEAU'S SIGN (CARPAL SPASM) WITH HYPOCALCAEMIA

**trophoblast** the layer of cells surrounding the blastocyst at the time of and responsible for implantation.

**tropia** a manifest squint, one that is present when both eyes are open.

**tropical** relating to the areas within 23.5° north and south of the equator, termed the tropics. *T. medicine* that concerned with diseases that are more prevalent in hot climates.

**tropism** an affinity or attraction of one cell to another.

**Trousseau's sign** *A. Trousseau, French physician, 1801–1867.* 1. spontaneous peripheral venous thrombosis. 2. a sign for tetany in which carpal spasm can be elicited by compressing the upper arm and causing ischaemia to the nerves distally (*see* Figure).

**truancy** absence of a child from school without leave. A disorder of conduct which may result from emotional insecurity or a feeling of unfairness.

**truncus** a trunk; the main part of the body, or a part of it, from which other parts spring. *T. arteriosus* the arterial trunk connected to the fetal heart which develops into the aortic and pulmonary arteries.

*Trypanosoma* a genus of protozoan parasites which pass some of their life cycle in the blood of vertebrates, including humans. *T. gambiense* and *T. rhodesiense* are transmitted by

the bite of the tsetse fly, and are the cause of sleeping sickness.

**trypanosomiasis** a disease caused by infestation with *Trypanosoma*. Sleeping sickness.

**trypsin** a digestive enzyme that converts protein into amino acids.

**trypsinogen** the precursor of trypsin. It is secreted in the pancreatic juice and activated by the enterokinase of the intestinal juices into trypsin.

**tryptophan** one of the essential amino acids.

**tsetse fly** a fly of the genus *Glossina* which transmits the parasite *Trypanosoma* to humans, causing trypanosomiasis.

**TSH** thyroid-stimulating hormone.

**tsutsugamushi disease** scrub typhus, which occurs in Japan and is transmitted by the bite of a mite.

**tubal** relating to a tube. *T. ligation* tying of the fallopian tubes as a method of female sterilization. *T. pregnancy* extrauterine pregnancy where the embryo develops in the uterine tube. Ectopic pregnancy.

**tube feeding** administration of liquid and semisolid foods through a nasogastric, gastrostomy or enterostomy tube. Tube feeds are administered to patients who are unable to take foods by mouth.

**Tubegauz** a proprietary brand of woven circular bandage available in a variety of sizes and applied with a special applicator.

**tubercle** 1. a small nodule or a rounded prominence on a bone. 2. the specific lesion (a small nodule) produced by the tubercle bacillus.

**tubercular** pertaining to tubercles.

**tuberculin** the filtrate from a fluid medium in which *Mycobacterium tuberculosis* has been grown and which contains its toxins. *Old t.* prepared from the human bacillus and used in skin tests in diagnosing tuberculosis. *See* MANTOUX TEST and HEAF TEST.

**tuberculosis** abbreviated TB. Chronic, recurrent notifiable infection, most commonly occurring in the lungs, caused by *Mycobacterium tuberculosis* or (rarely in the UK) *M. bovis* or *M. africanum*; transmission is usually by inhalation of bacilli in airborne droplets. *Bovine TB* endemic in cattle and some other animals and transmissible to humans by ingestion of meat or unpasteurized milk; causes extrapulmonary (non-respiratory) TB of the tonsils, abdominal organs, joints and bones and lymph nodes (also lymphadenitis in immunosuppressed patients). *Miliary TB* severe form occurring when tubercle bacilli are spread acutely throughout the bloodstream causing extrapulmonary TB. *Open TB* any type of TB in which infectious patients are excreting bacilli from the body, most often in the sputum. *Pulmonary TB* the most common form of TB, affecting the lungs. *TB of the spine* also known as Pott's disease.

**tuberosity** an elevation or protuberance on a bone to which tendons are attached.

**tuberous** covered with tubers. *T. sclerosis* a familial disease with tumours on the surfaces of the lateral ventricles of the brain and sclerotic patches on its surface; marked by mental deterioration and epileptic attacks.

**tubule** a small tube. *Renal* or *uriniferous t.* the essential secreting tube of the kidney.

**tularaemia** a plague-like disease of rodents, caused by *Francisella* (*Pasteurella*) *tularensis*, which is transmissible to humans. The illness can be contracted by handling diseased animals or their hides, eating infected wild game or being bitten by insects that have fed on infected animals. It causes fever and headache; the lymph glands enlarge and may suppurate.

**tumefaction** a swelling or the process of becoming swollen. *See* TUMESCENCE.

**tumescence** 1. a swelling or enlarging of a part. 2. a swollen condition. 3. a penile erection.

**tumour** an abnormal swelling. The term is usually applied to a morbid growth of tissue which may be benign or malignant. A neoplasm. *Benign* or *innocent t.* one that does not infiltrate or cause metastases, and is unlikely to recur if removed. *Malignant t.* one that invades and destroys tissue and can spread to neighbouring tissues, and to more distant sites via the blood and the lymphatic systems.

**tunica** a coat, a covering, or the lining of a vessel. *T. adventitia, t. media, t. intima* the outer, middle and inner coats of an artery, respectively. *T. vaginalis* the membrane covering the front and sides of the testis.

**tunnel** in anatomy, a canal through a structure. *Carpal t.* the osteofibrous channel in the wrist between the carpal bones and tissue covering the flexor tendons. *C. tunnel syndrome* pain and tingling in the hand and fingers caused by compression of the median nerve in the carpal tunnel. *T. vision* vision that is restricted to the central field. Occurs in chronic glaucoma and in retinitis pigmentosa.

**turbinate** scroll-shaped. *T. bone* one of the three long thin plates that form the walls of the nasal cavity.

**turgid** swollen or distended.

**Turner's syndrome** H.H. *Turner, American physician, 1892–1970.* A chromosomal defect in females, causing short stature. Classically, an absence of one X chromosome. Affects 1 in 3000 live female births. The majority have streak ovaries leading to an absence of puberty and infertility. Other features may include webbing of the neck, cubitus valgus, nail abnormalities and coarctation of the aorta. Intelligence is usually normal.

**twilight state** partial disturbance of consciousness, a state that may follow an epileptic fit and may be associated with alcoholism and some confusional states. The person can still carry out some routine activities but has no awareness or memory of doing so.

**twin** one of a pair of individuals who have developed in the uterus together. *Binovular (dizygotic) t.* each twin has developed from a separate ovum; fraternal, or non-identical, twins. *Uniovular (monozygotic) t.* both twins have developed from the same cell; identical twins.

**tympanectomy** excision of the tympanic membrane.

**tympanites** distension of the abdomen by accumulation of gas in the intestine or the peritoneal cavity.

**tympanitis** inflammation of the middle ear; otitis media.

**tympanoplasty** an operation to reconstruct the eardrum and restore conductivity to the middle ear. *See* MYRINGOPLASTY.

**tympanosclerosis** fibrosis and the formation of calcified deposits in the middle ear which lead to deafness.

**tympanum** 1. the middle ear. 2. the eardrum or tympanic membrane.

**type** the general or prevailing character of any particular case of disease, person, substance, etc. *Asthenic t.* a type of physical constitution, with long limbs, small trunk, flat chest and weak muscles. *Athletic t.* a type of physical constitution with broad shoulders, deep chest, flat abdomen, thick neck and good muscular development. *Blood t's see* BLOOD GROUPS. *Phage t.* a subgroup of a bacterial species susceptible to a particular bacteriophage and demonstrated by phage-typing (*see* PHAGE). Also called lysotype and phagotype. *Pyknic t.* a type of physical constitution marked by rounded body, large chest, thick shoulders, broad head and short neck.

**type A behaviour** a behaviour pattern associated with the development of coronary heart disease, characterized by excessive competitiveness and aggression and a fast-paced lifestyle. Research has shown that this type of behaviour is associated with coronary artery disease and myocardial infarction. The opposite type of behaviour, exhibited by individuals who are relaxed, unhurried and less aggressive, is called type B and is associated with a lower risk of heart disease.

**typhoid fever** enteric fever. A notifiable infectious disease caused by *Salmonella typhi*, which is transmitted by water, milk or other foods, especially shellfish, that have been contaminated. There is high fever, a red rash, delirium and sometimes intestinal haemorrhage. Recovery usually begins during the fourth week of the disease. A person who has had typhoid fever gains immunity from it but may become a carrier. Although perfectly well, the person harbours the bacteria and passes them out in the faeces. The typhoid bacillus often lodges in the gallbladder of carriers.

**typhus** an acute, notifiable, infectious disease caused by species of the parasitic microorganism *Rickettsia*. There is high fever, a widespread red rash and severe headache. Typhus is likely to occur where there is overcrowding, lack of personal cleanliness and bad hygienic conditions, because the infection is spread by bites of infected lice or by rat fleas. *Scrub t.* a form spread by mites and widespread in the Far East. Tsutsugamushi disease.

**tyramine** an enzyme present in cheese, game, broad-bean pods, yeast extracts, wine and strong beer, which has a similar effect in the body to that of adrenaline.

Foodstuffs containing tyramine should be avoided by patients taking monoamine oxidase inhibitors.

**tyrosine** an essential amino acid that is the product of phenylalanine metabolism. In some diseases, especially of the liver, it is present as a deposit in the urine. It is a precursor of catecholamines, melanin and thyroid hormones.

**tyrosinosis** a congenital condition in which there is an error of metabolism and phenylalanine cannot be reduced to tyrosine. Hepatic failure may occur.

**UK NHS Blood and Transplant (NHSBT)** special health authority set up for the purpose of providing a reliable and efficient supply of blood, haemopoietic stem cell donations and organs for transplantation throughout the NHS.

**ulcer** an erosion or loss of continuity of the skin or of a mucous membrane, often accompanied by suppuration. *Arterial u.* caused by arterial insufficiency, usually with a deep punched out appearance and is painful at rest with the legs elevated. *Decubitus u.* a pressure sore caused by lying immobile for long periods of time. *Duodenal u.* a peptic ulcer in the duodenum. *Gastric u.* one in the lining of the stomach. *Gravitational u.* a varicose ulcer of the leg which heals with difficulty because of its dependent position and the poor venous return. *Indolent u.* one that is painless and heals slowly. *Peptic u.* one that occurs on the mucous membrane of either the stomach or duodenum. *Perforating u.* one that erodes through the thickness of the wall of an organ. *Rodent u.* a slow-growing epithelioma of the face which may cause much local destruction and ulceration, but does not give rise to metastases. *See* BASAL CELL CARCINOMA. *Venous u.* gravitational ulcer. A shallow ulcer usually on the lower leg between the knee and the ankle that is linked with varicose veins resulting in a poor circulation to and from the area. Initially, often there is an area of eczematous skin and the ulcer forms with large amounts of exudate and oozing.

**ulcerative** characterized by ulceration (the formation of ulcers). *U. colitis* inflammation and ulceration of the colon and rectum of unknown cause.

**ultrasonic** relating to sound waves having a frequency range beyond the upper limit perceived by the human ear. These waves are widely used instead of X-rays, particularly in the examination of structures not opaque to X-rays.

**ultrasonogram** an echo picture obtained from using ultrasound.

**ultrasonography** a radiological technique in which deep structures of the body are visualized by recording the reflections (echoes) of ultrasonic waves directed into the tissues.

**ultrasound** ultrasonic waves used to examine the interior organs of the body. These waves can also be used in the treatment of soft-tissue pain, and to break up renal calculi or the crystalline lens when cataract is present. *U. screening* a method of body imaging based on the reflectivity of sound. Ultrasound scanning is non-invasive and is widely used in obstetrics to detect the site of the placenta, the presence of fetal abnormalities and the sex of the fetus; it will reveal a multiple pregnancy at an early stage.

**ultraviolet rays** short wavelength electromagnetic rays. They are present in sunlight and cause tanning and sunburn.

**ultra vires** a change made beyond powers. An NHS organization must behave reasonably and in accordance with its powers. If an organization acts beyond its powers (ultra vires), it lays itself open to judicial review.

**umbilical cord** arises from the placenta and enters the fetus at the site of the future navel, providing the nutritional, hormonal and immunological link between mother and fetus during pregnancy.

**umbilicus** the navel; the circular depressed scar in the centre of the abdomen where the umbilical cord of the fetus was attached.

**unconditioned response** an unlearned response, i.e. one that occurs naturally.

**unconscious** 1. insensible; incapable of responding to sensory stimuli and of having subjective experiences. 2. that part of mental activity which includes primitive or repressed wishes, concealed from consciousness by the psychological censor. *Collective u.* in Jungian psychology, the portion of the unconscious which is theoretically common to human beings.

**unconsciousness** the state of being unconscious. This may vary in depth from deep unconsciousness, when no response can be obtained, through to lesser degrees of unconsciousness when the patient can be roused by painful stimuli, to a level when the patient can be roused by speech or non-painful stimuli. Deep prolonged unconsciousness is known as coma.

**undine** a glass flask with a spout used for irrigation of the eye.

**undulant** rising and falling like a wave. *U. fever see* BRUCELLOSIS.

**unguentum** an ointment.

**uniform resource locator** abbreviated URL. In a computer a web browser that is used in the location of specific website, e.g http://www.medscape.com.

**unilateral** on one side only.

**union** 1. a joining together. 2. the repair of tissue after separation by incision or fracture. *See* CALLUS and HEALING.

**uniovular** from one ovum. *U. twins* identical twins, developed from one ovum.

**unipara** a woman who has had only one child.

**unit** 1. a single thing. 2. a standard of measurement. *Intensive care u.* a hospital department reserved for those with severe medical or surgical disorders. *International insulin u.* a measurement of the pure crystalline insulin arrived at by biological assay. *SI u.* one of the various units of measurement making up the Système International d'Unités (International System of Units).

**universal precautions** abbreviated UP. A concept developed by nurses during the mid-1980s (largely as a response to human immunodeficiency virus, or HIV, epidemics) that assumes all patients are potentially infected with BLOOD-BORNE VIRUSES; consequently, universal blood and body fluid infection control precautions are used for all patients, all the time. This concept has been further developed and is known as STANDARD PRECAUTIONS. *See also* BODY SUBSTANCE ISOLATION, INFECTION (CONTROL) and Appendices.

**urachal** referring to the urachus. *U. cyst* a congenital abnormality in which a small cyst persists along the course of the urachus. *U. fistula* one that forms when the urachus fails to close. Urine may leak from the umbilicus.

**urachus** a tubular canal existing in the fetus, connecting the bladder with the umbilicus. In the adult it persists in the form of a solid fibrous cord.

**uraemia** 1. an excess in the blood of urea, creatinine and other nitrogenous endproducts of protein and amino acid metabolism; sometimes referred to as azotaemia. 2. in current usage, the entire complex of signs and symptoms of chronic renal failure. Depending upon the cause it may or may not be reversible. Uraemia leads to vomiting and nausea, headache, weakness, metabolic disturbances, convulsions and coma (*see* RENAL (FAILURE)).

**urate** a salt of uric acid. *Sodium u.* a compound generally found in concentration around joints in cases of gout.

**urea** carbamide. A white crystalline substance which is an end product of protein metabolism and the chief nitrogenous constituent of urine. It is a diuretic. The normal daily output is about 33 g. *Blood u.* that which is present in the blood. Normal value is 20–40 mg/100 ml.

**ureter** one of the two long narrow tubes that convey the urine from the kidney to the bladder.

**ureterectomy** the surgical removal of a ureter.

**ureteric** relating to the ureter. *U. catheter see* CATHETER. *U. transplantation* an operation in which the ureters are divided from the bladder and implanted in the colon or loop of ileum. Congenital defects or malignant growth may make this necessary.

**ureterocele** a cystic enlargement of the wall of the ureter at its entry into the bladder.

**ureterolith** a calculus in a ureter.

**ureterolithotomy** removal of a calculus from the ureter.

**ureterostomy** the surgical creation of a permanent opening through which the ureter discharges urine.

**ureterovaginal** relating to the ureter and vagina. *U. fistula* an opening

into the ureter by which urine escapes via the vagina.

**urethra** the canal through which the urine is discharged from the bladder. The male urethra is about 18 cm long and the female about 3.5 cm.

**urethritis** inflammation of the urethra. The condition is frequently a symptom of gonorrhoea but may be caused by other infectious organisms. *Non-specific u.* abbreviated NSU. A sexually transmitted inflammation of the urethra caused by a variety of organisms other than gonococci. *See* NON-SPECIFIC (URETHRITIS).

**urethrocele** a prolapse of the female urethral wall which may result from damage to the pelvic floor during childbirth.

**urethrography** radiographic examination of the urethra. A radio-opaque contrast medium is inserted by catheter.

**urethroscope** an instrument for examining the interior of the urethra.

**uric acid** lithic acid, the end product of nucleic acid metabolism, a normal constituent of urine. Its accumulation in the blood produces uricacidaemia. Renal calculi are frequently formed of it.

**urinalysis** the bacteriological or chemical examination of the urine.

**urinary** relating to urine. *U. tract* the system that conducts urine from the kidneys to the exterior, including the ureters, the bladder and the urethra.

**urination** micturition. The act of passing urine.

**urine** the clear fluid of a varying straw colour secreted by the kidneys and excreted through the bladder and urethra. It is composed of 96% water and 4% solid constituents, the most important being urea and uric acid. Specific gravity = 1.017–1.020; slightly acidic. *Residual u.* that which remains in the bladder after micturition. **U. retention** the inability to urinate voluntarily or to empty a full bladder.

**urinometer** an instrument used for measuring the specific gravity of urine.

**URL** uniform resource locator.

**urobilin** the main pigment of urine, derived from urobilinogen.

**urobilinogen** a pigment derived from bilirubin which, on oxidation, forms urobilin.

**urochrome** the yellow pigment that colours urine.

**urodynamics** the dynamics of the propulsion and flow of urine in the urinary tract.

**urogenital** relating to the urinary and genital organs. Urinogenital.

**urography** radiographic examination of the urinary tract after the injection of a radio-opaque, water-soluble, iodine-containing medium.

**urokinase** an enzyme in urine which is secreted by the kidneys and causes fibrinolysis. In certain diseases it may cause bleeding from the kidneys.

**urolith** a calculus in the urinary tract.

**urology** the study of diseases of the urinary tract.

**urostomy** an artificial urinary conduit for deflecting urine from the ureters to the abdominal wall.

**urticaria** nettle-rash or hives. An acute or chronic skin condition characterized by the recurrent appearance of an eruption of weals, causing great irritation. The cause may be certain foods, infection, drugs or emotional stress. *See* ALLERGY.

**uterine** relating to the uterus. **U. tubes** see FALLOPIAN TUBES.

**uterosalpingography** radiographic examination of the uterus and the uterine tubes.

**uterovesical** referring to the uterus and bladder. **U. pouch** the fold of peritoneum between the two organs.

THE UTERUS AND ADNEXA

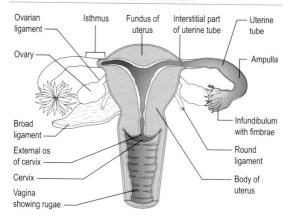

**uterus** the womb; a triangular, hollow, muscular organ situated in the pelvic cavity between the bladder and the rectum (*see* Figure on p. 405). Its function is the nourishment and protection of the fetus during pregnancy and its expulsion at term. *Bicornuate u.* one having two horns. A congenital malformation; see BICORNUATE. *Gravid u.* the pregnant uterus.

**utilitarianism** a philosophical or ethical view which holds that utility entails the greatest happiness of the greatest number of people and therefore that an action should always produce more benefits than harm.

**utricle** the delicate membranous sac in the bony vestibule of the ear.

**uvea** uveal tract. The pigmented layer of the eye, consisting of the iris, ciliary body and choroid.

**uveitis** inflammation of the uveal tract.

**uvula** the small fleshy appendage which is the free edge of the soft palate, hanging from the roof of the mouth.

**vaccination** the introduction of vaccine into the body to produce immunity to a specific disease.

**vaccine** a suspension of killed or attenuated organisms (viruses, bacteria or rickettsiae), administered for prevention, amelioration or treatment of infectious diseases. *Attenuated v.* one prepared from living organisms which, through long cultivation, have lost their virulence. *Bacille Calmette–Guérin v.* an attenuated bovine bacillus vaccine giving immunity from tuberculosis. *Sabin v.* an attenuated poliovirus vaccine that can be administered by mouth, in a syrup or on sugar. *Salk v.* one prepared from an inactivated strain of poliomyelitis virus. *TAB v.* a sterile solution of the organisms that cause typhoid and paratyphoid A and B. Paratyphoid C may now be included. *Triple v.* one that protects against diphtheria, tetanus and whooping cough.

**vaccinia** cowpox; a virus infection of cows, which may be transmitted to humans by contact with the lesions. A local pustular eruption is produced. Also known as cowpox.

**vacuum** a space from which air or gas has been extracted. *V. bag* a sealed plastic bag containing small expanded polystyrene spheres, the patient is positioned on the bag which has the air pressure inside reduced until it is hardened. This mould is used in radiotherapy to accurately immobilize the patient and to reproduce the position on a daily basis prior to treatment. *V. extractor* an instrument known as a Ventouse is used to assist delivery of the fetus. A suction cup is attached to the head and a vacuum created slowly. Gentle traction is applied, which is synchronized with the uterine contractions. *V. wound drainage system* a closed suction drainage system used following surgery for wound exudates.

**vagal** relating to the vagus nerve.

**vagina** the canal, lined with mucous membrane, that leads from the cervix of the uterus to the vulva.

**vaginismus** a painful spasm of the muscles of the vagina, occurring usually when the vulva or vagina is touched, resulting in painful sexual intercourse or dyspareunia.

**vaginitis** inflammation of the vagina caused by microorganisms. *Atrophic* or *post-menopausal v.* inflammation caused by degenerative changes in the mucous lining of the vagina and insufficient oestrogen secretion. Adhesions may occur, partially closing the vagina. *Trichomonas v.* infection caused by *T. vaginalis*, a protozoon that causes a thin, yellowish discharge, giving rise to local tenderness and pruritus.

**vagotomy** surgical incision of the vagus nerve or any of its branches.

A treatment for gastric or duodenal ulcer. **Highly selective *v*.** division of only those vagal fibres supplying the acid-secreting glands of the stomach. **Medical *v*.** interruption of impulses carried by the vagus nerve by administration of suitable drugs.

**vagus** the tenth cranial nerve, arising in the medulla and providing the parasympathetic nerve supply to the organs in the thorax and abdomen. *V*. **resection** vagotomy.

**valgus** a displacement outwards, particularly of the feet. *See* GENU, HALLUX, TALIPES.

**validity** the extent to which a measure, indicator or method of data collection possesses the quality of being sound or true, as far as can be judged. **Construct *v*.** the extent to which an instrument is said to measure a theoretical construct or trait. **Content *v*.** the degree to which the content of the measure represents the universe of content, or the domain of a given behaviour. **External *v*.** the degree to which findings of a study can be generalized to other populations or environments. **Face *v*.** a type of content validity that uses an expert's opinion to judge the accuracy of an instrument. **Internal *v*.** the degree to which it can be inferred that the experimental treatment, rather than an uncontrolled condition, resulted in the observed effects.

**valine** an essential amino acid formed by the digestion of dietary protein.

**Valsalva's manoeuvre** *A.M. Valsalva, Italian anatomist, 1666–1723.* Technique for increasing the intrathoracic pressure by closing the mouth and nostrils and blowing out the cheeks, thereby forcing air back into the nasopharynx. When the breath is released, the intrathoracic pressure drops and the blood is quickly propelled through the heart, producing an increase in the heart rate (tachycardia) and the blood pressure. Immediately after this event a reflex bradycardia ensues. Valsalva's manoeuvre occurs when a person strains to defecate or urinate, uses the arm and upper trunk muscles to move up in bed, or strains during coughing, gagging or vomiting. The increased pressure, immediate tachycardia and reflex bradycardia can bring about cardiac arrest in vulnerable heart patients.

**valve** 1. a means of regulating the flow of liquid or gas through a pipe. 2. a fold of membrane in a passage or tube, so placed as to permit passage of fluid in one direction only. Valves are important structures in the heart, in veins and in lymph vessels. **Semilunar *v*.** either of two valves at the junction of the pulmonary artery and aorta, respectively, with the heart.

**valvotomy** valvulotomy. A surgical operation to open up a fibrosed valve, e.g. mitral valvotomy to relieve mitral stenosis.

**valvulitis** inflammation of a valve, particularly of the heart.

**vaporizer** an apparatus for producing a very fine spray of a liquid.

**variable** a research term that describes any factor or circumstance that is part of the study. **Confounding *v*.** one that affects the conditions of the independent variables unequally. **Dependent *v*.** one that depends upon the experimental conditions. **Independent *v*.** the variable conditions of an experimental situation, e.g. control or experimental. **Random *v's*** background factors that may affect any conditions of the independent variables equally.

**variance** used in statistics. The distribution range of a set of results around a mean. *See* STANDARD DEVIATION.

**varicella** chickenpox. An infectious disease of childhood with an incubation period of 12–20 days. There is slight fever and an eruption of transparent vesicles on the chest, on the first day of disease; these appear in successive crops all over the body. The vesicles soon dry up, sometimes leaving shallow pits in the skin. The disease is usually mild, but may be severe in neonates, adults and those who are immunocompromised. Chickenpox is a notifiable disease in Scotland.

**varicella zoster virus** abbreviated VZV. A human herpes virus that causes chickenpox during childhood and may reactivate later in life to cause shingles.

**varices** alternative name for enlarged, distorted varicose veins or lymphatic vessels.

**varicose** swollen or dilated. *V. ulcer* gravitational ulcer. *See* ULCER. *V. veins* a dilated and twisted condition of the veins (usually those of the leg) caused by structural changes in the walls or valves of the vessels.

**varus** a displacement inwards. *See* GENU, HALLUX, TALIPES.

**vas** *pl.* vasa. A vessel or duct. *V. deferens* one of a pair of excretory ducts conveying the semen from the epididymis to the urethra. *V. efferens* one of the many small tubes that convey semen from the testis to the epididymis. *Vasa vasorum* the minute nutrient vessels that supply the walls of the arteries and veins.

**vascular** relating to, or consisting largely of, blood vessels. *V. system* the cardiovascular system.

**vascularization** the development of new blood vessels within a tissue that occurs during healing.

**vasculitis** angiitis; inflammation of a blood vessel. *Allergic v.* a severe allergic response to drugs or to cold. Arising in small arteries or veins, with fibrosis and thrombi formation.

**vasectomy** excision of a part of the vas deferens. If performed bilaterally, sterility results. Employed as a method of contraception.

**vasoconstrictor** any agent that causes contraction of a blood vessel wall, and therefore a decrease in the blood flow and a rise in the blood pressure.

**vasodilator** any agent that causes an increase in the lumen of blood vessels, and therefore an increase in the blood flow and a fall in the blood pressure.

**vasomotor** controlling the muscles of blood vessels, both dilator and constrictor. *V. centre* nerve cells in the medulla oblongata controlling the vasomotor nerves. *V. nerves* sympathetic nerves regulating the tension of the blood vessels.

**vasopressin** antidiuretic hormone (ADH). A hormone from the posterior lobe of the pituitary gland which causes constriction of plain muscle fibres and reabsorption of water in the renal tubules. Used in the treatment of diabetes insipidus and bleeding from oesophageal varices.

**vasovagal** vascular and vagal. *V. attack* fainting or syncope, often evoked by emotional stress associated with fear and pain. There is postural hypotension.

**VDU** visual display unit.

**vector** 1. an animal that carries organisms or parasites from one host to another, either to a member of the same species or to one of another species. 2. a quantity with magnitude and direction. *Electrocardiographic v.* the area of the heart that is monitored during electrocardiographic investigation.

**vegan** a vegetarian who excludes all animal protein from the diet.

**vegetarian** a person who eats only food of vegetable origin. *V. diet* one in which no meat is eaten. A *lacto-vegetarian* diet prohibits the intake of meat, poultry, fish and eggs.

An *ovo-lacto-vegetarian* diet allows all foods from plants plus eggs, milk and other dairy products. An *ovo-vegetarian* diet allows eggs and foods of plant origin, but prohibits all animal and dairy products.

**vegetation** in pathology, a plant-like outgrowth. *Adenoid v.* overgrowth of lymphoid tissue in the nasopharynx.

**vegetative** 1. the non-sporing stage of a bacterium. 2. profoundly lethargic and passive. *V. state* a type of deep coma that may follow severe head injuries. The patient's eyes may be open with some associated random movements of the head and limbs, but there are no other signs of consciousness or response to stimuli. Only basic functions such as breathing and heart beat are maintained

**vehicle** in pharmacy, a substance or medium in which a drug is administered.

**vein** a vessel carrying blood from the capillaries back to the heart. It has thin walls and a lining endothelium from which the venous valves are formed.

**venepuncture** the insertion of a needle into a vein for the introduction of a drug or fluid or for the withdrawal of blood.

**venereal** pertaining to or caused by sexual intercourse. *V. disease* a disease transmitted by sexual intercourse or other genital contact. In the UK, GONORRHOEA, SYPHILIS and CHANCROID are defined in law as venereal diseases. The term venereal disease (VD) has now been replaced by the term SEXUALLY TRANSMITTED INFECTION.

**venereology** the study and treatment of venereal diseases.

**venesection** phlebotomy. Surgical blood-letting by opening a vein or most usually by introducing a wide-bore needle. A procedure used to collect blood from blood donors and occasionally to relieve venous congestion.

**venogram** 1. a graphic recording of the pulse in a vein. 2. a radiograph taken during venography.

**venography** radiographic examination of a vein after the instillation of a contrast medium to trace its pathway.

**venom** a poison secreted by an insect, snake or other animal. *Russell's viper v.* the venom of the Russell viper (*Vipera russelli*), which acts in vitro as an intrinsic thromboplastin and is useful in defining deficiencies of clotting factor X.

**venous** pertaining to the veins. *See* CENTRAL VENOUS PRESSURE. *V. sinus* one of 14 channels, similar to veins, by which blood leaves the cerebral circulation. *V. ulcer see* ULCER (VARICOSE).

**ventilation** 1. the process or act of supplying a house or room continuously with fresh air. 2. in respiratory physiology, the process of exchange of air between the lungs and the ambient air. *Pulmonary v.* (usually measured in litres per minute) refers to the total exchange, whereas *alveolar v.* refers to the effective ventilation of the alveoli, where gas exchange with the blood takes place. 3. in psychiatry, the free discussion of one's problems or grievances.

**ventilator** an apparatus designed to qualify the air that is breathed through it either intermittently or continuously. Ventilators provide an intermittent flow of air and/or oxygen under pressure and are connected to the patient by a tube inserted through the mouth, the nose or an opening in the trachea.

**Ventimask** an oxygen mask that provides oxygen enrichment of the inspired air while eliminating the need to rebreathe the expired carbon dioxide.

**Ventouse** *see* VACUUM EXTRACTOR.

**ventricle** a small pouch or cavity; applied especially to the lower chambers of the heart and to the four cavities of the brain.

**ventricular** pertaining to a ventricle. *V.* **folds** the outer folds of mucous membrane forming the false vocal cords. *V.* **septal defect** abbreviated VSD. Congenital abnormality in which there is communication between the two ventricles of the heart as a result of maldevelopment of the intraventricular septum. *V.* **fibrillation** *see* FIBRILLATION.

**ventriculography** 1. radiographic examination of the ventricles of the heart using a radio-opaque contrast medium. 2. radiographic examination of the ventricles of the brain after the injection of air or a contrast medium through a burr hole.

**Venturi mask** *G.B. Venturi, Italian physicist, 1746–1822.* A type of disposable mask used to deliver a controlled oxygen concentration to a patient. The flow of 100% oxygen through the mask draws in a controlled amount of room air (21% oxygen). Commonly available masks deliver 24%, 28%, 35% or 40% oxygen. At concentrations above 24%, humidification may be required.

**Venturi nebulizer** a type of nebulizer used in AEROSOL therapy. The pressure drop of gas flowing through the nebulizer draws liquid from a capillary tube. As the liquid enters the gas stream it breaks up into a spray of small droplets.

**venule** a minute vein which collects blood from the capillaries.

**verbigeration** the monotonous repetition of phrases or meaningless words.

**vermicide** an agent that destroys intestinal worms; an anthelmintic.

**vermiform** worm-shaped. *V.* **appendix** the worm-shaped structure attached to the caecum.

**vermifuge** an agent that expels intestinal worms; an anthelmintic.

**verminous** infested with worms or other animal parasites, such as lice.

**vernix** [L.] *varnish*. *V.* **caseosa** the fatty covering on the skin of the fetus during the last months of pregnancy. It consists of cells and sebaceous material.

**verruca** a wart. Condyloma. Hypertrophy of the prickle cell layer of the epidermis and thickening of the horny layer. A virus is the causative organism. *V.* **acuminata** a venereal wart that appears on the external genitalia. *V.* **plana** a small, smooth, usually skin-coloured or light-brown, slightly raised wart, sometimes occurring in great numbers; seen most often in children. *V.* **plantaris** a viral epidermal tumour on the sole of the foot. *See* CONDYLOMATA.

**version** the turning of a part; applied particularly to the turning of a fetus in order to facilitate delivery. *External v.* manipulation of the uterus through the abdominal wall in order to change the position of the fetus. *Internal v.* rotation of the fetus by means of manipulation with one hand in the vagina. *Podalic v.* turning of the fetus so that the head is uppermost and the feet presenting. *Spontaneous v.* one that occurs naturally without the application of force.

**vertebra** one of the 33 irregular bones forming the spinal column: 7 cervical, 12 thoracic, 5 lumbar, 5 sacral (sacrum) and 4 coccygeal (coccyx) vertebrae.

**vertebral** pertaining to a vertebra. *V.* **column** the spine or backbone.

**vertebrobasilar** pertaining to the vertebral and the basilar arteries. *V.* **insufficiency** abbreviated VBI. A condition affecting the flow of blood through the vertebral and basilar arteries which may cause recurrent attacks of nausea, ataxia, diplopia, vertigo, dysarthria and hemiparesis.

**vertex** the crown of the head. *V. presentation* position of the fetus such that the crown of the head appears in the vagina first.

**vertical transmission** transmission of an infection from an infected mother to her newborn child during pregnancy, delivery or in the post-partum period through breast milk. Also called perinatal or mother-to-child transmission.

**vertigo** a feeling of rotation or of going round, in either oneself or one's surroundings, particularly associated with disease of the cerebellum and the vestibular nerve of the ear. It may occur in diplopia or Menière's syndrome.

**vesicle** 1. in anatomy, a small bladder, usually containing fluid. 2. a very small blister, usually containing serum. *Seminal v.* one of a pair of sacs which arise from the vas deferens near the bladder and contain semen.

**vesicoureteric** relating to the urinary bladder and the ureters. *V. reflux* the passing of urine backwards up the ureter during micturition. A cause of pyelonephritis in children.

**vesicovaginal** relating to the bladder and vagina. See FISTULA.

**vesicular** relating to or containing vesicles. *V. breathing* the soft murmur of normal respiration, as heard on auscultation. *V. mole* hydatidiform mole.

**vesiculitis** inflammation of a vesicle, particularly the seminal vesicles.

**vessel** a tube, duct or canal for conveying fluid, usually blood or lymph.

**vestibular** relating to a vestibule. *V. glands* those in the vestibule of the vagina, including Bartholin's glands. *V. nerve* a branch of the auditory nerve supplying the semicircular canals and concerned with balance and equilibrium.

**vestibule** a space or cavity at the entrance to another structure. *V. of the ear* the cavity at the entrance to the cochlea. *V. of the vagina* the

space between the labia minora at the entrance to the vagina.

**vestibulocochlear** pertaining to the vestibule of the ear and the cochlea. *V. nerve* the eighth cranial nerve. Also known as the auditory nerve.

**vestigial** rudimentary. Referring to the remains of an anatomical structure which, being of no further use, has atrophied.

**viable** capable of independent life.

**Vibrio** a genus of Gram-negative bacteria, curved and motile by means of flagellae. *V. cholerae* that which causes cholera.

**vicarious** 1. obtained or undergone at second hand through sympathetic participation in another's experiences. 2. substituted for another; used when one organ functions instead of another. *V. liability* the liability of an employer for the wrongful acts of an employee committed in the course of employment.

**villus** a small finger-like process projecting from a surface. *Chorionic v. see* CHORIONIC. *Intestinal villi* those of the mucous membrane of the small intestine, each of which contains a blood capillary and a lacteal.

**Vincent's angina** *J.H. Vincent, French physician, 1862–1950. See* ANGINA.

**viraemia** the presence of viruses in the blood.

**viral haemorrhagic fevers** a group of infectious diseases prevalent in Africa that cause fever, severe malaise and headache, diarrhoea and vomiting with severe bleeding and are commonly fatal. *See* EBOLA, LASSA and MARBURG FEVERS.

**virilism** masculine traits exhibited by a female owing to the production of excessive amounts of androgenic hormone either in the adrenal cortex or from an ovarian tumour. *See* ARRHENOBLASTOMA.

**virion** a fully developed complete infectious viral particle consisting of its nucleic acid and a surrounding coat of protein (capsid); the extracellular (cell-free) form of a virus.

**virology** the scientific study of viruses, their growth and the diseases caused by them.

**virulence** the power of a microorganism to produce toxins or poisons. This depends on (a) the number and power of the invading organisms, and (b) the power of the microorganism to overcome host resistance.

**virulent** dangerously infectious or poisonous.

**virus** any member of a unique class of infectious agents, which were originally distinguished by their smallness and their inability to replicate outside a living host cell; because these properties are shared by certain other microorganisms (rickettsiae, chlamydiae), viruses are now characterized by their simple organization and their unique mode of replication. A virus consists of genetic material, which may be either DNA or RNA, and is surrounded by a protein coat and, in some viruses, by a membranous envelope. They cause many diseases, including chickenpox (varicella), herpes zoster (shingles), herpes infections, measles (rubeola), German measles (rubella), mumps, infectious mononucleosis, hepatitis A and B, yellow fever, the common cold, acquired immune deficiency syndrome (AIDS), influenza, certain types of pneumonia and croup and other respiratory infections, poliomyelitis, and several types of encephalitis. There is evidence that certain viruses can cause cancer, e.g. cancer of the liver and cervix. *See* ORTHOMYXOVIRUS

**viscera** *pl.* of VISCUS.

**viscid** sticky and glutinous.

**viscosity** resistance to flowing. A sticky and glutinous quality.

**viscus** *pl.* viscera. Any of the organs contained in the body cavities, especially in the abdomen.

**vision** the faculty of seeing. Sight.

**visual** relating to sight. *V. acuity* sharpness of vision. It is assessed by reading test types. *V. cells* the rods and cones of the retina. *V. field* the area within which objects can be seen when looking straight ahead. *V. purple* the pigment in the outer layers of the retina. Rhodopsin.

**visual display unit** abbreviated VDU. The monitor screen attached to a computer.

**visualization** the technique of using the imagination and relaxation to create any desired changes in an individual's life.

**vital** relating to life. *V. capacity* the amount of air that can be expelled from the lungs after a full inspiration. *V. signs* the signs of life, namely pulse, respiration and temperature. *V. statistics* the records kept of births and deaths among the population, including the causes of death, and the factors that seem to influence their rise and fall.

**vitallium** a metal alloy used in dentistry and for prostheses in bone surgery.

**vitamin** any of a group of accessory food factors which are contained in foodstuffs and are essential to life, growth and reproduction. *See* Appendix 1.

**vitiligo** a skin disease marked by an absence of pigment, producing white patches on the face and body. Leukoderma.

**vitrectomy** surgical extraction of the vitreous humour and its replacement by a physiological solution in the treatment of vitreous haemorrhage in diabetic retinopathy.

**vitreous** glassy. *V. humour* the transparent jelly-like substance filling the posterior of the eye, from lens to retina.

**vocal** pertaining to the voice, or the organs that produce the voice. *V. cords* the two folds of tissue in the larynx, formed of fibrous tissue covered with squamous epithelium. *V. resonance* the normal sounds of speech heard through the chest wall by means of a stethoscope.

**volatile** having a tendency to evaporate readily.

**volition** the conscious adoption by the individual of a line of action.

**Volkmann's ischaemic contracture** *R. von Volkmann, German surgeon, 1830–1889.* Contraction of the fingers and sometimes of the wrist or of analogous parts of the foot, with loss of power, after severe injury or improper use of a tourniquet or cast.

**volume** the space occupied by a substance. *Minute v.* the total volume of air breathed in or out in 1 minute. *Packed cell v.* that occupied by the blood cells after centrifuging (about 45% of the blood sample). *Residual v.* the amount of air left in the lungs after breathing out fully.

**voluntary** under the control of the will. *See* INVOLUNTARY. *V. admission* a patient who voluntarily agrees to enter a psychiatric unit or hospital as an inpatient. *V. muscle* a striated muscle. *See* MUSCLE. *V. organizations* a group of people who join together with a shared common purpose or cause to provide a service to others. Many of these groups are registered charities and may also have grants from local or central government. Some employ professional and managerial staff but most remain dependent upon voluntary help. Many of these organizations provide considerable support to patients, their carers and families.

**volvulus** twisting of a loop of bowel causing obstruction. Most common in the sigmoid colon.

**vomer** a thin plate of bone forming the posterior septum of the nose.

**vomit** 1. matter ejected from the stomach through the mouth (vomitus). 2. to eject material in this way. *Bilious v.* vomit mixed with bile. The vomit is stained yellow or green. *Coffee-ground v.* ejected matter that contains small quantities of altered blood, which has the appearance of coffee grounds. *Faecal* or *stercoraceous v.* vomit mixed with faeces. Occurs in intestinal obstruction when the contents of the upper intestine regurgitate back into the stomach. It is dark brown with an unpleasant odour.

**vomiting** a reflex act of expulsion of the stomach contents via the oesophagus and mouth. It may be preceded by nausea and excess salivation if the cause is local irritation in the stomach. *Cyclical v.* recurrent attacks of vomiting often occurring in children and associated with acidosis. *Projectile v.* the forcible ejection of the gastric contents, usually without warning. Present in hypertrophic pyloric stenosis and in cerebral diseases. *V. of pregnancy* vomiting occurring in the months of pregnancy. Morning sickness.

**von Willebrand's disease** *E.A. von Willebrand, Finnish physician, 1870–1949.* A bleeding disorder inherited as an autosomal dominant trait (rarely recessive), characterized by a prolonged bleeding time, deficiency of coagulation factor VIII, and associated with epistaxis and increased bleeding after trauma or surgery, menorrhagia and postpartum bleeding.

**voyeurism** sexual deviation, whereby a person gains sexual satisfaction from covertly watching others who are naked or involved in sexual activity.

**VSD** ventricular septal defect.

**vulnerability** weakness. Susceptibility to injury or infection.

**vulva** the external female genital organs.

**vulvectomy** excision of the vulva.

**vulvitis** inflammation of the vulva.

**vulvovaginitis** inflammation of the vulva and vagina.

**VZV** varicella zoster virus.

**Waldeyer's ring** *H.W.G. von Waldeyer-Hartz, German anatomist, 1836–1921.* The circle of lymphoid tissue in the pharynx formed by the lingual, faucial and pharyngeal tonsils.

**walk-in centres** informal establishments that deliver accessible health care services on a drop-in basis. They offer free consultations and provide treatment for minor injuries and illnesses, general health information, self-treatment advice, information about out-of-hours general practitioner/dental services and local pharmacy services, and are situated in major towns and cities. They operate during the day and at weekends, in times and places that people find convenient. They are nurse-led, though a number of other health professionals and social care staff may be involved. Centres are managed by an NHS body or general practitioner cooperative and endorsed by the local health economy.

**Wangensteen tube** *O.H. Wangensteen, American surgeon, 1898–1981.* A gastrointestinal aspiration tube with a tip that is opaque to X-rays.

**wart** an elevation of the skin, often of a brownish colour, caused by hypertrophy of papillae in the dermis due to a virus infection. *See* VERRUCA *and* CONDYLOMA.

**Wassermann test (reaction)** *A.P. von Wassermann, German bacteriologist,* 1866–1925. A complement-fixation test used in the diagnosis of syphilis.

**water** a clear, colourless, tasteless liquid composed of hydrogen and oxygen ($H_2O$). *W. balance* fluid balance. That between the fluid taken in by all routes and the fluid lost by all routes. *W.-borne* descriptive of certain diseases that are spread by contaminated water. *W.-brash* the eructation of dilute acid from the stomach to the pharynx, giving a burning sensation. Pyrosis. Heartburn. *W. intoxication* a condition that results from excessive water retention in the brain, resulting in headaches, dizziness and confusion. In severe cases may cause seizures and unconsciousness. Water intoxication can also result from the use of the drug ecstasy, which may be taken by young people in night clubs and discos, leading to excessive quantities of water being drunk. *W.-seal drainage* a closed method of drainage from the pleural space allowing the escape of fluid and air but preventing air entering because the drainage tube discharges under water.

**Waterhouse–Friderichsen syndrome** *R. Waterhouse, British physician, 1873–1958; C. Friderichsen, Danish physician,1886–1979.* Meningococcal MENINGITIS marked by sudden onset and short course, fever, coma, cyanosis, haemorrhages from the skin and mucous membranes, severe shock and haemorrhage into the adrenal glands.

**Waterlow scale** *See* PRESSURE ULCER ASSESSMENT SCALES.

**waxy flexibility** a cataleptic state in which a patient's limbs are held indefinitely in any position in which they have been placed. *See* CATATONIA.

**weal** a raised stripe on the skin or small blister, as is caused by the lash of a whip. Typical of urticaria.

**wean** 1. to discontinue breast or bottle-feeding and substitute other feeding habits, e.g. solid foods. This should be effected gradually at about the 6th month. 2. in respiratory therapy, to gradually decrease dependence on assisted ventilation until the patient is able to breathe spontaneously.

**wear and tear theory** the concept of ageing that equates the human body with a machine, and that as parts wear out physiological functions deteriorate affecting the quality of life.

**web** a network or complex system of interconnected elements. *W. space* the soft tissue between the bases of the fingers and the toes. *W. site* in computing, one or more pages that can be accessed through the internet to the World Wide Web (WWW) that allows the browser to obtain specific information on the site.

**webbing** the state of being connected by a membrane or a fold of skin. *W. of the hands* or *feet* congenital abnormality in which the digits are not separated from each other. Syndactyly. *W. of the neck* folds of skin in the neck, giving it a webbed appearance. Occurs in certain congenital conditions, e.g. Turner's syndrome.

**Weil's disease** *A. Weil, German physician, 1848–1916.* Spirochaetal jaundice. The organism, *Leptospira icterohaemorrhagiae*, is harboured and excreted by rats and enters through a bite or skin abrasion, or infected food or water.

**Weil–Felix reaction** *E. Weil, Austrian physician, 1880–1922; A. Felix, Czech bacteriologist, 1887–1956.* An agglutination test of blood serum used in the diagnosis of typhus.

**well-baby clinic** mothers are encouraged to bring their infants to these clinics for assessment and monitoring of the child's health. Immunization is available and there are opportunities for 'family' health promotion.

**well-man clinic** a health promotion clinic available for men to screen for health problems and to promote health, e.g. self-examination of the testicles. *See* TESTICULAR SELF-EXAMINATION.

**well-woman clinic** a health promotion clinic available to screen women for breast and cervical cancer, anaemia, diabetes and hypertension and to promote health, e.g. self-examination of the breasts. *See* BREAST.

**wellness** the development of a personal lifestyle that promotes feelings of wellbeing, achieves the highest level of health within one's capability, and minimizes chances of becoming ill. It is guided by a developing sense of self-awareness and self-responsibility encompassing emotional, mental, physical, social, spiritual and environmental health.

**wen** a small sebaceous cyst; a steatoma.

**Werdnig–Hoffmann disease** *G. Werdnig, Austrian neurologist, 1844–1919; J. E. Hoffmann, German neurologist, 1857–1919.* A genetic condition characterized by progressive spinal muscular atrophy affecting the shoulder, neck, pelvis and eventually the respiratory muscles of infants.

**Wernicke–Korsakoff syndrome** *K. Wernicke, German neurologist, 1848–1905; S.S. Korsakoff, Russian neurologist, 1854–1900.* A disorder of the central nervous system, usually associated with chronic alcoholism, nutritional deficiency and severe deficiency of vitamin B₁. It is characterized by a combination of motor and sensory disturbances and disordered memory function. One form is Wernicke's encephalopathy, a neurological condition due to vitamin B₁ deficiency. Untreated, it progresses from mental confusion and double vision to lethargy and coma.

**Wertheim's operation** *E. Wertheim, Austrian gynaecologist, 1864–1920.* See HYSTERECTOMY.

**wet nurse** a lactating woman who breast feeds another woman's child.

**Wharton's jelly** *T. Wharton, English physician, 1614–1673.* The connective tissue of the umbilical cord.

**wheezing** breathing with a rasp or whistling sound. It results from constriction or obstruction of the throat, pharynx, trachea or bronchi.

**whiplash injury** injury to the spinal cord, nerve roots, ligaments or vertebrae in the cervical region due to a sudden jerking back of the head and neck. Common in road traffic accidents where there is sudden acceleration or deceleration of the vehicle.

**whiplash shake syndrome** a constellation of injuries to the brain and eye that may occur when a young child is shaken vigorously with the head unsupported. This causes stretching and tearing of the cerebral vessels and brain substance, commonly leading to subdural haematomas and retinal haemorrhages. It may result in paralysis, blindness and other visual disturbances, convulsions and death. See SHAKEN BABYSYNDROME.

**Whipple's operation** *A.O. Whipple, American surgeon, 1881–1963.* Radical pancreatoduodenectomy performed for carcinoma of the head of the pancreas.

**whipworm** *see* TRICHURIS.

**white leg** milk leg. *See* PHLEGMASIA.

**whitlow** a felon; a suppurating inflammation of a finger near the nail. *Melanotic w.* a malignant tumour of the nail bed characterized by formation of melanotic tissue. *Subperiosteal w.* one in which the infection involves the bone covering. *Superficial w.* a pustule between the true skin and cuticle. *See* PARONYCHIA.

**WHO** World Health Organization.

**whole system planning** strategic planning and commissioning across a range of services and organizational boundaries. Deals with the impact that changes in one part of the system, whether health and social care or housing, are likely to have on other parts.

**whole systems approach** the consideration of the interrelatedness of various elements, which come together for a common purpose and continually have impact upon one another. The comprehension of complex systems, e.g. health care and social care, requires understanding of a diverse range of perspectives, and an appreciation that change will often be required across a number of areas to meet needs.

**whole time equivalent** total weekly contracted hours of full- and part-time staff expressed as a multiple of the standard working week.

**whooping cough pertussis** a notifiable infectious disease characterized by catarrh of the respiratory tract and paroxysms of coughing, ending in a prolonged whooping respiration; called also pertussis. The causative organism is *Bordetella pertussis*. Whooping cough is a serious disease; most cases occur in children. All babies should be immunized against whooping cough unless there is a sound medical objection.

**Widal reaction** *G.F.I. Widal, French physician, 1862–1929.* A blood agglutination test for typhoid fever.

**Wilms' tumour** *M. Wilms, German surgeon, 1867–1918.* A highly malignant tumour of the kidney occurring in young children. A nephroblastoma.

**Wilson's disease** *S.A.K. Wilson, British neurologist, 1878–1937.* Hepatolenticular degeneration. A congenital abnormality in the metabolism of copper, leading to neurological degeneration.

**wiring** the fixing together of a broken or split bone by the use of a wire. Commonly used for the jaw, the patella and the sternum.

**wisdom teeth** the back molar teeth, the eruption of which is often delayed until maturity.

**wish fulfilment** a desire, not always acknowledged consciously by the person, which is fulfilled through dreams or by day-dreaming.

**withdrawal** 1. a pathological retreat from reality. 2. abstention from drugs or activities to which one is habituated or addicted; also denoting the symptoms occasioned by such withdrawal. *W. symptoms* symptoms brought about by abrupt withdrawal of the substance to which a person has become addicted; called also abstinence syndrome. The usual reactions to withdrawal may include anxiety, weakness, gastrointestinal symptoms, nausea and vomiting, tremor, fever, rapid heartbeat, convulsions and delirium.

**Wolff–Parkinson–White syndrome** *L. Wolff, American cardiologist, 1898–1972; Sir J. Parkinson, British physician, 1885–1976; P. D. White, American cardiologist, 1886–1973.* Abnormal heart rhythm caused by an accessory bundle between the atria and ventricles. A congenital disorder.

**womb** the uterus.

**Wood's light** *R.W. Wood, American physicist, 1868–1953.* Ultraviolet light transmitted through a glass filter containing nickel oxide. It produces fluorescence of infected hairs when placed over a scalp affected with ringworm.

**woolsorter's disease** pulmonary anthrax.

**word blindness** *see* DYSLEXIA.

**word salad** a colloquial term for rapid speech in which the words are strung together without meaning.

**World Health Organization** abbreviated WHO. The specialized agency of the United Nations that is concerned with health at an international level. WHO organizes health compaigns against infectious diseases and sponsors research in medical laboratories. It also provides expert advice on all matters directly or indirectly concerned with physical or mental health to all member states.

**World Wide Web** abbreviated WWW. Information that is stored on computer web sites and accessed via the internet.

**worm** any one of a number of groups of long soft-bodied invertebrates, some of which are parasitic to humans.

**wound** a cut or break in continuity of any tissue, caused by injury or operation. It is classified according to its nature. *Abrased w.* the skin is scraped off, but there is no deeper injury. *Contused w.* with bruising of the surrounding tissue. *Incised w.* usually the result of operation, and produced by a knife or similar instrument. The edges of the wound can remain in apposition, and it should heal by first intention. *Lacerated w.* one with torn edges and tissues, usually the result of accident or injury. It is often septic and heals by second intention. *Open w.* a gaping wound on the body surface. *Penetrating w.* often made by gunshot, shrapnel, etc. There may be an inlet and outlet hole and vital organs are often penetrated by the missile. *Punctured w.* made by a pointed or spiked instrument. *Septic w.* any type into which infection has been introduced, causing suppurative inflammation. It heals by second intention. *W. drain. See* DRAIN. *W. dressing* material applied to a surgical or medical wound to provide protection and assist healing. Dressings are made from a variety of materials with or without medication, e.g. hydrocellular or alginate dressings used in the management of cavities or exuding wounds, and low-adherent absorbent dressings used for clean wounds. The aim is that the dressing should be comfortable, permit the exchange of gases but be impermeable to bacteria, prevent adherence to the wound, and therefore reduce damage to new tissue when it is removed. *W. healing* the

restoration of integrity to injured tissues by replacement of dead tissue with viable tissue. In wound healing there are four stages – haemostasis, inflammation, proliferation and maturation – which may take several months to complete. Wound healing may be delayed by physical stress, inadequate blood supply or by more general factors that include malnutrition, ageing, drugs such as corticosteroids, etc. The process starts immediately after an injury and may continue for months or years. *See* HEALING.

**wrist** the point of the carpus and bones of the forearm. *W. drop* loss of power in the muscles of the hand. It may be due to nerve or tendon injury, but can result from lack of sufficient support by splint or sling.

**writer's cramp** a colloquial term for painful spasm of the hand and forearm, caused by excessive writing and poor posture.

**wryneck** *see* TORTICOLLIS.

*Wuchereria* a genus of nematode worms which are the principal vectors of filariasis. *W. bancrofti* the most common species in tropical and subtropical areas.

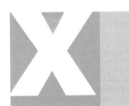

**X chromosome** the female sex chromosome, being present in all female gametes and only half the male gametes. When union takes place two X chromosomes result in a female child (XX) but one of each results in a male child (XY). *See* Y CHROMOSOME.

**X-linked** pertaining to the genes, or the effect of these genes, situated on the X chromosome. X-linked disorders are those caused by the genes on the X chromosome.

**X-rays** electromagnetic waves of short length which are capable of penetrating many substances and of producing chemical changes and reactions in living matter. They are used both to aid diagnosis and to treat disease. Also called Röntgen rays.

**xanthelasma** a disease marked by the formation of flat or slightly raised yellow cholesterol deposits on the eyelids.

**xanthine** a compound found in plant and animal tissues; the forerunner of uric acid in nucleoprotein metabolism.

**xanthochromia** 1. the presence of yellow patches on the skin. 2. the yellow colouring of cerebrospinal fluid seen in patients who have had a subarachnoid haemorrhage.

**xanthoma** the presence in the skin of flat areas of yellowish pigmentation due to deposits of lipids. There are several varieties. *X. palpebrarum* xanthelasma.

**xanthosis** a yellow skin pigmentation, seen in some cases of diabetes and poliomyelitis.

*Xenopsylla* a genus of fleas, some of which are vectors of plague. *X. cheopis* the rat flea, which transmits bubonic plague.

**xeroderma** a hereditary condition in which there is excessive dryness of the skin. A mild form of ichthyosis. *X. pigmentosum* a rare hereditary and often fatal disease in which there is extreme sensitivity of the skin and eyes to light. It begins in childhood and rapidly progresses. The formation of malignant neoplasms is common.

**xerophthalmia** a condition in which the cornea and conjunctiva become horny and necrosed owing to a deficiency of vitamin A. Xeroma.

**xerosis** a condition of dryness, especially of the eyes, mouth, vagina or skin.

**xerostomia** dryness of the mouth due to a failure of salivary gland secretion.

**xylose** a pentose sugar, found in connective tissue and sometimes in urine, which is not metabolized in the body. *X. absorption test* an investigation for malabsorption.

**XYY syndrome** an extremely rare condition in males in which there is an extra Y chromosome, making a total of 47 chromosomes in each body cell. *See* KLINEFELTER'S SYNDROME.

# Y

**Y chromosome** the male sex chromosome, being present in half the male gametes and none of the female. It carries few major genes. *See* X CHROMOSOME.

**yawning** an involuntary act in which the mouth is opened wide and air is drawn in and exhaled. It may accompany tiredness or boredom.

**yaws** framboesia. A skin infection common in tropical countries. Caused by *Treponema pertenue*, it is common among people, especially children, who live under primitive conditions in equatorial Africa, South America, and the East and West Indies.

**yeast** any of the fungi of the genus *Saccharomyces*. They produce fermentation in malt and in sweetened fruit juices, resulting in the formation of alcoholic solutions such as beer and wines.

**yellow card scheme** a system of reporting side effects from taking or using any prescription medicine, herbal remedy of an over-the-counter (OTC) medicine. A patient, parent, carer or health care professional can report a suspected side effect by completing a yellow card, either electronically or by completing a paper card. This reporting scheme is available in the UK and is monitored and managed by the Medicines and Healthcare Products Agency (MHRA).

**yellow fever** an acute, notifiable, infectious disease of the tropics caused by a virus and transmitted by a mosquito (*Aedes aegypti*). The virus attacks the liver and kidneys and the symptoms include rigor, headache, pain in the back and limbs, high fever and black vomit. Haemorrhage from the intestinal mucous membrane may occur. There is a high mortality rate. A vaccine is available.

**Yersinia** a genus of Gram-negative bacteria containing the pathogen *Y. pestis* responsible for the bubonic plague. *Yersinia* is also responsible for a variety of other infections, e.g. gastroenteritis in the young and septicaemia in adults.

**yin and yang** the two complementary principles of Chinese philosophy incorporated into traditional Chinese medicine. Yin is feminine, dark and negative; yang is masculine, bright and positive. Together, the Yin–Yang interaction and balance is believed to maintain the harmony of the body and, in a healthy person, maintain a state of dynamic balance (*see* Figure on p. 422).

**yoga** one of the six systems of Indian philosophy which emphasizes personal physical preparation using isometric exercises, relaxation, breathing techniques and the attainment of defined body positions to achieve relaxation, with physical and emotional harmony and wellbeing.

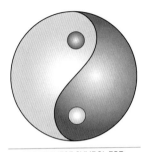

THE CHINESE SYMBOL FOR
YIN–YANG

**yolk sac** one of the two spaces which occurs in the inner cell mass of the trophoblast (the other space being the amniotic cavity). It is surrounded by entodermal cells, whereas the amniotic cavity is surrounded by ectodermal cells and between the two is an intervening layer of mesoderm. The embryo is formed from the area where the three tissues, ectoderm, mesoderm and entoderm, lie in apposition.

**yttrium** a rare metal which in its radioactive form is sometimes used in cancer therapy and the treatment of severe arthritis.

**Z-plasty** a plastic operation for removing and repairing deformity resulting from a contraction scar (*see* Figure).

**Z track injection** an intramuscular injection technique which allows a medication, e.g. an iron preparation, to be given but which prevents the leakage and the staining of tissues surrounding the site. *See* INJECTION.

**Zen** Zen Buddhism is the teaching that a form of meditation consisting of the contemplation of one's essential nature to the exclusion of everything else is the way to true enlightenment.

**zenith** the highest point. The opposite is NADIR.

**zero** nought; *symbol* 0. In the Celsius thermometer 0°C is the melting point of ice; in the Fahrenheit thermometer, 0°F is 32° below the melting point of ice. *See* CELSIUS and FAHRENHEIT.

**Ziehl–Neelsen method** *F. Ziehl, German bacteriologist, 1857–1926; F.K.A. Neelsen, German pathologist, 1854–1894.* A method of staining tubercle bacilli for microscopic study.

**Zimmer** the trade name of a metal, lightweight walking aid, commonly applied to other products of similar design and weight. Predominantly used by the elderly to assist in rehabilitation.

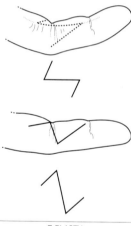

Z-PLASTY

**zinc** *symbol* Zn. A trace element which is essential in the body for cell growth and multiplication. The recommended daily intake of zinc is 15 mg for an adult. A severe deficiency of zinc can retard growth in children, cause a low sperm count in adult males, and retard wound healing.

**Zn** symbol for *zinc*.

**zona** a zone. *Z. facialis* herpes of the face. *Z. pellucida* the membrane surrounding the ovum.

**zonulysin** a proteolytic enzyme that may be used in eye surgery to dissolve the suspensory ligament.

**zoonosis** a disease of animals that is transmissible to humans, e.g. anthrax, cat-scratch fever, etc.

**zoster** *see* HERPES.

**zygoma** the arch formed by the union of the temporal bone with the malar bone in front of the ear.

**zygote** a single fertilized cell formed from the union of a male and a female gamete.

**zymosis** fermentation.

# Appendices

# Nutrition

CAROLINE KING, GARY FROST AND LINDA CARTER

Nutrition is the study of food in relation to health. It is defined in this dictionary as the sum of the processes involved in taking in nutrients and assimilating and utilizing them.

Nutrients are necessary for growth, maintenance and repair of the human body. The five main groups of nutrients in food are: protein, carbohydrate, fat, vitamins and minerals. In this section it should be noted that rich sources of particular nutrients are given as examples but that foods almost always contain a mixture of many nutrients.

## Protein

Protein is required for the body's growth and repair. Any excess protein consumed will be used as energy by the body. Protein provides 4 kcal per gram when used for energy and should provide about 10% of the day's energy needs for healthy adults.

When eaten, protein foods are broken down into amino acids. There are 20 amino acids. The body can make only 12 of the amino acids itself. The remaining eight are known as the essential amino acids and must come from food.

Protein from animal sources such as meat, fish, eggs and milk usually contains all the essential amino acids; most proteins from vegetable sources are deficient in some essential amino acids. Plant foods need to be combined together if no animal protein is included in the diet, such as baked beans and toast or cereal with nuts.

Most people in the Western world eat more protein than their body requires and deficiency is rare. In times of protein catabolism such as surgery, trauma and burns, the body's requirements for protein may increase.

Foods high in protein: meat, fish, eggs, milk, cheese, nuts, beans.

## Carbohydrate

The main function of carbohydrates is to provide energy. Some carbohydrates are also essential components of cells and other parts of the body. Carbohydrate provides approximately 4 kcal per gram. It comes in three forms: sugars, starches and non-starch polysaccharides.

Sugar carbohydrates are either monosaccharides (simple sugars) such as glucose, or disaccharides such as sucrose. They provide quick energy but virtually no nutrients as they are usually refined removing the other nutritious parts of the plant they come from. Only 10% of our total energy requirements should be from this type of carbohydrate.

Starch carbohydrates are made up of large numbers of glucose units joined together, and are found in foods such as rice, bread, pasta, cereals, potatoes and pulses. Starch has to be converted back to glucose during digestion in order for it to be used as energy by the body. Starch carbohydrates provide energy plus vegetable protein and some vitamins and minerals.

There are two types of non-starch polysaccharides (also known as dietary fibre). These are insoluble and soluble. Insoluble fibre is an indigestible carbohydrate that when ingested stimulates peristaltic movement and helps prevent constipation. It is found in cereal grains such as wheat, maize and rice. Soluble fibre such as pectin and guar gum is found in oats, peas, beans and lentils. Evidence shows that soluble fibre can help to reduce levels of cholesterol in the blood and help keep blood sugar levels even.

Approximately 50% of our total energy intake should be derived from carbohydrate with the majority from starchy carbohydrates.

Foods high in sugar: sweets, cakes, biscuits, soft drinks, honey and jam.

Foods high in starchy carbohydrate: breakfast cereals, rice, pasta, potatoes and pulses.

Foods high in non-starch polysaccharides: fruit, vegetables, breakfast cereals, oats.

# Fat

Fat is the most concentrated source of energy. It provides 9 kcal per gram. It is a carrier of fat-soluble vitamins, provides a store of concentrated heat and energy, protects vital organs and adds palatability and satiety value to the diet. Essential fatty acids are needed for optimal cell function.

Fat is made up of triglycerides, each of which is made up of three fatty acids and a unit of glycerol. Differences in fat are the result of the different fatty acids found in each. Fats may be saturated, monounsaturated or polyunsaturated. Saturated fatty acids tend to increase the amount of cholesterol in the blood and are usually solid at room temperature. Monounsaturated and polyunsaturated fatty acids have been shown to help reduce cholesterol in the blood. Polyunsaturated fatty acids also play a role in immune function, fat transport and metabolism, and maintenance of the integrity of cell membranes. Essential fatty acids cannot be made by the body, they have to be provided by the diet. Currently there is a lot of interest in 'omega 3 long chain polyunsaturates'. These are derived mainly from fatty fish and are found in high levels in brain and neuronal tissue; they are also important components of the immune system. Many claims are made as to their role in health and disease, however the most persuasive ones are with respect to heart disease and the immune system.

Approximately 30% of our total energy should be derived from fat: with approximate ratios of 10% from saturated fat, 5% from polyunsaturated fats and 15% from monounsaturated fats.

Foods high in saturated fat: butter, cheese, lard, suet.

Foods high in polyunsaturated fat: corn oil, grapeseed oil, sunflower oil, safflower oil, sesame oil, oily fish such as salmon, sardines, mackerel and fresh tuna.

Foods high in monounsaturated fat: olives, olive oil, peanuts, cashew nuts and avocados.

# Vitamins

These are found in small amounts in foods and are required by the body for normal biochemical function. Vitamins can be divided into two groups. These are fat-soluble (A, D, E, K) and water-soluble (vitamin B complex and C).

Water-soluble vitamins are not stored by the body, but fat-soluble vitamins are stored and if taken in excess over a long period of time can be toxic.

**Vitamin A**

There are two forms: retinol and carotenes.

Function: needed for growth and normal development of the retina in the eye, healthy skin and surface tissues. Antioxidant.

*Retinol*

Foods high in retinol: animal foods such as milk, cheese, eggs, fish liver oils, margarine and butter.

*Carotene*

Can be turned into retinol by the body.

Foods high in carotene: cabbage, carrots, peaches and apricots.

**Vitamin B Complex**

Function of all B vitamins (except vitamin $B_{12}$ and folate): help the body obtain energy from food. They take part in the way the body metabolizes fat and carbohydrate for energy. Requirements for these B vitamins are calculated in relation to energy need. Pyridoxine (vitamin $B_6$) plays an important role in protein metabolism.

Foods high in B vitamins are: meat, fish, milk, eggs, cereal grains and fortified cereals.

Deficiencies:

Vitamin $B_1$ (thiamine): beri beri.

Vitamin $B_2$ (riboflavin): sore mouth.

Niacin (nicotinic acid): pellagra.

Biotin: dermatitis, fatigue, nausea and depression.

*Vitamin $B_{12}$*

Function: essential for making red blood cells. Required for the correct formation of nerve sheaths. Only absorbed in the presence of intrinsic factor which is produced in the upper GI tract and is reduced as stomach acidity reduces with age.

Deficiency: pernicious anaemia, damage to the nerve sheaths.

Foods high in vitamin $B_{12}$: found only in animal foods – liver, oily fish, meat and eggs. However there is some evidence that a healthy gut flora produces $B_{12}$ which can be used by the host.

*Folate (folic acid)*

Function: involved in production of healthy blood cells. Folate plays a major role in the prevention of neural tube defects such as spina bifida.

Deficiency: megaloblastic anaemia.

Foods high in folate: liver, spinach, brussels sprouts, fortified breakfast cereals, eggs (levels reduced by heat during cooking).

### Vitamin C (ascorbic acid)

Function: forms a major part of the connective tissue which binds all cells together. Helps tissue to heal and thus is vital for wound healing. Aids absorption of iron from non-animal sources. Antioxidant.

Deficiency: scurvy, wounds not healing, bruising, low resistance to infections.

Foods high in vitamin C: fruit (particularly citrus fruits) and vegetables (if not overcooked as vitamin C is destroyed by heat).

### Vitamin D

Function: works to aid the absorption of calcium for the formation and growth of bones and teeth. Unlike other nutrients, food is not the main source of this vitamin. It is produced by the action of sunshine on the skin.

Deficiency: rickets and osteomalacia.

Foods high in vitamin D: margarine (if fortified, which is a statutary obligation in the UK at the moment), some fish such as kippers, mackerel, sardines.

### Vitamin E

Function: thought to be necessary for healthy muscles and good blood circulation. It is found in all cell structures and protects polyunsaturated fatty acids both in food and in the body from losing their properties through oxidation (antioxidant).

Foods high in vitamin E: polyunsaturated margarines, wheatgerm, nuts, fish such as tuna and salmon.

### Vitamin K

Function: needed for normal blood clotting.

Deficiency: delayed blood clotting, haemorrhagic tendency.

Foods high in vitamin K: green vegetables, cereals and pulses. Also made by a healthy gut flora.

## Minerals

Minerals are an essential part or carrier of enzymes, hormones and proteins such as haemoglobin. They are used by the body's nervous system to transport messages and are essential for strong bones and teeth.

Some minerals (also known as trace elements) are required by the body in very small quantities – zinc, selenium, copper, manganese, chromium, cobalt, fluorine, iodine, molybdenum. They are antioxidants which help to prevent damage to cells from free radicals or cofactors for enzyme systems.

## Iron
Function: carries oxygen from the lungs to all cells of the body. Over half of iron is in the form of haemoglobin.
  Deficiency: iron-deficiency anaemia.
  Foods high in iron: red meat, offal, fortified breakfast cereals, dried fruit, chocolate, nuts.

## Calcium
Function: needed for the development and maintenance of the skeleton, good muscle function, nerve functioning and normal clotting of blood.
  Deficiency: rickets, osteomalacia.
  Foods high in calcium: cheese, yoghurt, milk, dark-green leafy vegetables, white bread, sardines.

## Phosphorus
Function: together with calcium it provides the strength of bones and teeth. Required to form adenosine triphosphate and in enzyme systems for energy metabolism.
  Deficiency: unknown in humans.
  Foods high in phosphorus: milk, cheese, wholegrain cereals.

## Sodium
Function: regulation of body fluid and transmitting nerve impulses. Also important for energy release, muscle contraction and regulation of blood pressure.
  Deficiency: hyponatraemia with symptoms of cramps, weakness, fatigue, nausea and thirst.
  Foods high in sodium: salt, bacon, ham, soy sauce.

## Potassium
Function: maintenance of acid–base and water balances, osmotic equilibrium, muscle and nerve irritability and normal blood pressure.

Deficiency: rare, secondary deficiency may occur after excessive losses through vomiting, chronic diarrhoea or use of some diuretics, leading to loss of appetite, nausea, muscle weakness, mental disorientation and cardiac arrhythmias.

Foods high in potassium: vegetables including potatoes, fruits and fruit juices, chocolate and instant coffee.

# Artificial Nutritional Support
### Liesl Wandrag

### Indications

- An inability to meet nutritional requirements with normal food.
- For prevention or treatment of malnutrition.

Effective nutritional support is capable of treating malnutrition. Nutritional screening tools, such as the Malnutrition Universal Screening Tool, has been developed by the Malnutrition Advisory Group to help identify patients at risk of malnutrition. For details refer to web address.

### Artificial Nutritional Support

There are two types of artificial nutritional support:

- Enteral nutrition, e.g. nutritional supplements (sip feeds) or tube feeding.
- Parenteral nutrition (PN).

Enteral nutrition should be the first-line route for the provision of nutritional support. If the patient is able to absorb food enteral feeding should be used.

## Enteral Nutrition
Refer to dictionary entry for definition

### Enteral Nutrition Modalities
*Oral Diet*
Additional snacks or high-protein/energy diets. In addition to normal meals, glucose polymers, protein or milk powder or fat (such as cream or butter) may be added to food to increase its energy and protein content.

*Nutritional Supplements*

There are a wide variety of sweet supplements (milk shake/yoghurt/mousse/fruit juice style drinks) and savoury supplements (soups) that may be given. If a patient is reliant on the sip feed as the sole source of nutrition, it is important that the supplements are complete in macronutrients (carbohydrates, fat and protein) for energy, and micronutrients (vitamins, minerals and trace elements). A full list of prescribable products can be found in the appendix for borderline substance published in the British National Formulary (BNF).

*Tube Feeding*

- Prepyloric, e.g. nasogastric, oro-gastric, gastrostomy (surgical, radiological or endoscopic).
- Postpyloric, e.g. nasoduodenal/jejunal and jejunostomy. Some postpyloric tubes are placed blindly, others rely on endoscopic, radiological or surgical placement. A jejunal extension set can be placed through some gastrostomy tubes to facilitate postpyloric feeding. Naso-jejunal feeding tubes are available with a gastric port to facilitate concomitant gastric aspiration with jejunal feeding.

Tube feeding requires a team decision to select the most appropriate route and insertion method. It is important that the date, type of tube, feed exit point (gastric, duodenal, jejunal) and method of tube insertion is documented. This information is vital as it may alter feed and drug administration (refer to drug administration section on p. 437), and the daily management of the tube.

**Indications for Enteral Tube Feeding**

See Box 1.1.

| BOX 1.1 Indications for enteral tube feeding | |
|---|---|
| Increased nutritional requirements | • e.g. sepsis, burns, trauma, postoperative stress, head injuries, critically ill |
| Inadequate oral intake | • Anorexia |
| | • Unable to eat safely due to swallowing difficulties, e.g. cerebral vascular accident, (CVA), impaired consciousness, oesophageal carcinoma |
| | • Patients not meeting requirements via the oral route alone |

## Contraindications for Enteral Tube Feeding

Patients with a non-functioning gut (refer to Parenteral Nutrition section).

## Composition of Enteral Tube Feeds

All enteral feeds contain protein, carbohydrate, fat, electrolytes, vitamins and minerals.

- Standard feeds: 1 kcal per ml (available with or without fibre).
- High-energy feeds: 1.5 kcal per ml (available with or without fibre).

A variety of specialist feeds are also available for the management of a range of acute and chronic medical conditions. These include renal failure, malabsorption, acute respiratory disorders, chronic pulmonary disease, cancer and inflammatory bowel disease. The feed selected will depend on the clinical condition of the patient and their nutritional requirements.

## Tube Feeding Regimen

The regimen will depend upon the route of tube feeding, the clinical condition of the patient and the aims of nutritional support. Most prepyloric regimens have a rest period in order to allow the stomach to re-acidify, however this is not required for feeds administered postpylorically. Feed is either administered using a pump or as a bolus regimen. Bolus regimens should not be used in patients that are deemed at high risk of aspiration.

## Check Tube Position Prior to Initiating Feed

The position of the feeding tube should be checked daily prior to feeding as per guidance from the National Patient Safety Agency. Accepted methods for confirming the position of nasogastric tubes include either gastric aspirate checks with Universal pH paper (pH < 5.5) or chest X-ray if aspirates cannot be obtained. (Please refer to NPSA, MHRA, NNNG websites). Nasal tubes can be easily dislodged; those at high risk are patients who are retching, vomiting or coughing severely or who require frequent nasotracheal suctioning. Gastrostomy and jejunostomy tube sites also need to be checked regularly. These tubes can migrate, leak, kink or become embedded into the lumen wall and result in skin ulceration.

## Complications of Enteral Tube Feeding

See Table 1.1

| Table 1.1 Complications of enteral tube feeding | |
|---|---|
| **Complication** | **Recommendation** |
| **Diarrhoea (listed below are possible causes)** | Monitor bowel frequency; establish a definition, e.g. include frequency and consistency |
| • Infective diarrhoea | Send stool sample; ensure a cleaning frequency with consistency and the appropriate handling feeds |
| • Medication, e.g. motility agents, antibiotics, medication | Review medication containing sorbitol |
| • Bacterial overgrowth | Hydrogen breath test |
| • Constipation | Review history of bowel function |
| • Malabsorption | Check for pancreatic, biliary or gastrointestinal disease |
| • Too rapid infusion of feed | Check rate of feed matches regimen, check for pump malfunction |
| • Hypoalbuminaemia | Discuss with dietitian |
| • Hyperosmolar feeds | Discuss with dietitian |
| N.B. Most feeds are lactose- and gluten-free | |
| **Constipation** | |
| • Inadequate fluid intake | Check fluid intake |
| • Drug therapy, e.g. opiates | Review medications; consider laxative prescription; consider fibre-based feed |
| **Mucosal erosion and oesophageal strictures** | Use fine-bore feeding tubes instead of wide-bore PVC tubes, e.g. ryles |
| **Regurgitation/aspiration** | |
| • Delayed gastric emptying | Rate of feed must not exceed the patient's absorption. Consider use of prokinetic agents, e.g. metoclopramide or erythromycin |
| • Tube misplacement: | |
|   —On insertion | Tilt the bed head by 45 degrees when tube feeding supine patients |
|   —During nutritional support | Check tube position prior to commencing feed |
| **Tube occlusion** | |
| • Viscous feeds and drugs | Use liquid drug preparations; dilute viscous drugs; flush tube regularly, before/after the feed/drug is administered; if multiple drugs are given at one time water should be flushed between each drug administered |
| • Crushed tablets | Flush the tube after aspiration |
| • Inadequate flushing | Flush regularly, ideally every 4–6 hours |
| **Psychological problems** | Where possible involve the patient and carers in the care of the tube feed |
| • Altered body image | |
| • Hunger | |
| • Loss of autonomy | |
| • Loss of the pleasure of eating | |

## Other Tube Feeding Considerations

*Feed Administration Sets*

Many plastics are single-use. Scrupulous attention should be paid to hygiene in the handling and administration of feeds. Syringes used to flush tubes should be 50 ml as the pressure exerted by smaller syringes may rupture the tube lumen. All enteral syringes need to comply with National Patient Safety Agency guidance where they no longer adapt to IV administration sets and are all purple in colour.

*Drug Administration*

- The route of administration corresponds to absorption site.
- Interactions between drugs and feed must be identified prior to administration. Common interactions between feed and drugs occur with NG administration of phenytoin, warfarin, penicillins, ciprofloxacin and rifampicin.

N.B. Please discuss with local pharmacist and refer to local policies, drug information departments and BAPEN guidelines (refer to website addresses).

*Water*

The use of sterile or tap water varies according to local policy, patient's condition and location (home or hospital patient).

*Home Tube Feeding*

Tube feeding at home needs to be adapted to the home environment and must take into account carer/patient capabilities and social considerations. Feed and its administration set may be delivered by home care companies or collected from a pharmacy.

*Monitoring*

Effective monitoring can reduce the complications associated with artificial nutritional support. It is very important to:

- Check accurate tube position/inspect tube site prior to commencing feed daily.
- Flush the tube regularly.
- Monitor gastrointestinal function, e.g.:

—Bowel movements.
—Vomiting.
—Bloating.
—Gastric distension.
• Identify drug–nutrient interactions.

# Parenteral Nutrition (PN)

Refer to dictionary for definition. Parenteral nutrition (PN) should be used to prevent or treat malnutrition when the gastrointestinal tract is unavailable, or gastrointestinal function is inadequate.

## Possible Indications for Parenteral Nutrition
See Box 1.2.

## Routes Used for Parenteral Nutrition
The perceived length of feeding will influence the route of nutritional support.

*Central Access*
• Short-term: multilumen lines.
• Intermediate duration: peripherally inserted central catheter (PICC) >15 cm long (>5 days–4 weeks).
• Long-term: e.g. Hickman line or Portacath.

| Box 1.2   Possible indications for parenteral nutrition | |
| --- | --- |
| Failure to tolerate enteral nutritional support | • E.g. paralytic ileus, vomiting, profuse diarrhoea, radiation enteritis, chronic idiopathic pseudo-obstruction. |
| Intestinal failure | • Intestinal atresia, short bowel syndrome, motility disorders |
| Severe malabsorption | • Cannot be managed by an elemental diet<br>• Large output enterocutaneous fistula |
| Inflammatory bowel disease | • Crohn's disease, unable to tolerate elemental/semi-elemental diet |
| Severe mucositis | • Unable to pass enteral tube |
| Bowel rest | • Post-gastrointestinal surgery, which cannot be achieved by an elemental diet |

Note that full nutritional requirements cannot be met via the enteral route

*Peripheral Access*

Peripheral access should not be used for PN due to risk of thrombophlebitis.

## Composition of Parenteral Nutrition Feeds

PN is usually administered in an all-in-one preparation (1.5–3 litres) which contains:

- 10%, 20%, 50% glucose.
- 0%, 10%, 20% lipid.
- Amino acids.
- Electrolytes.
- Water.
- Fat- and water-soluble vitamins.
- Trace elements.

A variety of standard preparations are usually available to meet patients' requirements. These may be in a multi-chamber format, in which the separate macronutrient chambers are combined by rolling the bag to break the inner membrane seal prior to administration. The clinical condition of a patient may warrant an individually compounded preparation, such as lipid-free preparations for patients with liver funtion derangement and cholestasis.

## Feeding Regimens

- In all cases the lumen should be **dedicated** to the use of PN only.
- Strict flow control is essential. This can be done with volumetric pumps fitted with occlusion and air-in-line alarms.
- PN is usually administered continuously over 24 hours, however this can be reduced in certain cases.

## Glutamine

It is now common practice to use intravenous glutamine preparations for critically ill and bonemarrow transplant patients who require PN.

## Complications

See Table 1.2.

Careful monitoring detects most of the complications associated with nutritional support. Multidisciplinary team management is essential.

Table 1.2  Complications of parenteral nutrition

| Complication | Comment |
|---|---|
| **Catheter-related** | |
| Catheter-related infection | Meticulous care of the line and catheter site can prevent sepsis; follow protocols; use a dedicated line for feeding |
| Insertion-related<br>• Air embolism<br>• Pneumothorax<br>• Catheter malposition | Adhere to policies; experienced staff only to insert; confirm position by X-ray before commencing feed |
| Catheter occlusion and damage | Discuss with medical team |
| Central venous thrombosis | Discuss with medical team |
| **Nutritional and metabolic** | |
| Dehydration | Monitor abnormal losses, e.g. fistulae or diarrhoea. N.B. Additional IV fluids may be required |
| Over-hydration | Monitor all other IV fluids that are administered, e.g. antibiotics, chemotherapy |
| Hyperglycaemia | Discuss carbohydrate content of PN with dietitian<br>Discuss blood sugar management with medical team |
| Hypoglycaemia | Can occur if PN is stopped immediately. PN infusion rate should be decreased slowly. If this is not possible provide an IV glucose solution and monitor blood glucose 4-hourly for 24 hours. |
| Lipaemia | At-risk patients include critically ill or septic patients or those with renal failure. |
| Electrolyte imbalance | Over- or under-administration of electrolytes |
| **Effect on other organ systems** | |
| Hepatobiliary disease | Consider impact of underlying disease and PN composition |
| Metabolic bone disease | Consider poor nutritional status and exposure to corticosteriod therapy |

### Basic Monitoring for Enteral (Tube Feeding) and Parenteral Nutrition

N.B. The frequency of monitoring can be reduced for stable patients; refer to figures in brackets in Table 1.3.

Table 1.3 Monitoring for enteral and parenteral nutrition

| Parameter | Parameters to assess | Frequency enteral | Parenteral |
|---|---|---|---|
| Clinical | Temperature, pulse, respiration and blood pressure | 4-hourly | 4-hourly |
| | Ward urine analysis | Daily | Daily |
| Fluid balance | Fluid balance | At each bottle change | Hourly |
| | Serum urea | Daily (2 x week once stable) | Daily |
| Biochemistry | Full serum electrolyte profile | Daily (2 x week once stable) | Daily |
| | Glucose | Daily (2 x week once stable) | 4-hourly blood (urinalysis) |
| | Liver function chemistry | 2 x weekly | 2 x weekly |
| | Zinc, copper and selenium | Monthly | Monthly. Assessment is NM in patients on long term PN |
| Nutritional status | Nutrient intake | Daily | Daily |
| | Body weight | Weekly | Weekly (daily if fluid balance information required) |
| Haematology | Full blood count | 2 x weekly | Daily |
| | Prothrombin time | As indicated | Weekly |
| Lipaemia | Cholesterol and triacylglycerol | As indicated | On initiation and then weekly |

BIBLIOGRAPHY

American Gastroenterological Association 1999 American Gastroenterology Association technical review on tube feeding for enteral nutrition. Gastroenterology 1208:1282–1301

Department of Health 2001 Essence of care. The Stationary Office, London

Fawcett, H, MacFie, J, McWhirter, J, Sizer, T, Whitney, S 1996 Current perspectives on parenteral nutrition in adults. Pennington, C R (ed). ADM, Biddenden, Kent

Green, C J 1999 Existence, causes and consequences of disease-related malnutrition in the hospital and the community, and clinical and financial benefits of nutritional intervention. Clinical Nutrition 18(suppl 2):3–28

Lipman T O 1998 Grains or veins: is enteral nutrition really better than parenteral nutrition? A look at the evidence. Journal of Enteral and Parenteral Nutrition 22:167–182

Pancorbo-Hidalgo P L, Garcia-Fernandez F P, Ramirez-Perez C 2001 Complications associated with enteral nutrition by nasogastric tube in an internal medicine unit. Journal of Clinical Nursing 10(4):482–490

Royal College of Physicians 2002 Nutrition and patients: a doctor's responsibility. RCP, London

Saunders C 1993 Surgical nutrition: a review. Journal of the Royal College of Surgeons of Edinburgh 38:195–204

Stratton R J, Elia M A 1999 Critical, systematic analysis of the use of oral nutritional supplements in the community. Clinical Nutrition 18(Suppl 2):29–84

Stroud M et al 2003 Guidelines for enteral feeding in adult hospital patients. GUT 52 (suppl VII): vii1–vii12

---

USEFUL WEBSITE ADDRESSES

---

www.bapen.org.uk (for access to nurse nutrition site, nutrition policies and drug administration)
www.betterhospitalfood.com
www.mhra.gov.uk
www.nice.org.uk (Nutrition Support in Adults, Feb 2006)
www.nnng.org
www.npsa.nhs.uk
www.peng.org.uk

# Nutritional Management of Coronary Heart Disease
### CAROLINE KING

## Introduction

In a similar way to obesity and diabetes, coronary heart disease (CHD) is a major cause of mortality and morbidity within the UK. Nutritional advice plays a key role in its prevention and treatment.

A healthy diet and lifestyle can reduce the risks of many of the major diseases of later life. There is a clear relationship between too much saturated fat, hypertension, obesity, insufficient exercise and CHD.

# What Is a Healthy Diet?

A healthy, well-balanced diet provides enough energy for the body to function optimally and a mixture of foods to include all the main nutrient groups: protein, fat, carbohydrate, vitamins and minerals. It is based on starchy foods, fruit and vegetables and is low in fat. So it does not have to be more expensive as larger portions of starchy foods such as whole-grain bread and cereals, rice and pasta are recommended and smaller portions of meat, cheese and dairy foods. This is often seen as similar to the 'mediterranean diet' (de Lorgeril & Salen 2008).

# Total Energy

A healthy diet should provide enough energy to maintain a healthy weight. Weight gain occurs when the amount of energy going in is greater than that which is being expended.

The nutrients which contribute to total energy intake are fat, carbohydrate and protein. These need to be consumed in foods in the right proportions for a healthy diet.

### Fat

The link between total fat and saturated fat intake with CHD is well established. So the recommendations are that fat should contribute no more than 30% of total energy. All types of fat are high in calories containing 9 kcal per gram, compared with 4 kcal per gram for protein and carbohydrate. In addition diets high in fat are often very palatable and likely to lead to over-consumption and therefore increase risk of obesity. Saturated fat, found mainly in animal and dairy foods, should be reduced and replaced with a mixture of polyunsaturated and monounsaturated oils where there is a need to add fat (see below – Cholesterol and see Box 1.3). Saturated fat raises the blood cholesterol while unsaturated fat lowers blood cholesterol. There is sometimes confusion about chosing margarine or butter; butter is high in saturated fat and calories and margarine (polyunsaturated) has the same amount of calories but contains a better type of fat.

### Oily Fish

Oily fish include salmon, mackerel, herring, trout and pilchards. They are high in fat but it is a good type of fat (polyunsaturated). They are also rich in omega-3 fatty acids. It has been proposed that these fatty acids reduce the risk of a second heart attack after a first. There is

| Box 1.3   Types of fat in foods |
| --- |
| **Saturated fat**<br>    Lard, butter, cheese, fat on red meat, cream, suet, meat produce<br>**Polyunsaturated**<br>    Sunflower oil<br>    corn oil<br>    Soya oil<br>**Monounsaturated**<br>    Olive oil<br>    Rapeseed oil<br>**Good sources of omega 3**<br>    Fish oil |

evidence that they make blood less likely to clot and less viscous. Oily fish should be included in the diet at least twice a week. Some tasty examples are tinned fish on sandwiches or in a baked potato or fresh fish baked or grilled.

**Cholesterol**

Blood cholesterol is made in the body from the saturated fat found in the diet. Cholesterol found in food (e.g. eggs, shellfish) is thought to make only a small contribution to actual blood cholesterol levels. The main focus of a cholesterol-lowering diet is (a) reducing all fat in the diet and (b) changing fat from saturated to polyunsaturated and monounsaturated fats. Thus a cholesterol-lowering diet is different from a low-cholesterol diet. Blood cholesterol itself, in normal amounts, has many important body functions.

**Carbohydrate**

Carbohydrates should provide 50% of total energy. To achieve this starchy carbohydrates should be included in every meal. There is no evidence that high-carbohydrate diets are linked to CHD or diabetes. Sugar is also a carbohydrate, however it contributes no vitamins and minerals, just 'empty calories', so intake should be limited. It is also makes foods and drinks palatable and can encourage overconsumption.

**Fibre**

Fibre can be divided into two categories: insoluble and soluble. Insoluble fibre which is found in bran, wholemeal bread and cereals is good for bowel health, to prevent constipation and reduce the risk of bowel cancer. Soluble fibre is good for the heart and is found in foods such as beans, pulses and oats. Many studies show that this type of fibre lowers cholesterol and also improves blood sugar control. Many high-fibre starchy foods contain a mixture of the two.

## Minerals Vitamins and Antioxidants

These are mainly found in fruit and vegetables, and the wider the range of different types consumed the better for the balance of nutrients.

The current target is for people to eat at least five portions of fruit and vegetables (excluding potatoes) a day.

## Salt

Research suggests that on average we consume ten times more salt than is required. In people at risk of hypertension salty foods can increase blood pressure. This in turn increases the risk of heart disease, kidney disease and stroke. So a healthy diet is a low-salt diet where salt is added to food at the table but not during cooking and processed foods are limited. Herbs and spices can be added to flavour food.

## Alcohol

The recommended safe limits of alcohol are 21 units a week for men and 14 units a week for women. However these amounts can be ammended by government bodies – particularly for vunerable groups – so it is important to check for current guidelines. It is healthier to spread alcohol consumption through the week. Alcohol is another form of empty calories, so should be restricted if weight loss is desirable. Drinking alcohol is not recommended during pregnancy.

Some research has suggested that red wine contains antioxidants that have a protective effect against heart disease. So it may be better to have red wine if alcohol is taken rather than other drinks.

## Novel foods

There are now a range of foods containing plant sterols which can act to reduce blood cholesterol levels. These are effective but work best as part of a healthy diet and lifestyle as they only address the problem of raised cholesterol.

REFERENCES AND BACKGROUND READING

Van Horn et al 2008 The evidence for dietary prevention and treatment of cardiovascular disease. Journal of the American Dietetic Association 108(2):287

de Lorgeril & Salen 2008 The mediterrranean diet:rationale and evidence for its benefit. Current Atherosclerosis Reports 10(6):518

Retelnv et al 2008 Nutrition protocols for the prevention of cardiovascular disease. Nutrition in Clinical Practice 23(5):468

# Nutritional Management of Obesity
## JOANNE BOYLE

## Definition

The definition of obesity in adults is usually based on the Body Mass Index (BMI)

$$NB:\ Body\ Mass\ Index\ (Quetelet\ Index) = \frac{Weight\ (kg)}{Height\ (m^2)}$$

The international consensus on BMI ranges classifies them as in Table 1.4 (WHO 1998).

## Prevalence

In 2006, 38% of adults were overweight and 24% were obese in the UK. This reflects a doubling of the number of overweight individuals and a trebling of those who are obese since 1980. Overall, 67% of men and 56% of women are either overweight or obese (The Information Centre 2008). Analysis by the government's Foresight programme (2007) shows that over half of the UK adult population could be

| Table 1.4 | BMI classification |
|---|---|
| **BMI (kg/m²)** | **Classification** |
| <18.5 | Underweight |
| 18.5–24.9 | Healthy weight |
| 25–29.9 | Pre-obese (overweight) |
| 30–34.9 | Obese class 1 (moderately obese, commonly referred to as 'fat') |
| 35–39.9 | Obese class 2 (severely obese, commonly referred to as 'very fat') |
| >40 | Obese class 3 (morbidly obese) |

obese by 2050 (McPherson et al 2007). The economic implications are substantial since obesity is related to many different diseases. The NHS costs attributable to overweight and obesity are projected to double to £10 billion per year by 2050. The wider costs to society and business are estimated to reach £49.9 billion per year (at today's prices) (McCormack and Stone 2007).

Our environment has changed drastically over the last 50 years with a reduction in active occupations, a rise in more sedentary occupations and increased car ownership. This has been coupled with changes in food production and an increased availability of high calorie and cheap food. These changes have corresponded with the increasing levels of obesity. Being overweight or obese increases the risk of a number of chronic diseases including type 2 diabetes, hypertension, heart disease, stroke and certain types of cancers. This is especially true if the weight is carried around the waist (known as apple shape or trunkal obesity) rather than around the hips (known as pear shaped obesity).

## Waist Circumference

Waist circumference measurements are also an important in risk factor assessment, indicating the accumulation of excess intra-abdominal fat. Evidence suggests that an accumulation of fat in the upper body area is associated with an increased risk for developing heart disease and non-insulin dependent diabetes more than the same amount of fat distributed subcutaneously below the waist (Carpenter 1997, Chan et al 1994). These two distinct distributions of body fat are commonly referred to as 'apple-shaped' and 'pear-shaped' respectively.

Populations differ in the level of risk associated with a particular waist circumference. South Asians have higher levels of abdominal obesity, although they might not be considered obese by conventional BMI criteria (McKeigue et al 1991). The WHO Report (2000) suggested lower cut-off points for South Asians.

Increased risk levels are shown in Table 1.5 (Han et al 1995, WHO 2000):

| Table 1.5 | Increased risk levels associated with waist circumference | |
| --- | --- | --- |
| | **At risk** | **High risk** |
| Men | ≥94 cm/37 in | ≥102 cm/40 in |
| South Asian Men | | ≥90 cm/35.5 in |
| Women | ≥80 cm/31 in | ≥88 cm/34 in |
| South Asian Women | | ≥80 cm/31 in |

# Why Should Individuals Who are Overweight Lose Weight?

Research shows that losing between 5% and 10% of your current body weight can vastly improve your health (SIGN 1996). Weight loss is of particular benefit in diabetes, high blood pressure, shortness of breath, joint problems, sleep apnoea and raised cholesterol.

# What Does Losing Weight Involve?

An individual's body weight represents the balance between all the energy taken in from what they eat and drink and all the energy used up in daily life. To lose weight energy intake needs to be reduced and energy output or activity increased. The only way to lose weight and keep it off is to change one's eating and physical activity habits permenantly. Crash or 'fad' diets may reduce weight in the short-term, however, they are unsustainable and usually result in weight regain. The best approach to weight loss is sensible, healthy eating where weight loss is approximately ½ –1 kg (1–2 lbs) each week. This is equivalent to a reduction in energy intake of approximately 500 kilocalories each day.

# Practical Guidelines for Weight Loss

- Regular meals.
- Avoidance of high calorie snacks.
- Starchy food at each meal with a focus on wholegrain varieties rather than white.
- 2–3 servings of vegetables and salads each day.
- 2–3 servings of fruit each day.
- At meal times, the vegetables/salad should take up about half the plate.
- Choose low fat foods wherever possible, and eat smaller portions of fat rich food.
- Avoid sugar and sugary foods.
- Alcohol contains kilocalories – keep to limits of 14 units/week for women and 21 units/week for men.
- Monitor body weight, but not more than once/week.
- Regular activity.

See also Box 1.5 for distribution of energy intake in the diet.

# Prevention is Better than Cure

All the current reviews of obesity management agree that there should be a greater focus on the prevention of obesity. However, the best way of achieving this is still a topic of current research.

REFERENCES

Carpenter M 1997 Taking account of a fat distribution in the assessment of obese patients. Practice Nurse 14(7)

Chan J M, Rimm E B, Colditz G A, Stampfer M J, Willett W C 1994 Obesity, fat distribution and weight gain as risk factors for clinical diabetes in men. Diabetes Care 17:961–969

Han T S, Van Leer E M, Seidell J C, Lean M E J 1995 Waist circumference action levels in identification of cardiovascular risk factors. BMJ 311:158–161

The Information Centre 2008 Statistics on Obesity, Physical Activity and Diet. Retrieved on 23.02.2009 from http://www.ic.nhs.uk/webfiles/publications/opan08/OPAD

McCormack B, Stone I 2007 Economic costs of obesity and the case for government intervention. Short Science Review. Foresight Tackling Obesities: Future Choices. Obesity Reviews 8(s1):161–164. Retrieved on 23.02.2009 from http://www.foresight.gov.uk

McKeigue P M, Shah B, Marmot M G 1991 Relation of central obesity and insulin resistance with high diabetes prevalence and cardiovascular risk in South Asians. Lancet 337–382

McPherson K, Marsh T, Brown M 2007 Modelling future trends in obesity and the impact on health. Foresight Tackling Obesities: Future Choices. Retrieved on 23.02.2009 from http://www.foresight.gov.uk

SIGN 1996 Obesity in Scotland; integrating prevention with weight management: a National Clinical Guideline recommended for use in Scotland. SIGN, Edinburgh

WHO 1998 Obesity: preventing and managing the global epidemic. Report of a WHO consultation on obesity. World Health Organization, Geneva

WHO 2000 The Asia-Pacific perspective: redefining obesity and its treatment. World Health Organization, Geneva

# Nutritional Management of Diabetes

Nicola Bandaranayake

## Nutritional Advice for People with Diabetes

There are two main categories of diabetes: type 1, previously called insulin-dependent or juvenile onset diabetes, and type 2, which used to be called non-insulin-dependent diabetes. The main reason for the change is that many people with type 2 diabetes require insulin to treat their diabetes. In both cases dietary management is an essential part of the treatment and unless the diet is right it is impossible to meet the glycaemic control targets. Dietary treatment is not just about controlling blood glucose levels but also about preventing the long-term complications of diabetes such as heart disease and renal disease.

The recommendations for the nutritional management of diabetes remain those from Diabetes UK in 2003 given in Table 1.6.

These nutritional recommendations are translated into practical advice that will help the person with diabetes to adapt their diet, working towards the following ideal that will help to control their diabetes and reduce the risk of long-term complications.

## Dietary Goals

The phrase 'diabetic diet' is no longer promoted. Instead, the goal is a healthy balanced diet that is sustainable for life and incorporates:

- A regular meal pattern. People who eat small, frequent meals/ snacks tend to have better glycaemic control. At a minimum this would mean breakfast, lunch and an evening meal. Some people may be encouraged to snack between meals or at bedtime depending on which medications are taken.
- Starchy carbohydrate in each meal/snack, especially low glycaemic index carbohydrates. The slowly absorbed or low glycaemic index starchy foods will improve blood glucose levels especially those which contain soluble fibre. These include foods like oats and wholegrain cereals, beans and pulses and pasta.
- A reduction in total fat intakes, replacing saturated fat with mono-unsaturated rich fats and oils, like rapeseed or olive oil.
- At least five portions of fruit and vegetables each day.
- Limiting excess sugar (sucrose) intake, and replacing it with sweeteners.

Table 1.6  Nutritional advice for people with diabetes: 2003

| Diet element | Comment |
|---|---|
| • Keep body mass index (BMI) in healthy range | |
| • Control total energy intake | |
| Carbohydrate | 45–60% total energy intake |
| Sucrose | <10% of total energy intake as part of a healthy diet |
| Total fat | <35% of total energy intake |
| — saturated and trans fatty acids (or if LDL cholesterol elevated) | <10% of total energy intake <8% of total energy intake |
| — polyunsaturated fat | <10% of total energy intake |
| — monounsaturated fat | 10–20% of total energy intake |
| — monounsaturated fat + carbohydrate | 60–70% of total energy intake |
| • Soluble fibre | Has beneficial effects on glycaemic and lipid profiles |
| • Oily fish | 2 servings per week |
| • Protein | 10–20% of total energy intake or not more than 1 g per kg body weight |
| • Vitamins and antioxidants | Encourage foods naturally rich in vitamins and antioxidants (in chronic renal failure these might need to be restricted). There is no evidence to support the use of supplements and some evidence that they are harmful. |
| • Salt | ≤6 g per day |
| • Alcohol | 14 units per weeks for women 21 units per week for men 1–2 alcohol-free days per week |
| • Specially formulated diabetic foods | There are no known grounds for encouraging the use of specially formulated foods for people with diabetes |

- Two portions of oily fish each week. Including oily fish like sardines, herrings, salmon, trout and mackerel regularly in the diet can help reduce cardiovascular disease risk.
- Aim for a 'no added salt diet'. A reduction in salt intake by limiting processed foods and using herbs and spices instead of salt can help reduce blood pressure.
- Moderate alcohol consumption, with a maximum of one to two drinks per day (unless medically contraindicated).

- A reduction in energy intake by 500 kcal per day, where appropriate to aid weight loss. If the individual with diabetes is overweight then losing even a few pounds can improve blood glucose control and improve overall health.

These points can be summarized by imagining a plate. At mealtimes most people's plates consist of large portions of meat, fish, eggs or cheese. These foods are often high in fat and cover half of the plate, leaving very little room for vegetables and starchy foods such as rice, pasta, chapattis, yam and potatoes. It is recommended that the amount of starchy foods and vegetables or salad take up most of the plate so that the smallest portion is the meat or alternative protein rich foods. In this way the fatty foods are reduced.

## Why Should People with Diabetes Reduce their Fat Intake?

Probably the most important recommendation for people with diabetes is to reduce their fat and oil intake. Two of the major aims of the diet are to reduce the risk of heart disease and reduce weight. Fats and oils (regardless of type used) increase the risk of heart disease and weight gain. As they are all high in calories reducing intakes will help with weight loss.

## Which Foods are High in Fat?

There are visible fats – the fat that can be seen in or on foods such as cooking oils including all the vegetable oils, ghee, lard, butter, margarine, meat fat and dripping. The fat from meat should be removed and less butter, margarine and oil should be used. There are also foods that have hidden fats such as biscuits, cakes, pies and pastries, where the high-fat content is not so obvious. As they are high in fat they should only be eaten very occasionally. It is also advisable to cut down on fried foods, snacks such as samosas, crisps and high-fat foods that come from take-aways.

## It is Important to Remember

Diabetes is not just a disease involving sugar and cutting out sugar from the diet. It is about adding foods to the diet that will help control blood glucose levels, limiting the amount of fat and increasing the amount of vegetables and fresh fruit that are eaten. This involves enjoying a wide variety of foods and adopting a healthier diet and lifestyle.

# Nutrition in Paediatrics

CAROLINE KING

## Nutrient Requirements

Nutrient requirements mirror growth rates, hence children have higher requirements than adults per kg body weight, with the highest being during infancy and adolescence (see Table 1.7).

## Infant Feeding

Breast milk is the optimal food for the vast majority of infants whether well or sick, with recent government guidelines recommending exclusive breast feeding for 6 months before the introduction of solid food. This recommendation brings UK guidelines into line with World Health Organization recommendations.

When breast milk is unavailable proprietary infant formulas are the next choice as their composition follows agreed nutritional guidelines. Specialized formulas include preterm, nutrient-dense, thickened, soya-based, semi-elemental, elemental, lactose-free, low-calcium and those catering for inborn errors of metabolism. Their use is best kept to that supervised by a dietitian.

## Nutritional Deficiencies

Preschool children are the most vulnerable group. Those who are socioeconomically disadvantaged and those from some ethnic groups are at highest risk of suboptimal intake of some nutritents.

| Table 1.7 Estimated average requirements/kg body weight* | | | |
|---|---|---|---|
| Age | Fluid (ml) | Energy (kcal) | Protein (g) |
| Preterm | 150–200 | 120 | 3.5 |
| 0–3 months | 150 | 115–100 | 2.1 |
| 4–6 months | 130 | 95 | 1.6 |
| 7–9 months | 120 | 95 | 1.5 |
| 10–12 months | 110 | 95 | 1.5 |
| 1–3 years | 95 | 95 | 1.1 |
| 4–6 years | 85 | 90 | 1.1 |
| 7–10 years | 75 | 85 | No COMA rec |
| 11–14 years | 55 | 65 | No COMA rec |
| 15–18 years | 35–50 | 40 | 0.6 |

Note: The higher fluid requirements result in an increased risk of dehydration during illness.
* Committee on Medical Aspects of Food (COMA) 1991 DOH report on health and social subjects, no. 41. HMSO, London. ISBN 0–11–321397–2.

Those from the Asian subcontinent are at high risk of iron and vitamin D deficiency. Large national surveys are carried out periodically to give an insight into childhood eating habits and nutritional intake. See National Diet and Nutrition Surveys (London, HMSO).

## Obesity

Obesity is increasing in all sectors of industrialized societies but the socially disadvantaged seem to be at highest risk. If the UK continues to follow the childhood obesity trend seen in the USA there will be an increase in short-term morbidity, e.g. diabetes, abnormal liver function tests, weight-bearing-joint problems and psychological issues. In addition childhood obesity does not bode well for adult health and is likely to lead to increased risk of diabetes and heart disease as these children grow up. Research is ongoing to try and tease out the relative roles of reduced exercise vs increased intake. There are indications that energy intake has not increased sufficiently to explain the rise in obesity, however there has been a very rapid increase in sedentary behaviour, e.g. computer games and television viewing, coupled with less playing outdoors, which could underpin the increased weight of children today. In addition there is evidence that those who are not obese may still be developing an abnormal body composition due to lack of exercise, with an increased proportion of the body's weight being fat compared to several years ago.

## Allergies

There is evidence that food allergies are on the increase in industrialized countries with diagnosis occurring primarily in infancy and early childhood. However, perceived prevalence is probably much lower than clinically established disease; therefore when exclusion of a nutritionally important food is suggested, there should be a trial period after which the food is added back into the diet if no improvement is seen. Children on cows'-milk-free diets are at risk of poor growth and poor bone mineralization.

## Chronic Diseases of Childhood

There are many chronic diseases of childhood that require major nutritional or dietetic intervention. For many there is associated poor appetite and supplementation of the diet with tube feeding is necessary; if this is likely to be necessary for an indefinite period a gastrostomy should be considered. For others a fundamental change in the diet is necessary, e.g. coeliac condition, renal and liver disease, cystic fibrosis and many of the inborn errors of metabolism. A lifetime change in diet is often needed which requires monitoring and support of the child and family from medical professionals.

## Useful Resources

British Dietetic Association www.bda.uk.com/

Cochrane Database of Systematic Reviews. www.nelh.nhs.uk/cochrane.asp

Scottish Intercollegiate Guidelines Network. www.sign.ac.uk

Shaw V, Lawson M (eds) 2007 Clinical paediatric dietetics, 3rd edn. Blackwell, Oxford

# Appendix 2

# Resuscitation
### LINDSAY CREEK

## Introduction/Overview
The act of resuscitation is usually separated into two component parts: basic life support (BLS) and advanced life support (ALS). This appendix concentrates purely on basic life support, and is based on the 2005 guidelines published by the European Resuscitation Council, and the Resuscitation Council (UK).

Resuscitation guidelines are reviewed and revised every 5 years, and are a result of international consensus between various resuscitation experts with access to the latest international research. Further information on current guidelines and on relevant publications can be gained by visiting the Resuscitation Council (UK) website www.resus.org.uk. Information can also be found on this site on the range of more advanced courses coordinated by the Resuscitation Council (UK), such as Immediate Life Support (ILS), Advanced Life Support (ALS), Paediatric Immediate Life Support (PILS) and European Paediatric Life Support (EPLS).

This chapter concentrates on adult and paediatric basic life support for nurses and health care workers. It is not intended to replace practical training, (which as a minimum should be attended on an annual basis), but is designed to provide a useful aide-mémoire. The paediatric section is directed at those working within paediatrics, and therefore with a duty of care to respond to this client group. As always, the focus in both adults and paediatrics remains the prevention of cardiac arrest if at all possible, by responding to early warning signs from these patients.

# *The 2005 Resuscitation Guidelines*
## Adult Cardiac Arrest
### Ensure Safety
Check it is safe to approach – if necessary dealing with any hazards prior to approaching the person.

### Shout for Help
In many cases it is obvious there is a problem necessitating help before any kind of response has been ascertained from the person, and therefore a shout for help can be made to attract attention. Within hospital environments there is often the additional benefit of an emergency buzzer system, and this should be utilized if present.

### Check for Response/Stimulate the Person
Shout at and gently shake the person ensuring you cause no further harm with the stimuli you apply.

### Open the Airway
Look in the mouth for foreign bodies (dentures can be left in place if they fit well). If anything is seen, remove it carefully.

To open the airway perform a head tilt/chin lift manoeuvre. To do this, place one hand on the forehead and tilt the head back; at the same time, with two fingers of the other hand, lift the chin. This action will lift the tongue from the back of the throat, thus opening the airway (Fig. 2.1).

### Check for Breathing and Circulation
Whilst maintaining the airway position, check for breathing by bringing your cheek over the mouth and nose of the casualty and looking along the line of the chest:

- Look for chest movement.
- Listen for breath sounds.
- Feel for breathing on your cheek.

In addition, observe for signs of a circulation being present such as *regular* breathing, movement, swallowing, coughing, etc. If you have been trained to do so check for a carotid pulse at this point using the combined technique illustrated here (Fig. 2.2).

Check breathing and circulation for up to 10 seconds and no longer. If you are still unsure at this point about the circulation, but there

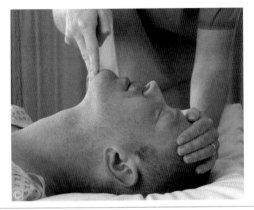

**Fig. 2.1**  Opening the airway

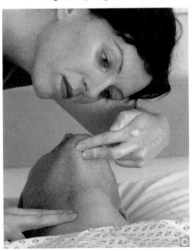

**Fig. 2.2**  Combined check for breathing and pulse

is no adequate breathing, assume cardiac arrest as the most likely option and treat accordingly.

### Obtain Help/Ensure Phone Call is Made

In hospital it is highly unlikely that you would still be on your own at this point in time (especially if the emergency buzzer system has been used), however, if this is the case, leave the casualty and call the cardiac arrest team yourself.

It is more likely that several people will have responded. Ensure you focus on one person and ask them clearly what you wish them to do, to avoid the situation of everyone thinking someone else has performed this task.

In most hospitals the emergency number to activate the cardiac arrest team has been standardized to 2222. It is important when starting in a new Trust that you familiarize yourself with the calling system in place, including the variety of teams available to you, i.e. obstetric/paediatric/adult, to ensure the correct team is activated. In addition, some larger Trusts may provide a guide for describing the location of the arrest, to direct team members to the area. Most hospitals have a Resuscitation Officer who will cover this as part of training, and a resuscitation policy which should give this information, including the calling system for car parks, etc.

If you are in the community rather than a hospital environment, ensure an ambulance has been called via the 999/112 system. In all cases stay on the phone until all the essential information has been received by the operator.

### Start Chest Compressions

To perform chest compressions effectively you must ensure that the person is lying on their back on a firm flat surface (hospital mattresses are designed for this purpose, but pressure relieving mattresses will need to be deflated). If necessary, expose the chest to enable you to find the correct hand position. Place two fingers on the xiphisternum and the heel of your other hand beside them (if this can't be done quickly then place your hands in the centre of the chest to avoid delaying the compressions). Place the heel of your other hand over the first, and interlock your fingers pulling them clear of the chest. This will ensure that pressure is delivered solely by the heel of your hand.

Keep your elbows straight and bring your shoulders over the person's chest (Fig. 2.3). Commence 30 chest compressions, aiming to

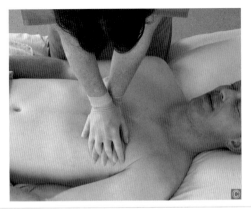

**Fig. 2.3**  Chest compressions

depress the sternum by 4–5 cm. The compressions should be delivered smoothly with equal time spent on compression and relaxation,
at an approximate rate of 100 per minute.

### Attempt Two Ventilations

As a minimum the clinical area should have a pocket mask available
to deliver these ventilations, and training in its use will be provided
during annual BLS sessions. Ensure the airway is open, and aim only
to achieve a chest rise – overdoing the volume of air will lead to a
higher chance of gastric regurgitation. If the first ventilation fails to
achieve a chest rise re-position the airway, if the second fails, return to
chest compressions – you only have 2 attempts at ventilations.

  If you are willing to perform mouth to mouth ventilation ensure
you are aware of your Trust's Resuscitation policy, as many do not
advocate this technique when dealing with unknown patients who
present a potential infection risk.

### Continue Resuscitation

Continue resuscitation with a ratio of 30 compressions to 2 ventilations, until competent help arrives and tells you to stop, you are too
exhausted to continue (although hopefully in hospital you will regularly

be rotating the person doing chest compressions to avoid this), or you notice signs of life – in which case stop and reassess the patient.

What else you do will depend on your skill level, training experience, and local trust policy.

Please refer to Figure 2.4 for a flow diagram summarizing the approach to an adult in cardiac arrest.

**Fig. 2.4** Adult cardiac arrest

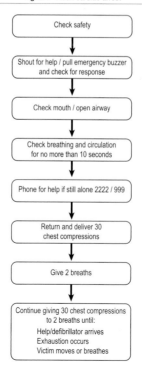

## Other Situations
*Obstetric Arrests*
In addition to the resuscitation techniques previously described, a women over 20 weeks of pregnancy should be tilted towards the left side, to remove some of the pressure of the uterus on the inferior vena cava, thus improving circulating blood flow. Aim to achieve at least 15 degrees of tilt by placing objects such as a Cardiff wedge, pillows, blankets, etc. under the right side/hip.

*Respiratory Arrests*
This will be discovered at the point of checking for breathing and circulation. Ensure an arrest call is put out, then whilst waiting for help to arrive, provide ventilations over 1 minute before assessing the circulation for a further 10 seconds. If a circulation remains present, continue breathing, stopping only for circulation checks every minute. If you are ventilating a patient at the correct rate, you should achieve 10–12 breaths per minute.

*Tracheostomy Patients*
Remember to ventilate these patients via the stoma in their neck. Pocket mask valves can often fit onto these stomas if no bag valve mask device is present.

*Unconscious Breathing Patient*
Consider placing the person in the recovery position. The use of the recovery position should achieve two things – the maintenance of a patent airway, and, if they vomit, the prevention of aspiration of gastric contents.

- Before moving them remove any glasses (if worn), and any keys or bulky objects from the pockets. To remove items safely from a stranger's pocket, gently pull the linings out, thus avoiding personal injury from sharp objects.
- Kneel beside the person. Place the arm nearest you at right angles to their body. Bend the elbow, keeping the palm uppermost.
- Bring the far arm across their chest, and hold the back of their hand against the nearest cheek.
- With your other hand grasp the far knee and pull it up, keeping the foot on the ground. Using the knee as a lever, pull the person towards you and on to his or her side.

- Adjust the upper leg aiming to achieve right-angle bends of both the hip and knee. Open the airway.

**Please note that if the patient is to be in this position for longer than 30 minutes, turn them onto their other side to prevent circulation problems to the lower arm.**

*Paediatric Cardiac Arrest (for people not working in paediatrics)*
Adapt the adult approach – if possible trying to remember to give an initial 5 breaths. Continue resuscitation with a ratio of 30 compressions to 2 ventilations, and if you have to leave to phone for help, ensure you perform 1 minute of resuscitation first.

## Adult Choking

There are three possible situations as far as choking is concerned – partial/mild, complete/severe and collapsed.

**Partial Obstructions/Mild Obstructions**
*Recognition*
The person is able to speak, cough adequately and clear the obstruction themselves.

*Treatment*
Stay with them and be prepared to intervene should the situation deteriorate.

**Complete Obstructions/Severe Obstructions**
*Recognition*
The person is unable to move any air past the obstruction and therefore is unable to cough, talk, breathe, or clear the object – often they will clutch at their throat. If in doubt on the cause, confirm the person is choking, and then having received confirmation treat it.

*Treatment*
Support the chest with one hand and lean the person forward to ensure that if dislodged the obstruction comes out of the mouth. Deliver up to 5 back slaps between the shoulder blades, checking each time to see if the obstruction has been relieved.

If these fail to work, move on to deliver up to 5 abdominal thrusts (previously known as the Heimlich manoeuvre). With the person still leaning forwards, stand behind them and bring your arms underneath theirs. Form a fist with one hand and place this on the abdomen between the umbilicus and sternum. Place the other hand over the first, and pull the fist inwards and upwards. If the abdominal thrusts fail, attempt a futher 5 back slaps, and continue alternating 5 back slaps and 5 abdominal thrusts until the obstruction is removed, help arrives or the person collapses.

### Collapsed as a Result of a Choking Episode You Have Been Treating

There is no point assessing this patient as you know what the problem is already. As a result, the advice is to commence BLS starting with 30 compressions. It is possible that the pressures generated within the chest may shift the obstruction to a point where you are able to blow air past it, or it may break up slightly. Attempt 2 ventilations as normal, although they may or may not be successful. Continue resuscitation until assistance arrives. Be aware of your Trust policy relating to do not resuscitate orders, as many of these treat choking as a reversible cause, and therefore advise full treatment in this situation.

## Paediatric Cardiac Arrest

Children have a tendency to arrest as a result of respiratory difficulties rather than a primary cardiac dysfunction, and as a result they more commonly arrest into a non-shockable rhythm.

The resuscitation guidelines for children – complete with the fundamental differences in techniques – are summarized in Table 2.1.

## Other Situations

### Children with a Known Cardiac History

It is more likely that a defibrillator may be required for this group of patients. For that reason, if you are a lone rescuer, leave and phone for help as soon as you discover there is no breathing.

### Respiratory Arrest

An adequate pulse will have been discovered at the point of checking for circulation. Provide ventilations over 1 minute before assessing the circulation for a further 10 seconds. If a circulation remains present, continue breathing, stopping only for circulation checks every minute. If you are ventilating a child at the correct rate, you should achieve approximately 12–20 breaths per minute.

### Unconscious Breathing Children

It may be appropriate to consider using the recovery position (see pp. 462–463 in this section for technique). In infants roll them onto their side and support with rolled up bedding.

### Tracheostomy Patients

*See* p. 462 in adult section.

## Paediatric Choking

The same classifications exist as defined in the adult choking section, but techniques vary for removing a complete obstruction depending on the age/size of the child. An advantage in smaller children is that gravity can be used very effectively in a choking episode.

### Infants (under 1 year of age)

Support the infant's head with one of your hands along the bony part of their jaw, then turn them head down over your lap so their bottom is higher than their head, and they are face down. If the object hasn't already fallen out at this point deliver up to 5 back slaps. If these fail to work, continue to support the head and turn the child over, delivering up to 5 chest thrusts (in the same place as chest compressions but slower and with more force). Continue in cycles of 5 back slaps and 5 chest thrusts until the object comes out or help arrives. If they lose consciousness commence basic life support from the intial 5 ventilations (see Table 2.1).

### Child (above 1 year of age)

Use the adult techniques of 5 back slaps and 5 abdominal thrusts with less force than in adults. If physically possible, turning the child over your lap for the back slaps will be helpful for extra gravitational force. If the child collapses commence BLS at the point of attempting 5 ventilations (see Table 2.1).

Table 2.1    Paediatric resuscitation

| Infant (baby under 1 year of age) | | Child (1 year to puberty) |
|---|---|---|
| Approach and assess the the situation | **Safe approach** | Approach and assess the the situation |
| Shout at and gently stimulate the infant | **Assess for response** | Shout at and gently stimulate the child |
| Ensure an early 2222 call can be made by colleagues and essential equipment and assistance provided | **Shout for help/pull emergency buzzer** | Ensure an early 2222 call can be made by colleagues and essential equipment and assistance provided |
| Head tilt/chin lift into a neutral position | **Open the airway** | Head tilt/chin lift into a 'sniffing' position |
| Look listen and feel for breathing for up to 10 seconds | **Check breathing** | Look listen and feel for breathing for up to 10 seconds |
| Ideally use a paediatric pocket mask to deliver these. If performing mouth to mouth place your mouth over the mouth and nose of the infant | **Deliver 5 rescue breaths** | Ideally use a pocket mask. If performing mouth to mouth place your mouth over the mouth and occlude the nose |
| Look for signs of a circulation such as regular breathing, moving, swallowing or coughing. In addition, if you are a trained health care provider, check the brachial pulse. If the pulse is 60 or below with signs of poor perfusion, or is absent, commence chest compressions | **Assess for signs of a circulation for up to 10 seconds** | Look for signs of a circulation such as regular breathing, moving, swallowing or coughing. In addition, if you are a trained health care provider check the carotid pulse. If the pulse is 60 or below with signs of poor perfusion or is absent commence chest compressions |
| Place 2 fingers on the sternum 1 finger's breadth up from the xiphisternum. Aim to compress the chest by a third of its depth at a rate of 100 per minute | **Commence 15 chest compressions** | Place the heel of 1 hand (possible 2 handed technique in larger children) 1 finger up from the xiphisternum. Aim to compress the chest by a third of its depth at a rate of 100 per minute |

Table 2.1  Paediatric resuscitation—*cont'd*

| Infant (baby under 1 year of age) | | Child (1 year to puberty) |
|---|---|---|
| Continue in cycles of 2 breaths to 15 compressions | **Continue resuscitation** | Continue in cycles of 2 breaths to 15 compressions |
| This is more likely in the community where assistance is less readily available and lone working more possible | **Leave and phone for help after 1 minute of resuscitation if a lone rescuer. Dial 999 or 2222 depending on location** | This is more likely in the community where assistance is less readily available and lone working more possible |

BIBLIOGRAPHY

Resuscitation Council (UK) 2006 Advanced life support course provider manual, 5th edn. Resuscitation Council (UK), London
Resuscitation Council (UK) 2006 European Paediatric Life Support course provider manual, 2nd edn. Resuscitation Council (UK), London

ILLUSTRATION REFERENCES

Figures 1, 2 and 3:
Resuscitation Council (UK) 2006 Advanced life support course provider manual, 5th edn. Resuscitation Council (UK), London Figures 2.1, 2.2 and 2.3 are reproduced with kind permission of Michael Scott and the Resuscitation Council (UK)
Figure 2.4:
Resuscitation Services, Cambridge University Hospitals NHS Foundation Trust (Addenbrooke's Hospital) 2006

# Appendix

# Medicines and their Control
CHRIS EVANS

## Definitions

A medicinal product is: 'Any substance or combination of substances presented for treating or preventing disease in human beings or in animals. Any substance or combination of substances which may be administered to human beings or animals with a view to making medical diagnosis or to restoring, correcting, or modifying physiological functions in human beings or animals is likewise considered a medicinal product' (Council Directive 65/65/EEC).

### Medicines Management:

> The clinical, cost effective and safe use of medicines to ensure patients get the maximum benefit from the medicines they need, while at the same time minimising potential harm. (MHRA 2004)

*Use of the Word 'Registrant' Throughout this Appendix*
Where the word 'registrant' is used this refers to nurses, midwives and specialist community public health nurses who are registered on the Nursing and Midwifery Council Register.

The two Acts that control the manufacture, supply and use of medicines are the *Medicines Act 1968* and the *Misuse of Drugs Act 1971*.

## The Medicines Act 1968

This was the first comprehensive legislation on medicines in the United Kingdom. The combination of this primary legislation and the various statutory instruments (secondary legislation) on medicines produced since 1968 provides the legal framework for the manufacture, licensing, prescription, supply and administration of medicines.

Among recent statutory instruments of particular relevance to registered nurses and midwives is The Prescription Only Medicines (Human Use) Order 1997, SI No 1830. This consolidates all previous secondary legislation on prescription-only medicines and lists all of the medicines in this category. It also sets out who may prescribe them. The sections on exemptions are of particular relevance to midwives, including those in independent practice, and to nurses working in occupational health settings.

The *Medicines Act 1968* classifies medicines into the following categories:

**Prescription-only Medicines (POMs)**
These are medicines that may only be supplied or administered to a patient on the instruction of an appropriate practitioner. An appropriate practitioner is a doctor, dentist, supplementary prescriber or nurse or pharmacist independent prescriber. For more information on the appropriate use of medicines and the relevant legislation it is advisable to consult with the pharmacist.

**Pharmacy-only Medicines (P)**
These can be purchased from a registered primary care pharmacy, provided that the sale is supervised by the pharmacist.

**General Sale List Medicines (GSLs)**
These need neither a prescription nor the supervision of a pharmacist and can be obtained from retail outlets.

# The Misuse of Drugs Act 1971
The Misuse of Drugs Act (MDA) 1971 and its associated regulations provide the statutory framework for the control and regulation of Controlled Drugs. The primary purpose of the MDA is to prevent the misuse of controlled drugs. The MDA 1971 makes it unlawful to possess or supply a controlled drug unless an exception or exemption applies. A controlled drug is defined as any drug listed in Schedule 2 of the Act.

# Misuse of Drugs Regulations 2001 (MDR)

The use of controlled drugs in medicine is permitted by the Misuse of Drugs Regulations (MDR). The MDR classifies the drugs in five schedules according to the different levels of control required. Schedule 1 controlled drugs are subject to the highest level of control, whereas Schedule 5 controlled drugs are subject to a much lower level of control. For practical purposes, health care staff need to be aware of the current legislation.

As a registrant, you should be particularly familiar with the regulations concerning schedule 2 medicines such as morphine, diamorphine and pethidine, and schedule 3 drugs such as barbiturates.

Following the Shipman Inquiry, there has been legislative change and new governance arrangements for controlled drugs. These additional statutory measures for the management of controlled drugs are laid down in the Health Act 2006 and its associated regulations. This Act is primarily legislation and applies to the whole of the UK although the regulations may differ in each devolved administration. Registrants should be familiar with the DH guide *Safer management of controlled drugs 2006*.

If you are responsible for the storage or administration of controlled drugs (this will also include receipt, key holding and access, record keeping and stock checks), you should be aware of the content of the *Misuse of Drugs Regulations 2001* and the *Misuse of Drugs (Safe Custody) Regulations 1973* and the *NMC Standards for medicines management 2008*.

Queries are often raised in relation to prescriptions for schedule 2 medicines (controlled drugs).

Prescriptions for schedule 2 or 3 controlled drugs must comply with the following requirements:

- drug name
- route and dose
- name of patient and their address
- age of patient (if under 12 years)
- state (in words and figures) the total quantity of the drug to be supplied
- specify the dose to be taken and, in the case of a prescription containing a controlled drug which is a preparation, the form and, where appropriate, the strength of the preparation
- signature of the prescriber in their own handwriting.

In hospitals, requisitioning, receipt, storage and record keeping of controlled drugs is subject to tight control:

- They must be stored separately in a locked cupboard (which may be within a second outer cupboard) to which access is restricted. Cupboards must be locked when not in use and the lock must not be common to any other lock in the hospital.
- The nurse in charge of the ward is responsible for the CD key and should know its whereabouts at all times. Key holding may be delegated to other suitably trained members of staff but the legal responsibility rests with the nurse in charge.
- Supply from the pharmacy is made to a ward or department only on receipt of a written order signed by a responsible nurse.
- A record is kept of stock held and details of doses given. A special register is used for this and no other purpose, and it is usually the case that each entry is countersigned by two nurses. The records should be regularly checked by the nurse in charge and by a pharmacist, according to Trust policy.

If you have any queries in relation to the misuse of drugs, or if you are aware of illicit substances being in the possession of a patient, you must refer to and act on local policy and/or appropriate Department of Health guidance.

## Unlicensed medicines

An unlicensed medicine is the term used to refer to a medicine that has no marketing authorization. If an unlicensed medicine is administered to a patient, the manufacturer may not have liability for any harm that ensues. The person who prescribes and dispenses/supplies the medicine carries the liability. This may have implications for you in obtaining informed consent. A registrant may administer an unlicensed medicinal product with the patient's informed consent against a patient-specific direction but NOT against a patient group direction.

Medication which is licensed but used outside its licensed indications (commonly known as 'off-label') may be administered under a patient group direction only where such use is exceptional, justified by best practice, and the status of the product is clearly described. As a registrant you should be satisfied that you have sufficient information to administer a medicine prescribed 'off-label' safely and whenever possible that there is acceptable published evidence for the use of that product for the intended indication. In addition you should be satisfied that you have sufficient information to administer an unlicensed or 'off-label' medicine safely and, wherever possible, that there is acceptable evidence for the use of that medicine for the intended indication. Liability for prescribing an 'off-label' medicine sits with the prescriber and the dispenser/supplier.

The British National Formulary for children provides useful information for the administration of 'off-label' medication for children. More information on unlicensed and 'off-label' medicines can be found in the NMC publication *Standards of Proficiency for Nurse Midwife Prescribers 2006*.

## Abbreviations Used in Prescriptions

Abbreviations of Latin are being replaced by English versions, which are considered safer; however, the nurse may still meet the Latin abbreviations given in Table 3.1.

## NMC: Standards for Medicine Management 2008

*Guidelines for the administration of medicines* was first published by the former United Kingdom Central Council for Nursing, Midwifery and Health Visiting (UKCC) in October 2000. In April 2002, this revised

Table 3.1   Abbreviations and prescriptions

| Abbreviation | Latin | English |
|---|---|---|
| a.c. | ante cibum | before food |
| ad lib | ad libitum | to the desired amount |
| b.d. or b.i.d. | bis in die | twice a day |
| c. | cum | with |
| o.m. | omni mane | every morning |
| o.n. | omni nocte | every night |
| p.c. | post cibum | after food |
| p.r.n. | pro re nata | whenever necessary |
| q.d. | quaque die | every day |
| q.d.s. | quaque die sumendum | four times daily |
| q.i.d. | quarter in die | four times a day |
| q.q.h. | quarter quaque hora | every four hours |
| R | recipe | take |
| s.o.s. | si opus sit | if necessary |
| stat | statim | at once |
| t.d.s. | ter die sumendum | three times a day |
| t.i.d. | ter in die | three times a day |

edition was published by the new Nursing and Midwifery Council (NMC) and these were again revised in 2004.

*The Standards for medicines management 2008* replace the Guidelines for the administration of medicines 2004. The main body of the paper is reproduced in this appendix.

As the regulatory body for nursing and midwifery, the primary function of the NMC is public protection through professional standards. One of the most important ways of serving the public interest is through providing advice and guidance to registrants on professional issues. The new document includes standards that cover the process from prescribing, through to dispensing, storage, administration and disposal of medicines. It also incorporates guidance on controlled drugs and provides helpful links to a range of documents on medicines management.

As many changes have taken place in relation to medicines management and the way health care is developed in the United Kingdom, it has been necessary to review the advice previously given by the regulatory body on the administration of medicines.

> *The administration of medicines is an important aspect of the professional practice of persons whose names are on the Council's register. It is not solely a mechanistic task to be performed in strict compliance with the written prescription of a medical practitioner. It requires thought and the exercise of professional judgement ....*

Many government and other agencies are involved in medicines management, from manufacture, licensing, prescribing and dispensing, to administration. An extensive range of guidance on these issues is provided by the relevant bodies. Sources of information are listed in the references. One of the best sources of advice locally is usually your pharmacist.

As with all NMC guidance, this booklet is neither intended to be a rule book nor a manual. Nor is it intended to cover every single situation that you may encounter during your career. Instead, it sets out a series of standards that we hope will enable you to think through the issues and to apply your professional expertise and judgement in the best interests of your patients. It will also be necessary to develop and refer to additional local policies or protocols to suit local needs. Within the document, the word 'patient' is used for convenience to refer to a person receiving medication, irrespective of the environment in which they are residing.

# Standards for Practice of Administration of Medicines

As a registrant, you are accountable for your actions and omissions. In administering any medication, or assisting or overseeing any self-administration of medication, you must exercise your professional judgement and apply your knowledge and skill in the given situation.

Having initially checked the 'direction to supply or administer' that a medicinal product is appropriate for your patient you may then administer the medication.

As a registrant, in exercising your professional accountability in the best interests of your patients, you must:

- be certain of the identity of the patient to whom the medicine is to be administered
- check that the patient is not allergic to the medicine before administering it
- know the therapeutic uses of the medicine to be administered, its normal dosage, side effects, precautions and contra-indications
- be aware of the patient's care plan/pathway
- check that the prescription, or the label on medicine dispensed by a pharmacist, is clearly written and unambiguous
- have considered the dosage, method of administration, route and timing of the administration in the context of the condition of the patient and co-existing therapies
- check the expiry date of the medicine to be administered
- contact the prescriber or another authorized prescriber without delay where contra-indications to the prescribed medicine are discovered, where the patient develops a reaction to the medicine, or where assessment of the patient indicates that the medicine is no longer suitable
- make a clear, accurate and immediate record of all medicine administered, intentionally withheld or refused by the patient, ensuring that any written entries and the signature are clear and legible; it is also your responsibility to ensure that a record is made when delegating the task of administering medicine
- administer or withhold in the context of the patient's condition (e.g. digoxin not usually to be given if pulse below 60) and co-existing therapies (e.g. physiotherapy)
- where supervising a student nurse or midwife in the administration of medicines, clearly countersign the signature of the student.

Some drug administrations can require complex calculations to ensure that the correct volume or quantity of medication is administered. In these situations, it may be necessary for a second practitioner to check the calculation in order to minimize the risk of error. The use of calculators to determine the volume or quantity of medication should not act as a substitute for arithmetical knowledge and skill.

It is unacceptable to prepare substances for injection in advance of their immediate use or to administer medication drawn into a syringe or container by another practitioner when not in their presence. An exception to this is an already established infusion which has been instigated by another practitioner following the principles set out above, or medication prepared under the direction of a pharmacist from a central intravenous additive service and clearly labelled for that patient.

In an emergency, where you may be required to prepare substances for injection by a doctor, you should ensure that the person administering the drug has undertaken the appropriate checks as indicated above.

Instruction by telephone to a practitioner to administer a previously unprescribed substance is not acceptable. In exceptional circumstances, where the medication has been previously prescribed and the prescriber is unable to issue a new prescription, but where changes to the dose are considered necessary, the use of information technology (such as fax or e-mail) is the preferred method. This should be followed up by a new prescription confirming the changes within a given time period. The NMC suggests a maximum of 24 hours. In any event, the changes must have been authorized before the new dosage is administered.

Text messaging is an increasing possibility in the process of an order to administer a medicine. However, you must ensure there are protocols in place to ensure patient confidentiality and that local policies and procedures are in place to provide robust audit trail and clinical governance, in order to support such practice.

## Prescribing

Detailed guidance on prescribing is contained in the *British National Formulary* (BNF) and in *Medicines, Ethics and Practice: A Guide for Pharmacists*. Until 1992, prescribing was essentially restricted to doctors and dentists. Any qualified and registered independent prescriber may prescribe all Prescription-only Medicines for all medical conditions. In addition Nurse Independent Prescribers may also prescribe some controlled drugs. Supplementary prescribers may prescribe in accordance with a clinical management plan in a tripartite arrangement with a doctor or dentist, the patient and the supplementary prescriber.

## Prescribing by Nurses, Midwives and Specialist Community Public Health Nurses

The *Medicinal Products: Prescription by Nurses Act 1992* and subsequent amendments to the pharmaceutical services regulations allow nurses and midwives, who have recorded their qualification on the NMC register, to become nurse or midwife prescribers. There are two levels of nurse and midwife prescribers:

### Community Practitioner Nurse Prescribers

These are registrants who have successfully undertaken a programme of preparation to prescribe from the Community Practitioner Nurse Prescribers Formulary. They can prescribe the majority of dressings and appliances, and a limited range of Prescription-only Medicines. The Community Nurse Prescribers Formulary can be found on the *British National Formulary* website: www.bnf.org.

### Independent/Supplementary Nurse and Midwife Prescribers

These are nurses and midwives who are trained to make a diagnosis and prescribe the appropriate treatment (independent prescribing). They may also, in cases where a doctor has made an initial diagnosis, go on to prescribe or review the medication and change the drug, dosage, timing, frequency or route of administration of any mediation as appropriate as part of a clinical management plan (supplementary prescribing).

Nurse or Midwife Independent Prescribers can prescribe Prescription-only Medicines including some controlled drugs and all medication that can be supplied by a pharmacist or purchased over the counter. They must only prescribe drugs that are within their area of expertise and level of competence, and should only prescribe for children if they have the expertise and competence to do so.

Nurse, midwife and specialist community public health nurse prescribers must comply with current prescribing legislation and are accountable for their practice.

For Department of Health guidance go to www.dh.gov.uk and search: nurse independent prescribing.

## Patient Group Directions (PGDs)

Patient group directions (PGDs) are specific written instructions for the supply or administration of a licensed named medicine including vaccines to specific groups of patients who may not be individually identified before presenting for treatment. Guidance on the use of PGDs is contained within *Health Care Circular (HSC) 2000/026*.

Patient group directions are drawn up locally by senior doctors or, if appropriate, by dentists, pharmacists and other health professionals. They must be signed by a doctor or dentist and a senior pharmacist, both of whom should have been involved in developing the direction, and must be approved by the appropriate health care organization. The NMC would consider it good practice that a lead practitioner from the professional group using the PGD and senior manager where possible, are also involved and sign off a PGD.

## Dispensing

If, under exceptional circumstances, you are required to dispense, there is no legal barrier to this practice. However, this must be in the course of the business of a hospital and in accordance with a doctor's written instructions. In a dispensing doctor's practice, nurses may supply to patients under a particular doctor's care, when acting under the directions of a doctor from that practice.

Dispensing includes such activities as checking the validity of the prescription, the appropriateness of the medicine for an individual patient, assembly of the product, labelling in accordance with legal requirements, advising in its safe and effective use and providing information leaflets for the patient.

If you, as a registrant, are engaged in dispensing, this represents an extension to your professional practice. The patient has the legal right to expect that the dispensing will be carried out with the same reasonable skill and care that would be expected from a pharmacist.

## Aids to Support Concordance (compliance aids)

Registrants must assess the patient's suitability and understanding of how to use an appropriate compliance aid safely.

Before considering the use of compliance aids, you should explore with the patient other possible solutions, for example reminder charts, large print labels, non-child-proof tops. Self-administration from dispensed containers may not always be possible for some patients. If an aid to concordance is considered necessary, careful attention should be given to the assessment of the patient's suitability and understanding of how to use an appropriate aid safely. However, all patients will need to be regularly assessed for continued appropriateness of the aid. Ideally, any concordance aid, such as a monitored dose container or a daily/weekly dosing aid, should be dispensed, labelled and sealed by a pharmacist.

Where it is not possible to get a concordance aid filled by a pharmacist, you should ensure that you are able to account for its use. The patient has a right to expect that the same standard of skill and care will be applied by you in dispensing into a compliance aid as would be applied if the patient were receiving the medication from a pharmacist. This includes the same standard of labelling and record keeping. Compliance aids, which are able to be purchased by patients for their own use, are aids that are filled from containers of dispensed medicines. If you choose to repackage dispensed medicines into compliance aids, you should be aware that their use carries a risk of error. You should also be aware the properties of the drug might also change when re-packaged and so may not be covered by their product licence.

## Self-administration of Medicines

Access to professional support and advice is available in the *Standards for medicines management (standard 9: standards for practice of administration of medicines)*, published by the Nursing & Midwifery Council (NMC) in 2008. The NMC welcomes and supports the self-administration of medicines and the administration of medication by carers wherever it is appropriate. However, the essential safety, security and storage arrangements must be available and, where necessary, agreed procedures must be in place.

For the hospital patient approaching discharge, but who will continue on a prescribed medicines regime on the return home, there are obvious benefits in adjusting to the responsibility of self-administration while still having access to professional support. It is essential, however, that where self-administration is introduced, arrangements are in place for the safe and secure storage of the medication, access to which is limited to the specific patient.

Where self-administration of medicines is taking place, you should ensure that records are maintained appropriate to the environment in which the patient is being cared for.

It is also important that, if you are delegating this responsibility, you ensure that the patient or carer/care assistant is competent to carry out the task. This will require education, training and assessment of the patient or carer/care assistant and further support if necessary. The competence of the person to whom the task has been delegated should be reviewed periodically.

## Complementary and Alternative Therapies

Complementary and alternative therapies are increasingly used in the treatment of patients.

Registrants must have successfully undertaken training and be competent to practise the administration of complementary and alternative therapies (please refer to *The NMC Code of professional conduct: standards for conduct, performance and ethics*). You must have considered the appropriateness of the therapy to both the condition of the patient and any co-existing treatments. It is essential that the patient is aware of the therapy and gives informed consent.

Complementary and alternative therapies may interact with other types of medicinal products and laboratory tests. You need to ensure that your employer has accepted vicarious liability for any complementary/alternative therapy you may undertake or that you have indemnity insurance to cover your practice.

## Management of Adverse Events (Errors or Incidents) in the Administration of Medicines

It is important that an open culture exists in order to encourage the immediate reporting of errors or incidents in the administration of medicines.

If you make an error, you must take any action to prevent any potential harm to the patient and report as soon as possible the prescriber, your line manager or employer (according to local policy) and document your actions. Midwives should also inform their named supervisor of midwives. Registered nurses and midwives who have made an error, and who have been honest and open about it to their senior staff, appear sometimes to have been made the subject of local disciplinary action in a way that might discourage the reporting of incidents and, therefore, be potentially detrimental to patients and the maintenance of standards.

The NMC believes that all errors and incidents require a thorough and careful investigation at a local level, taking full account of the context and circumstances and the position of the practitioner involved. Such incidents require sensitive management and a comprehensive assessment of all the circumstances before a professional and managerial decision is reached on the appropriate way to proceed. If a practising midwife makes or identifies a drug error or incident, she should also inform her supervisor of midwives as soon as possible after the event.

The NMC supports the use of a thorough, open and multi-disciplinary approach to investigating adverse events, where improvements to local practice in the administration of medicines can be discussed, identified and disseminated.

When considering allegations of misconduct arising from errors in the administration of medicines, the NMC takes great care to distinguish between those cases where the error was the result of reckless or incompetent practice or was concealed, and those that resulted from other causes, such as serious pressure of work, and where there was immediate, honest disclosure in the patient's interest. The NMC recognizes the prerogative of managers to take local disciplinary action where it is considered to be necessary but urges that they also consider each incident in its particular context and similarly discriminate between the two categories described above.

## Reporting Adverse Reactions

As a registrant, if a patient experiences an adverse drug reaction to a medication you must take any action to remedy harm caused by the reaction. You must record this in the patient's notes, notify the prescriber (if you did not prescribe the drug) and notify via the Yellow Card Scheme immediately.

Yellow cards are found in the back of the British National Formulary and online on www.yellowcard.gov.uk.

# Information on New and Developing Pharmacy Services and Extended Roles of Pharmacists

## Repeat Dispensing Schemes

A repeat medication service is a service operated in co-operation with local prescribers, in which pharmacists will provide professional support to assist in the rational, safe, effective and economic use of medicines.

- The pharmacy must operate a patient medication record (PMR) system notified to the Information Commissioner, and ensure that an audit trail exists to identify each request and supply.
- The pharmacist must establish at the time of each request, which items the patient or carer considers are required and ensure that unnecessary supplies are not made. At this stage the pharmacist must also use his/her professional judgement to decide whether concordance or other problems encountered by the patient may require early reference to the prescriber.
- The pharmacist must not request a repeat prescription from the surgery before obtaining the patient or carer's consent. The pharmacist, may however, institute a patient reminder system.
- At the time of each request the pharmacist must establish which items the patient or their carer considers are required and ensure that unnecessary supplies are not made. At this stage pharmacists must also use their professional judgement to decide whether concordance or other problems encountered by the patient may require early reference to the prescriber.
- Records of all interventions should be kept in order to be able to deal with any queries that may arise and to advise the prescriber.

## The Supply of Emergency Hormonal Contraception as a Pharmacy Medicine

Pharmacists in personal control of a pharmacy must ensure that the following standards are observed in the supply of emergency hormonal contraception as a pharmacy medicine. As with all medicines, pharmacists must have sufficient knowledge of the product to enable them to make an informed decision when requests are made.

- Pharmacists must deal with the request personally and decide whether to supply the product or make a referral to an appropriate health care professional.
- Pharmacists must ensure that all necessary advice and information is provided to enable the patient to assess whether to use the product.

- Requests for emergency hormonal contraception must be handled sensitively with due regard being given to the patient's right of privacy.
- Only in exceptional circumstances should pharmacists supply the product to a person other than the patient.
- Pharmacists should whenever possible take reasonable measures to inform patients of regular methods of contraception, disease prevention and sources of help.

### Health Care Information and Advice

Pharmacists are encouraged to contribute to the promotion of healthy lifestyles. By increasing public awareness of health promotion issues and participating in disease prevention strategies pharmacists can work actively towards improving the nation's health.

The public and other health care professions are entitled to expect pharmacists and their staff to be able to provide up to date, accurate and reliable advice and information on a wide range of health care issues. Pharmacists and staff providing information and advice on health related issues must:

- have an adequate level of current knowledge and information about relevant subjects
- ensure that all advice is independent and not compromised by commercial considerations
- seek appropriate and sufficient information from the enquirer to enable them to provide informed advice
- continually review their knowledge and keep up to date regarding new products and new policies for health promotion
- be aware of local and major national and topical health promotion initiatives
- work in partnership with patients and other health care professionals in seeking to promote healthy lifestyles and respect patients' rights to be involved in decisions about their health.

### Diagnostic Testing and Health Screening

Pharmacists working in primary care are well placed to provide diagnostic testing and health screening services to the public, who would expect any such service to be safe and accurate. Services include: blood pressure/hypertension management, cholesterol testing, obesity management, anti-smoking guidance and pregnancy testing.

## Advisory Services to Nursing and Residential Homes

This service specification applies to any service intended to facilitate the safe, effective and appropriate usage of medicines, dressings and appliances, their storage, stock control or disposal, and the associated record keeping in nursing and residential homes and hospices. Pharmacists providing advisory services must ensure that:

- they have undertaken adequate training relevant to the services being provided
- they visit the home regularly by appointment; all staff visiting the home should carry identification
- they have contact, regularly and as frequently as needed with medical and nursing personnel responsible for the care and medical treatment of residents
- they undertake professional assessments to ensure appropriate usage of medicines in the home
- they assess and advise on procedures to ensure safe and accurate administration of medicines
- all necessary supplementary information, e.g. patient information leaflets, is available in the home
- they advise on the safe disposal of unwanted medicines supplied by the pharmacy and of other pharmaceutical and clinical waste, in compliance with legal requirements
- adequate records are maintained to enable them to deal with any queries that may arise and to enable audit of the service
- where they do not supply the medicines to the home they liaise with the pharmacy that does.

## Needle and Syringe Exchange Schemes

Needle and syringe exchange schemes involve the provision of clean syringes and needles and the collection of contaminated equipment used by substance and drug misusers.

- Pharmacists must be aware of local facilities for drug misusers and have established contacts with other health care professionals involved in the care of drug misusers.
- All staff who may be involved in the service must be instructed on procedures to be followed to minimize risks.
- Supplies of syringes and needles must be made by pharmacists or trained staff.

- Individuals must be encouraged to return used contaminated equipment in approved disposal containers, but a supply of clean equipment must not be refused if they omit to do so.
- Used equipment must be disposed of, preferably by the individual, into a properly designed sharps container available in the pharmacy.
- Suitable arrangements must be made for the disposal of full sharps containers.

REFERENCES/BIBLIOGRAPHY

Department of Health 2003 Mechanisms for Nurse and Pharmacist Prescribing and Supply of Medicines: Medicines Pharmacy and Industry Group. Department of Health, London

Great Britain (1972) Medicines Act 1968 (as amended). HMSO, London

Great Britain (1984) Misuse of Drugs Act 1971 (as amended). HMSO, London

Great Britain (2001) Misuse of Drugs Regulations 2001 SI No 3938. HMSO, London

National Prescribing Centre (NPC) 2004 A guide to good practice in the management of controlled drugs in primary care (England)

Nursing and Midwifery Midwives Rules and Standards 2004 NMC, London

Nurse Prescribers' Formulary 2008 British National Formulary, September 2008 BMA/RPS Publishing, London

Nursing & Midwifery Council 2008 Standards for medicines management. NMC, London

Royal Pharmaceutical Society of Great Britain 2005 The safe and secure handling of medicines: a team approach. A revision of the Duthie Report (1988). RPSGB, London

Royal Pharmaceutical Society of Great Britain. Medicines, Ethics and Practice: A guide for pharmacists – is published annually and is available from www.rpsgb.org.uk

FURTHER INFORMATION

Adverse reactions to drugs and yellow card scheme: www.yellowcard. gov.uk

The British National Formulary online: www.bnf.org/

Departments of Health's prescribing pages, including a list of the medicines that can be prescribed at: www.doh.gov.uk/ nurseprescribing

Drug safety update, a monthly newsletter from MHRA is available at: www.mhra.gov.uk/mhra/drugsafetyupdate

Information on controlled drugs: www.dh.gov.uk/controlleddrugs

Supplementary prescribing at: www.doh.gov.uk/supplementary-prescribing

Nurse Independent Prescribing and Non-medical Prescribing: www. dh.gov.uk/nonmedicalprescribing

Nurse and Midwifery Council: www.nmc-uk.org

Nurse Practitioner: www.nursepractitioner.org.uk

Nurse Prescriber: www.nurseprescribing.com

Patient Group Directions: www.pgd.nhs.uk

# Appendix

## The Legal and Professional Framework of Nursing

JONATHAN GREEN

### Accountability

Health care is regulated in a number of ways. The most important of these for nurses are:

- professional regulation
- Acts of Parliament
- civil law
- contracts of employment
- ethical standards.

The Nursing and Midwifery Council sets the minimum standard of accountability through the Code of Conduct. The latest version of the code was launched on 7 April 2008 (and can be found at www.nmc-uk.org and Appendix 5). The code interprets the boundaries set by Acts of Parliament which may set limits on nursing practice in areas such as prescribing or abortion. Where there is no Act of Parliament, the courts will interpret the law in the civil courts on health issues such as the right to refuse life-saving treatment, where there are problems regarding patients who appear to lack capacity to make judgments for themselves or cases where no agreement can be reached on what treatment is in a patient's best interests, and the code will reflect these judgments.

Contracts of employment set out the rights, responsibilities and expectations of the nurse in the context of his/her employment and may also require that protocols are followed by nursing staff. This is a fourth area of accountability, while a fifth area relates to the ethical scope and practice of nursing, from a professional and a personal perspective. Consent, for example, is an ethical principle.

## Law

The laws of the land bind nurses as citizens and professionals, comprising both criminal and civil law. Criminal law is generally contained in statutes (Acts of Parliament), violation of which may arise either from performing a prohibited action or omitting to perform a required act. A crime is a wrong punishable by the State. Successful prosecution by the Crown will result in a variety of penalties, from fines to imprisonment.

Table 4.1 lists the statutes which relate directly to the clinical and health care environment. They describe clearly what types of behaviour Parliament considers to be unacceptable, responding to the perceived demands of society in general.

## Professional Negligence

'Negligence' is a tort (or civil wrong), created by the courts, the definition of which has evolved over the years. In contrast to the criminal law, the law of tort regulates the behaviour (in terms of rights and duties) of one individual towards another.

Negligence is centred around the concept of a 'duty of care' or 'responsibility', owed by one individual/organization to another and the subsequent harm that can be caused to an individual if this duty or responsibility is broken. To establish liability in negligence, three key elements must be present, as follows:

- Did a duty of care exist?
- Was that duty breached?
- Was the subsequent harm caused by the breach?

A critical part of the test for negligence is to show that harm was caused directly by the negligent (or careless) act or omission of the nurse or health care provider, although it does not have to be the sole or main cause. If all the elements are present, the claimant will be financially compensated, the amount awarded being decided by the court, unless the parties to a claim can reach agreement between themselves.

| Table 4.1    Health law statutes | |
|---|---|
| **Statute** | **Year** |
| Offences against the Person Act | 1861 |
| Perjury Act | 1911 |
| Venereal Diseases Act | 1917 |
| Infant Life (Preservation) Act | 1929 |
| Children and Young Persons Act | 1933 |
| National Assistance Act | 1948 |
| Sexual Offences Act | 1956 |
| Human Tissue Act | 1961 |
| Suicide Act | 1961 |
| Abortion Act | 1967 |
| Medicines Act | 1968 |
| Family Law Reform Act | 1969 |
| Misuse of Drugs Act | 1971 |
| Congenital Disabilities (Civil Liability) Act | 1976 |
| National Health Service Act | 1977 |
| Unfair Contract Terms Act | 1977 |
| Vaccine Damage Payments Act | 1979 |
| Mental Health Act | 1983 |
| Medical Act | 1983 |
| Public Health (Control of Disease) Act | 1984 |
| Data Protection Act | 1984 |
| Enduring Powers of Attorney Act | 1985 |
| Prohibition of Female Circumcision Act | 1985 |
| Surrogacy Arrangements Act | 1985 |
| Family Law Reform Act | 1987 |
| Human Organ Transplant Act | 1989 |
| Children Act | 1989 |
| NHS and Community Care Act | 1990 |
| Human Fertilization and Embryology Act | 1990 |
| Medicinal Products: Prescription by Nurses Act | 1992 |
| Data Protection Act | 1998 |
| Health Act | 1999 |
| Care Standards Act | 2000 |
| Health and Social Care Act | 2001 |
| National Health Service Reform & Health Care Professions Act | 2002 |
| Health and Social Care (Community Health and Standards) Act | 2003 |
| Health Act | 2006 |
| National Health Service Act | 2006 |
| National Health Service (Wales) Act | 2006 |
| NHS Redress Act | 2006 |

Source: Kennedy & Grubb (1994), updated and Halsbury's Statutes

When a Court is making an assessment as to whether a patient has been the subject of negligent treatment, a Judge will make an assessment by comparison with two standards:

The nurse must deliver the standard of care expected from a reasonably competent nurse exercising that professional skill.

The nurse must act in accordance with practice accepted by a relevant body of responsible and skilled nursing opinion (see the decision in Bolam v Friern Hospital Management Committee (1957) and the comments of Lord Scarman in Sidaway v Governors of Bethlem Royal Hospital (1985).

If the practitioner has departed from either standard, then negligence can be inferred. It is essential to recognize here the importance of adherence to the Code of Professional Conduct and all local policies relating to the clinical environment because both will offer legal protection. The patient will not generally be able to prove professional negligence where the nurse has followed commonly accepted and up-to-date nursing clinical practice.

## Legal Issues Affecting Clinical Practice

An objective of this appendix is to present a concise guide to legal controls on commonly encountered nursing procedures and situations. In so doing, it is essential to bear in mind, firstly, any relevant statutes (see Table 4.1) and, secondly, the Code of Professional Conduct (see Appendix 5). Where there is no specific statute to cover any particular area, compliance with professional regulations and protocols from the employer will contribute to a defence in the face of any legal claims under civil law, specifically negligence.

## Consent

At the heart of the law on consent lies the fundamental principle that every person has a right to control what happens to his or her body. Consent issues generally arise in relation to patients giving consent for physical procedures.

This subject is covered by both criminal law (e.g. Offences against the Person Act 1861) and the judgments of the courts in civil cases (usually in cases involving the torts of battery and negligence). The basic rule is possibly best summed up in the case of Malette v Shulman (1990) where a Judge directed 'any intentional non-consensual touching which is harmful or offensive to a person's reasonable sense of dignity, is actionable'. Clearly securing consent, makes that interference lawful. To proceed without consent renders the nurse liable for a claim for assault (an attempt to apply force to another, such as to put him or her in fear of physical violence) or battery (the actual application of physical force). The physical force does not have to be substantial and damage does not have to be caused, but intent to carry out the non-consensual contact must be present.

As the major legal defence against assault and battery is consent, the verbal or written agreement of the patient must be sought before any physical treatment can be given. However, the presence of a signed consent form alone is not sufficient. It is a legal requirement that an effective consent must satisfy the following criteria to ensure that it is a true consent (Montgomery 2003):

- The procedure for which consent is sought must have been explained adequately to the patient. It may be negligent to withhold important information. What must be disclosed is an issue of clinical judgement, but must be sufficient to enable a patient to weigh up the risks and advantages of undergoing the procedure, and appreciate any alternative treatments
- The patient must be able to understand the choices he or she is required to make.
- Consent must then be given freely and voluntarily.
- Consent must not be obtained by duress or deceit.

The Department of Health sets out a patient's rights in relation to consent in its Health Circular HC(90)22 *A Guide to Consent for Examination or Treatment*. The Department has included within its Guidance specimen Consent Forms.

To take account of the nature of medical and nursing practice, three exceptions to the principles above relating to obtaining consent are recognized but practitioners should still proceed with caution.

Firstly, as outlined previously, an informal explanation and verbal agreement between patient and nurses are often sufficient to allow routine clinical care and treatment to be performed, e.g obtaining bloods or carrying out routine observations.

Secondly, the principle of 'necessity' will justify treatment of a patient where consent cannot be given, primarily in an emergency situation, perhaps where the patient is unconscious. As such, this exception permits life-saving treatment without a patient's consent. (See Re F (1990)) but should be applied in extreme situations only.

The treatment would have to satisfy the 'Bolam' test, being acceptable to a responsible and relevant body of professional opinion, and must go no further than is required to safeguard life. Further, the treatment will be unlawful if the patient had clearly communicated his or her objection to such treatment, before becoming 'incompetent'.

Thirdly, and similarly to the above, an 'implied consent' can be relied upon if there is sufficient certainty that the patient would have requested or acceded to the treatment had it been offered in more controlled circumstances. Again, this applies to emergency events where either an initiation of a new treatment or an extension of an existing one is needed. In such events, it is ethically correct to consider that the treatment should be of obvious benefit to the patient, that it would be unreasonable to withhold it, and that no express objection has previously been given.

Children who have reached the age of 16 years are able to consent to treatment in their own right. Children under 16 years of age can still legally give their own consent if they have sufficient intelligence and understanding of what is involved, and the consent is valid. The Guide to Consent for Examination or Treatment referred to above specifies that full notes should be kept of all interactions with the child, attempts made to persuade the child to involve their parents and if there is any doubt that the child does not have sufficient understanding, parental consent should be obtained (save in emergency situations).

Relatives and close friends are frequently involved in care and consultation about patients, although they cannot (save in accordance with the provisions of the Mental Capacity Act) legally give consent on behalf of the patient. This is governed by the legal rule that one adult does not have the authority to give consent for another adult.

## Confidentiality

In the course of their duties, nurses handle confidential information about patients. The control of such sensitive details is regulated by statute, specifically the Data Protection Act 1998, and also by the Code of Professional Conduct. Written information is accessible to an individual to whom the information refers, however, access to it can be restricted if certain exclusions specified in the Act apply. Information entered and stored on a computer is controlled by the Act (not just computer data but also written information).

Nurses are required to prioritize the protection of all confidential information and only to disclose it under specific conditions.

---

Box 4.1   Principles of holding personal data (Data Protection Act 1998)

1. Data are obtained fairly and lawfully
2. Data are held for one or more lawful purpose only (specified in the Data User's register entry—a legal requirement)
3. Data are used or disclosed only in accordance with the Data User's register entry
4. Data are adequate, relevant and not excessive for the purpose
5. Data are accurate and up to date
6. Data are not kept longer than necessary for a specific purpose
7. Data are made available to data subjects upon request
8. Data are properly protected against loss or disclosure

---

Box 4.1 lists the principles concerning the collection and storage of confidential patient data.

Breach of confidentiality can lead to three penalties. Firstly, failing to secure confidential information could lead to prosecution under the Data Protection Act 1998.

Secondly, the Nursing and Midwifery Council (NMC) has power to consider whether a charge of professional misconduct applies, risking removal from the register. The NMC Code expressly states that a Nurse must respect people's right to confidentiality, ensure people are informed about how and why information is shared by those who will be providing their care and finally, authorises disclosure of information if a Nurse believes someone may be at risk of harm.

Thirdly, a breach of confidentiality may constitue a breach of contract, leading to disciplinary action and possible dismissal.

Four clear exceptions to maintaining confidentiality are recognized, as follows:

1. Where the patient consents to disclosure.
2. Where the information is required to continue a patient's care.
3. Where the law (Act of Parliament) requires disclosure, e.g. accidents, firearm incidents, drug-related activities, reporting of notifiable diseases.
4. Where the public interest in disclosure is deemed of greater importance than the public interest in maintaining confidentiality, e.g. child abuse.

Nurses should abide strictly by the rules of confidentiality unless one of these exceptions clearly applies. The reason for disclosure should be well documented in a patient's records.

# Drug Administration

The responsibility of the nurse for storage and administration of medicines is discussed in Appendix 3.

# Safety

Nurses have a comprehensive responsibility for the safety of patients in their care under the NMC Code of Professional conduct – Nurses 'must have the knowledge and skills for safe and effective practice …' – and this duty is shared clinically with doctors and environmentally with employers.

Nurses are also legally bound by the civil 'duty of care' principle set out above, which formalizes in law the responsibility that nurses have to their patients. As stated above, breach of that duty may entitle the injured patient to make a claim of negligence.

In the general ward environment, safety is maintained by attention to three main areas. Firstly, by formal identification of the patient and the implementation of a system ensuring correct identification throughout the patient's treatment on the ward, which usually includes the use of non-removable identity bands for patients. The personal details recorded on the bands should be consistent with all documents. Secondly, the careful compilation of admission, inpatient and discharge charts and care planning documents should ensure that patient safety is not compromised. Thirdly, the full and conscientious dissemination of information between the patient and all members of the medical multidisciplinary team is essential. This also allows the patient to have an understanding of the plan of care.

Application of these safety principles will be enhanced in certain acute and specialist environments. In these areas, identification of the patient and the passing on of accurate and detailed information is critical. Nurses trained working in extended roles will of course be accountable for all of their actions in this respect. Nurses should also be aware of their own practical limitations, as encouraged in the Code of Professional Conduct (the Code expressly states that a nurse 'must recognize and work within the limits of [their] competence'). A nurse should not assume roles or undertake tasks that compromise their clinical ability and the patient's safety.

The responsibility for safety within the physical environment of care and the facilities is allocated to health care management and the health care provider although, under Health and Safety Regulations, all employees must act responsibly in relation to their own health and safety, and that of others. Within the ward, the relevant management team has specific responsibility for providing adequate basic safety measures, e.g. fire precautions or the control of hazardous substances.

Nurses are instructed in the Code of Professional Conduct to evaluate the safety of the environment and to take action if this is jeopardized. The Code states that a nurse must report any concerns in writing if problems in the environment of care are putting people at risk. Nursing staff are also required to be professionally aware of other factors affecting safety, particularly quality of care and availability of resources. This applies, for example, to potentially unsafe staffing levels, inappropriate skill mix of staff, or a combination of demanding patients and clinical conditions.

## Documentation

The range of documentation requiring nursing attention is often voluminous, wide-ranging and detailed. Occasionally, some of it is not directly related to nursing activities. As a result some documents will have a legal significance while others will not. The purpose of documentation is fourfold, as follows:

1. Legal or non-legal record-keeping.
2. Ease of administration.
3. Maintaining standards.
4. Ensuring continuity and safety.

Legal record-keeping infiltrates the nursing environment in several areas, e.g. administration of medicines, recording usage of controlled drugs, and contracts of employment between nurses and employing authorities. Nursing records can ultimately become legal documents; their main function being to evidence the care planned, treatment received and outcomes of a patient's stay. As a comprehensive record of the patient's visit, they form an important defence against allegations of misconduct or negligence. The time within which potential legal actions can be initiated (until a child reaches 21 years or 3 years from the date a victim became aware that he or she had been the victim of potentially negligent treatment) makes the necessity for accurate documentation clear and obvious.

A strong defence is much more likely from the basis of clear, precise documentation written at the time of the incident or treatment. The Code of Practise requires that a practitioner must complete records as soon as possible after an event has occurred and it also states that any records must include 'clear and accurate records of the discussions you have, the assessments you make, the treatment and medicines you give and how effective these have been'.

Of equivalent importance to patient records are documents affecting staff, visitors and members of the public that could subsequently acquire a legal significance, e.g. accident reporting forms. Employers are legally required to report accidents, injuries and dangerous incidents to the Health and Safety Executive, and are required to act under the Reporting of Injuries, Diseases and Dangerous Occurrences Regulations 1985 and the Occupiers Liability Act 1957 and 1984.

## Decisions Made by Patients

A potentially problematic area for health care providers arises where patients choose to make a decision contrary to the professional advice they have received. Having received a full description of proposed treatment, a patient may still exercise their right to refuse to undertake the recommended course of action. The individual patient has an absolute and inviolable right under civil law to decline treatment. Doctors and nurses must ensure that these decisions are recorded (along with details of the action taken/discussions leading to the patient's decision). The NMC Code declares that all nurses must 'be able to demonstrate that you have acted in someone's best interests if you have provided care in an emergency'. Only this will prevent a practitioner from leaving themself wide open to a possible negligence action if the outcome of declining treatment is unfavourable.

Secondly, patients may choose to discharge themselves from medical care against the advice of doctors and nurses. Patients cannot be legally detained (unless subject to various sections of the Mental Health Act 1983) and are free to leave at their will. A 'discharge against medical advice' form is valuable as a record of a discussion with a patient and as a place to note that the unplanned and unadvised discharge is the patient's choice. The form should be witnessed by the clinical staff involved, although the patient cannot be legally compelled to sign it.

## Patients' Property

Handling of a patient's property requires careful attention from nurses at all stages during a patient's hospitalization – from admission, while an inpatient, during any transfers between clinical areas, and on discharge.

The actions taken to safeguard property are to protect the patient from losing potentially valuable personal property in terms of sentimental as well as financial value. Failure to adequately protect patient's property during an admission may also lead a practitioner facing an allegation of theft.

If conscious and capable, the patient will automatically retain control of any property although some facilities for the safekeeping of valuables may be offered by a health care provider. In many cases the patient will be required to sign a disclaimer form, which will absolve the hospital during the patient's stay. If any items are retained for security by the hospital a patient will receive a signed receipt.

If the patient is unable to take responsibility for personal property while unconscious, confused or mentally incapacitated, the nurse will be required to take charge of it. The nurse's legal responsibility in this position assumes that of an 'involuntary bailee' (technically a person to whom goods are entrusted with no intention of transferring ownership). This demands that the nurse takes care of the property and exercises the same degree of care as the patient would have done had he or she been able.

The well-established procedure of written documentation, double-checking and witnessing with another member of staff, as well as signing in duplicate for property received, is vital to ensure protection against accusations of theft by a patient. Accurate and careful description of all property held is prudent. On discharge all property must be returned to the patient (and on death to authorized receivers). In both cases, this must be in exchange for a signed receipt.

The penalties for inadequate or careless control of a patient's property are individual prosecutions for theft or activation of the health authority's liability for negligence. A nurse may also potentially face dismissal and be reported to the NMC for professional misconduct.

References

Kennedy I, Grubb A 1994 Medical law. Butterworth, London

Montgomery J 2003 Health care law. Oxford University Press, Oxford

Further Reading

Brazier M 1992 Medicine, patients and the law. Penguin, London

Dyer C (ed) 1992 Doctors, patients and the law. Blackwell, Oxford

McCall Smith A, Mason J K 1994 Law and medical ethics. Butterworth, London

Rumbold G 1999 Ethics in nursing practice, 3rd edn. Baillière Tindall, London

Tingle J, Cribb A (eds) 2002 Nursing law and ethics. Blackwell Scientific, Oxford

Tschudin V 1991 Ethics in nursing. Heinemann, London

# Appendix

# Standards of Conduct, Performance and Ethics

## Section 1
### Nursing and Midwifery Council (NMC)

The Code: Standards of conduct, performance and ethics for nurses and midwives.

The people in your care must be able to trust you with their health and wellbeing.

To justify that trust, you must:

- make the care of people your first concern, treating them as individuals and respecting their dignity.
- work with others to protect and promote the health and wellbeing of those in your care, their families and carers, and the wider community.
- provide a high standard of practice and care at all times.
- be open and honest, act with integrity and uphold the reputation of your profession.

As a professional, you are personally accountable for actions and omissions in your practice and must always be able to justify your decisions.

You must always act lawfully, whether those laws relate to your professional practice or personal life.

Failure to comply with this Code may bring your fitness to practise into question and endanger your registration.

This Code should be considered together with the Nursing and Midwifery Council's rules, standards, guidance and advice available from www.nmc-uk.org.

# Make the Care of People Your First Concern, Treating Them as Individuals and Respecting Their Dignity

### Treat People as Individuals
- You must treat people as individuals and respect their dignity.
- You must not discriminate in any way against those in your care.
- You must treat people kindly and considerately.
- You must act as an advocate for those in your care, helping them to access relevant health and social care, information and support.

### Respect People's Confidentiality
- You must respect people's right to confidentiality.
- You must ensure people are informed about how and why information is shared by those who will be providing their care.
- You must disclose information if you believe someone may be at risk of harm, in line with the law of the country in which you are practising.

### Collaborate with Those in Your Care
- You must listen to the people in your care and respond to their concerns and preferences.
- You must support people in caring for themselves to improve and maintain their health.
- You must recognize and respect the contribution that people make to their own care and wellbeing.
- You must make arrangements to meet people's language and communication needs.
- You must share with people, in a way they can understand, the information they want or need to know about their health.

### Ensure You Gain Consent
- You must ensure that you gain consent before you begin any treatment or care.
- You must respect and support people's rights to accept or decline treatment and care.
- You must uphold people's rights to be fully involved in decisions about their care.
- You must be aware of the legislation regarding mental capacity, ensuring that people who lack capacity remain at the centre of decision making and are fully safeguarded.

- You must be able to demonstrate that you have acted in someone's best interests if you have provided care in an emergency.

### Maintain Clear Professional Boundaries

- You must refuse any gifts, favours or hospitality that might be interpreted as an attempt to gain preferential treatment.
- You must not ask for or accept loans from anyone in your care or anyone close to them.
- You must establish and actively maintain clear sexual boundaries at all times with people in your care, their families and carers.

## Work with Others to Protect and Promote the Health and Wellbeing of Those in Your Care, their Families and Carers, and the Wider Community

### Share Information with Your Colleagues

- You must keep your colleagues informed when you are sharing the care of others.
- You must work with colleagues to monitor the quality of your work and maintain the safety of those in your care.
- You must facilitate students and others to develop their competence.

### Work Effectively as Part of a Team

- You must work cooperatively within teams and respect the skills, expertise and contributions of your colleagues.
- You must be willing to share your skills and experience for the benefit of your colleagues.
- You must consult and take advice from colleagues when appropriate.
- You must treat your colleagues fairly and without discrimination.
- You must make a referral to another practitioner when it is in the best interests of someone in your care.

### Delegate Effectively

- You must establish that anyone you delegate to is able to carry out your instructions.
- You must confirm that the outcome of any delegated task meets required standards.
- You must make sure that everyone you are responsible for is supervised and supported.

**Manage Risk**

- You must act without delay if you believe that you, a colleague or anyone else may be putting someone at risk.
- You must inform someone in authority if you experience problems that prevent you working within this Code or other nationally agreed standards.
- You must report your concerns in writing if problems in the environment of care are putting people at risk.

# Provide a High Standard of Practice and Care at All Times

### Use the Best Available Evidence

- You must deliver care based on the best available evidence or best practice.
- You must ensure any advice you give is evidence based if you are suggesting health care products or services.
- You must ensure that the use of complementary or alternative therapies is safe and in the best interests of those in your care.

### Keep Your Skills and Knowledge Up To Date

- You must have the knowledge and skills for safe and effective practice when working without direct supervision.
- You must recognize and work within the limits of your competence.
- You must keep your knowledge and skills up to date throughout your working life.
- You must take part in appropriate learning and practice activities that maintain and develop your competence and performance.

### Keep Clear and Accurate Records

- You must keep clear and accurate records of the discussions you have, the assessments you make, the treatment and medicines you give and how effective these have been.
- You must complete records as soon as possible after an event has occurred.
- You must not tamper with original records in any way.
- You must ensure any entries you make in someone's paper records are clearly and legibly signed, dated and timed.

- You must ensure any entries you make in someone's electronic records are clearly attributable to you.
- You must ensure all records are kept confidentially and securely.

# Be Open and Honest, Act with Integrity and Uphold the Reputation of Your Profession

## Act with Integrity
- You must demonstrate a personal and professional commitment to equality and diversity.
- You must adhere to the laws of the country in which you are practising.
- You must inform the NMC if you have been cautioned, charged or found guilty of a criminal offence.
- You must inform any employers you work for if your fitness to practise is impaired or is called into question.

## Deal with Problems
- You must give a constructive and honest response to anyone who complains about the care they have received.
- You must not allow someone's complaint to prejudice the care you provide for them.
- You must act immediately to put matters right if someone in your care has suffered harm for any reason.
- You must explain fully and promptly to the person affected what has happened and the likely effects.
- You must cooperate with internal and external investigations.

## Be Impartial
- You must not abuse your privileged position for your own ends.
- You must ensure that your professional judgement is not influenced by any commercial considerations.

## Uphold the Reputation of Your Profession
- You must not use your professional status to promote causes that are not related to health.
- You must cooperate with the media only when you can confidently protect the confidential information and dignity of those in your care.
- You must uphold the reputation of your profession at all times.

# Information About Indemnity Insurance

The NMC recommends that a registered nurse, midwife or specialist community public health nurse, in advising, treating and caring for patients/clients, has professional indemnity insurance. This is in the interests of clients, patients and registrants in the event of claims of professional negligence.

Whilst employers have vicarious liability for the negligent acts and/or omissions of their employees, such cover does not normally extend to activities undertaken outside the registrant's employment. Independent practice would not be covered by vicarious liability. It is the individual registrant's responsibility to establish their insurance status and take appropriate action.

In situations where an employer does not have vicarious liability, the NMC recommends that registrants obtain adequate professional indemnity insurance. If unable to secure professional indemnity insurance, a registrant will need to demonstrate that all their clients/patients are fully informed of this fact and the implications this might have in the event of a claim for professional negligence.

**Contact:**
Nursing & Midwifery Council
23 Portland Place
London W1B 1PZ
020 7333 9333
advice@nmc-uk.org
www.nmc-uk.org
*This Code was approved by the NMC's Council on 6 December 2007 for implementation on 1 May 2008.*

# Section 2
# Health Professions Council (HPC)
### Standards of Conduct, Performance and Ethics

The Independent body currently responsible for the regulation of thirteen health professions: art therapists, biomedical scientists, chirpodists/podiatrists, clinical scientists, dieticians, occupational therapists, operating department practitioners, prosthetists & orthotists, radiographers, speech and language therapists.

As a registered member you are must continue to meet the standards set for your profession as a demonstration of your fitness to practice.

The standards of conduct, performance and ethics you must keep to state:

1. You must act in the best interests of service users.
2. You must respect the confidentiality of service users.
3. You must keep high standards of personal conduct.
4. You must provide (to us and any other relevant regulators) any important information about your conduct and competence.
5. You must keep your professional knowledge and skills up to date.
6. You must act within the limits of your knowledge, skills and experience and, if necessary, refer the matter to another practitioner.
7. You must communicate properly and effectively with service users and other practitioners.
8. You must effectively supervise tasks that you have asked other people to carry out.
9. You must get informed consent to give treatment (except in an emergency).
10. You must keep accurate records.
11. You must deal fairly and safely with the risks of infection.
12. You must limit your work or stop practising if your performance or judgement is affected by your health.
13. You must behave with honesty and integrity and make sure that your behaviour does not damage the public's confidence in you or your profession.
14. You must make sure that any advertising you do is accurate.

This document sets out the standards of conduct, performance and ethics we expect from the health professionals we register. The standards also apply to people who are applying to become registered.

### 1. You Must Act in the Best Interests of Service Users

You are personally responsible for making sure that you promote and protect the best interests of your service users. You must respect and take account of these factors when providing care or a service, and must not abuse the relationship you have with a service user. You must not allow your views about a service user's sex, age, colour, race, disability, sexuality, social or economic status, lifestyle, culture, religion or beliefs to affect the way you treat them or the professional advice you give. You must treat service users with respect and dignity. If you are providing care, you must work in partnership with your service users and involve them in their care as appropriate.

You must not do anything, or allow someone else to do anything, that you have good reason to believe will put the health or safety of a service user in danger. This includes both your own actions and those of other people. You should take appropriate action to protect the rights of children and vulnerable adults if you believe they are at risk, including following national and local policies.

You are responsible for your professional conduct, any care or advice you provide, and any failure to act. You are responsible for the appropriateness of your decision to delegate a task. You must be able to justify your decisions if asked to.

You must protect service users if you believe that any situation puts them in danger. This includes the conduct, performance or health of a colleague. The safety of service users must come before any personal or professional loyalties at all times. As soon as you become aware of a situation that puts a service user in danger, you should discuss the matter with a senior colleague or another appropriate person.

## 2. You Must Respect the Confidentiality of Service Users

You must treat information about service users as confidential and use it only for the purposes they have provided it for. You must not knowingly release any personal or confidential information to anyone who is not entitled to it, and you should check that people who ask for information are entitled to it.

You must only use information about a service user:

- to continue to care for that person; or
- for purposes where that person has given you specific permission to use the information.

You must also keep to the conditions of any relevant data protection laws and always follow best practice for handling confidential information. Best practice is likely to change over time, and you must stay up to date.

## 3. You Must Keep High Standards of Personal Conduct

You must keep high standards of personal conduct, as well as professional conduct. You should be aware that poor conduct outside of your professional life may still affect someone's confidence in you and your profession.

**4. You Must Provide (to Us and Any Other Relevant Regulators) Any Important Information About Your Conduct and Competence**

You must tell us (and any other relevant regulators) if you have important information about your conduct or competence, or about other registrants and health professionals you work with. In particular, you must let us know straight away if you are:

- convicted of a criminal offence, receive a conditional discharge for an offence, or if you accept a police caution;
- disciplined by any organization responsible for regulating or licensing a health care or social care profession; or
- suspended or placed under a practice restriction by an employer or similar organization because of concerns about your conduct or competence.

You should co-operate with any investigation or formal inquiry into your professional conduct, the conduct of any other health care provider or the treatment of a service user, where appropriate. If anyone asks for relevant information in connection with your conduct or competence, and they are entitled to it, you should provide the information.

We can take action against you if you are convicted of a criminal offence or have accepted a police caution. We will always consider each case individually to decide whether we need to take any action to protect the public.

However, we will consider rejecting an application for registration, or removing you from the Register if you are already registered, if you are convicted of a criminal offence or accept a police caution that involves one of the following types of behaviour.

- Violence.
- Abuse.
- Sexual misconduct.
- Supplying drugs illegally.
- Child pornography.
- Offences involving dishonesty.
- Offences for which you received a prison sentence.

This is not a full list. We will always look at any convictions or cautions we find out about, and we have arrangements in place to be told about convictions and cautions involving registrants.

## 5. You Must Keep Your Professional Knowledge and Skills Up To Date

You must make sure that your knowledge, skills and performance are of a good quality, up to date, and relevant to your scope of practice.

You must be capable of meeting the standards of proficiency that apply to your scope of practice. We recognize that your scope of practice may change over time.

We acknowledge that our registrants work in a range of different settings, including education, research and clinical practice. You need to make sure that whatever your area of practice, you are capable of practising safely and effectively.

Our standards for continuing professional development link your learning and development to your continued registration. You also need to meet these standards.

## 6. You Must Act Within the Limits of Your Knowledge, Skills and Experience and, If Necessary, Refer the Matter to Another Practitioner

You must keep within your scope of practice. This means that you should only practise in the areas in which you have appropriate education, training and experience. We recognize that your scope of practice may change over time.

When accepting a service user, you have a duty of care. This includes the duty to refer them for further treatment if it becomes clear that the task is beyond your own scope of practice. If you refer a service user to another practitioner, you must make sure that the referral is appropriate and that the service user understands why you are making the referral.

In most circumstances, a person is entitled to be referred to another practitioner for a second opinion. In these cases, you must accept the request and make the referral as soon as you can.

If you accept a referral from another practitioner, you must make sure that you fully understand the request. You should only provide the treatment if you believe that this is appropriate. If this is not the case, you must discuss the referral with the practitioner who made the referral, and also the service user, before you begin any treatment or provide any advice.

## 7. You Must Communicate Properly and Effectively With Service Users and Other Practitioners.

You must take all reasonable steps to make sure that you can communicate properly and effectively with service users. You must communicate appropriately, co-operate, and share your knowledge and expertise with other practitioners, for the benefit of service users.

## 8. You Must Effectively Supervise Tasks You have Asked Other People to Carry Out

People who consult you or receive treatment or services from you are entitled to assume that a person with appropriate knowledge and skills will carry out their treatment or provide services. Whenever you give tasks to another person to carry out on your behalf, you must be sure that they have the knowledge, skills and experience to carry out the tasks safely and effectively. You must not ask them to do work which is outside their scope of practice.

You must always continue to give appropriate supervision to whoever you ask to carry out a task. You will still be responsible for the appropriateness of the decision to delegate. If someone tells you that they are unwilling to carry out a task because they do not think they are capable of doing so safely and effectively, you must not force them to carry out the task anyway. If their refusal raises a disciplinary or training issue, you must deal with that separately, but you should not put the safety of the service user in danger.

## 9. You Must Get Informed Consent to Give Treatment (Except in an Emergency)

You must explain to the service user the treatment you are planning on carrying out, the risks involved and any other possible treatments. You must make sure that you get their informed consent to any treatment you do carry out. You must make a record of the person's decisions for treatment and pass this on to other members of the health care or social care team involved in their care. In emergencies, you may not be able to explain treatment, get consent or pass on information to other members of the health care or social care team. However, you should still try to do all of these things as far as you can.

A person who is capable of giving their consent has the right to refuse treatment. You must respect this right. You must also make sure that they are fully aware of the risks of refusing treatment, particularly if you think that there is a significant or immediate risk to their life.

You must keep to your employers' procedures on consent and be aware of any guidance issued by the appropriate authority in the country you practise in.

## 10. You Must Keep Accurate Records

Making and keeping records is an essential part of care and you must keep records for everyone you treat or who asks for your advice or services. You must complete all records promptly. If you are using paper-based records, they must be clearly written and easy to read, and you should write, sign and date all entries.

You have a duty to make sure, as far as possible, that records completed by students under your supervision are clearly written, accurate and appropriate.

Whenever you review records, you should update them and include a record of any arrangements you have made for the continuing care of the service user.

You must protect information in records from being lost, damaged, accessed by someone without appropriate authority, or tampered with. If you update a record, you must not delete information that was previously there, or make that information difficult to read. Instead, you must mark it in some way (for example, by drawing a line through the old information).

## 11. You Must Deal Fairly and Safely With the Risks of Infection

You must not refuse to treat someone just because they have an infection. Also, you must keep to the rules of confidentiality when dealing with people who have infections. For some infections, such as sexually transmitted infections, these rules may be more restrictive than the rules of confidentiality for people in other circumstances. We discussed confidentiality in more detail earlier in this document.

You must take appropriate precautions to protect your service users and yourself from infection. In particular, you should protect your service users from infecting one another. You must take precautions against the risk that you will infect someone else.

This is especially important if you suspect or know that you have an infection that could harm other people. If you believe or know that you may have this kind of infection, you must get medical advice and act on it. This may include the need for you to stop practising altogether, or to change your practice in some way in the best interests of protecting your service users.

## 12. You Must Limit Your Work or Stop Practising if Your Performance or Judgement is Affected by Your Health.

You have a duty to take action if your physical or mental health could be harming your fitness to practise. You should get advice from a consultant in occupational health or another suitably qualified medical practitioner and act on it. This advice should consider whether, and in what ways, you should change your practice, including stopping practising if this is necessary.

### 13. You Must Behave With Honesty and Integrity and Make Sure that Your Behaviour Does Not Damage the Public's Confidence in You or Your Profession.

You must justify the trust that other people place in you by acting with honesty and integrity at all times. You must not get involved in any behaviour or activity which is likely to damage the public's confidence in you or your profession.

### 14. You Must Make Sure that Any Advertising You Do is Accurate

Any advertising you do in relation to your professional activities must be accurate. Advertisements must not be misleading, false, unfair or exaggerated. In particular, you should not claim your personal skills, equipment or facilities are better than anyone else's, unless you can prove this is true.

If you are involved in advertising or promoting any product or service, you must make sure that you use your knowledge, skills and experience in an accurate and responsible way. You must not make or support unjustifiable statements relating to particular products. Any potential financial reward should not play a part in the advice or recommendations of products and services you give.

*These standards apply from 1 July 2008*

**Appendix 6**

# Useful Addresses
### Compiled by Sandra Horn

**Action for Sick Children**
National Children's Bureau
36 Jacksons Edge Road
Disley
Stockport
SK12 2JL
Tel. 01663 763 004
E-mail enquiries@actionforsickchildren.org
Web http://www.actionforsickchildren.org

**Action on Smoking and Health**
First Floor
144-145 Shoreditch High Street
London
E1 6JE
Tel. 0207 739 5902
E-mail enquiries@ash.org.uk
Web http://www.ash.org.uk

**Age Concern England**
Astral House
1268 London Road
London
SW16 4ER
Tel. 0800 00 99 66
E-mail ace@ace.org.uk
Web http://www.ageconcern.org.uk

**Alcohol Concern**
64 Leman Street
London
E1 8EU
Tel. 0207 264 0510
E-mail contact@alcoholconcern.org.uk
Web http://www.alcoholconcern.org.uk

**Alcoholics Anonymous**
PO Box 1
10 Toft Green
York
YO1 7ND
Tel. 01904 644026
See web page for e-mail
Web http://www.alcoholics-anonymous.org.uk

**Alzheimer's Society**
Devon House
58 St Katharine'sWay
London
E1W 1JX
Tel. 0207 423 3500
E-mail info@alzheimers.org.uk
Web http://www.alzheimers.org.uk

**Arthritis Research Campaign (ARC)**
Copeman House
St Mary's Court
St Mary's Gate
Chesterfield
Derbyshire
S41 7TD
Tel. 0870 850 5000
E-mail info@arc.org.uk
Web http://www.arc.org.uk

**Association for Improvements in the Maternity Services (AIMS)**
5 Ann's Court
Grove Road
Surbiton
Surrey
KT6 4BE
Tel. 0870 765 1453
E-mail chair@aims.org.uk
Web http://www.aims.org.uk

**Association for Perioperative Practice**
Daisy Ayris House
6 Grove Park Court
Harrogate
North Yorkshire
HG1 4DP
Tel. 01423 508079
E-mail hq@afpp.org.uk
Web http://www.afpp.org.uk

**Association of British Paediatric Nurses (ABPN)**
34 Primrose Hill Green
Swillington
Leeds
LS26 8XP
Tel. 0113 232 0234
E-mail j.a.pettitt@leeds.ac.uk
Web http://abpn.org.uk

**Association of Radical Midwives**
Sarah Montagu
16 Wytham Street
Oxford
OX1 4SU
Tel: 01865 2481597
E-mail sarahmontagu@gmail.com
Web http://www.radmid.demon.co.uk

**BackCare**
16 Elmtree Road
Teddington
Middlesex
TW11 8ST
Tel. 0208 977 5474
E-mail info@backcare.org.uk
Web http://www.backpain.org

**Breast Cancer Care**
5–13 Great Suffolk Street
London
SE1 0NS
Tel. 0845 092 0800
E-mail info@breastcancercare.org.uk
Web http://www.breastcancercare.org.uk

**British Colostomy Association**
15 Station Road
Reading
Berkshire
RG1 1LG
Tel. 0118 939 1537
E-mail sue@bcass.org.uk
Web http://www.colostomyassociation.org.uk

**British Deaf Association**
10th Floor
Coventry Point
Market Way
Coventry
CV1 1EA
Tel. 02476 550936
E-mail midlands@bda.org.uk
Web http://www.bda.org.uk

**British Dietetic Association**
5th Floor Charles House
148/9 Great Charles Street Queensway
Birmingham
B3 3HT
Tel. 0121 200 8080
E-mail info@bda.uk.com
Web http://www.bda.uk.com

**British Geriatric Society**
Marjory Warren House
31 St John's Square
London
EC1M 4DN
Tel. 0207 608 1369
E-mail generalinformation@bgs.org.uk
Web http://www.bgs.org.uk

**British Heart Foundation**
14 Fitzhardinge Street
London
W1H 6DH
Tel. 0207 935 0185
E-mail internet@bhf.org.uk
Web http://www.bhf.org.uk

**British Nutrition Foundation**
High Holborn House
52–54 High Holborn
London
WC1V 6RQ
Tel. 0207 404 6504
E-mail postbox@nutrition.org.uk
Web http://www.nutrition.org.uk

**British Pregnancy Advisory Service**
20 Timothys Bridge Road
Stratford Enterprise Park
Stratford-upon-Avon
Warwickshire
CV37 9BF
Tel. 0845 365 5050
E-mail info@bpas.org
Web http://www.bpas.org

**British Red Cross Society**
Bradbury House
Central Park
Ohio Avenue
Salford
M50 2GT
Tel. 0844 871 8000
E-mail firstaidtraining@redcross.org.uk
Web http://www.redcrossfirstaidtraining.co.uk

**British Renal Society**
26 Oriental Road
Woking
Surrey
GU22 7AW
Tel. 01483 764114/724472
E-mail brs@britishrenal.org
Web http://www.britishrenal.org

**Care Quality Commission CQC National Correspondence**
PO Box 1258
Newcastle upon Tyne
NE99 5AU
E-mail enquiries@cqc.org.uk
Web http://www.cqc.org.uk

**Carers National Association**
20 Great Dover Street
London
SE1 4LX
Tel. 0207 378 4999
E-mail info@carersuk.org
Web http://www.carersuk.org

**ChildLine**
Studd Street
London
N1 0QW
Tel. 0207 239 1000
Helpline 0800 1111
Web http://www.childline.org.uk

**Coeliac UK**
Suites A-D Octagon Court
High Wycombe
Buckinghamshire
HP11 2HS
Tel. 01494 437278
E-mail contact@coeliac.co.uk
Web http://www.coeliac.org.uk

**Commission for Racial Equality**
St Dunstans House
201-211 Borough High Street
London
SE1 1GZ
Tel. 0207 939 0000
E-mail info@cre.gov.uk
Web http://www.webmentorlibrary.com

**Community Practitioners' and Health Visitors' Association**
33-37 Moreland Street
London
EC1V 8HA
Tel. 0207 505 3000
E-mail InfoCPHVA@amicustheunion.org
Web http://www.rdfunding.org.uk

**Council of Deans and Heads of UK University Faculties for Nursing, Midwifery and Health Visiting**
Woburn House
20 Tavistock Square
London
WC1H 9HD
Tel. 0207 419 5520
E-mail Janice.Durbridge@chms.ac.uk
Web http://www.councilofdeans.org.uk

**Council for Healthcare Regulatory Excellence**
11 Strand
London
WC2N 5HR
Tel. 0207 389 8030
E-mail info@chre.org.uk
Web http://www.chre.org.uk

**Cruse Bereavement Care**
PO Box 800
Richmond
Surrey
TW9 1RG
Tel. 020 8939 9530
E-mail helpline@cruse.org.uk
Web http://www.crusebereavmentcare.org.uk

**Department of Health**
Richmond House
79 Whitehall
SW1A 2NS
Tel. 0207 210 4850
E-mail dhmail@dh.gsi.gov.uk
Web http://www.dh.gov.uk

**Diabetes UK**
10 Parkway
London
NW1 7AA
Tel. 0207 424 1000
E-mail info@diabetes.org.uk
Web http://www.diabetes.org.uk

**Disabled Living Foundation**
380–384 Harrow Road
London
W9 2HU
Tel. 0845 130 9177
E-mail advice@dlf.org.uk
Web http://www.dlf.org.uk

**Epilepsy Action**
New Anstey House
Gate Way Drive
Yeadon
Leeds
LS19 7XY
Tel. 0113 210 8800
E-mail helpline@epilepsy.org.uk
Web http://www.epilepsy.org.uk

**Epilepsy Bereaved**
PO Box 112
Wantage
Oxfordshire
OX12 8XT
Tel. 01235 772850
E-mail info@epilepsybereaved.org.uk
Web http://www.sudep.org

**Equality and Human Rights Commisssion**
(formerly Equal Opportunities Commission, Commission for Racial
Equality and Disability Rights Commission)
3 More London
Riverside
Tooley Street
London
SE1 2RG
Tel. 020 3117 0235
E-mail info@equalityhumanrights.com
Web http://www.equalityhumanrights.com

**Family Planning Association (FPA)**
50 Featherstone Street
London
EC1Y 8QU
Tel. 0207 608 5240
See web page for email
Web http://www.fpa.org.uk

**Foresight Preconception Head Office**
178 Hawthorn Road
West Bognor
West Sussex
PO21 2UY
Tel. 01243 868001
See web page for email
Web http://www.foresight-preconception.org.uk

**Gamblers Anonymous**
PO Box 88
London
SW10 0EU
Tel. 08700 50 88 80
E-mail info@gamblersanonymous.org.uk
Web http://www.gamblersanonymous.org.uk

**General Medical Council**
Regents Place
350 Euston Road
London
NW1 3JN
Tel. 0845 357 8001
E-mail gmc@gmc-uk.org
Web http://www.gmc-uk.org

**Haemophilia Society**
1st Floor Petersham House
57A Hatton Garden
London
EC1N 8JG
Tel. 020 7831 1020
E-mail info@haemophilia.org.uk
Web http://www.haemophilia.org.uk

**Health and Safety Executive**
Rose Court
2 Southwark Bridge
London
SE1 9HS
Tel. 0845 345 0055
E-mail hse.infoline@natbrit.com
Web http://www.hse.gov.uk

**Health Professions Council**
Park House
184 Kennington Park Road
London
SE11 4BU
Tel. 0207 582 0866
E-mail info@hpc-uk.org
Web http://www.hpc-uk.org

**Help the Aged**
207–221 Pentonville Road
London
N1 9UZ
Tel. 0207 278 1114
E-mail info@helptheaged.org.uk
Web http://www.helptheaged.org.uk

**Hospice Information Service**
St Christopher's Hospice
51–59 Lawrie Park Road
Sydenham
London
SE26 6DZ
Tel. 020 8768 4500
E-mail info@stchristophers.org.uk
Web http://www.stchristophers.org.uk

**Ileostomy and Internal Pouch Support Group**
Peverill House
1–5 Mill Road
Ballyclare
County Antrim
BT39 9DR
Tel. 0289 334 4043
E-mail info@iasupport.org
Web http://www.iasupport.org

**Institute for Complementary Medicine**
PO Box 194
London
SE16 1QZ
Tel. 0207 231 5855
E-mail info@icnm.org.uk
Web http://www.i-c-m.org.uk

**International Confederation of Midwives**
Laan van Meerdervoort 70
2517AN
The Hague
The Netherlands
Tel. +31 70 3060520
E-mail info@internationalmidwives.org
Web http://www.internationalmidwives.org

**International Council of Nurses**
3 Place Jean Marteau
1201 Geneva
Switzerland
Tel. +41 22 908 01 00
E-mail icn@icn.ch
Web http://www.icn.ch

**International Office Royal College of Nursing**
20 Cavendish Square
London
W1G 0RN
Tel. 0207 647 3597
E-mail international.office@rcn.org.uk
Web http://www.rcn.org.uk

**Invalids at Home**
Bamford Cottage
South Hill Avenue
Harrow
Middlesex
HA1 3PA
Tel. 0208 864 3818
No e-mail or web page

**King's Fund**
11–13 Cavendish Square
London
W1G 0AN
Tel. 0207 307 2400
E-mail Libweb@kingsfund.org.uk
Web http://www.kingsfund.org.uk

**Leukaemia Society (UK)**
PO Box 6831
London
N22 8XG
Tel. 0208 374 4821
E-mail info@leukaemiasociety.org.uk
Web http://www.leukaemiasociety.org

**Macmillan Cancer Support**
(includes CancerBACUP and Cancerlink)
89 Albert Embankment
London
SE1 7UQ
Tel. 0207 840 7840
E-mail contactus@macmillan.org.uk
Web http://www.macmillan.org.uk

**Marie Curie Cancer Care**
89 Albert Embankment
London
SE1 7TP
Tel. 0207 599 7777
E-mail info@mariecurie.org.uk
Web http://www.mariecurie.org.uk

**MedicAlert**
1 Bridge Wharf
156 Caledonian Road
London
N1 9UU
Tel. 0207 833 3034
E-mail info@medicalert.org.uk
Web http://www.medicalert.org.uk

**Medicines and Healthcare Products Regulatory Agency**
10-2 Market Towers
1 Nine Elms Lane
London
SW8 5NQ
Tel. 0207 084 2000
E-mail info@mhra.gsi.gov.uk
Web http://www.mhra.gov.uk

**MIND**
15–19 Broadway
London
E15 4BQ
Tel. 020 8519 2122
E-mail contact@mind.org.uk
Web http://www.mind.org.uk

**Multiple Sclerosis Society**
372 Edgware Road
London
NW2 6ND
Tel. 0208 438 0700
E-mail pothen@mssociety.org.uk
Web http://www.mssociety.org.uk

**Narcotics Anonymous**
202 City Road
London
EC1V 2PH
Tel. 0207 251 4007
E-mail nahelpline@ukna.org
Web http://www.ukna.org

**National Asthma Campaign**
Summit House
70 Wilson Street
London
EC2A 2DB
Tel. 020 7786 4900
E-mail info@asthma.org.uk
Web http://www.asthma.org.uk

**National Childbirth Trust**
Alexandra House
Oldham Terrace
London
W3 6NH
Tel. 0300 33 00 770
E-mail enquiries@nct.org.uk
Web http://www.nct.org.uk

**National Council for One Parent Families**
255 Kentish Town Road
London
NW5 2LX
Tel. 0207 428 5400
E-mail info@oneparentfamilies.org.uk
Web http://www.oneparentfamilies.org.uk

**National Health Service (NHS) in Wales**
Second Floor
Cathays Park
Cardiff
CF10 3NQ
E-mail hplibrary@wales.gsi.gov.uk
Web http://wales.gov.uk

**National Institute for Health and Clinical Excellence (NICE)**
Mid City Place
71 High Holborn
London
WC1V 6NA
Tel. 0845 003 7780
E-mail nice@nice.org.uk
Web http://www.nice.org.uk

**National Kidney Federation**
The Point
Coach Road
Shireoaks
Worksop
S81 8BW
Tel. 01909 544999
E-mail nkf@kidney.org.uk
Web http://www.kidney.org.uk

**National Patient Safety Agency**
4–8 Maple Street
London
WIT 5HD
Tel. 0207 927 9500
E-mail enquiries@npsa.nhs.uk
Web http://www.npsa.nhs.uk

**National Society for Epilepsy**
Chesham Lane
Chalfont St Peter
Buckinghamshire
SL9 0RJ
Tel. 01494 601300
See web page for e-mail
Web http://www.epilepsynse.org.uk

**National Society for the Prevention of Cruelty to Children**
Weston House
42 Curtain Road
London
EC2A 3NH
Tel. 0207 825 2500
E-mail help@nspcc.org.uk
Web http://www.nspcc.org.uk

**Neonatal Nurses Association**
PO Box 8708
Nottingham
NG2 9BJ
Tel. 07974 416919
E-mail nnaoffice@nna.org.uk
Web http://www.nna.org.uk

**The NHS Confederation**
29 Bressenden Place
London
SW1E 5DD
Tel. 0207 074 3200
E-mail enquiries@nhsconfed.org
Web http://www.nhsconfed.org

**NHS Education for Scotland**
Thistle House
91 Haymarket Terrace
Edinburgh
EH12 5HE
Tel. 0131 313 8000
E-mail enquiries@nes.scot.nhs.uk
Web http://www.nes.scot.nhs.uk

**Northern Ireland Practice and Education Council
for Nursing and Midwifery**
Centre House
79 Chichester Street
Belfast
BT1 4JE
Tel. 0289 023 8152
E-mail enquiries@nipec.n-i.nhs.uk
Web http://www.nipec.n-i.nhs.uk

**Nursing and Midwifery Council**
23 Portland Place
London
W1B 1PZ
Tel. 0207 637 7181
E-mail advice@nmc-uk.org
Web http://www.nmc-uk.org

**Parkinson's Disease Society**
215 Vauxhall Bridge Road
London
SW1V 1EJ
Tel. 0207 931 8080
E-mail enquiries@parkinsons.org.uk
Web http://www.parkinsons.org.uk

**Parliamentary and Health Service Ombudsman**
Millbank Tower
Millbank
London
SW1P 4QP
Tel. 0207 217 4000
E-mail phso.enquiries@ombudsman.org.uk
Web http://www.ombudsman.org.uk

**Qualification and Curriculum Authority**
83 Picadilly
London
W1J 8QA
Tel. 0207 509 5555
E-mail info@qca.org.uk
Web http://www.qca.org.uk

**Rethink**
89 Albert Embankment
London
SE1 7TP
Tel. 0845 456 0455
E-mail info@rethink.org
Web http://www.rethink.org

**Royal Association for the Deaf**
18 Westside Centre
London Road
Stanway
Colchester
Essex
CO3 8PH
Tel. 0845 688 2525
E-mail info@royaldeaf.org.uk
Web http://www.royaldeaf.org.uk

**Royal Association for Disability and Rehabilitation**
12 City Forum
250 City Road
London
EC1V 8AE
Tel. 0207 250 3222
E-mail radar@radar.org.uk
Web http://www.radar.org.uk

**Royal College of Midwives (RCM)**
15 Mansfield Street
London
W1G 9NH
Tel. 0207 312 3535
E-mail info@rcm.org.uk
Web http://www.rcm.org.uk

**RCM UK Board for England**
2nd Floor
King's House
King Street
Leeds
LS1 2HH
Tel. 0113 244 4310
E-mail carol.windmill@rcm.org.uk
Web http://www.rcm.org.uk

**RCM UK Board for Northern Ireland**
58 Howard Street
Belfast
BT1 6PJ
Tel. 0289 024 1531
E-mail breedagh.hughes@rcm.org.uk
Web http://www.rcm.org.uk

**RCM Board for Scotland**
37 Frederick Street
Edinburgh
EH2 1EP
Tel. 0131 225 1633
E-mail sharon.allison@rcm.org.uk
Web http://www.rcm.org.uk

**RCM UK Board for Wales**
4 Cathedral Road
Cardiff
CF11 9LJ
Tel. 0292 022 8111
E-mail helen.rogers@rcm.org.uk
Web http://www.rcm.org.uk

**Royal College of Nursing (RCN)**
20 Cavendish Square
London
W1G 0RN
Tel. 0207 409 3333
E-mail london.region@rcn.org.uk
Web http://www.rcn.org.uk

**RCN Northern Ireland**
17 Windsor Avenue
Belfast
BT9 6EE
Tel. 028 90 384 600
E-mail ni.board@rcn.org.uk
Web http://www.rcn.org.uk

**RCN Scotland**
42 South Oswald Road
Edinburgh
EH9 2HH
Tel. 0131 662 1010
E-mail scottish.board@rcn.org.uk
Web http://www.rcn.org.uk

**RCN Wales**
Ty Maeth
King George V Drive East
Cardiff
CF14 4XF
Tel. 0292 075 1373
E-mail welsh.board@rcn.org.uk
Web http://www.rcn.org.uk

**Royal Commonwealth Society**
25 Northumberland Avenue
London
WC2N 5AP
Tel. 0207 930 6733
E-mail info@rcsint.org
Web http://www.rcsint.org

**Royal National Institute of Blind People**
105 Judd Street
London
WC1H 9NE
Tel. 0207 388 1266
E-mail helpline@rnib.org.uk
Web http://www.rnib.org.uk

**Royal National Institute for the Deaf**
19–23 Featherstone Street
London
EC1Y 8SL
Tel. 0808 808 0123
E-mail informationline@rnid.org.uk
Web http://www.rnid.org.uk

**Royal National Pension Fund for Nurses (part of Liverpool Victoria Friendly Society Limited)**
County Gates
Bournemouth
BH1 2NF
Tel. 01202 292333
See web page for e-mail
Web http://www.lv.com/rnpfn

**Royal Society for the Prevention of Accidents**
Edgbaston Park
353 Bristol Road
Edgbaston
Birmingham
B5 7ST
Tel. 0121 248 2000
E-mail help@rospa.com
Web http://www.rospa.com

**Royal Society for Public Health**
(formerly Royal Institute of Public Health and Royal Society
of Health)
3rd Floor Market Towers
1 Nine Elms Lane
London
SW8 5NQ
Tel. 0203 177 1600
E-mail info@rsph.org.uk
Web http://www.rsph.org.uk

**Royal Society of Medicine**
1 Wimpole Street
London
W1G 0AE
Tel. 0207 290 2900
See web page for e-mail
Web http://www.rsm.ac.uk

**St John Ambulance**
27 St John's Lane
London
EC1M 4BU
Tel. 020 7324 4000
See web page for e-mail
Web http://www.sja.org.uk

**Samaritans**
The Upper Mill
Kingston Road
Ewell
Surrey
KT17 2AF
Tel. 0208 394 8300
E-mail admin@samaritans.org
Web http://www.samaritans.org

**Sargent Cancer Care for Children**
Griffin House
161 Hammersmith Road
London
W6 8SG
Tel. 020 8752 2800
E-mail helpline@clicsargent.org.uk
Web http://www.clicsargent.org.uk

**SCOPE**
6 Market Road
London
N7 9PW
Tel. 0808 800 3333
E-mail response@scope.org.uk
Web http://www.scope.org.uk

**Scottish Government Health Directorates**
St Andrew's House
Regent Road
Edinburgh
EH1 3DG
Tel. 0131 556 8400
E-mail ceu@scotland.gov.uk
Web http://www.sehd.scot.nhs.uk

**Sickle Cell Society**
54 Station Road
Harlesden
London
NW10 4UA
Tel. 0208 961 7755
E-mail info@sicklecellsociety.org
Web http://www.sicklecellsociety.org

**Society and College of Radiographers**
207 Providence Square
Mill Street
London
SE1 2EW
Tel. 0207 740 7200
E-mail info@sor.org
Web http://www.sor.org

**Standing Conference on Drug Abuse**
Waterbridge House
32–36 Lomax Street
SE1 0EE
Tel. 0207 928 9500
E-mail info@24dr.com
Web http://www.24dr.com

**Stillbirth and Neonatal Death Society (SANDS)**
28 Portland Place
London
W1B 1LY
Tel. 0207 436 5881
E-mail helpline@uk-sands.org
Web http://www.uk-sands.org

**Sue Ryder Foundation**
2nd Floor
114–118 Southampton Row
London
WC1B 5AA
Tel. 020 7400 0440
See web page for e-mail
Web http://www.suerydercare.org

**Terence Higgins Trust**
314–320 Gray's Inn Road
London
WC1X 8DP
Tel. 020 7812 1601
E-mail info@tht.org.uk
Web http://www.tht.org.uk

**Twins and Multiple Birth Association**
2 The Willows
Gardner Road
Guildford
Surrey
GU1 4PG
Tel. 01483 302 483
E-mail enquiries@tamba.org.uk
Web http://www.tamba.org.uk

**UNISON**
1 Mabledon Place
London
WC1H 9AJ
Tel. 0845 355 0845
E-mail out@unison.co.uk
Web http://www.unison.org.uk

**Vegan Society**
Donald Watson House
21 Hylton Street
Hockley
Birmingham
B18 6HJ
Tel. 0121 523 1730
E-mail info@vegansociety.com
Web http://www.vegansociety.com

**Women's Health Concern**
4–6 Eton Place
Marlow
Buckinghamshire
SL7 2QA
Tel. 01628 478473
E-mail pshervington@womens-health-concern.org
Web http://www.womens-health-concern.org

**Women's Royal Voluntary Services (WRVS)**
Garden House
Milton Hill
Steventon
Abingdon
Oxfordshire
OX13 6AD
Tel. 01235 861166
E-mail enquiries@wrvs.org.uk
Web http://www.wrvs.org.uk

**World Health Organization**
Avenue Appia 20
1211 Geneva 27
Switzerland
Tel. +41 22 791 21 11
E-mail info@who.int
Web http://www.who.int

# Degrees, Diplomas and Organizations: Abbreviations in Nursing and Health Care

| AA | Alcoholics Anonymous |
| AC | Aromatherapy Council |
| ACPI | Audit Commission Performance Indicator |
| AHP | Allied Health Professional |
| APEL | Accreditation of Prior Experiential Learning |
| APEX | Association of Professional, Executive, Clerical and Computer Staff |
| ASC | Action for Sick Children |
| ASH | Action on Smoking and Health |
| BA | Bachelor of Arts |
| BACUP | British Association of Cancer United Patients |
| BDA | British Dental Association |
| BDSc | Bachelor of Dental Science |
| BEd | Bachelor of Education |
| BMAS | British Medical Acupuncture Society |
| BPOS | British Psychosocial Oncology Society |
| BRA | British Reflexology Association |
| BRC | British Red Cross |
| BSc | Bachelor of Science |
| BSMDH | British Society of Medical and Dental Hypnosis |
| CATS | Credit Accumulation Transfer Scheme |
| CCETSW | Central Council for Educational Training in Social Work |
| CDC | Center(s) for Disease Control and Prevention |

| CDNA | Community and District Nursing Association |
| CEMACH | Confidential Enquiry into Maternal And Child Health |
| CHAI | Commission for Healthcare Audit and Inspections |
| CI NAHL | Cumulative Index to Nursing and Allied Health Literature |
| CNF | Commonwealth Nurses Federation |
| COSHH | Control of Substances Hazardous to Health |
| CPHVA | Community Practitioners' and Health Visitors' Association |
| CRB | Criminal Records Bureau |
| CPR | Child Protection Register |
| CRHP | Council for the Regulation of Healthcare Professionals |
| CSM | Committee on Safety of Medicines |
| CSP | Chartered Society of Physiotherapy |
| DCH | Diploma in Child Health |
| DH | Department of Health |
| DipEd | Diploma in Education |
| DipHE | Diploma of Higher Education |
| DipN | Diploma in Nursing |
| DipNE | Diploma in Nursing Education |
| DPH | Department of Public Health |
| DPHHP | Department for Public Health and Health Professions (Wales) |
| DPhil | Doctor of Philosophy |
| DPM | Diploma in Psychological Medicine |
| DSc | Doctor of Science |
| DTM&H | Diploma in Tropical Medicine and Hygiene |
| ERASMUS | European Region Action Scheme for the Mobility of University Students |
| EWTD | European Working Time Directive |
| FCSP | Fellow of the Chartered Society of Physiotherapy |
| FPA | Family Planning Association |
| FRCN | Fellow of the Royal College of Nursing |
| FRSH | Fellow of the Royal Society of Health |
| FSA | Food Standards Agency |
| GMC | General Medical Council |
| GNVQ | General National Vocational Qualification |
| HDA | Health Development Agency |
| HFEA | Human Fertilization and Embryology Authority |
| HPW | Health Professions Wales |
| HV | Health Visitor |

| ICN | International Council of Nurses |
| IHF | International Hospital Federation |
| MA | Master of Arts |
| MAOT | Member of the Association of Occupational Therapists |
| MBA | Master of Business Administration |
| MCSP | Member of the Chartered Society of Physiotherapists |
| MHAC | Mental Health Act Commission |
| MHRA | Medicines and Healthcare Products Regulatory Agency |
| MIND | National Association for Mental Health |
| MPhil | Master of Philosophy |
| MRC | Medical Research Council |
| MRSH | Member of the Royal Society for the Promotion of Health |
| MRSHom | Member of the Royal Society of Homeopaths |
| MSc | Master of Science |
| MSoR | Member of the Society of Radiographers (Radiography) |
| MSR(T) | Member of the Society of Radiographers (Radiotherapy) |
| NAMH | National Association for Mental Health |
| NAO | National Audit Office |
| NATN | National Association of Theatre Nurses |
| NCEPOD | National Confidential Enquiry into Perioperative Deaths |
| NeLH | National Electronic Library for Health |
| NES | NHS Education for Scotland |
| NHS | National Health Service |
| NICE | National Institute for Clinical Excellence |
| NINR | National Index of Nursing Research |
| NIPEC | Northern Ireland Practice and Education Council |
| NMC | Nursing and Midwifery Council |
| NNEB | National Nursery Examination Board |
| NPSA | National Patient Safety Agency |
| NSF | National Service Frameworks |
| NVQ | National Vocational Qualification |
| ODA | Operating Department Assistant |
| OHE | Office of Health Economics |
| OT | Occupational Therapist |
| PCG | Primary Care Group |

| PCT | Primary Care Trust |
| PhD | Doctor of Philosophy |
| PHLS | Public Health Laboratory Service |
| PMRAFNS | Princess Mary's Royal Air Force Nursing Service |
| PPA | Prescription Pricing Authority |
| QARANC | Queen Alexandra's Royal Army Nursing Corps |
| QARNNS | Queen Alexandra's Royal Naval Nursing Service |
| QNI | Queen's Nursing Institute |
| RADAR | Royal Association for Disability and Rehabilitation |
| RCM | Royal College of Midwives |
| RCN | Royal College of Nursing |
| RGN | Registered General Nurse |
| RM | Registered Midwife |
| RMN | Registered Mental Nurse |
| RN | Registered Nurse |
| RNIB | Royal National Institute for the Blind |
| RNMH | Registered Nurse for the Mental Health |
| RSCN | Registered Sick Children's Nurse |
| SGHD | Scottish Government Health Directorates |
| StAAA | St Andrew's Ambulance Association |
| SJA | St John Ambulance |
| SHA | Strategic Health Authority |
| SMAC | Standing Medical Advisory Committee |
| SNMAC | Standing Nursing and Midwifery Advisory Committee |
| SNOMED | Systematized Nomenclature of Human Medicine |
| SSD | Social Services Department |
| SSI | Social Services Inspectorate |
| VSO | Voluntary Service Overseas |
| WHO | World Health Organization |
| WRVS | Women's Royal Voluntary Service |

# Units of Measurement and Tables of Normal Values

### Metric Measures, Units and SI Symbols

| Name | SI unit | Symbol |
|------|---------|--------|
| Length | metre | M |
| Mass | kilogram | kg |
| Amount of substance | mole | mol |
| Pressure | pascal | Pa |
| Energy | joule | J |

### Decimal Multiples and Submultiples of the Units are Formed by the Use of Standard Prefixes

| Multiple | Prefix | Symbol | Submultiple | Prefix | Symbol |
|----------|--------|--------|-------------|--------|--------|
| $10^6$ | mega | M | $10^{-1}$ | deci | d |
| $10^3$ | kilo | k | $10^{-2}$ | centi | c |
| $10^2$ | hecto | h | $10^{-3}$ | milli | m |
| $10^1$ | deca | da | $10^{-6}$ | micro | $\mu$ |
| | | | $10^{-9}$ | nano | n |
| | | | $10^{-12}$ | pico | p |
| | | | $10^{-15}$ | femto | f |

### Conversion Table for kPa $\leftrightarrow$ mmHg (e.g. for capillary pressures)

| | |
|---|---|
| 1 mmHg | = 0.13 kPa |
| 1 kPa | = 7.5 mmHg |
| 35 mmHg | = 4.7 kPa |
| 25 mmHg | = 3.3 kPa |
| 15 mmHg | = 2.0 kPa |
| 10 mmHg | = 1.3 kPa |

## Hydrogen Ion Concentration (pH)

Neutral = 7          Acid = 0 to 7          Alkaline = 7 to 14

| Normal pH of some body fluids | |
| --- | --- |
| Blood | 7.35 to 7.45 |
| Saliva | 5.4 to 7.5 |
| Gastric juice | 1.5 to 3.5 |
| Bile | 6.0 to 8.5 |
| Urine | 4.5 to 8.0 |

## Some Normal Plasma Levels in Adults

| Calcium | 2.12 to 2.62 mmol/l | (8.5 to 10.5 mg/100 ml) |
| --- | --- | --- |
| Chloride | 97 to 106 mmol/l | (97 to 106 mEq/l) |
| Cholesterol | 3.6 to 6.7 mmol/l | (140 to 260 mg/100 ml) |
| Glucose | 3.5 to 8 mmol/l | (63 to 144 mg/100 ml) |
| Fasting glucose | 3.6 to 5.8 mmol/l | (65 to 105 mg/100 ml) |
| Potassium | 3.3 to 4.7 mmol/l | (3.3 to 4.7 mEq/l) |
| Sodium | 135 to 143 mmol/l | (135 to 143 mEq/l) |
| Urea | 2.5 to 6.6 mmol/l | (15 to 44 mg/100 ml) |

## Arterial Blood Gases

| $Pao_2$ | 12 to 15 kPa | (90 to 110 mmHg) |
| --- | --- | --- |
| $Paco_2$ | 4.5 to 6.1 kPa | (34 to 46 mmHg) |
| Bicarbonate | 21 to 27.5 mmol/l | |
| $H^+$ ions | 36 to 44 nmol/l | (7.35 to 7.45 pH units) |

## Blood Pressure

Normal adult 120/80 mmHg

| Hypertension, i.e. above 'normal' maximum for age | |
| --- | --- |
| 20 years | 140/90 mmHg |
| 50 years | 160/95 mmHg |
| 75 years | 170/105 mmHg |

## Heart Rate

| At rest | 60 to 80/min |
| --- | --- |
| Sinus bradycardia | < 60/min |
| Sinus tachycardia | > 100/min |

## Respiration Rate

At rest 15 to 18/min

| | |
|---|---|
| Tidal volume | 500 ml |
| Dead space | 150 ml |
| Alveolar ventilation | 15 (500–150) = 5.21 l/min |

## Blood Count

| | | | |
|---|---|---|---|
| Leukocytes | $4 \times 10^9$/l | to | $11 \times 10^9$/l |
| Neutrophils | $2.1 \times 10^9$/l | to | $7.2 \times 10^9$/l |
| Eosinophils | $0.04 \times 10^9$/l | to | $0.44 \times 10^9$/l |
| Basophils | $0.015 \times 10^9$/l | to | $0.2 \times 10^9$/l |
| Monocytes | $0.2 \times 10^9$/l | to | $0.8 \times 10^9$/l |
| Lymphocytes | $1.5 \times 10^9$/l | to | $4.0 \times 10^9$/l |
| Erythrocytes | | | |
| Female | $3.8 \times 10^{12}$/l | to | $5 \times 10^{12}$/l |
| Male | $4.5 \times 10^{12}$/l | to | $6.5 \times 10^{12}$/l |
| Thrombocytes | $150 \times 10^9$/l | to | $440 \times 10^9$/l |

## Diet

1 kilocalorie (kcal) = 4.182 kilojoules (kJ)

1 kilojoule = 0.24 kilocalories

| Energy source | Energy released | Recommended proportion in diet |
|---|---|---|
| Carbohydrate | 1 g = 17 kJ = 4 kcal | 55–75% |
| Protein | 1 g = 17 kJ = 4 kcal | 10–15% |
| Fat | 1 g = 38 kJ = 9 kcal | 15–30% |

## Urine

| | |
|---|---|
| Specific gravity | 1.020 to 1.030 |
| Volume excreted | 1000 to 1500 ml/day |

Glucose is normally absent, but appears in urine when blood glucose levels exceed 9 mmol/l

## Body Temperatures

| | |
|---|---|
| Normal | 36.8°C (98.4°F): axillary |
| Hypothermia | 32°C (89.6°F): axillary |
| | 35°C (95°F): core temperature |

**Cerebrospinal Fluid Pressure**
Lying on the side 50 to 180 mmHg

**Intraocular Pressure**
1.3 to 2.6 kPa (10 to 20 mmHg)

Unless otherwise stated, reference ranges apply to adults; values in children may be different.

# Immunization and Vaccinations

Newborn babies have some temporary immunity to infections as a result of the passive transfer of maternal antibodies to the unborn infant in the last trimester of pregnancy. However, the duration of this protection varies as some antibodies to certain infections are more long-lasting than others.

As an example, a mother's antibodies to measles usually protect her baby against the disease for 6–12 months, but those against whooping cough and Hib only last a few weeks. This is why the immunization programme starts at 2 months of age (see Table 9.1). Every effort should be made to ensure that all children are immunized, even if they are older than the recommended age range; no opportunity to immunize should be missed. **If any course of immunization is interrupted, it should be resumed and completed as soon as possible. There is no need to start any course of immunization again.**

It is important that premature infants have their immunizations at the appropriate chronological age, according to the schedule. There is no evidence that premature infants are at increased risk of adverse reactions from vaccines.

However, individual considerations always need to be borne in mind – both in terms of possible contraindications and adverse reactions. These concerns can be discussed with the family doctor, the practice nurse, health visitor or by contacting NHS Direct, the number of which can be obtained from the local telephone directory.

| Table 9.1   Childhood immunization programme (UK) | | |
| --- | --- | --- |
| **When to immunize** | **What vaccine is given** | **How it is given** |
| 2 months old | Diphtheria, tetanus, pertussis, polio and *Haemophilus influenzae* type B (DTaP/IPV/Hib) | One injection |
| | Pneumococcal meningitis (PCV) | One injection |
| 3 months old | Diphtheria, tetanus, pertussis, polio and *Haemophilus influenzae* type B (DTaP/IPV/Hib) | One injection |
| | Meningococcus - Men-C | One injection |
| 4 months old | Diphtheria, tetanus, pertussis, polio and *Haemophilus influenzae* type B (DTaP/IPV/Hib) | One injection |
| | MenC | One injection |
| | PCV | One injection |
| 12 months old | Hib/MenC | One injection |
| Around 13 months | Measles, mumps, rubella (MMR) | One injection |
| | PCV | One injection |
| Children aged 3 years 4 months to 5 years old but before nursery school | Diphtheria, tetanus, pertussis and Hib (DTaP/IPV or dTaP/IPV) | One injection |
| | Measles, mumps and rubella (MMR) | One injection |
| Girls 12–13 years old | Human papillomavirus (cervical cancer) | One injection |
| 13–18 years old | Tetanus, diphtheria and polio (Td/IPV) | One injection |

## Immunization Aftercare and Side-effects
### Polio, Diphtheria, Tetanus, Pertussis, Hib and Men-C
Some children become irritable and may develop a slight fever, with drowsiness and anorexia, between 6 and 24 hours after immunization; there may also be erythema, induration and a palpable nodule at the injection site.

### Measles, Mumps and Rubella
A week to 10 days after the injection, the child may become pyrexial for 1–2 days, and there may also be a rash. Lymphadenopathy in the neck may occur 2–3 weeks after immunization.

# Hepatitis A

The risks of this disease for children under the age of 1 year are low, and vaccines are not licensed for their use at this age. Care should be taken to prevent exposure to hepatitis A infection through food and water.

Vaccination is recommended for:

- Patients with severe liver disease
- Patients with haemophilia
- Men who have sex with men
- Injecting drug users
- Travellers to those countries where the disease is endemic, preferably 2 weeks before departure
- Health care staff and laboratory personnel who may be exposed to hepatitis A in the course of their work
- Sewage workers
- People who work with primates.

Vaccination may also be considered under certain circumstances for:

- Food handlers and packagers
- Staff working in day care facilities.

After the primary immunization a booster dose should be given at 6–12 months and a further booster is recommended at 20 years for those at ongoing risk.

# Hepatitis B

This vaccine is given to all babies including those who are preterm or low birth weight, whose mothers or close family contacts have been infected with hepatitis B. The first dose is given within 2 days of birth, followed by a second dose at 1 month, and a third at 2 months. A blood test to ascertain immunity status and a booster dose are given at 1 year of age.

The most common side-effects are temporary pain at the injection site and a slight fever.

Vaccination is recommended for:

- Injecting drug users and partners (even if not injectors) and their children
- Men having sex with men

- Families adopting children from countries with a high or intermediate prevalence of hepatitis B
- Those likely to be in close contact with carriers or at occupational risk, e.g. health care workers, laboratory staff, staff of residential accommodation and other settings working with people with learning difficulties
- Prison inmates and service staff in regular contact with prisoners.
- People travelling or going to reside in areas of high or intermediate prevalence.

A schedule of three doses usually at 0, 1 and 2 months, with a fourth dose after 12 months.

## Polio
This is included in the childhood immunization schedule therefore all adults should be protected against polio, to those who are not already protected it should be offered. 10-yearly boosters are only necessary for those at risk, e.g. health care workers in laboratories and clinical infectious disease units.

## Rubella (German measles)
Women of child-bearing age should be tested for rubella antibodies: if negative, the MMR vaccine should be offered and they should be advised to guard against pregnancy for 1 month. MMR vaccine should not be given to women known to be pregnant.

## Tetanus
If no previous immunization, three doses should be given 4 weeks apart. A booster dose is recommended every 10 years following initial course, particularly for those at occupational risk of soil-contamination wounds.

## Tuberculosis
The Bacillus–Calmette–Guerin (BCG) immunization should not be given to the following:

- Those who have already had a BCG vaccination
- Those with a past history of TB
- Those with an induration of 6 mm or more following Mantoux tuberculin skin testing

- Neonates in a household where an active TB case is suspected or confirmed
- Immuno-compromised people, including those infected with human immunodeficiency virus (HIV)
- Those suffering from malignant conditions, e.g. lymphoma, leukaemia.

For all those at higher risk of tuberculosis BCG immunization should be offered:

- Health service staff who have contact with infectious patients or their specimens
- Veterinary and other staff who handle animal species known to be susceptible to tuberculosis, e.g. simians
- Staff of prisons, old people's homes, refugee hostels and hostels for the homeless
- Contacts of cases known to be suffering from active tuberculosis
- New entrants to the UK, including students, refugees and asylum seekers from countries with a high prevalence of tuberculosis unless there is definite evidence of a BCG scar; infants born subsequently should be immunized within a few days of birth
- Those intending to stay in Asia, Africa, Central or South America for more than a month.

## Influenza

Vaccination is offered every autumn to protect people who are at risk of serious illness, e.g. those with chronic heart or respiratory disease, diabetes, etc., should they catch influenza. It is also advised for everyone over the age of 65 and to those living in residential and nursing homes. Health care workers are also encouraged to take up the vaccination. Repeated annual flu vaccination in October/early November is necessary due to the development of changing strains of the virus.

## Pneumococcal Vaccination

This prevents pneumonia caused by the *Pneumococcus* bacterium. The vaccine is recommended for those over the age of 65 years, those with health problems which include renal disease, liver disease, diabetes, gluten intolerance, those with immunodeficiency or immunosuppression due to disease or treatment including HIV infection at all stages of the disease and severe dysfunction of the spleen, and for those children considered to be at risk due to their health status.

## Travel Vaccinations

These vary widely according to the destination of the traveller. Contact the local primary health care centre several weeks before departure, for up-to-date information regarding which immunizations will be required, particularly if visiting tropical or developing areas of the world.

Further details about all immunizations can be found on: http://www. dh.gov.uk/en/Publichealth/Healthprotection/Immunisation/Greenbook/dh_4097254.

# Occupational Health and Safety
JUDY RIVETT

The Health and Safety at Work etc. Act 1974 provided the structure for all modern health and safety legislation. The foundation Act placed duties on employers for the health, safety and welfare of their employees while at work as far as is reasonably practicable. It also placed a duty on the employees to cooperate with their employers in adhering to the safe systems of work implemented by the employers and not to interfere with or misuse anything provided for this purpose.

## Health and Safety Commission and Health and Safety Executive

The Act also established the Health and Safety Commission and the Health and Safety Executive. The role of the Commission is to advise the appropriate ministers on the need for new health and safety regulations. It is a tripartite body comprising representatives from the Confederation of British Industry (CBI), the Trades Union Congress (TUC), local authorities and the Health and Safety Executive (HSE), and invited representatives from independent and local authorities. The HSE is a separate statutory body appointed by the Commission and undertakes the work required by the Commission. The Executive is the enforcing body for health and safety law and provides an advisory service to both sides of industry and commerce.

In April 2008, the Health and Safety Commission merged with the Health and Safety Executive to become a unitary body which retains the name Health and Safety Executive.

Since 1974 an enormous tranche of regulations controlling more specific aspects of industry and commerce have become law. The Control of Substances Hazardous to Health Regulations 1988 (amended 1998) and the 'Six Pack' of 1992 (see below), driven by the European Parliament, have had a tremendous impact on improving conditions at work for the nation's workforce.

## The Control of Substances Hazardous to Health Regulations 1988 (amended 1998)

These regulations introduced the idea of risk assessment in the workplace. Employers are required to assess the substances used in their workplace for their potential as health hazards under the categories 'very toxic', 'toxic', 'harmful', 'corrosive' or 'irritant'. The assessment should also include the measures required to control the risks, whether by eliminating the substances from the work process; containing the substances in an enclosed system thus preventing exposure; or safeguarding the individual with protective equipment or workwear. Whichever control measure is introduced, the system must be monitored and reviewed continuously.

## Health Surveillance

As part of the monitoring system, health surveillance should be undertaken if appropriate. The health of employees exposed to hazardous substances can be affected through absorption into the body. The absorption route can be by inhalation, by ingestion, through the skin or a combination of these. When inside the body the substances are metabolized. Metabolites can target various organs of the body which can thereby be harmed. A classic example of this is exposure to asbestos. The small fibres are breathed in and lodge in the lungs and pleura. Asbestosis, mesothelioma and lung cancer can be fatal outcomes. Health surveillance therefore requires biological monitoring. At its simplest this could be a skin inspection ensuring no dermatitic changes have occurred as a result of exposure to an irritant, through to lung function tests and urine, breath or blood analysis. The criteria used to decide which type of surveillance is appropriate depend on whether a test is available. Tributyl tin oxide was once used as a timber preservation treatment; however, it was not known how it was metabolized in the body and therefore no appropriate test existed. The potential for it to cause harm could not be eradicated and, as many occupational diseases have a long latency period – up to 40 years for asbestosis, for example – tributyl tin oxide was withdrawn from use.

## Environmental Monitoring

Monitoring the work environment is imperative to ensure that all control measures are effective. This may include checking that local exhaust ventilation systems are functioning properly; checking that noise levels are not above legal limits; or asking people to wear passive air samplers to ensure they are not inhaling possible contaminants.

## Records

Results of all monitoring must be recorded. Health surveillance records must be treated in confidence although a 'fitness to work' certificate should be given to the employer. As health surveillance records have to be kept for 40 years, the appropriate place for storing these documents is with an occupational health service. Records for environmental monitoring should be designed so that data can be read alongside data from fitness certificates. This will help to identify any failing control measures at a glance.

## The Reporting of Injuries, Disease and Dangerous Substances Regulations 1985

Employers are required to report to the HSE (or local authority for retail premises) certain injuries, diseases or dangerous occurrences that have stemmed from work activities. The enforcing authority must be notified immediately. This is now available by a number of methods including by telephone, 0845 300 9923, or e-mail: riddor@ batbrit.com to the Incident Contact Centre.

The aim of the regulations is to provide information to the HSE for epidemiological purposes. Analysis of the information may suggest a pattern of disease or injury associated with a particular industry. Action can be taken to establish the cause of the risk and its prevention. A free guidance leaflet is available on the HSE website at www. hse.gov.uk.

## The 'Six Pack' 1992

Six new sets of regulations were produced in 1992 in response to the European Parliament Framework Directive. These are:

- Management of Health and Safety at Work
- Manual Handling Operations
- Personal Protective Equipment at Work
- Health and Safety (Display Screen Equipment)
- Provision and Use of Work Equipment
- Workplace (Health, Safety and Welfare).

While each set of regulations focuses on specific aspects of the workplace, they all have a common theme. They reinforce the need for risk assessments, introducing control measures and follow-up monitoring and review systems. However, for the first time the idea of a 'competent person' is introduced. The employer is required to appoint one or more competent persons to assist in undertaking the measures needed to comply with the relevant statutory provisions. In small businesses this may be the employer in person or a colleague. In larger organizations it is likely to be a full occupational health and safety service. Whoever it is, the person must be knowledgeable about the risks to health and safety within that workplace.

Another important aspect of the 'Six Pack' is the need to provide information, instruction and training for employees. In practice this means providing factual information about the risks and the measures used to control them, telling people what they must do for their protection and training them how to do it (see Box 10.1).

## Working Time Regulations 1998

As a general guide, these regulations state that workers cannot be forced to work for more than 48 hours a week on average, and limits young workers' hours to 8 hours a day or 40 hours a week. From 1 August 2004, junior doctors' hours were also restricted. The number of hours should be averaged out over a 17-week period. Besides

---

| Box 10.1   A step-by-step guide |
| --- |

- The employer has duty for assessing risks in the workplace.
- Is anyone at work knowledgeable about health and safety?
- Appoint a person to carry out health risk assessment.
- Refer to the Health and Safety Regulations and HSE guidance for help in health risk identification.
- Could employees be harmed?
- What can be done about the risks?
- Has the appointed person sufficient specialist knowledge about controlling the risks?
- Is expert help needed?

working time limits, the regulations cover working at night, health assessments for night workers, time off, rest breaks at work and paid annual leave.

There are provisions for workers to come to an 'opt-out' agreement with their employers for defined periods, should the nature of the work make this necessary. For detailed information about the regulations, access the Department of Trade and Industry website on: www.dti.gov.uk/er/work_time_regs/wtr2.htm.

## Hazard and Risk

Frequently, there is confusion about the terms 'hazard' and 'risk'. 'Hazard' is something which will cause harm if not controlled. 'Risk' is the potential for harm when control measures are in place. An unguarded guillotine, for example, poses a tremendous hazard to health – certainly it did for many French aristocrats! Guarded industrial guillotine machines, which can only be operated from a safe distance, pose little risk.

## Failing to Safety as Opposed to Failing to Danger

It is a fact of life that things break down. All systems introduced to protect the health, safety and welfare of employees need to be assessed for their potential to fail to safety – not to danger. A simple example of this is hand-washing. Where there is a risk of employees ingesting a toxic residue on their hands, one of the control measures associated with the work process would be to ask them to wash their hands before eating. People in general will not go out of their way to find washing facilities so it is imperative to ensure there are adequate facilities adjacent to the area in which they will be eating. On a building site, construction workers burning lead paint from girders were absorbing high levels of lead. They had been provided with protective air-fed helmets, gloves and overalls. Their work site was opposite the Portakabin used as a canteen. The lavatory and washing facilities were on the opposite side of the site. Clearly, they just removed their helmets and gloves before going into the canteen. Not only did they remove their helmets and gloves but they stored the dust-laden gloves neatly tucked into the breathing zone of their helmets – a natural act for the many bikers among them! The obvious solution to this problem was to install a second Portakabin with washing facilities and storage for the gloves and the helmets in front of the canteen. Their lead levels subsequently reduced.

## Safe Systems of Work and Human Factors

Safe systems of work are not achieved by writing a policy document and putting it in a manual in a cupboard. They involve understanding how people go about their work and incorporating their natural behaviour into the system. In the hand-washing example given previously, guiding the construction workers through the washing facilities to gain access to the canteen made it quite natural for them to wash their hands. Yes, even bikers!

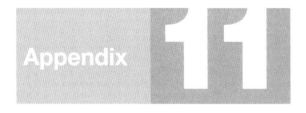

# Nursing on the Internet
CHRISTINE BISHOP

For the health care professional, the internet provides a veritable treasure chest of information, but mixed in with the nuggets of gold is a vast amount of irrelevant or useless data. Many hours can be wasted searching for the precise information you require, so the trick is to learn to navigate the internet without too much frustration.

The various types of information accessible via the World Wide Web include:

- Details about professional organizations, academic institutions and hospitals, e.g. the Royal College of Nursing.
- Full text or abstracts of many published articles available through Medline. In addition many journals are now accessible online, either free of charge or on a subscription basis.
- Purely electronic journals, not available in printed format.
- Facts about disease states, e.g. AIDS Insite– http://hivinsite.ucsf.edu
- Interactive learning resources.
- Textbooks on line.
- Discussion lists, e.g. http://www.jiscmail.ac.uk
- Data on drugs.
- Support groups for parents.
- Notices of conferences.
- News services.
- Educational material.
- Job vacancies.

In fact, information on almost any topic is probably now available electronically if you know where to find it. If you don't know the URL of the address of the web page you want to access, then a quick search on a search engine such as Google (www.google.co.uk) or Yahoo (http://uk.yahoo.com/), should point you in the right direction. Choosing precise keywords will enable you to restrict the list to the most relevant websites. Using a specialist internet search tool designed for health professionals, such as that found on the Intute site (see below), will direct you to high-quality resources. Always consider the date of publication, authorship and the origin of the information as well as the type of website, when evaluating the information provided. Once you have found a site which interests you make sure you bookmark it so that you can find it again. Many sites include links to related websites and these are a good source of high-quality information.

To help you find your way around the World Wide Web, listed below are some nursing sites that you may find useful, but do bear in mind that sites are constantly being added and deleted, so you will need to do your own research.

### Allnurses (http://allnurses.com)

A valuable site with an extensive compilation of links to online nursing sites and journals, colleges and universities, lists of employment vacancies and nursing humour.

### American Association of Colleges of Nursing (AACN) (http://www.aacn.nche.edu/)

Web homepage of the AACN, the national voice of America's university and higher degree nursing education programmes. For members only there is an interactive issues forum.

### BBC News Health (http://news.bbc.co.uk/hi/english/health/default.stm)

Updated daily, this free news service has a UK bias and features health news as well as articles on various health topics.

### Community Practitioners' and Health Visitors Association (CPHVA) (http://www.amicus-cphva.org/)

The UK professional body that represents registered nurses and health visitors in primary or community health settings.

**Cumulative Index of Nursing and Allied Health Literature (CINAHL) (http://www.ebscohost.com/cinahl/)**
An index of the nursing and allied health literature from 1982 to the present, including over 1500 nursing and allied health journals. Abstracts are included for some journal titles.

**Current Controlled Trials (http://www.controlled-trials.com/)**
Provides access to a searchable database of ongoing UK-funded trials, reports of controlled trials and trial protocols and links to other online registers of controlled trials. The site is free but requires registration.

**Department of Health (http://www.dh.gov.uk)**
Information about the work of the Department of Health, as well as health and social care guidance, publications and policy.

**eBNF (http://www.bnf.org/)**
The British National Formulary provides UK healthcare professionals with authoritative and practical information on the selection and clinical use of medicines. This site is a freely searchable online version of the book widely used throughout the NHS. Published jointly by the British Medical Association and the Royal Pharmaceutical Society of Great Britain. Registration required.

**e-journals.org (http://www.e-journals.org/)**
Providing links to the world's electronic journals.

**Electronic Medicines Compendium (http://emc.medicines.org.uk/)**
Information on thousands of licensed medicines with summaries of product characteristics including side-effects, dosage and treatment possibilities, as well as patient information leaflets. It is freely accessible and also fully searchable.

**Health and Care Northern Ireland (http://www.n-i.nhs.uk/)**
Provides advice and information on health and social care services in Northern Ireland, with links to all local acute and community hospital trusts, general practitioner surgeries and central government health care services.

**Healthcare Republic (http://www.healthcarerepublic.com)**
Website for healthcare professionals working in primary care. Contains a nurse prescribing area produced in conjunction with the Association for Nurse Prescribing.

**Health of Wales Information Service (HOWIS)(http://www.wales.
nhs.uk/)**
HOWIS is the official website of the NHS in Wales providing information about the health and lifestyle of the population of Wales. It
includes an e-library with a range of free and licensed resources for
staff, including ejournals.

**Health Protection Agency (http://www.hpa.org.uk/infections/)**
Details on the work of the Health Protection Agency and searchable
information about common infections, including incubation period,
route of entry and transmission.

**Intute: Health and Life Services – Nursing Midwifery and Allied
Health (http://www.intute.ac.uk/healthandlifesciences/nursing/)**
This excellent free resource provides quality nursing, midwifery and
allied health information on the internet. All sites found through this
gateway have been evaluated and indexed and come with a brief
description that enables you to assess their usefulness before you
visit. Each month an extensive directory of websites and databases
on a designated hot topic is produced.

**Medscape (http://www.medscape.com)**
Permits free access to the full text of a selection of peer-reviewed journals as well as the latest news in different specialties. Registration is
required. Also gives free access to Medline.

**Medscape Drug Information (http://search.medscape.com/
drug-reference-search)**
Information on more than 200 000 prescriptions and over-the-counter drugs including indications, interactions and precautions. The
site also enables you to find drugs to treat a disease and includes an
online medical dictionary.

**National Library for Health (NLH) (http://www.library.nhs.uk/
Default.aspx)**
This digital library provides access to a range of resources including
pathways and guidelines, evidence-based reviews (e.g. Bandolier,
Cochrane library) health care databases, knowledge sources and
latest key documents applicable for NHS staff, patients and the
public. It also includes branch libraries for various conditions and

professional portals for different professional groups including nursing, midwifery and community practitioners.

### NHS Careers (http://www.nhscareers.nhs.uk/)
Information on more than 300 careers available within the NHS, including details of qualifications required, pay and benefits, flexible working hours and how to apply.

### NHS Choices (http://www.nhs.uk/)
The official site of the National Health Service providing expert information on conditions, treatment, local services and healthy living, and a local NHS information database. It incorporates information from the NHS Direct website.

### NHS Education for Scotland Nursing, Midwifery and Health Visiting (http://www.nes.scot.nhs.uk/nursing/)
Responsible for standards of education and training for nurses, midwives and health visitors in Scotland. Provides career information for these professions.

### NHS Jobs (http://www.jobs.nhs.uk/)
Comprehensive listing of vacancies from NHS employers across England and Wales. Sign up to Jobs by Email to receive information on new vcancies to suit your profile.

### NICE – National Institute for Health and Clinical Excellence (http://www.nice.org.uk/)
Independent organization responsible for providing national guidance on the use of medicines, appraisal of new drugs and information regarding appropriate treatment of specific diseases and conditions. Contains a link to NHS evidence – a search engine providing access to high quality clinical and non-clinical evidence and best practices regarding drug treatment.

### Nurses Reconnected (http://www.nursesreconnected.com/)
Easy-to-use global service that aims to help nurses renew old friendships. Registration is free and provides access to searchable database of personnel at hospitals and other health care sites.

### PubMed (http://www.ncbi.nlm.nih.gov/PubMed/)
The National Library of Medicine's free search service with access to 9 million citations in Medline with links to participating online journals.

**Royal College of Nursing Conference and Exhibition Unit (http://www.rcn.org.uk/newsevents/events)**
A listing of conferences organized by the RCN in the UK and Europe.

**Royal College of Nursing UK (http://www.rcn.org.uk)**
The RCN is the world's largest professional union for registered nurses, midwives and health visitors. The site provides information about the organization and a service for members who require professional, legal and educational advice.

# Infection Control

CAROL PELLOWE

Preventing health-care-associated infections (HCAI) is a major Government priority since the rates of HCAI in the 1990s grew to intolerable levels. At that time, 9% of inpatients had a HCAI and over 100 000 inpatients a year acquired one or more infections (Taylor et al 2001). As many as 5000 inpatient deaths were directly attributable to HCAI and a further 15 000 deaths occured in which HCAI was a contributing factor (Department of Health 2001, Taylor et al 2001). The economic burden of HAI in England alone was estimated to be £1 billion per annum, yet 15–30% of these infections were thought to be preventable (Plowman et al 1999). A more recent HCAI prevalence survey in England (Hospital Infection Society (HIS) 2007) showed an overall HCAI prevalence of 8.2%.

Following the National Audit Office report (Taylor et al 2001), HCAI became a health service priority and the Department of Health (DH) has responded in several ways. In *Getting Ahead of the Curve* (DH 2002), the Chief Medical Officer proposed a clear strategy to make sweeping changes throughout the service, including the creation of the Health Protection Agency (HPA) to prevent, investigate and control infectious diseases threats and address health protection more widely. The following year, *Winning Ways* (DH 2003) outlined seven action areas including active surveillance and investigation, reducing reservoirs of infection and management and organization. This included the appointment of a Director of Infection Prevention and Control in each trust reporting directly to the Chief Executive. By making the chief executive overall responsible for preventing HCAI the importance of the issue was emphasized.

The National Patient Safety Agency (NPSA) launched the 'clean-**your**hands' campaign in 2004 which aims to minimize the risk to patient safety of low compliance with hand hygiene by NHS staff through a national strategy of improvement. The campaign targets hand hygiene improvement and uses both a multi-modal approach and the promotion and provision of near-patient alcohol hand rub as the corner stone for improvement. An assessment undertaken on behalf of the NPSA by the DH, exploring the costs of implementing the campaign, has found it to be cost saving even if the reduction in HCAI rates were as low as 0.1% (NPSA 2004).

In 2005 the DH published the self assessment and action planning toolkit *Saving Lives* (DH 2005). This was designed to help acute trusts work towards reducing HCAI by embedding best practice in infection prevention and control across every ward, department and unit. Since then there has been an additional publication, *Going Further Faster* (DH 2006a). The purpose of this guidance is to enable Trusts to make significant progress towards achieving the meticillin resistant *Staphylococcus aureus* (MRSA) target by making more rapid year on year improvement. To assist in reducing MRSA, *Essential Steps* (DH 2006b), a toolkit published by the DH, is based on root cause analysis, designed for particular clinical areas.

The Healthcare Act 2006 introduced a Code of Practice, commonly known as the 'Hygiene Code', that outlines how organizations should ensure patient safety. All NHS bodies are subject to inspection by the Healthcare Commission to check compliance with the Code.*

Infection prevention is not a new issue for the health service. With the advent of the emerging AIDS pandemic in the early 1980s, an infection control system known as Blood and Body Fluid Precautions was introduced primarily to protect health care personnel (Pratt 2003). These precautions were used for patients known or suspected to be infected with HIV or another blood-borne pathogen, e.g. hepatitis B virus (HBV), and focused on preventing needlestick or sharps injuries and the use of protective clothing to prevent exposure to blood and body fluids. By 1985 it was recognized that such precautions should be applied to all patients and the concept of Universal Precautions was introduced into health care practice throughout the world

---

*Following a period of consultation a new regulator, the Care Quality Commission for England, will replace the Commission for Social Care Inspection (CSCI), the Mental Health Act Commission (MHAC) and the Healthcare Commission in April 2009.

(Pratt 2003). This approach was later modified to Body Substance Isolation, which primarily extended the use of gloves before contact with all body fluids, mucous membranes or non-intact skin (Pratt 2003).

In 1996, the Centers for Disease Control and Prevention (CDC) published a further revision of their guidance that introduced a two-tier system of precautions (Garner et al 1996). The first tier known as Standard Precautions are to be used for all patients regardless of diagnosis or infection status and are a synthesis of Universal Precautions and Body Substance Isolation. The second tier, Transmission-based Precautions, are to be taken in addition to Standard Precautions when a patient is known or suspected of being infected with a pathogen transmissible by air, droplet or contact with dry skin or contaminated surfaces.

In England, evidence-based infection prevention guidelines have been published for acute care and primary and community care settings (Pellowe et al 2003, Pratt et al 2001). Standard Principles reflect the guidance from CDC and include new evidence published since 1996 (Table 12.1). Standard Principles cover hand hygiene, the use of personal protective equipment, the safe use and disposal of sharps, and education of patients, carers and their health care personnel. In addition, the acute care guidelines include hospital environmental hygiene. As Standard Principles are broad statements of good practice, they need to be incorporated into local protocols to reflect individual circumstances. They must be observed by all health care personnel and should provide a uniform response to infection prevention regardless of setting. In order to reflect current evidence, both sets of guidelines are subject to review and updating every 5 years. In 2007 the acute care infection prevention guidelines were updated and reissued as the epic2 guidelines (Pratt et al 2007).

Additional evidence-based guidelines have been developed and published which make recommendations for preventing health-care-associated infections when using a variety of medical devices, e.g. urinary catheters, enteral feeding systems or central venous catheters. These precautions are to be used in addition to the Standard Principles (Pellowe et al 2003, Pratt et al 2007).

To assist organizations to meet the education demands of the Code of Practice, a national e-learning education programme has been developed for clinical and non-clinical staff which explains the infection prevention guidelines and is available at http://www.corelearning.nhs.uk.

Table 12.1    Standard principles for preventing health-care-associated infections

| Standard area number (SP) | Principle | Action required |
|---|---|---|
| SP1 | The hospital environment must be visibly clean, free from dust and soilage and acceptable to patients, their visitors and staff | *Class C* |
| SP2 | Increased levels of cleaning should be considered in outbreaks of infection where the pathogen concerned survives in the environment and environmental contamination may be contributing to spread | *Class D* |
| SP3 | The use of hypochlorite and detergent should be considered in outbreaks of infection where the pathogen concerned survives in the environment and environmental contamination may be contributing to spread | *Class D* |
| SP4 | Shared equipment used in the clinical environment must be decontaminated appropriately after each use | *Class D* |
| SP5 | All health care workers need to be aware of their individual responsibility for maintaining a safe care environment for patients and staff. Every health care worker needs to be clear about their specific responsibilities for cleaning equipment and clinical areas (especially those areas in close proximity to patients). They must be educated about the importance of ensuring that the hospital environment is clean and that opportunities for microbial contamination are minimized. | *Class D* |

Table 12.1   Standard principles for preventing health-care-associated infections—*cont'd*

| Standard area number (SP) | Principle | Action required |
|---|---|---|
| SP6 | Hands must be decontaminated immediately before each and every episode of direct patient contact/care and after any activity or contact that potentially results in hands becoming contaminated | *Class C* |
| SP7 | Hands that are visibly soiled or potentially grossly contaminated with dirt or organic material (i.e. following the removal of gloves) must be washed with liquid soap and water | *Class A* |
| SP8 | Hands should be decontaminated between caring for different patients or between different care activities for the same patient. For convenience and efficacy an alcohol-based handrub is preferable unless hands are visibly soiled | *Class A* |
| SP9 | Hands should be washed with soap and water after several consecutive applications of alcohol handrub. Local infection control guidelines may advise an alternative product in some outbreak situations | *Class D/GPP* |
| SP10 | Before a shift of clinical work begins, all wrist and ideally hand jewellery should be removed. Cuts and abrasions must be covered with waterproof dressings. Fingernails should be kept short, clean and free from nail polish. False nails and nail extensions must not be worn by clinical staff | *Class D* |

*(Continued)*

Table 12.1   Standard principles for preventing health-care-associated infections—cont'd

| Standard area number (SP) | Principle | Action required |
|---|---|---|
| SP11 | An effective handwashing technique involves three stages: preparation, washing and rinsing, and drying. Preparation requires wetting hands under tepid running water <u>before</u> applying the recommended amount of liquid soap or an antimicrobial preparation. The handwash solution must come into contact with <u>all</u> of the surfaces of the hand. The hands must be <u>rubbed</u> together vigorously for a minimum of 10–15 seconds, paying particular attention to the tips of the fingers, the thumbs and the areas between the fingers. Hands should be rinsed thoroughly prior to drying with good quality paper towels | *Class D* |
| SP12 | When decontaminating hands using an alcohol-based handrub, hands should be free of dirt and organic material. The handrub solution must come into contact with all surfaces of the hand. The hands must be rubbed together vigorously, paying particular attention to the tips of the fingers, the thumbs and the areas between the fingers, and until the solution has evaporated and the hands are dry | *Class D* |
| SP13 | Clinical staff should be aware of the potentially damaging effects of hand decontamination products. They should be encouraged to use an emollient hand cream regularly, for example, after washing hands before a break or going off duty and when off duty, to maintain the integrity of the skin | *Class D* |

Table 12.1  Standard principles for preventing health-care-associated infections—cont'd

| Standard area number (SP) | Principle | Action required |
|---|---|---|
| SP14 | If a particular soap, antiseptic hand wash or alcohol-based product causes skin irritation, review methods as described in Recommendation SP11 and 12 before consulting the occupational health team | *Class D* |
| SP15 | Near patient alcohol-based hand rub should be made available in all health care facilities | *Class D* |
| SP16 | Hand hygiene resources and individual practice should be audited at regular intervals and the results fed back to health care workers | *Class D* |
| SP17 | Education and training in risk assessment, effective hand hygiene and glove use should form part of all health care workers' annual updating | *Class D* |
| SP18 | Selection of protective equipment must be based on an assessment of the risk of transmission of microorganisms to the patient or to the carer, and the risk of contamination of the health care practitioners' clothing and skin by patients' blood, body fluids, secretions or excretions | *Class D/ H&S* |
| SP19 | Everyone involved in providing care should be educated about standard principles and trained in the use of protective equipment | *Class D/ H&S* |
| SP20 | Adequate supplies of disposable plastic aprons, single use gloves and face protection should be made available wherever care is delivered. Gowns should be made available when advised by the infection control team | *Class D/ H&S* |

*(Continued)*

Table 12.1  Standard principles for preventing health-care-associated infections—*cont'd*

| Standard area number (SP) | Principle | Action required |
|---|---|---|
| SP21 | Gloves must be worn for invasive procedures, contact with sterile sites, and non-intact skin or mucous membranes, and all activities that have been assessed as carrying a risk of exposure to blood, body fluids, secretions and excretions; and when handling sharp or contaminated instruments | *Class D/ H&S* |
| SP22 | Gloves must be worn as single use items. They are put on immediately before an episode of patient contact or treatment and removed as soon as the activity is completed. Gloves are changed between caring for different patients, or between different care/treatment activities for the same patient | *Class D/ H&S* |
| SP23 | Gloves must be disposed of as clinical waste and hands decontaminated, ideally by washing with liquid soap and water after the gloves have been removed | *Class D/ H&S* |
| SP24 | Gloves that are acceptable to health care workers and CE marked must be available in all clinical areas | *Class D/ H&S* |
| SP25 | Sensitivity to natural rubber latex in patients, carers and health care workers must be documented and alternatives to natural rubber latex must be available | *Class B/ H&S* |
| SP26 | Neither powdered nor polythene gloves should be used in health care activities | *Class C/ H&S* |

Table 12.1 Standard principles for preventing health-care-associated infections—*cont'd*

| Standard area number (SP) | Principle | Action required |
|---|---|---|
| SP27 | Disposable plastic aprons must be worn when close contact with the patient, materials or equipment are anticipated and when there is a risk that clothing may become contaminated with pathogenic microorganisms or blood, body fluids, secretions or excretions, with the exception of perspiration | *Class D/ H&S* |
| SP28 | Plastic aprons/gowns should be worn as single-use items, for one procedure or episode of patient care, and then discarded and disposed of as clinical waste. Non-disposable protective clothing should be sent for laundering | *Class D/ H&S* |
| SP29 | Full-body fluid-repellent gowns must be worn where there is a risk of extensive splashing of blood, body fluids, secretions or excretions, with the exception of perspiration, onto the skin or clothing of health care workers (for example when assisting with childbirth) | *Class D/ H&S* |
| SP30 | Face masks and eye protection must be worn where there is a risk of blood, body fluids, secretions or excretions splashing into the face and eyes | *Class D/ H&S* |
| SP31 | Respiratory protective equipment, i.e. a particulate filter mask, must be correctly fitted and used when recommended for the care of patients with respiratory infections transmitted by airborne particles | *Class D/ H&S* |

References

Department of Health 2002 Getting Ahead of the Curve. Department of Health, London

Department of Health 2003 Winning Ways: working together to reduce healthcare associated infection in England. A report by the Chief Medical Officer. Department of Health, London

Department of Health 2005 Saving Lives: a delivery programme to reduce healthcare associated infection (HCAI) including MRSA. Department of Health, London

Department of Health 2006a Going Further Faster: implementing the Saving Lives delivery programme. Sustainable change for cleaner, safer care. Department of Health, London

Department of Health 2006b Essential Steps to Safe Clean Care. Department of Health, London

Department of Health 2006c The Health Act 2006. Code of Practice for the prevention and control of health care associated infections. Department of Health, London

Garner JS, Hospital Infection Control Practices Advisory Committee 1996 Guideline for isolation precautions in hospital. Infection Control and Hospital Epidemiology 1996;17:53–80.

Hospital Infection Society 2007 The third prevalence study of healthcare associated infections in acute hospitals in England. A report for the Department of Health. Available at http://www.nric.org.uk/IntegratedCRD.nsf/NRIC_All?SearchView&Query=HCAi%20prevalence (accessed 2 June)

National Patient Safety Agency 2004 The Economic Case: implementing near-patient alcohol handrub in your trust. NPSA, London

Pellowe CM, Pratt RJ, Harper P et al 2003 Evidence-based guidelines for preventing healthcare-associated infections in primary and community care in England. Journal of Hospital Infection 55(suppl): S1–S127. Available: http://www.richardwellsresearch.com

Plowman R, Graves N, Griffin M et al 1999 The socio-economic burden of hospital acquired infection. Public Health Laboratory Service, London

Pratt RJ, 2003 HIV/AIDS: a foundation for nursing and healthcare practice, 5th edn. Arnold, London

Pratt RJ, Pellowe C, Loveday HP et al 2001 The Epic Project: developing national evidence-based guidelines for preventing healthcare associated infections. Phase 1: Guidelines for preventing hospital-acquired infections. Journal of Hospital Infection 47(suppl):S1–S82. Online. Available: http://www.doh.gov.uk/hai/epic.htm

Pratt RJ, Pellowe CM, Wilson JA, Loveday HP, Harper PJ, Jones SRLJ, McDougall C, Wilcox MH 2007 epic2: National evidence-based guidelines for preventing healthcare-associated infections in NHS hospitals in England. Journal of Hospital Infection **65**(1): supplement 1:S1-69 (Available at: http://www.richardwellsresearch.com)

Taylor K, Plowman R, Roberts JA 2001 The challenge of hospital acquired infection. National Audit Office, London

# 13 Appendix

## Practice Development
BOB BROWN AND JOHN DRISCOLL

## Introduction

Practice development (PD) is a term that has been used to describe particular approaches to supporting change in health care (predominantly nursing) for over 20 years. It has been a broadly based term that has been defined and conceptualized from several different points of view (Kitson 1994, Gerrish & Ferguson 2000, McSherry & Bassett 2002, Garbett & McCormack 2002, McCormack et al 2004a, McCormack et al 2007a,b) and includes a wide range of activities aimed at continually developing and improving practice in health care settings. Whilst change has always been a cultural feature within the health service, UK government modernization and service improvement reforms during recent decades, as well as an emerging theory base for practice development, has led to an increasing recognition of the term and its values as actively supporting a continuous process of developing more effective person-centred care.

Practice development was primarily introduced into the UK by the nursing profession in the late 1970s and early 1980s. Nursing at the time was shifting from a traditionalist approach to clinical practice that was based on tasks, rituals and the division of labour (skill-mix and profiling) to a more patient-centred approach to care through the development of quality, standards and evaluation of practice (McCormack et al 1999). The 1990s saw the emergence of a more humanistic approach to caring and a move toward more patient focused developments in practice with a greater emphasis on clinical effectiveness and patient outcomes. Since then, various improvement focused reforms and the modernization of health services through the framework of Clinical and Social Care Governance (Department of Health in England 1998, 1999) now not only places a statutory organizational commitment under the United Kingdom Health Act (1999) for the provision of high quality health care, but endorses practice development activities through inter-professional team working and placing the service user at the centre of care.

Over the past ten years significant conceptual, theoretical and methodological advances have been made in the development of frameworks to guide practice development activities. Of most significance has been an increased understanding of key concepts underpinning PD work, for example workplace culture (Manley 2004), person-centredness (Dewing 2004), practice context (McCormack et al 2002), evidence (Rycroft-Malone et al 2003), values (Manley 2001, Wilson et al 2005) and approaches to learning for sustainable practice (Hardy et al 2006).

## Defining Practice Development

It is important to differentiate practice development from a wide range of educational, research and audit activities also intended to promote and support change in health care such as implementing evidence-based practice and other quality initiatives such as The Essence of Care (Department of Health in England 2001a) and the development of integrated care pathways or National Service Frameworks (e.g. NSF for Older People, Department of Health in England 2001b). These other activities are often referred to as ways of developing practice, and although they share some of the characteristics of PD work, i.e. aimed at improving the quality of delivered services, they are not underpinned by the conceptual, theoretical or evidence-based outcomes of practice development.

Early work undertaken by Garbett and McCormack (2004) to examine the activities and approaches of practice developers identified four key themes which outlined the purpose of practice development as:

• a means of improving patient/service user care
• transforming the contexts and cultures in which nursing/health care takes place

- employing a systematic approach to effect changes in practice
- involving various types of facilitation for change to take place.

In a concept analysis of practice development, Garbett and McCormack (2004) further articulated the interconnected and synergistic relationships between the development of knowledge and skills, enablement strategies, facilitation and systematic, rigorous and continuous processes of emancipatory change in order to achieve the ultimate purpose of evidence-based person-centred care. The original definition of Practice Development offered by Garbett and McCormack (2002) has recently been updated to reflect the emerging theoretical and research knowledge base of the discipline, and thus a new definition of practice development is proposed as:

> ... a continuous process of developing person-centred cultures. It is enabled by facilitators who authentically engage with individuals and teams to blend personal qualities and creative imagination with practice skills and practice wisdom. The learning that occurs brings about transformations of individual and team practices. This is sustained by embedding both processes and outcomes in corporate strategy.

Manley, McCormack and Wilson (2008)

Clearly, the unique nature of practice development is that change happens within the professional's 'own' practice setting (Page & Hamer 2002) and such activities or processes contribute to the quality of care by using as its focus patients'/service users' needs.

For practice development to continue to flourish, there also needs to be an organizational framework in which it can occur (Eve 2004, McSherry & Driscoll 2004), thus the importance of connecting PD work with local team and organizational strategy, as reflected in the above definition. In a recent systematic review of the evidence underpinning practice development, McCormack et al (2007a,b) identified methodological principles that underpin all PD work (collaboration, inclusion and participation), as well as 18 methods that are systematically used in the development of practice. These methods include, clarifying the development focus and workplace culture, analysing stakeholder roles and ways of engaging stakeholders, developing a shared vision, developing critical intent, facilitating participatory engagement and shared ownership, undertaking continuous reflective learning and evaluation.

## Characteristics, Qualities and Skills of Practice Developers

Practice development is a systematic approach which aims to help practitioners and health care teams to look critically at their practice and identify how it can be improved. Its purpose is to develop effective workplace cultures that have embedded within them person-centred processes, systems and ways of working. Unique to PD is its explicit person-centred focus and it has become clear that the enabling role of skilled facilitation is vital to successfully undertaking PD work. Thus person centredness is a key concept underpinning every aspect of facilitation practice. In the PD literature the facilitation role is seen to be a key element in PD frameworks (Manley 2004) and to enabling PD to achieve its purpose and goals, such as the transformation of practitioners and practices (McCormack et al 2007a). Successful practice developers are most likely to be effective at utilizing the 'enabling' skills of facilitation, characteristics understood better through undertaking a concept analysis of 'enabling and enablement', demonstrated in the work of Shaw et al (2008). The study indicates that facilitators display strong attributes in knowing their own beliefs and values; demonstrating authentic ways of working such as through a sense of personal integrity and realness in order to achieve personal development, learning and transformation in self and others. Facilitators are also effective at building person-centred relationships on a one-to-one and group level and have an ability to establish vision and ownership. They tend to understand and have the ability to utilize a range of PD methods and processes, work effectively in differing context and cultures and know how to access and use different types of evidence and resources.

## Evaluating the Outcomes of Practice Development

As practice development is intended to support clinicians to change their perspectives about what is possible in practice, a systematic approach to evaluation is important. Systematic evaluation of PD activities and programmes is important for demonstrating to key stakeholders outcomes in terms of learning achieved, value for money and quality monitoring. McCormack et al (2004b) articulated the need for a clear evaluation strategy to underpin PD initiatives in order for it to be both systematic and rigorous. Wilson, Hardy and Brown (2008) have built on the above work by developing a framework for 'praxis evaluation' which they contend reflects the six core components of effective evaluation of PD work: purpose, reflexivity, approaches, context, intent and stakeholders. The first component focuses on understanding the purpose of PD work and how this shapes the evaluation. Next, the importance of undertaking critical questioning and reflection about the evaluation process itself is an essential component and supports critical consideration, regarding which approaches best 'fit' the evaluation. Further deliberation should be given to the context in which the PD work is taking place and the potential impact of the context on the evaluation. Finally, there is a clear need to identify and work with the stakeholders for whom the PD work holds significance.

The evidence base for practice development suggests that outcome measurement in PD is complex (Wilson et al 2008) and does not lend itself to traditional methods of outcome evaluation. It is suggested that outcome measurement needs to be consistent with the values of 'participation, collaboration and inclusivity' where data collection and analysis is an integral component of the development itself. In the international systematic review of the evidence underpinning practice development, McCormack et al (2007a,b) identified a wide range of outcomes arising from development initiatives undertaken, including, implementation of patient care knowledge utilization projects, development of facilitation skills among staff; development of new services; increased effectiveness of existing services or expansion of more effective services; changes in workplace cultures to ones that are more person-centred; development of learning cultures; increased empowerment of staff. Future PD work should aim to build on current understandings of evaluation by testing such frameworks as praxis evaluation while ensuring that all evaluation is both process and outcome orientated, creative in its application and aimed at understanding better the experience of being engaged in PD work as well as through capturing the outcomes that aim towards improvements in health care practice.

## The Future for Practice Development

From quiet beginnings during the 1980s, the practice development movement in health care is now recognized for making a direct impact on improving patient/service user experience as well as outcomes of health care provision, whether in the hospital or community setting. Practice developer's often working in teams are employed in many health care settings, contributing to the development of and disseminating excellence in practice. In future years it has however been seen as necessary to discontinue the dominant focus on PD roles per se and instead develop transferable principles based on the methodological perspectives of practice development, to guide the facilitation of PD within and across organizations (McCormack et al 2007a,b). The increasing amount of published materials related to practice development, e.g. the journal *Practice Development in Healthcare,* ensures the advancement of a practice developer's knowledge and expertise through debate and rigorous scrutiny. Further research is however needed to advance the development and testing of PD methods in order to transform outcome measurement. There is also a need to further evaluate the methods of PD such as models of facilitation.

The challenge for practice development is to extend the transforming culture of improvement in the patient/service user experience of health care into all arenas of care provision. This will include the need to engage key policy and strategy stakeholders in order to develop a strategic way forward for connecting practice development methods with service and system developments, set within the modernization agenda of health and social care.

## REFERENCES

Department of Health in England 2001a The essence of care. Department of Health, Leeds, UK

Department of Health in England 2001b The National Service Framework for older people. HMSO, London

Department of Health in England 1998 A first class service – quality in the New NHS. HMSO, London

Department of Health in England 1999 Clinical Governance: quality in the new NHS. Department of Health, Leeds, UK

Dewing J 2004 Concerns relating to the application of frameworks to promote person-centredness in nursing with older people. International Journal of Older People Nursing 13(3a):39–44

Eve JD 2004 Sustainable practice: how practice development frameworks can influence team work, team culture and philosophy of practice. Journal of Nursing Management 12:124–130

Garbett R, McCormack B 2002 A concept analysis of practice development. Nursing Times Research 7(2):87–100

Garbett R, McCormack B 2004 A concept analysis of practice development. In: Practice development in nursing (eds McCormack B, Manley K, Garbett R), pp 10–32. Blackwell, Oxford

Gerrish K, Ferguson A 2000 Nursing development units: factors influencing their progress. British Journal of Nursing 9(10):109–118

Hardy S, Garbarino L, Titchen A, Manley K 2006 A framework for work-based learning. In: Royal College of Nursing, workplace resources for practice development, pp 8–56. RCN, London

Kitson A 1994 Clinical nursing practice development and research activity in the Oxford region. Centre for Practice Development and Research, Institute of Nursing, Oxford

Manley K 2001 Consultant nurse: concept, processes, outcomes. University of Manchester/RCN Institute, London

Manley K 2004a Transformational culture: a culture of effectiveness. In: Practice development in nursing (eds McCormack B, Manley K, Garbett R), pp 51–82. Blackwell, Oxford

Manley K 2004b Workplace culture: is your culture effective? How would you know? Nursing in Critical Care 9(1):1–3

Manley K, McCormack B, Wilson V 2008 International practice development in nursing and healthcare. Blackwell, Oxford

McCormack B, Manley K, Kitson A, Titchen A, Harvey G 1999 Towards practice development – a vision in reality or a reality without vision? Journal of Nursing Management 7:255–264

McCormack B, Kitson A, Harvey G, Rycroft-Malone J, Titchen A, Seers K 2002 Getting evidence into practice: the meaning of 'context'. Journal of Advanced Nursing 38(1):94–104

McCormack B, Manley K, Garbett R 2004a Practice development in nursing. Blackwell, Oxford

McCormack B, Manley K, Wilson V 2004b Evaluating practice developments. In: Practice development in nursing (eds McCormack B, Manley K, Garbett R), pp 83–117. Blackwell, Oxford

McCormack B, Wright J, Dewar B, Harbey G, Ballantine K 2007a A realist synthesis of evidence relating to practice development: findings from the literature review. Practice Development in Healthcare 6:25–55

McCormack B, Wright J, Dewar B, Harbey G, Ballantine K 2007b A realist synthesis of evidence relating to practice development: interviews and synthesis of data. Practice Development in Healthcare 6:56–75

McSherry R, Bassett C (eds) 2002 Practice development in the clinical setting: a guide to implementation. Nelson Thornes, Cheltenham, UK

McSherry R, Driscoll JJ 2004 Practice development: promoting quality improvements in orthopaedic care … as well as ones' self! Journal of Orthopaedic Nursing 8:171–178

Page S, Hamer S 2002 Practice development – time to realise the potential. Practice Development in Health Care 1(1):2–17

Rycroft-Malone J, Seers K, Titchen A, Harvey G, Kitson A, McCormack B 2003 What counts as evidence in evidence-based practice. Journal of Advanced Nursing 47(1):81–90

Shaw T, Dewing J, Young R, Devlin M, Boomer C, Legius M 2008 Enabling practice development: delving into the concept of facilitation from a practitioner perspective. In: (eds Manley K, McCormack B, Wilson V), International practice development in nursing and healthcare, pp 147–169. Blackwell, Oxford

Wilson V, McCormack B, Ives G 2005 Understanding the workplace culture of a special care nursery. Journal of Advanced Nursing 50(1):27–38

Wilson V, Hardy S, Brown R 2008 An exploration of practice development evaluation: unearthing praxis. In: (eds Manley K, McCormack B, Wilson V), International practice development in nursing and healthcare, pp 126–146. Blackwell, Oxford

---

USEFUL WEBSITES

*http://www.bournemouth.ac.uk/ihcs/practicedevelopment*

An academic centre for practice development supporting practice development activities in health care.

*http://www.fons.org/dp/default.asp*

The Foundation of Nursing Studies: a registered charity actively supporting a network for health professionals interested in or already engaged in practice development in health care.

*www.ppdnf.org/index.html*

A forum bringing together nurses and allied health professionals interested in professional and practice development issues to influence clinical practice throughout Scotland.

*http://www.rcn.org.uk/development/researchanddevelopment/completed/practice_development*

A professional organization for nurses and health professionals actively supporting practice development.

*http://www3.interscience.wiley.com/journal/112094320/home*

Access to *Practice Development in Health Care,* a journal specifically aimed at health professionals working in practice development.

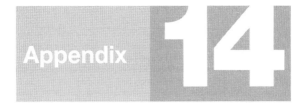

# Clinical Governance

JOHN DRISCOLL AND LORNA TELFORD

## Introduction

Clinical governance places a statutory duty on all NHS organizations across all four countries of the UK under the *Health Act 1999* to ensure the delivery of quality care and develop ways in which that care can be continually improved to meet the evolving needs of service-users. Prior to 1999 the main statutory responsibilities of NHS Trust Boards was to ensure proper financial management of the organization and an acceptable level of patient safety but with no requirement to ensure a particular level of quality. Maintaining and improving the quality of patient care was understood then to be the responsibility of the relevant clinical professions.

In an early definition clinical governance is described as:

> *A framework through which NHS organisations are accountable for continuously improving the quality of their services and safeguarding high standards of care by creating an environment in which excellence in clinical care will flourish (Scally & Donaldson 1988, Welsh Office 1999).*

A number of factors led to the need for a clinical governance framework being introduced throughout the NHS in the late 1990s (DHSSPS 2001, DOH 1998, 1999, Scottish Executive 1997, Welsh Office 1999). Two key concerns at that time were the need to tackle perceived differences in the quality of health care in the UK, as well as address public concerns and lack of confidence in previously well-publicized cases of poor professional and organizational performance.

Whilst there are differences in the way that clinical governance has been implemented in the different countries of the UK, the provision of high quality health care through the development of common organizational purposes and goals remains a key tenet (Lugon 2007). Although clinical governance is a complex organizational concept, it does contain core elements. The term 'clinical' governance specifically applies to health and social care organizations in relation to the delivery of *clinical* care. However the term *integrated* governance has since emerged (DOH 2006a) that refers jointly to both the corporate and clinical governance responsibilities and duties of health care organizations. Therefore adoption of a more integrated approach to governance in health care is redefining clinical governance and emphasizing individual accountability of:

> *A governance system for health care organizations that promotes an integrated approach towards management of inputs, structures and process to improve the outcome of health care service delivery where health staff work in an environment of greater accountability for clinical quality (Vanu Som 2004)*

Ensuring both individual and corporate accountability for quality health care has been through the development of specific standards in which there is a statutory responsibility for its monitoring and regulation.

## Ensuring Effective Cinical Governance in UK Health Care

The '7 domains' of clinical governance have superseded the 'seven pillars' of clinical governance' forming the basis for the Department of Health's *Standards for Better Health* (DOH 2004, updated 2006). This outlinines a performance framework setting out the quality standards all organizations providing NHS care are expected to meet, or aspire to across the NHS in England;

- Safety
- Clinical and cost effectiveness
- Governance
- Patient focus
- Accessible and responsive care
- Care environment and amenities
- Public health.

The development of measureable standards provides a common set of requirements that apply to all health care organizations both in state provision and the private health care sector to ensure that the health services provided are both safe and of an acceptable quality. Secondly, it is expected that the publication of standards provide a framework for continuous improvement in the overall quality of care people receive.

Similar standards have also been agreed following consultation for the HPSS in Northern Ireland (DHSSPS 2006), Wales (WAG 2005) and Scotland (NHS QIS 2005). The Royal College of Nursing (RCN 2007) in a review of all the health care standards in the UK published by each of the four countries that form the basis for monitoring clinical governance, identify five broad themes relating to effective clinical governance:

- Patient focus – ways in which health care services are based on patient needs.
- Information focus – how information is utilized for the benefit of service users and to improve care.
- Quality improvement – how standards are reviewed and evidence used to support quality health care practice.
- Staff development – developing knowledge and skills, assessing competence, ongoing support and supervision and career development.
- Leadership – ways in which health care can be transformed in practice, e.g. an emphasis on teamworking, being patient focused and being politically aware.

All four countries in the UK are subject to inspection and regulatory arrangements which provide an independent asssessment of that health care provider's ability to deliver effective clinical governance arrangements. All the regulators have a statutory duty to report upon and publish the performance of health service providers against published Government standards. In addition the following organizations also investigate serious failings and produce an annual report on that country's health care performance;

## Healthcare Commission[*] (Previously the Commission for Health Improvement) – England

The Healthcare Commission replaced the Commission for Health Improvement in 2004 and the statutory responsibilities and private

---

[*]Following a period of consultation a new regulator, the Care Quality Commission for England, will replace the Commission for Social Care Inspection (CSCI), the Mental Health Act Commission (MHAC) and the Healthcare Commission in April 2009.

and voluntary functions of the National Care Standards Commission and the Audit Commission. From 2006, the Healthcare Commission developed the Annual Health Check replacing the use of star ratings and league tables with a four point scale to demonstrate quality that include both Core and Developmental standards for each of seven domains alluded to earlier (DOH 2004, updated 2006). As part of the periodic monitoring, audit and inspection activities a number of Concordats (organizational voluntary agreements) led by the Healthcare Commission support the improvement of health services for the public.

The responsibility for local inspection and investigation of NHS bodies in Wales rests with the new Healthcare Inspectorate Wales (WAG 2005), while the private health care sector is regulated by the Care Standards Inspectorate for Wales. The Healthcare Commission does undertake national thematic reviews in Wales and the annual state of health care report covers both England and Wales. Equivalent bodies to the Healthcare Commission in Scotland and Northern Ireland, respectively, are NHS Quality Improvement Scotland (NHSQIS 2005) and the Health & Personal Social Services Regulation and Improvement Authority (DHSSPS 2006) in Northern Ireland. For more details on the health care standards in these countries and how these are monitored, the reader should refer to the appropriate websites at the end of this appendix.

In addition to the publication and monitoring of health care standards in health care organizations across the UK, effective clinical governance also relates to the ongoing reforms in professional regulation and registration requirements to enhance public and professional confidence as part of the Government's response to the Shipman Inquiry (Smith 2002–2005).

## Supporting Effective Clinical Governance in UK Health Care

A number of NHS linked bodies have been established to assist health care organizations and staff to deliver safe and effective care through a range of initiatives designed to support the statutory regulations and functions.

## National Institute for Health and Clinical Excellence (NICE)

The National Institute for Health and Clinical Excellence (NICE) is the independent organization responsible for providing national guidance on the promotion of good health and the prevention and treatment of ill health. NICE produces robust and authoritative guidance to the NHS in England and Wales in a number of ways that includes:

- **Clinical guidelines** for the appropriate treatment and care of patients with specific diseases and conditions.
- **Technology appraisals** for the use of new and existing medicines and treatments.
- **Interventional procedures** covering the safety and efficacy of interventional procedures used for diagnosis or treatment.
- **Public health guidance** through giving advice, providing services and support.

In line with the NHS Plan to develop a patient led NHS (DOH 2007), NICE actively encourages patient and public involvement for all its work and has developed a Patient and Public Involvement Programme. Northern Ireland joined England, Scotland and Wales as full participants in NICE Interventional Procedures Programme (recommendations on whether specific procedures are safe and efficacious for routine use in the NHS) in 2006.

## NHS Evidence

Following publication of the Darzi report, *High Quality Care for All* (DOH 2008), NICE was asked to establish NHS Evidence – a web-based service to help people find, access and use high-quality clinical and non-clinical evidence and best practice (NICE 2008). It is envisaged that NHS Evidence should be the 'first point of contact' for NHS staff to access evidence and related information that will include sources of research evidence and information on local experience, e.g. evidence-based practice.

## National Service Frameworks (NSFs)

NSFs are templates or blueprints for care in major service areas that have been developed nationally by NICE to be used locally by the NHS Executive and other health care organizations to review and reshape local service provision. The need to establish National Service Frameworks in the NHS is to be able to:

- set national standards and identify key interventions for a defined service or care group

- put in place strategies to support implementation in the NHS
- establish ways to ensure progress within an agreed timescale.

As a consequence not every NSF will apply to each country of the NHS, however the current programme of National Service Framework's in England and Wales (DOH undated) are:

- blood pressure
- cancer
- children
- chronic obstructive pulmonary disease
- coronary heart disease
- long term conditions
- long term neurological conditions
- mental health
- older people
- renal
- vascular.

## Essence of Care

The *Essence of Care* (DOH 2006a) provides a benchmarking tool to help practitioners take a patient-focused and structured approach to sharing and comparing practice. It has enabled health care personnel to work with patients to identify best practice and to develop and review action plans where appropriate to improve care in the following care situations:

- continence and bladder and bowel care
- personal and oral hygiene
- food and nutrition
- pressure ulcers
- privacy and dignity
- record keeping
- safety of clients with mental health needs in acute mental health and general hospital settings
- principles of self-care
- communication
- promoting health (DOH 2006b).

This new benchmark for promoting health provides a framework for shifting the focus from treating ill health to ensuring promoting healthier life choices is firmly embedded in all good patient care. It is intended to be part of the Essence of Care toolkit for benchmarking the fundamentals of care.

## The National Patient Safety Agency (NPSA)

The NPSA is one of a number of 'Arms Length Bodies' of the Department of Health that covers the NHS through three divisions – *National Reporting and Learning Service* aiming to reduce risks to patients receiving NHS care and improve safety, *National Clinical Assessment Service* supporting the resolution of concerns about the performance of individual practitioners to ensure their practice is safe and valued, *National Research Ethics Service* protecting the rights, safety, dignity and well being of research participants within the NHS.

## Clinical Governance Support Units

Clinical Governance Support Units (CGSUs) have existed in all countries of the UK to establish and sustain improvement projects in their local services. Although some support websites have since been discontinued, both Scotland and Wales provide expert resources supporting clinical governance.

- Clinical Governance and Patient Safety Support Unit (Scotland): http://www.clinicalgovernance.scot.nhs.uk
- Clinical Governance Support and Development Unit (CGSDU) (Wales): http://www.wales.nhs.uk/sites3/home.cfm?orgid=419

## Clinical Governance: A Commitment to Quality Healthcare Through Continuous Improvement

In summary, clinical governance along with the other NHS modernizing reforms remains a dominant influence in health policy. It provides a framework and infrastructure for the provision and delivery of high-quality health care. For it to work, clinical governance not only needs a firm organizational commitment that places patients at the heart of care and involves them in decision-making, but also galvanizes multi-professional team working and accepts both individual as well as corporate accountability for quality health care in the UK.

An integrated governance approach brings together the corporate organization to focus on clinical issues and provide a quality framework. This in turn draws together initiatives, processes, systems and ways of working that ensures patients/service users are at the centre of health care. Clinical governance activities are fast becoming a core function of every nurse's daily practice and nurses can be considered to be at the very forefront of its realization in practice.

Whilst there is an expectation that health care organizations will change and evolve through the monitoring of rigorous standards emerging from within practice itself, professional practitioners must also be willing to change and have a direct influence on an increasingly patient/service user driven National Health Service.

REFERENCES

DHSSPS 2001 Best practice – best care. Department of Health, Social Services and Public Safety, Belfast

DHSSPS 2006 The quality standards for health and social care. Department of Health, Social Services and Public Safety, Belfast

DOH 1998 A first class service: quality in the new NHS. Department of Health, Leeds, UK

DOH 1999 Clinical governance: quality in the new NHS. Department of Health, Leeds, UK

DOH 2004, updated 2006 Standards for better health. Department of Health, London

DOH 2006a Essence of care: benchmarks for promoting health. Department of Health [online]. http://www.dh.gov.uk/en/Publicationsandstatistics/Publications/PublicationsPolicyAndGuidance/DH_075613 accessed 07/01/09

DOH 2006b Integrated Governance Handbook: a handbook for executives and non-executives in healthcare organisations. Department of Health, London

DOH 2007 Creating a patient led NHS – delivering the NHS improvement. Department of Health, London

DOH 2008 (Darzi Report) High quality care for all: NHS next stage review final report. Department of Health, London

DOH (undated) National Service Frameworks Department of Health [online]. http://www.dh.gov.uk/en/Healthcare/NationalServiceFrameworks/index.htm accessed 050109

Lugon M 2007 Editorial: Challenging Times for the NHS' Clinical Governance Bulletin 6(4) p. 1 [online] http://www.rsmpress.co.uk/cgbaug06.pdf accessed 10/12/08

NHSQIS 2005 Standards for Clinical Governance & Risk Management NHS Quality Improvement Scotland [online] http://www.nhshealthquality.org/nhsqis/files/CGRM_CSF_Oct05.pdf accessed 07/01/09

NICE 2008 NHS Evidence Briefing Document National Institute for Health and Clinical Excellence [online] http://www.nice.org.uk/media/AA1/CA/NHSEvidenceBriefingDocument.pdf accessed 09/01/09

RCN 2007 Clinical Governance [online]. http://www.rcn.org.uk/development/practice/clinical_governance (Royal College of Nursing) accessed 07/01/09

Scally G, Donaldson L 1998 Clinical governance and the drive for quality improvement in the new NHS in England. British Medical Journal 317:61–65

Scottish Executive 1997 Designed to care: renewing the National Health service in Scotland. Scottish Executive Health Department, Edinburgh

Smith J 2002–2005 Shipman Inquiry Reports (6) [online]. http://www.the-shipman-inquiry.org.uk/reports.asp (accessed 09/01/09)

Vanu Som C 2004 Clinical governance: a fresh look at its definition. Clinical Governance: An International Journal 9(2):87–90

WAG 2005 Healthcare standards for Wales; making the connections designed for life. Welsh Assembly Government, Cardiff

Welsh Office 1999 Quality care and clinical excellence. Welsh Office, Cardiff

Useful Websites

Concordat website: www.concordat.org.uk

Care Quality Commission: http://www.cqc.org.uk

National Institute for Health and Clinical Excellence: http://www.nice.org.uk

National Patient Safety Agency: (NPSA) www.npsa.nhs.uk

NHS Institute for Improvement and Innovation: www.institute.nhs.uk/

NHS Quality Improvement Scotland: http://www.nhshealthquality.org/nhsqis/CCC_FirstPage.jsp

Regulation and Quality Improvement Authority (RQIA): http://www.rqia.org.uk/home/index.cfm

Welsh Assembly Government Clinical Governance Support and Development Unit (2008) Clinical Governance in Wales: http://www.wales.nhs.uk/sites3/docmetadata.cfm?orgid=419&id=108050